The Evolution of Psychotherapy

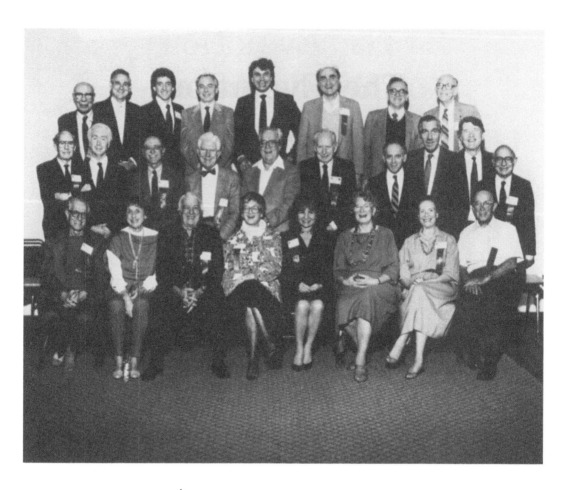

FRONT ROW (from left to right): Albert Ellis, Mary Goulding, Robert Goulding, Zerka Moreno, Cloé Madanes, Virginia Satir, Miriam Polster, and Carl Rogers. SECOND ROW: Rollo May, Arnold Lazarus, Judd Marmor, Aaron Beck, Carl Whitaker, Murray Bowen, Thomas Szasz, Paul Watzlawick, Jay Haley, and Joseph Wolpe. BACK ROW: Bruno Bettelheim, James Masterson, Jeffrey Zeig, Ronald D. Laing, Ernest Rossi, Erving Polster, Salvador Minuchin, and Lewis Wolberg.

The Evolution of Psychotherapy

Edited by

Jeffrey K. Zeig, Ph.D.

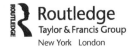
Routledge
Taylor & Francis Group
New York London

Library of Congress Cataloging-in-Publication Data

Evolution of Psychotherapy Conference (1985 : Phoenix, Ariz.)
    The evolution of psychotherapy.

    "Dedicated to the faculty of the Evolution of
Psychotherapy Conference"—T.p. verso.
    Conference held Dec. 11–15, 1985 in Phoenix, Arizona.
    Includes bibliographies and index.
    1. Psychotherapy—Congresses. I. Zeig, Jeffrey K.,
1947–   II. Title. [DNLM: 1. Psychotherapy—trends
—congresses. WM 420 E925e 1985]
RC475.5.E96   1985   616.89′14   86–23263
ISBN 0–87630–440–4

Copyright © 1987 by The Milton H. Erickson Foundation

First published 1987 by BRUNNER\MAZEL, INC.

This edition published 2013 by Routledge
711 Third Avenue, New York, NY 10017
27 Church Road, Hove East Sussex BN3 2FA

First issued in paperback 2015

Routledge is an imprint of the Taylor & Francis Group, an informa business

ISBN 13: 978-1-138-86903-5 (pbk)
ISBN 13: 978-0-87630-440-2 (hbk)

This book is dedicated to the faculty of
The Evolution of Psychotherapy Conference
whose brilliance, compassion, and tireless efforts
have shaped the practice of modern
psychotherapy.

About The Milton H. Erickson Foundation

The Milton H. Erickson Foundation, Inc. is a federal nonprofit corporation. It was formed to promote and advance the contributions made to the health sciences by the late Milton H. Erickson, M.D., during his long and distinguished career. The Foundation is dedicated to training health and mental health professionals. Strict eligibility requirements are maintained for attendance at our training events or to receive our educational materials. The Milton H. Erickson Foundation, Inc. does not discriminate on the basis of race, color, national, ethnic origin, handicap or sex. Directors of the Milton H. Erickson Foundation, Inc. are: Jeffrey K. Zeig, Ph.D., Kristina K. Erickson, M.D., Sherron S. Peters, and Elizabeth M. Erickson.

ERICKSON ARCHIVES

In December 1980, the Foundation began collecting audiotapes, videotapes, and historical material on Dr. Erickson for the Erickson Archives. Our goal is to have a central repository of historical material on Erickson. More than 300 hours of videotape and audiotape have already been donated to the Foundation.

The Erickson Archives are available to interested and qualified professionals who wish to come to Phoenix to independently study the audiotapes and videotapes that are housed at the Foundation. There is a nominal charge for use of the Archives. Please write if you are interested in details.

PUBLICATIONS OF THE ERICKSON FOUNDATION

BOOKS

The following books, in addition to the present volumes, are published by Brunner/Mazel, Publishers:

A Teaching Seminar with Milton H. Erickson (J. Zeig, Ed. & Commentary) is a transcript, with commentary, of a one-week teaching seminar held for professionals by Dr. Erickson in his home in August, 1979.

Ericksonian Approaches to Hypnosis and Psychotherapy (J. Zeig, Ed.) contains the edited proceedings of the First International Erickson Congress.

Ericksonian Psychotherapy, Volume I: Structures, Volume II: Clinical Applications (J. Zeig, Ed.) contains the edited proceedings of the Second International Erickson Congress.

NEWSLETTER

The Milton H. Erickson Foundation publishes a newsletter for professionals three times a year to inform its readers of the activities of the Foundation. Articles and notices that relate to Ericksonian approaches to hypnosis and psychotherapy are included and should be sent to the editor, Bill O'Hanlon, M.S., P.O. Box 24471, Omaha, NE 68124.

THE ERICKSONIAN MONOGRAPHS

The Foundation has initiated the publication of *The Ericksonian Monographs*, which appears on an irregular basis, up to three issues per year. Edited by Stephen Lankton, M.S.W., the *Monographs* publishes only the highest quality articles on Ericksonian hypnosis and psychotherapy, including technique, theory, and research. Manuscripts should be sent to Stephen Lankton, P.O. Box 958, Gulf Breeze, Florida 32561. For subscription information, contact Brunner/Mazel, Publishers.

AUDIO AND VIDEO TRAINING TAPES

The Milton H. Erickson Foundation has available for purchase professionally recorded audiotapes from its meetings. Professionally produced videocassettes of one-hour clinical demonstrations by members of the faculty of the 1981, 1982, and 1984 Erickson Foundation Seminars and the 1983 and 1986 Erickson Congresses can also be purchased from the Foundation.

Audio and videocassettes from The Evolution of Psychotherapy Conference are also available from the Foundation.

AUDIOTAPES OF MILTON H. ERICKSON

The Erickson Foundation distributes tapes of lectures by Milton Erickson from the 1950s and 1960s when his voice was strong. Releases in our audiotape series are announced in the *Newsletter*.

TRAINING VIDEOTAPES FEATURING HYPNOTIC INDUCTIONS CONDUCTED BY MILTON H. ERICKSON

The Process of Hypnotic Induction: A Training Videotape Featuring Inductions Conducted by Milton H. Erickson in 1964.

Jeffrey K. Zeig, Ph.D., discusses the process of hypnotic induction and describes the microdynamics of technique that Erickson used in his 1964 inductions. Length: 2 hours.

Symbolic Hypnotherapy. Jeffrey K. Zeig, Ph.D., presents information on using symbols in psychotherapy and hypnosis. Segments of hypnotherapy conducted by Milton Erickson with the same subject on two consecutive days in 1978 are shown. Zeig discusses the microdynamics of Erickson's symbolic technique. Length: 2 hours, 40 minutes.

Videotapes are available in all U.S. formats, as well as in the European standard.

TRAINING OPPORTUNITIES

The Erickson Foundation organizes the International Congress on Ericksonian Approaches to Hypnosis and Psychotherapy. These meetings are held triennially in Phoenix, Arizona; the first two meetings were held in 1980 and 1983. Each was attended by over 2,000 professionals. The 1986 International Congress is scheduled for December 3–7.

In the intervening years, the Foundation organizes national seminars. The seminars are limited to approximately 450 attendees, and they emphasize skill development in hypnotherapy. The 1981, 1982 and 1984 seminars were held in San Francisco, Dallas and Los Angeles respectively.

Regional workshops are held regularly in various locations.

Programs held at the Foundation for local therapists include beginning and advanced ongoing training in hypnotherapy and strategic family therapy.

All training programs are announced in the Foundation's *Newsletter*.

ELIGIBILITY

Training programs, the newsletter, audiotapes, and videotapes are available to professionals in health-related fields, including physicians, doctoral level psychologists, and dentists who are qualified for membership in, or are members of their respective professional organizations (AMA, APA, ADA). They are also available to professionals with graduate degrees in areas related to mental health (M.S.W., M.S.N., M.A., or M.S.) from accredited institutions. Full-time graduate students in accredited programs in the above fields must supply a letter from their department certifying their student status if they wish to attend training events, subscribe to the newsletter, or purchase tapes.

Acknowledgments

$\blacklozenge$

The assistance of a great many individuals was instrumental in the success of The Evolution of Psychotherapy Conference. I would like to take this opportunity to thank them.

Deserving special recognition are Mrs. Elizabeth Erickson and Kristina Erickson, M.D., members of the Board of Directors of the Milton Erickson Foundation, who gave generously of their time and energy to make many executive decisions about the Conference. They have worked tirelessly on behalf of the Foundation.

On behalf of the Board of Directors of the Erickson Foundation, I want to take this additional opportunity to thank the distinguished faculty of the meeting. The extra efforts of the faculty were certainly noticed and appreciated by all concerned.

The Staff of the Erickson Foundation worked endless hours in handling the registration, meeting arrangements and administrative tasks. Led by Sherron Peters, Administrative Director of the Foundation, the following staff deserves special recognition: Sylvia Cowen, bookkeeper; Greg Deniger, computer operator; Sally Northrup, receptionist; Joy Patzer, secretary; Joyce Walker, secretary; Lori Weiers, M.S., secretary.

A number of volunteers helped, both prior to and at the Conference, including Brent Geary, M.S.; Michael Munion, M.A.; Martin Zeig; and Ruth Zeig. In addition there were more than 160 student volunteers who served as monitors and who staffed the registration and continuing education desks.

A Steering Committee consisting of senior Arizona clinicians was formed and met on a regular basis to develop policy and procedure relating to The Evolution of Psychotherapy Conference. The Steering Committee was invaluable to the administration of the Conference. Warm appreciation is extended to: Aaron Canter, Ph.D.; Sharon Cottor, M.S.W.; John Racy, M.D.; F. Theodore Reid, M.D.; Ann Wright-Edwards, M.A.; and Stuart Gould, M.D.

The Evolution was cosponsored by the Department of Psychiatry, University of Arizona Medical School and the Department of Psychology, Arizona State University, and their efforts are gratefully acknowledged.

Jeffrey K. Zeig, Ph.D.
Director
Milton H. Erickson Foundation

Table of Contents

$\blacklozenge$

SECTION I. FAMILY THERAPISTS

SECTION VII. COUNTERPOINT

Introduction:
The Evolution of Psychotherapy— Fundamental Issues

—————————◆—————————

Jeffrey K. Zeig, Ph.D.

The Evolution of Psychotherapy Conference was a milestone in the history of psychotherapy. This landmark meeting featured leading clinicians each of whom has made seminal contributions to the field of psychotherapy. In this introductory chapter, I will discuss The Evolution of Psychotherapy Conference and distill from the experience of this Conference some important issues that psychotherapists face. Here is a list of what I will present:

1) I will describe The Evolution of Psychotherapy Conference and its history;
2) I will present some of the issues involved in defining psychotherapy;
3) I will delineate some historical trends in the way therapy has developed and indicate some unresolved issues;
4) I will remark about some of the commonalities in theory and practice of the faculty of the Evolution Conference;
5) I will discuss how therapy is evolving;
6) I will offer a communications viewpoint on how therapy works.

THE EVOLUTION OF PSYCHOTHERAPY CONFERENCE

The night before the convocation there was a pre-Conference meeting of the faculty. After the meeting, I watched as Carl Rogers introduced himself to Joseph Wolpe. Rogers observed, "Well, I don't think that we have ever met before." Wolpe agreed.

I was taken aback! Here meeting for the first time were two pioneers who have dominated their respective areas of psychotherapy.

A few months after the Conference, I told this story to Jay Haley, who said that he had not met Rogers before the meeting or even *at* the meeting. Haley added that at the Conference he talked with another Evolution faculty member who disparaged brief psychotherapy, apparently unaware of Haley's predilection for that approach. Later, I read an article about the Conference in *Time Magazine* where it was reported that Thomas Szasz and Bruno Bettelheim met at the convention for the first time.

I present these vignettes as a serious indictment of the field of psychotherapy. People of this caliber should have met before now. They should have participated together and shared their viewpoints on conference panels all along. Psychotherapy has needed—greatly—direct cross-fertilization of ideas.

Unfortunately, cross-fertilization is only starting now—after we enter the second century of the development of modern psychotherapy. Only recently are we beginning to take baby steps toward serious dialogues across schools in psychotherapy.

ABOUT THE EVOLUTION CONFERENCE

The Evolution Conference, held December 11–15, 1985, in Phoenix, Arizona, was described as being the "Woodstock" of psychotherapy, and in many ways it was. It represented who most would consider to be the leading practitioners and theorists in the field. In fact, it is hard to imagine an important work on psychotherapy that does not significantly reference the ideas of the Evolution faculty. They were: Aaron Beck, Bruno Bettelheim, Murray Bowen, Albert Ellis, Bob and Mary Goulding, Jay Haley, Ronald Laing, Arnold Lazarus, Cloé Madanes, Judd Marmor, James Masterson, Rollo May, Salvador Minuchin, Zerka Moreno, Erv and Miriam Polster, Carl Rogers, Ernest Rossi, Virginia Satir, Thomas Szasz, Paul Watzlawick, Carl Whitaker, Lewis Wolberg, Joseph Wolpe and myself, Jeffrey Zeig. The mean age of the faculty was well into the sixties. The age range was from 38 (myself) to 83 (Carl Rogers).

This was the very first comprehensive gathering of master clinicians and theorists from major contemporary disciplines. At the meeting, Rollo May indicated that the field of psychotherapy was made up of 300 distinct schools. The Conference represented 14 of them (not including Thomas Szasz, who is difficult to pigeonhole): Behavioral, Cognitive, Ericksonian, Existential, Family (including six distinct approaches to family therapy), Gestalt, Humanistic, Jungian, Multimodal, Psychoanalytic, Rational-Emotive, Psychodrama, Rogerian, and Transactional Analysis.

The program was not devised for the faculty to describe commonalities across schools of psychotherapy. It was more akin to a psychological smorgasbord where people could sample something from the presented approaches. Attendees would make their own decisions about what was happening in the field of psychotherapy and how the field is evolving. They could follow two tracks:

In one track were *workshops* where participants could spend three hours with an individual faculty member learning more in-depth about that person's clinical approach. A second, more academic, track consisted of *addresses, panels* and *conversation hours*. Each faculty member presented an *invited address* which was followed by discussion and critique from another faculty member.* Faculty members chose their own topics. To promote cohesion in the program of invited addresses, faculty were given a series of suggested questions to answer. These were not meant to make the format rigid. The questions were:

1) How do you define psychotherapy? What are its goals? How do you define mental health?
2) How do people change in therapy? What are the basic premises and underlying assumptions in your approach to facilitate change?
3) What are seen as the benefits/limitations of your approach?
4) How do you train students? What are the qualities that are important in a psychotherapy trainee?
5) How do you evaluate the effectiveness of your approach? What is the place of therapy research?
6) How has your approach evolved and where do you see it evolving? Where do you see psychotherapy evolving?

Faculty also indicated whom they wished as a discussant and whose address they wished to critique. In only a few

---

* *Ed. Note:* It is the invited addresses and subsequent discussions and question and answer periods that are reported in this book. They are organized in a different order than they were presented at the meeting.

cases did scheduling problems make it impossible to give faculty members their desired choice.

There were three types of *panels:* (1) *case discussion panels* where panelists were presented with a written description of a case and asked for conceptualization and treatment plan. The case reports were submitted prior to the meeting by attendees and given to the faculty the first day of the conference; (2) *topical panels,* on themes such as schizophrenia, resistance, training; (3) *supervision panels* where attendees could present cases to the faculty for comment. Informal *conversation hours* were held at the end of the day.

THE HISTORY OF THE CONFERENCE

The Evolution of Psychotherapy Conference was organized by The Milton H. Erickson Foundation, a nonprofit corporation which has spearheaded the movement to promote strategic and hypnotic psychotherapy. The Foundation, led by its Board of Directors consisting of Jeffrey K. Zeig, Ph.D., Sherron S. Peters, Kristina K. Erickson, M.D., and Elizabeth M. Erickson, was founded in 1979 and then organized its initial meeting—the 1980 International Congress on Ericksonian Approaches to Hypnosis and Psychotherapy.* Shortly after the Congress, I conceived of the Evolution Conference. This would be in keeping with the philosophy of the Foundation since we did not want to establish a school of Ericksonian therapy. Rather, we intended to present and build on what Erickson accomplished as a step advancing the development of effective treatment.

In late 1984, it was decided that the time was ripe for the Evolution meeting. We convened the Steering Committee, consisting of senior Arizona clinicians, which met monthly to suggest policy to the Board. The Department of Psychology, Arizona State University, and the Department of

Psychiatry, University of Arizona School of Medicine, agreed to be nominal co-sponsors. The final faculty selections were made; it was decided to limit the meeting to psychotherapies that were currently influential. Biological approaches, "body therapists," and research methodologists were not to be included. The administration of the Conference was handled by Sherron S. Peters, Administrative Director of the Foundation, and her staff. Publicity was sent to members of major professional organizations.

The response was incredible. In the original proposal to the faculty, it was predicted that attendance would range between 3,000–6,000. The meeting was sold out at 7,000 on September 2, 1985. Subsequently, several thousand would-be registrants were turned away for lack of space. We even received some reports that registrations for the meeting were being scalped! The composition of attendees was approximately 2,000 doctoral practitioners (M.D.'s, Ph.D's, etc.), 3,000 masters level practitioners (M.A.'s, M.S.W.'s, etc.), and 2,000 graduate students. Professionals came from 29 countries and every state in the United States.

The Conference came off beautifully. Even though the sessions were large, most attendees could get to the ones that they wanted, and a special spirit of camaraderie developed (in spite of the fact that it snowed the first day of the meeting— the first measurable snow in Maricopa County in four decades). One small example of this spirit occurred in a workshop demonstration in which Miriam Polster worked with a young black woman whose mother was seriously ill back home in South Africa. She was deeply torn between returning there immediately to be with her—and living under the intolerable conditions—or remaining in the United States and continuing her graduate education before going back. One great source of sorrow was that she could not easily keep in touch with her mother, who had no telephone. Attendees spontaneously collected over $2,000 as a gesture of their

* Milton H. Erickson, M.D., was a member of the original board of directors. When he died on March 25, 1980, he was replaced by his daughter, Kristina.

support for the two women and to make it possible for the mother to install a phone. Not only did her mother do that but there was also enough left over to help pay her medical expenses.

The Conference occupied the entire Civic Plaza Convention Center. The largest rooms seated 7,000 and 3,500 respectively. Two other rooms seated 2,000. The smallest room seated 450. To enhance visibility, large screen projectors were used in three big meeting rooms.

Understanding that attendees could want to attend more sessions than was physically possible (up to seven were held simultaneously), tapes were made available for purchase. Much of the Conference was professionally videotaped and all of it was professionally audiotaped.

The Convention Center spanned two city blocks so a shuttle service of golf carts transported the faculty between hotels and meeting rooms. A staff of 160 graduate student volunteers monitored rooms and assisted attendees.

Because this was such a unique conference, a number of commemorative items were sold, including large posters with the Conference logo and names of the faculty, with profits being used to endow scholarships for graduate students. Faculty were regularly asked to autograph posters.

After it was clear that the program would be successful, a special event was organized. Grandchildren of Sigmund Freud and Carl Jung were contacted and invited to participate in a special conversation hour on "The Masters." Each would discuss what it was like to grow up in their households. Sophie Freud, Ph.D., Professor of Social Work at Simmons College, and Dieter Baumann, M.D. in private practice in Zurich, agreed to attend. Alfred Adler's son was also invited but could not participate. At the last minute, Adler's only grandchild, Margot Adler, agreed to join the panel. Margot works for public radio and happened to be covering the Conference as a member of the press!

This was a very moving and inspira-
tional experience held on two consecutive evenings. The first night Sophie Freud could not attend due to an air traffic delay and Bruno Bettelheim took part and discussed Freud's Vienna. These evening panels were meant to symbolize the mending of old rifts and the move toward integration which was a philosophical underpinning of the meeting.

Even the media recognized the importance of the psychological goings-on in Phoenix. Feature articles appeared in *Time Magazine*, *The New York Times* and *The Los Angeles Times*. A thought-provoking critique was published in the *Fessenden Review*, a literary magazine. Coverage was provided by trade papers, local press, local television and national radio. Special press conferences were held: Bruno Bettelheim and Virginia Satir on "Children and the Family," R.D. Laing and Carl Whitaker on "Schizophrenia and Mental Health," Carl Rogers on "Psychotherapy and Social Issues: South Africa," and Albert Ellis and Judd Marmor on "Human Sexuality."

DEFINING PSYCHOTHERAPY

The world's greats expounded on it for days at the Conference, and yet the question remains: What *is* psychotherapy?

Freud remarked that psychotherapy was a "talking cure" but I think some of the faculty would not concur. In fact, I do not believe there is any capsule definition of psychotherapy on which the 26 presenters could agree. For example, one could talk about psychotherapy as using communication to promote change, but I think that Carl Whitaker would say, "I am not up to promoting change, I am there to have an experience—to be more of who I can be." If one defined psychotherapy as using communication to access latent potentials, there still would be objections; some might say it has more to do with teaching new skills.

Here were reigning experts on psychotherapy and I could see no way they could agree on defining the territory! Can anyone dispute, then, that the field is in disarray? I suppose this inability to define psychotherapy can be reframed as something positive: It leaves practitioners free to come up with their own definitions. And it *is* necessary to have a definition, because if we claim expertise, we should be able to describe what we are doing.

There are many possible definitions of psychotherapy. Personally, I have never been one to think of it as being "Better living through chemistry," but there certainly are many experts who subscribe to that theory. I now think of psychotherapy as being that situation where the therapist helps the patient to empower himself to do something possible which he had been promising himself but had not had the wherewithal to do because he did not really believe it was possible. In that sense, psychotherapists make the improbable, possible—or make the improbable, doable.

Befitting my Ericksonian orientation, I define psychotherapy interpersonally. We all have degrees of responsiveness. Psychotherapy is about presenting ideas so that patients can respond constructively in and of their own accord. Paraphrasing Erickson, psychotherapy is creating a matrix for a reassociation of inner strengths. That is my bias, but psychotherapy has not been evolving entirely in accord with my bias. I like to think in terms of five different streams of evolvement, each with its own distinct goal.

HISTORICAL TRENDS

The first of the five streams from which psychotherapy evolved is an *analytic* tradition whose goal was uncovering and insight—in a word, "self-understanding." The roots of psychotherapy are grounded in a European mentality which is more theoretical and analytic than the pragmatic American approach. Because psychotherapy developed in Europe, it initially assumed an orientation to analyze the past, with self-understanding as its

goal. For example, in Europe an advertiser probably would not put the word "new" in front of a product—many Europeans place a pejorative connotation to that word. But in the United States "new" means good. In Europe, "tried-and-true" is associated with good; in the United States, there is a different orientation. Furthermore, European culture tends to be more private and past tradition has much value. In the United States, we tend to be extroverted and more oriented to the future.

Since World War II, psychotherapy has become an American export. Most of the world turns its head to the United States for the definitive word on matters of the mind. The streams that developed after World War II reflected American pragmatism and were oriented to intervention. Carl Rogers developed the client-centered approach which heralded the *humanistic* tradition. Psychotherapy was no longer based on understanding. Rather, the goal of psychotherapy was *awareness*. As a natural outcome, expression was encouraged—especially expression of feelings. What followed was the emergence of "growth-oriented" therapies such as Gestalt, encounter groups, emotive approaches and the touchy-feely human-potential movement of the 1960s where the main purpose was to be more aware of the here-and-now.

The 1950s saw the development of the *behavioral* stream of psychotherapy with its theoretical understandings based in the experimental work of B.F. Skinner, and with some of its clinical application developed by Wolpe and his followers. The goal of this methodology is to change behavior, rather than to increase understanding or awareness. This stream also spawned cognitive approaches, which aimed to change behavior, although the method was not strictly geared to behavior per se.

A fourth stream that developed and began to flourish in the 1960s was the idea of *systems*. No longer was the individual the unit of treatment; now a therapist would center on relational aspects—what happens between human beings, rather than inside them. The group psychotherapy movement was one of the antecedents of family approaches to psychotherapy. The goal was systemic change.

Unfortunately, for the most part, these four streams have remained discrete. The analysts speak to analysts; the behaviorists speak to behaviorists, and so forth. However, on a day-to-day basis, most psychotherapists use all of these streams, overtly and covertly. Therapeutic goals for patients take into consideration numerous factors including self-understanding, behavioral change, increased awareness, and sensitivity to the fact that we are very much influenced by our social context, especially the immediate environment in which we live.

I am going to be so bold as to suggest that what Milton Erickson did was discretely different from the other four streams. Erickson was the heralder of a *communications approach* to psychotherapy. He was a pioneer who explored the parameters of how communication, especially indirect communication, could be used to maximize therapeutic responsiveness.

Especially as initially devised, the first four streams of psychotherapy were based on uncovering deficits—deficits in the person's behavior, awareness, or understanding, or in the way the person reacted within a system. More than any other psychotherapist that I have seen, Erickson was dedicated to utilization: What does the patient bring to the therapy? What is present in the reality situation, and how can it be used? This communication approach is not based on deficits—it is based on taking the strength that the patient has and helping the patient develop and recombine resources in effective ways.

The first century of psychotherapy can be seen as one of theory. The second century elevates application. Erickson is a pivotal figure in this change.

Perhaps the five streams can be elucidated by using a metaphor of trees: The analytic approaches would be directed at uncovering and examining roots; the awareness method would subscribe to the philosophy of Joyce Kilmer—sit back and revel in the inherent beauty of the tree; the behavioral school would say, "If you don't like the way the tree's developing, shine light in the direction you want it to grow"; systems adherents would observe trees in their ecosystem; and some Ericksonians would maintain that you can best influence trees by beating around the bushes.

UNRESOLVED ISSUES

There are many unresolved issues in psychotherapy—perhaps too many. The following were distilled from the Evolution Conference. Roughly, this presents an overview of what we are trying to understand about the process of modern psychotherapy as we enter its second century. The issues can be divided in terms of technique and theory. I will first address technique.

We all know that psychotherapy is a process that should be individualized to the person; it should be based on the client's understanding of the world. But how and to what extent is really unclear.

It is common knowledge that when a person has a problem, it is important to divide the problem into surmountable bits. However, among major theorists, there is a disagreement as to the essence of these basic units. Some divide problems into behaviors, others use cognitions. Many therapists actively defend their choice of unit and are critical of other choices. It leads me to postulate that as far as the theorists of psychotherapy are concerned, the quarks to one are quirks to another.

A number of technique-related questions were discussed at the meeting: Is psychotherapy a right hemisphere art or is it a left hemisphere science? Do we use direct confrontation or do we use indirect suggestion? Should we be linear or metaphoric in our approach? Is insight a necessary precursor of change or is change independent of insight? And there are some people, especially from the existential schools, who would ask, "Should technique be a part of psychotherapy at all?"

What about inpatient treatment? There are some who maintain that inpatient treatment is not to be used except under dire circumstances. Should we help people to ventilate and express their emotional conflicts in order to have a corrective emotional experience, or should we encourage suppression of conflicts? Should patients be confronted to assume responsibility for their feelings, thoughts and behaviors, and to what extent can patients assume voluntary control?

There was no agreement as to the extent to which diagnosis should be emphasized versus taking concerted action. Neither was there agreement as to whether we should be treating the context or the patient, the conscious or the unconscious, the individual or the family; whether therapy should be symptom-based or if it should be a matter of growth facilitation. Also, it was not clear what direction psychotherapy should take. Is psychotherapy going to be directed to the past, will it be directed to the present, or should it be directed toward the future? As far as a general understanding about the application of technique, the major theorists presented few areas of agreement.

Theory was just as cloudy. There was disagreement about how theory should be emphasized and utilized in practice. Moreover, it was unclear whether there is a place at all for theory in psychotherapy because some maintained that theory unreasonably limited practitioners. Perhaps in reaction to Freud's monolithic orthodoxy, the trend among presenters was to deemphasize theory.

COMMONALITIES

In spite of polarization, there were a number of commonalities among the faculty. Basically the faculty consisted of extraordinarily sensitive, perceptive and bright people. They also are quite articulate and very persuasive. When I listened to the speakers at the Evolution Conference, they all seemed intrinsically right about their perspectives—especially their perspectives about how other theorists were wrong. The theories and methods that were presented all seemed eminently sound—emotionally, rationally and on the basis of research. And yet, something was a bit wrong; positions seemed too extreme.

But the extremism is understandable— all of the speakers had once swum upstream. Now they are mainstream. Swimming upstream forces provocativeness in order to make a counterpoint. Part of being provocative is limiting one's focus especially to one's own work and taking an extreme position.

Actually, all theories of therapy are adventures in extremism. These torchbearers took fresh and bold perspectives, often against dogma, and created models of their own. But I think it is most interesting how tenaciously theorists and students become committed to their own models. Probably it is twice as effective to have the courage of one's fantasies as it is to have the courage of one's convictions.

Certainly there has been a lot of proselytizing among the disciplines. Thomas Szasz speaks to this issue in his chapter when he makes some comparisons between religion and psychotherapy. He talks about the catholic position (catholic meaning "universal") where the true believer goes forth and proselytizes. Faiths have numerous models; some religions maintain that they are just one of a number of ways. They don't have *the* truth.

In teaching Ericksonian hypnosis and strategic models, I want to portray a similar understanding: This is just one of a number of ways of thinking about and doing psychotherapy. It is not *the* truth. Extreme positions often do injustice to the field.

Take, for example, Carl Whitaker whom I respect immensely. When asked, "When do you *not* do family therapy?" Whitaker's answer is, "You do not do family therapy when there are no family therapists available." Whitaker's orientation is always to do family therapy. But I think those of us in clinical practice on a daily basis use family therapy as just one approach.

There is also a positive side to the mentality that creates extreme positions. Perhaps because of having to swim outside of the mainstream of psychotherapy, most of the theorists who spoke at the meeting had a good ability to step aside—an ability to look past the prevailing norm and get a fresh perspective. Often this ability came out in clever turns of a phrase or pithy one-liners. Some of their genius seems tied to their ability to detach, create, reorganize and synthesize from an observer's position.

In fact, many practitioners complain that having a traditional education in psychotherapy is a detriment and that they have to unlearn a lot of things that were learned in graduate school. Dogma does become a limitation in psychotherapy. One becomes wedded to an approach and it becomes difficult to see the forest for the trees.

One of the other commonalities of the Evolution faculty was the degree of social activism and social awareness. This was especially evidenced by the fact that one night of the meeting, Virginia Satir and Mary Goulding organized a special session on world peace attended by 3,000 people. Subsequently, letters were written to Reagan and Gorbachev. This social perspective was not limited to any particular school; for example, Judd Marmor, R.D. Laing and Paul Watzlawick each spoke strongly to social issues, advocating positive action—not just hiding in the consulting room.

Another commonality was that faculty drew from fields other than therapy, quoting from physics, chemistry, the humanities, and the arts. One example will be found in Bruno Bettelheim's critique of Rollo May's paper. Both cited Greek and existential philosophers to make their points.

HOW THERAPY IS EVOLVING

How would one say that psychotherapy is evolving? Well, it continues to inch along in rather stumbling baby steps. Here are some notable trends:

1) We are moving psychotherapy off the couch. Therapy is more directed to the patient's immediate life situation—for example, by the use of therapeutic tasks and the involvement of the family.

2) Psychotherapy is using more humor. At one time it was taboo to think of using humor. There was serious discussion at scientific meetings about when and where humor should be used. Now theorists from disparate disciplines use humor regularly because it can be so effective in promoting change.

3) Psychotherapy has become more public. This is especially evidenced by the emergence of media psychologists. The aura of privacy that often led to secrecy is no longer as prevalent; now demonstrations of psychotherapy regularly happen at professional meetings and this allows more thorough scrutiny.

4) There was one surprising development in the area of technique. Across disciplines, there is an increasing use of symbols to influence patients. Symbolic hypnotherapy is a notable Ericksonian method. Erickson also used symbolic tasks outside of hypnosis, as for example instructing a couple to climb a local mountain (see Zeig's chapter). But across disciplines, faculty were using symbols, not only interpreting them, but using them in a directed fashion. For example, Bruno Bettelheim's (1976) book, *The Uses of Enchantment*, is a wonderful example of how symbolic fairy tales influence children. In her work with family reconstruction, Satir uses symbols. The Gouldings create transactional symbol dramas. Lazarus uses

guided imagery. In many therapies symbols are used to help patients change. Psychotherapy is moving away from explanations and toward creating constructive experiences. This is a recognition of a need for experiential learning as well as analytic understanding.

5) More and more, theorists emphasize mobilizing resources rather than uncovering pathology. Psychotherapy happens best when patients' strengths are identified and developed.

6) Systems approaches are becoming more popular. Some of the most well-attended sessions were on family therapy. More family therapists were represented at the Evolution Conference than any other schools—the family of origin school of Bowen, the strategic school of Haley and Madanes, the structural school of Minuchin, the interactional approach of Watzlawick, the experiential approach of Whitaker, and the Satir model.

7) Psychotherapy has become more results-oriented. Patients are expected to work for specified changes. Rather than delving into the past, therapy is directed toward the patient's future. As a consequence, psychotherapy has become briefer. This reflects sociological issues (there is a cultural call for a "quick fix") and also speaks to fiscal matters—patients and insurance companies are less willing to foot an extended bill.

8) Across psychotherapies, emphasis is on tailoring the therapy to the patient—meeting the patient at the patient's frame of reference. Carl Rogers made this point in relation to his person-centered method. Bruno Bettelheim argued for this perspective in his psychoanalytic work with children. It is certainly one of the central tenets of the Ericksonian approach.

9) There is movement to using the vernacular. Sesquipedalia is out. Simple language and observable and easily understood constructs are preferred.

10) There is increasing specialization. Many therapists treat only special diagnostic groups such as borderline patients, anorexics, and so forth; others treat only special classes of patients, such as children or families.

A COMMUNICATIONS VIEWPOINT ON HOW THERAPY WORKS*

Where does all this leave us in trying to sort out how therapy works? Let me offer a communications approach to provide some explanation.

Communication is an interpersonal process that can be conceived as being composed in both the sender and receiver of 12 discrete elements (cf. Zeig, 1980). There are four primary elements: *behavior, feeling, thought,* and a *sensory component* composed of two aspects, perceived sensory experience and imagined sensory experience.

For example, if a person says, "It is really a beautiful day," there is a *behavior* consisting of the actions surrounding the words. The expressed *feeling* could be pleasure, "I really feel good today." A *thought* is expressed about the composition of the day's weather. The *sensory* experience is perceived auditorially, visually, tactilely, chemically, and proprioceptively. There is also an internally represented sensory experience that may or may not coincide with the perceived sensory experience.

It would simplify psychotherapy if the primary elements were all there were to communication, because there would be less to pay attention to and fewer choices to be made as far as intervention is concerned. What makes things complicated is that there are eight secondary elements to communication, secondary in that they augment or modify the primary elements.

Concurrent with the primary elements are *attitudes* consisting of a new constellation of thoughts, feelings, behaviors, and sensory experience. Attitudes can be pos-

---

* With appreciation to Braulio Montalvo who read this section and provided comments that were included in the final draft.

itive, neutral or negative. Simultaneously with saying, "It is a really beautiful day," the speaker can have a positive attitude, "That was really a good thing to say," a neutral attitude, "Wasn't that interesting that I said that?" and a negative attitude,"Why did I say something so foolish?".

Communication is *ambiguous* because it can't be fully specified. If one says, "It is a really beautiful day" to a person from Washington, D.C., it is different from the meaning of a "really beautiful day" to a resident of Phoenix, Arizona. The speaker cannot fully indicate what is meant by his/her expression.

Communication is also *symbolic*. For example, it is a symbolic representation of experience. If one talks about a chair, the word "chair" is a symbol that stands for something.

There is a *relational* aspect to every communication. Gregory Bateson (1951) indicated that every communication contains a directive message about the ongoing relationship: "This is a kind of relationship where we can learn," "This is a kind of relationship where we can have fun," and so forth.

There is a *qualitative* aspect to communication in that it has intensity and/ or duration. "It is a really beautiful day" differs from "It is a *really* beautiful day."

Another element of communication is the *context*. Every communication happens in one particular time and one particular place. Therefore, every communication is unique. It never happens again. Moreover, the context in which the communication happens often is a major determinant of its meaning and effect.

Every communication is *biologically based;* it occurs because of a chemical reaction. Also, communications are *idiosyncratic* in that they are idiosyncratic representations of aspects of the history and goals of the participants.

Every communication consists of 12 elements that interplay with and modify each other. However, it should be remembered that every symptom is also a communi-

cation (Szasz, 1961; Haley, 1963). Therefore, every symptom is composed of these elements.

Patients presenting their complaint emphasize particular aspects of the communication complex. One person coming in with depression could emphasize the way that it feels to be depressed, while another person complaining of depression could emphasize the thinking process. Yet another depressed person could emphasize his/her dysphoric attitude.

It is not only the patients who emphasize a particular aspect of the communication. Theorists in psychotherapy also emphasize particular elements of communication. For example, behavioral therapists maintain that psychotherapy is about changing behavior. Feeling therapists (for example, the Rogerian schools and some Gestalt schools) say that psychotherapy is about expressing and changing feelings. Analytic schools can be based on thinking. There are even some sensory-based schools, for example, Neurolinguistic Programming (TM).

Cognitive approaches emphasize changing attitudes. For example, much of Ellis' work is directed to attitudinal change. Ericksonian therapists are often ambiguous; Jungians are symbolic. Family and group therapists emphasize relational aspects. There are even schools labeled "contextual." Biological approaches are used by some. Others delve into history.

So, if one is going to develop a school of psychotherapy, the only niche left is to establish the "qualitative" school of psychotherapy. (It might not be a bad idea; many complain that more quality is needed.)

When one considers the elements of communication from a systems point of view, it provides some understanding of effective and ineffective intervention. Every symptom is a system of 12 elements. If the therapist modifies the behavior of the symptom, the psychotherapy can be effective—because a behavioral change can modify the entire system. Changing an aspect of a system can have systemic reverberations; however, it might transpire that the system does not respond to a behavioral intervention. Then the therapist can work on modifying other elements or other combinations of elements. One can recognize that there can be multiple roads to home. It may be that symptom change can occur by modifying disparate elements or combinations thereof; the practitioner works to determine which element(s) are most responsive to change.

Psychotherapy is idiosyncratic by nature—the nature of the therapist as well as of the patient. I would say that psychotherapy is a mixture of common sense, communication skill and artistic talent. Like music, it should have a catchy beat and poetic lines. Jorge Colapinto (1979) said that the choice between one theory and another boils down in the end to a matter of taste. The same thing could be said about technique. It is often a matter of taste and perspective as to where one chooses to intervene.

Actually it might be best to start by pacing the element the client emphasizes, thereby meeting the patient at his model of the world. Subsequently, one can intervene by modifying a peripheral element because it is less defended and sufficiently different from the client's habitual experience to provide new perspective. The general rule of thumb is to work from the periphery in. Pick an element or elements that are not overtly emphasized or defended and promote minimally significant change. There often will be a snowballing effect.

CONCLUSIONS

There is no general reconciliation in sight for psychotherapy.

Little convergence can be expected in the immediate future. This is unfortunate because patients would benefit most from interdisciplinary cross-fertilization. The field will probably continue to lumber along on elephantine theories and soar into a fog bank of techniques. There will be mas-

sive generalizations in the from of "all therapy" statements, such as, all psychotherapy is re-education; all psychotherapy is re-parenting, it is reframing; it is changing roles; it is changing behaviors; it is changing hierarchies; it is changing attitudes; or it is changing cognitions. Actually, it would be easy to remedy this type of thinking. One would merely insert the words "more than," for example, "All therapy is *more than* reeducation," and so forth.

Besides encouraging integrationism, I would like to call for emphasis in two other directions. First, training should increase perceptiveness more than cognitive understanding; it should emphasize effective ways of diagnosing, developing and utilizing responsiveness. Students in training should be encouraged to understand redundant patterns that are positive as well as negative.

Second, basically therapy is an art of improvisation and we need more gifted therapists who are willing to demonstrate their gifts of improvisation publicly. It is hard to do therapy publicly. It entails being able to play many different instruments and play them well. Musicians have their own range; some are good at percussion, others at woodwinds. It is difficult business to respond constructively to all of the different kinds of people. But, I think we need fewer music theorists, art critics, stage directors and orchestra leaders. We need more composers, and we need to learn from their examples.

Having begun with an anecdote about Carl Rogers, it seems fitting to end the same way.

Carl Rogers championed the use of empathy, genuineness and unconditional positive regard in clinical practice. These are not mere techniques; they are an integral part of Rogers' lifestyle.

In August 1985, Rogers presented a conversation hour for undergraduate psychology students at a meeting of the American Psychological Association. He was gracious and generous in sharing with the young and eager students the accumulated wisdom of his five decades as a psychologist. The topics ranged from psychology to social issues to the quality of life. One attendee encouraged 83-year-old Rogers to speak about old age and death. After a few preliminary remarks he hesitated. Then, surveying the audience, his eyes twinkled as he replied in a thoughtful, measured voice, "When I was a child it was predicted that I would die young. Now that I am 83, I know that prediction will be true."

To me, that resounding phrase was therapeutic: It was filled with warm contact and focused on flowers rather than weeds. It called on me to respond out of my own accord with the best within me.

REFERENCES

Bettelheim, B. (1976). *The uses of enchantment: The meaning and importance of fairy tales.* New York: Alfred Knopf.

Bateson, G. & Ruesch, J. (1951). *Communication: The social matrix of psychiatry.* New York: W.W. Norton.

Colapinto, J. (1979). Quoted in J. Wilk & W. O'Hanlon, *Shifting contexts: The generation of effective psychotherapy.* New York: Guilford (in press).

Haley, J. (1963). *Strategies of psychotherapy.* New York: Grune & Stratton.

Szasz, T. (1961). *The myth of mental illness.* New York: Hoeber, Harper; Rev. Ed., New York: Harper & Row, 1974.

Zeig, J. (1980). Symptom prescription techniques: Clinical applications using elements of communication. *The American Journal of Clinical Hypnosis,* Volume 23, pp. 23–33.

Convocation

---◆---

My name is Jeffrey Zeig and I am the organizer of The Evolution of Psychotherapy Conference. In convening this meeting, there are some rumors that could be addressed. A number of people have wondered if there would be any oblique references to Woodstock. Certainly there will be none. Nor will we make any references to Star Wars.

But in a more serious vein, there are a number of reasons for convening this gathering, not the least of which is to honor some master clinicians and psychotherapists. The faculty consists of renowned experts who have influenced the development of twentieth-century clinical practice.

But this is not only a moment of honoring, it is also a moment of history that we now convene. Probably this meeting is the largest congress ever held that is solely devoted to the topic of psychotherapy. Certainly it is the first comprehensive meeting of leaders of major contemporary schools. Moreover, the Evolution Conference celebrates modern psychotherapy's 100th year. It was just a century ago that Freud initiated his interest into the psychological aspects of medicine (Alexander & Selesnick, 1966).

So, what can we expect at this great psychotherapeutic cafeteria? As you proceed through the lines, I hope that the emphasis is on "conciliance." Perhaps conciliance can be the watchword of the meeting. Because we are here to speak to commonalities—the commonalities that underlie successful clinical work. It would seem that one of our colleagues, Bradford Keeney (1983, p. 146), had the right idea when he talked about a mythical conference on family therapy indicating that it could be a ballet of differences, rather than a symmetrical battle of who is right and who is wrong. So, together let us orchestrate the Evolution Conference in this way.

In the evolution of the infant discipline of psychotherapy, the first 100 years have been divergent. It has been a period of growth, consisting both of flowers and of weeds. Especially in the last 40 years, there has been a proliferation of discrete schools. Perhaps we can begin this second century of modern psychotherapy in a way that is more convergent.

Psychotherapy has been a house divided. If we were to hold with tradition, the psychoanalysts would huddle together in one section of the room. The emotive therapists would be in their corner. The Ericksonians would meet atop Squaw Peak. Each group would have its special language and group leaders would persuasively argue the righteousness of their cause.

But in this auditorium, we sit shoulder to shoulder. And, I think that most people would agree that psychotherapy is about helping people to empower themselves—assisting them to surmount the "I can't" that they have in their minds and to actualize the idea, "I can."

Now there are many roads to home. To name a few, there is the empathy of Carl Rogers; the directives of Jay Haley; the rational approach of Albert Ellis; the interpretations of Bruno Bettelheim; the humor of Carl Whitaker; the desensitization of Joseph Wolpe; the cognitive methods of Aaron Beck; and the poetry of R.D. Laing. But it is important to remember that method is derived from goal. Method and theory are not written in stone in an exclusive and illusive esoteric language. So, let us share a common language at this meeting and that way we can learn *with* each other.

One of the characteristics that separates humans from other animal species is that unrelated humans use others to help themselves overcome feeling stuck. In the evolution of humanity, we only recently have reached the point where creative intelligence is valued over physical strength. So, don't you agree that psychotherapists should catalyze a revolution towards concilience? If that is what we want from our patients—if we want them to use their power to cooperate—it would be wise and fitting for us to lead the way.

Isn't it great that these leaders of psychotherapy have agreed to come together to share their understanding of the human situation? Each will be able to teach us something. No one has scope. I cannot keep up with the literature in my specific area of psychotherapy. Let us try to use this opportunity to begin to get some scope.

Some people have inquired about the history of the Evolution Conference: How is it possible to bring together all these great names? The answer quite simply is that they responded to the invitation.

That is not meant to be a flip reply. I think that the occurrence of this meeting is a matter of timing. The speakers and the attendees alike recognize that this time is one for constructive interdisciplinary dialogue, and that the time for such dialogue is long overdue.

Personally I hope that waves from this Conference reverberate and that they give impetus to a conciliance in the development of the second century of modern psychotherapeutic practice. Our common interest is in the experience of psychotherapy and out of that spirit I hope that you take away with you some vibrant and new ideas.

I am glad that you are here to make this opportunity happen. On behalf of the Board of Directors of The Milton H. Erickson Foundation and the Steering Committee of the Evolution Conference, I welcome you!

REFERENCES

Alexander, F.G., & Selesnick, S.T. (1966). *History of psychiatry: Evaluation of psychiatric thought and practice from prehistory to the present.* New York: Harper & Row.
Keeney, B. (1983). *Aesthetics of change.* New York: Guilford Press.

SECTION I

Family Therapists

My Many Voices

◆

Salvador Minuchin, M.D.

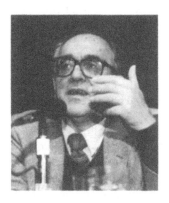

Salvador Minuchin, M.D.

Salvador Minuchin received his M.D. from the University of Cordoba in Argentina in 1947. For ten years, he served as Director of the Philadelphia Child Guidance Clinic.

Currently, he is Clinical Professor of Child Psychiatry at the University of Pennsylvania School of Medicine; research professor of Psychiatry at New York University; and resides in New York where he teaches and practices family therapy.

Minuchin has developed the structural approach to family therapy which is one of the major models in the field. He has authored two books and co-authored three, and there is also a volume about his approach. Additionally, he has over 30 original papers and journal contributions. He is recipient of the Distinguished Family Therapy Award from the American Association of Marriage and Family Therapy.

In presenting the evolution of his own approach to treating families, Minuchin discusses how other seminal family theorists and practitioners influenced him. He does not merely describe their impact; he also summarizes their essential positions, including strengths and shortcomings. If the family therapy approach can be seen as a quilt, this chapter is an artfully integrated patchwork. In viewing the quilt, one can see the particular patches, how they were embroidered by their designer, and how they comprise a significant part of the whole.

History, or "the past," is by definition a construction. There are facts, which are more or less objective; but their grouping, the way they are highlighted, and the shadows that are left are the product of the historian's present position. The mores of his time, the ideologies fashionable at the moment, and current constraints all contribute to the framing of the "proper" interpretation of recorded events— "proper" meaning, in this context, "correct at this historical juncture."

The field of family therapy, at least in its labeled version, is so new that my own experience as a child psychiatrist, analyst and family therapist very nearly encompasses it. Therefore, I am using myself as the "framer" of the memories I will recall for you. Perhaps my collection of framed memories, or (as I like to call it) my collection of "voices," can serve as a contribution to the oral history of family therapy.

Family therapy officially began in 1954 with John Elderkin Bell's monograph. For my own personal reasons, however, I would suggest that family therapy began in 1925 with the first case seen at the Philadelphia Child Guidance Clinic* under the auspices of Dr. Frederick Allen. The patient was a ten-year-old boy who lived in one of Philadelphia's ethnic neighborhoods with his mother, stepfather and a three-year-old half sister. The case started with a letter from the mother stating that her son was not doing well in school, misbehaved at home, and was getting beyond her.

A social worker was assigned to prepare the social history as an initial step in treatment. She interviewed all the family members at home, meeting with them separately and together. Her several home visits included contact with the neighbors. She visited the school with a social worker "patron" and the hospital where the mother was currently under medical care. As part of the study, the boy had psychological tests and two appointments with Dr. Allen, director of the clinic at the time. There was also a thorough physical examination at Children's Hospital. (By the way, there was no charge for the clinic's services.)

Allen, who became one of the leading child psychiatrists in the United States, reported that he found the child to be open with him. Although he thought the child was somewhat more impulsive and irresponsible in his behavior than the average ten-year-old, Allen did not consider him a seriously disturbed child. The boy spoke affectionately of his father, mother and aunt. He acknowledged that he ought to be a better boy, but he also thought that the grown-ups could stand improvement. It was hard to know what they expected, he said, because grown-ups, especially his mother, sometimes said contradictory things, or said one thing and did another.

The developmental history taken by the social worker revealed that the mother

* I am indebted to Dorothy Hankins for the use of her unpublished history of the Philadelphia Child Guidance Clinic.

had been rather promiscuous as a girl, and that the boy was illegitimate. He had been reared by his aunt until the mother married. She and her husband then took the child, but the aunt continued in the picture as an active and very critical member of the extended family.

The staffing conference decided that the problem resided primarily in the family. The treatment plan covered a wide span. The social worker, for instance, was to encourage the parents to have the boy's teeth treated and to have him seen by a pediatrician to treat a mild anemia revealed by the physical examination. The parents were to be helped to be more consistent in their expectations and their discipline. The school was to be encouraged to coordinate its expectations with those of the parents. The mother and aunt were to be helped to resolve their differences in relation to the child.

Accordingly, the social worker worked with the family for about a year. She saw the mother and aunt in the clinic and had occasional appointments at the home with the stepfather and child. During the second year, contact with the family was reduced and more widely spaced. The case was closed at the end of two years on the basis of an improved relationship between the mother and aunt and the improved behavior of the boy. The referring social worker in this case continued occasional follow-up contacts for the next 20 years. The last entry, dated 1944, reports that the client, now happily married, had just been promoted to captain's rank in the U.S. Army.

This was a remarkable case, treated by a procedure that would seem radically modern today. First, the clinic considered the child's problems to be supported by the conflicts between the parenting members of his family, that is, the mother and the aunt. Therapy included coordinating the parents' and the school's approach to the child. There was close cooperation with a pediatrician. The psychiatrist elicited the child's ideas about himself and about the world in which he lived. There were no references to fears or anxieties. The concern was with integration and competence.

What view of a child organized this kind of treatment? In 1925, a child was seen as a victim—primarily as done to rather than doing. The family, the school, or other aspects of a child's environment were the context to which a child responded. What was the view of parents? Here an interesting contradiction arises. Parents were presumed to have caused a child's problems. Nevertheless, it was expected that parents would be able to modify their relationship with a child once they understood the meaning of their input. Clearly this was an optimistic period, in which educational procedures directed toward the social context were considered necessary for helping children, and in many cases, sufficient. A brochure published by the clinic in 1930 stated, "Each individual child is part of the group setting, and to treat and help a child readjust his mental outlook he must be considered in terms of the whole family. It would hardly be wise," the pamphlet concluded, "to concentrate on the child alone. Our real philosophy is that both the parents and child are reacting to the given situation, and it is this interaction of each of them with the situation that generates the difficulty."

When I began working in the field of child psychiatry, 25 years after the initiation of this case, there was a very different focus. In my training, the emphasis was on the child's internalized pathology. The first DSM was a few years in the future, but I recall that our chief interest in the 1950s was diagnosis. Diagnostic categories were expanding, and the richness of labels was in itself entrancing and seductive. Services, on the other hand, were fragmented at best. In my training at Bellevue with Lauretta Bender, where I interviewed and diagnosed psychotic children, contact with the parents was not a significant part of the treatment. We saw the parents mostly as visitors, coming (probably unwillingly) to see their children on weekends. Occasionally we did observe their relationship to their children. We described it as "detached."

Some years later I worked in a residential institution for juvenile delinquents. Hawthorne Cedar Knolls School, part of the Jewish Board of Guardians, emphasized the youngster's individual dynamics and the creation of a therapeutic milieu. Parents were considered frankly destructive to the children. If they were seen at all, they were seen individually, in the "main office." During this time, Bettelheim, at the Orthogenic School in Chicago, was writing about the pathogenic influence of parents. His recommendation for very disturbed youngsters was "parentectomy"—for life.

It is clear that over these years, the profession's views of parents and families were changing along with the enormous social, economic, and cultural shifts of those decades. New understandings of the complexity of the human condition developed new therapeutic procedures. But the view of humans as somehow innately pathological and pathogenic gained more and more salience. In the 1940s David Levy discovered the overprotective mother. In the 1950s Frieda Fromm-Reichman's "schizophrenogenic mother" was popularized in a number of antifeminine forms, like Philip Wylie's "Momism" (the direct cause of the United States' withdrawal from Korea and the triumph of communism on that archipelago). In 1953 Johnson and Szurek described the superego lacunae in which children's acting out is a projection of parents' deficient superego.

It was about this time that family therapy began its entrance to the field. And consistent with its time, its first interventions followed constructs that looked at families in order to protect patients from them. Ronald Laing's organization of Kingsley Hall followed these premises. The purpose was the organization of an institution where adults could repair the damage they had sustained in their families. Murray Bowen's theories encouraged people to differentiate themselves from the undifferentiated family ego mass—a kind of psychological quicksand in which family members seemed to lose their capacity for individual movement. Nathan Ackerman's early papers dealt with the child as the family scapegoat. Bateson's double bind theories obviously contain the period's mistrust of families, even though systems theory should have prevented such linearity. It took a number of years for the family therapy movement to free itself from this ideology.

I began to work with the families of institutionalized children in the late 1950s. Juvenile delinquency was hitting the headlines in those years, along with the opening guns in what was to become one of the shorter wars in American history—the "War on Poverty." I came from an intense political commitment as a Socialist Zionist, having worked with displaced children from a wide variety of ethnic backgrounds in Israel. This oriented me to both cultural and social issues, so that when I began to work with black and Puerto Rican children and their families in the lower socioeconomic groups of New York City, my sense of their pathology was framed by my broader view of their lack of power within a social context that disorganized their lives. In some way, I think my own experience closed the circle, returning me to the concepts of Frederick Allen in 1925—the context of the child and of the family emerged once more as a significant component of both individual and family behavior.

At the time this was the stuff of Young Turks. Don Jackson's article, around 1954, gave us the theoretical rationale, as well as a rallying cry, for a frontal attack on the mental health establishment, with its overwhelming concern with internalized pathology.

By the late 1950s, we were doing family therapy at the Wiltwyck School for Boys. At the time we were using a three-stage interview, exploring how different family subsystems change when they interact alone and with other subsystems. In the course of each session we first saw the family together, then the parents in one subgroup and the sibling subsystem in another, and then the family regrouped once more. We wanted to see whether the relationship of family members changed in different contexts. But as we saw families in these contexts, the importance of authority—of hierarchy and power—became evident. We learned to look for the alliances and coalitions formed within the family and to explore the characteristics of the family's affective range and the way family members negotiated control. At the same time, a host of techniques evolved as a necessary analog to working with a number of people in a number of different contexts.

There were five of us on the Wiltwyck team: Dick Auerswald, Charlie King, Braulio Montalvo, Clara Rabinowitz, and myself. Braulio Montalvo is a voice I still hear from that time. He has a rare capacity for managing a combination of holistic thinking and a search for precision. During the Wiltwyck years, he was dreaming of a family therapy that would have specific, discrete interventions—an alphabet of skills. We used to study each other's work with this implausible goal in mind. His voice, as I hear it today, maintains its capacity for complexity. But it has softened over the years, melding with Carl Whitaker's voice in bringing me more acceptance of human frailty.

Dick Auerswald's is the other voice that still speaks urgently to me today. Whenever I use the words "epistemology" and "ecology," that is Dick talking. He used to play with this concept, giving "ecology" such resonance that finally it took meaning for us all. He also lived by it. In the 1960s he was dreaming strategies to change the way New York City politicians thought, as the only way to change mental health services for poor families. He wrote a classic paper on multiple agency impact on welfare families and the destruction caused by it. In the 1970s he left for Maui, where he has worked for 15 years on the mental health of a whole island, thereby giving ecology a real visibility in the field of family therapy.

In 1962 Dick Auerswald and I made a pilgrimage to the centers of family therapy. We traveled to Palo Alto to see Bateson, Satir, Jackson and Haley. In New Haven we met Lidz, Fletch and Cornelison, and we went to Washington to see Lyman Wynne's work. We knew of no one other than Nathan Ackerman doing family therapy at that time.

In Palo Alto we wanted to see a session with Bateson, but we were detoured by Jay Haley. He suggested we attend a class of Virginia Satir's instead, since Bateson's anthropological cast made his therapeutic sessions more a matter of gathering information than attempting change. Bateson was leery of change. His concern had a clear theoretical bias: When you focus on one corner of an ecological system, your perspective of the total system will distort and your intervention, which will be skewed, will chop the ecology.

I worked with Jay Haley for many years, and I also learned a lot from many other people who had worked with Bateson. Although I met Bateson personally only once, in a conference in 1982, in Topeka, clearly his voice has become part of my thinking, and the thinking of all family therapists. It is therefore with a sense of respect for his contributions that I want to focus on the constraints they introduced in the field. I myself have always felt uncomfortable with the cybernetic language that he used: "The family is a system." "The family therapist is caught in the feedback loops of the family." "The therapist cannot control a system of which he forms a part."

The descriptive language of cybernetics is demonstrably poor. Excluded are the sweat and tears and pain, the hopes, confusion, ambiguity, boredom, passion, and weariness that characterize human encounters. The world of systems thinking is a world of ideas. Ideas are organized at different levels. They can be reversible. Wrapped in language, they can be manipulated without breaking. They can deal with ideal types; they can conflict and cancel without bloodshed. They exist on infinite axes of time and space. Humans do not.

I think that when Bateson lent family therapy the cloak of systems thinking, we lost in the exchange. We lost drama. We lost understanding of the human being's emotional world. Storytelling became too predictable because the idiosyncratic gave way to the generic. We gained in understanding patterns, in seeing truth as perspective, in the ability to manipulate reality. But 30 years later, some family therapists are speaking with a dry, dehumanized, predictable babble all too similar to the language analysts used to speak (which is why I decided to leave the field of psychoanalysis). As a clinician I feel uncomfortable with the complexity of cybernetic language and the concomitant simplicity of its view of human beings. In focusing on logical systems, Bateson's thinking, as reflected in the field, eschews affect, doesn't give enough significance to the family as a complex system with subsystems with different agendas, and somehow makes the individual disappear. Its concern with the wholeness of systems also dismisses power in family dynamics because when what you are studying is a system, you see people as the way they participate in maintaining that system.

Let me return to 1962 and our meeting with Virginia Satir, the first family therapist I ever met in action. She was teaching then with a strictly communicational bias. In effect, the idea was that if a woman offers a cup of tea to her husband and the husband says, "I like the tea," and by that he means that he likes the tea, not that he loves her, a lot of the disharmony in the family can be resolved. Through the years, Virginia's theory became more complex, incorporating some of the thinking and techniques of Gestalt therapy and certainly saving the emotional life from its neglect in the cybernetic schools.

Although Virginia started with the Bateson school, affect and the blocks to intimacy became her main focus of exploration. Over the years her work with families moved in two directions—one toward the individual and his needs, the other toward social groups in conflict. I think this reflects her position as a single person whose family is all over the world. Our dialogues tend to become parallel monologues in which she emphasizes intimacy and cosmic union, and I reply with Talmudic order.

On that trip, we visited New Haven and the group of Lidz, Fleck and Cornelison, who had written some articles on the families of schizophrenics. We were surprised to find that the dynamics of the family they described had been collated from individual interviews with family members. At this particular time this group had not yet begun to do any intervention with the total family.

Our visit to the National Institute of Mental Health to see Lyman Wynne's work was also disappointing to a couple of beginners in search of new truth. Lyman was interviewing schizophrenics and members of their families, but his focus was on the individual patient's dynamics. Lyman's techniques of interviewing still had strong roots in psychoanalytic thinking. It seems now that Lyman remained in this position as a therapist for a number of years, coming only slowly to his own style, even while making significant new contributions in theory building. His research on the match of cognitive styles of the parents of schizophrenics and the identified patient was one of the early scientific supports for the existence of a family system. His interest in research with schizophrenics remained constant, demanding, and, of course, he had a critical view of the organization of institutions. His latest book on large systems, emphasizing the need to look at the family in context and study the interdigitation of family and large social systems, is a valuable signpost for the field.

But to go back once again, we returned from that 1962 trip feeling that, although we might be new kids on the block, we were ahead in making meaningful explo-

rations. In family therapy, the 1960s were characterized by great excitement, as well as by great competition between various practitioners, all rejecting psychoanalysis, but all enthusiastically exploring their own corners of the new world. Eventually this fervent exploration of small turfs was to coalesce into a much richer understanding of the entire area.

A couple of years later I again met Ackerman, who was directing the family program of Jewish Family Services. I had been in contact with Ackerman from 1950 to 1952, and he guided my early development as a child psychiatrist. But I had lost contact with him until 1964, at which point I was already a family therapist of four to five years' experience. Ackerman's influence, like that of Bateson, cannot be measured only by his thinking. A traditionally trained child psychiatrist and child analyst, Ackerman came to family therapy through an exploration of better ways of understanding children, adults and families and in search of better ways of helping people. His early period included strong criticism by his psychoanalytic colleagues, who felt he had betrayed the truth and embraced superficial behavioral techniques when he controlled a screaming child for half an hour in a demonstration to hundreds of his colleagues. His theoretical thinking evolved slowly from his traditional roots. Yet his courage of practicing and his teaching were certainly instrumental in the development of family therapy throughout the East Coast. I remember him sometimes when I use myself with a couple, creating a seductive triangle. He was a master of this technique. I think that, with Whitaker, one of his major contributions was in focusing on the therapist as a member of the system.

Bowen has been a puzzle to me for many years, since he responds to questions with a mysterious smile and seems satisfied to leave the responsibility of interpreting his smile to the other. This is a problem for a communicator like me.

Lately I have regained my respect for the complexity of Bowen's ideas and the

MY MANY VOICES   11

tenacity with which he has maintained and expanded his point of view. There is no family therapist today who will not deal with his concept of triangulation, the system of emotionality, his concern with intergenerational transmission of pathology (while in his therapeutic technique he sometimes works only with one individual) and, in some way, his idea of sending an individual to change his position in the family. All have been incorporated in some form or another into a variety of training systems as well as into therapeutic technique.

Nonetheless, Bowen's theory does not give room for the expansion of the individual when a couple forms. There is a determinism that restricts the individual to the organization of his family of origin, which he always carries regardless of the intensity of his relationship with significant others. It is as if the idea of lineage has been carried to its logical extreme.

I met Jay Haley in 1962 when he blocked my desire to watch a session by Bateson —to protect me from boredom, he said. He joined the Philadelphia Child Guidance Clinic in the late 1960s and was there for nine or ten years. Jay is a hybrid, though being Jay he would reject that label along with the rest. Evolving as a member of Bateson's team, with its strong theory building, he was attracted to the imagery and wizardry of Milton Erickson.

Jay and I worked together in Philadelphia. In the beginning, he acted as a researcher. He sat, watched and thought, and was bored. But then we developed a program of training for paraprofessionals. The team was composed of Jerry Ford, Rae Weiner, Braulio Montalvo, Carter Umbarger, Jay, myself, and later Marianne Walters. The project appealed to all of us in different ways.

For Jay, it was a chance to demonstrate that family therapists are handicapped by higher education and the influence of New York City, since supposedly the paraprofessionals had not been exposed to the taint of psychodynamic thinking. I was attracted to the project by its social im-

plications and by the educational challenge. In any case, for five years we worked together in what was probably the most intense training program ever developed in family therapy. One of the faculty members was always supervising the students, one to one. I think it was then that Jay Haley became a real supervisor, and, as a result, he developed a lot of his ideas on training. Among other things, he developed a format for a first interview that one can follow without previous training. It was at the Philadelphia Child Guidance Clinic, I think, that the reality of poor families intersected with his theoretical stance. It was necessary to think how the abstract theoretical concepts of the Bateson group could be meaningful in the development of techniques in working with poor populations. I think it was then that Jay locked horns with Bateson about the need to introduce power into thinking about families and family therapy. It was then, too, that he became interested in the development of supervisory techniques and the micro as well as macro movements of strategic therapy.

During this period Braulio, Jay and I were evolving together a way of working that first meshed and then diverged. One of the differences between Jay and me related to development. Having evolved as a child psychiatrist, I take developmental issues more into account. I also think that I am more concerned with the characteristics of family organization after the symptom has been alleviated. I pay more attention to the movements in the session, whereas Jay pays more attention to the goals of therapy and to the tasks to be performed outside of the session. For me a task defines a transactional field. I don't much care what people do with it. For Jay, the task is itself an important part of the way he directs people toward the alleviation of symptoms. Therefore, his tasks are paths in a certain direction, whereas mine are probes. His strategies seem much more coherent than mine. They are ingenious ways of dealing with a symptom in a particular way. And the symptom itself is the pathway to the production of change. To me, the symptom is more a by-product, and I try to finish with it in order to get on with the job. In my thinking about therapy, the therapist is an important part of the system. When I work in supervision, I pay attention to the therapist's personality and style and the need to expand his repertore. Jay deals with the therapist as a conveyer of significant strategies.

Yet, Jay's is a voice I hear rather frequently. At first I felt the artificiality of techniques like restraining, assigning symptoms at particular times, ordeal techniques, or prescribing the symptom, and I refused to use them. It seemed to me they were distancing and were not totally honest ways of transacting with people. I accepted them for other therapists, however, and slowly I myself began to incorporate these techniques and make them mine.

One of the puzzles about Jay is that while he maintains an aggressive and combative stance in his writings, the personal characteristics that he projected in his work with the staff in the clinic were a sort of shyness, a certain aloofness, and a tremendous respect for the patients and trainees.

I first met Cloé Madanes when she began to work at the Philadelphia Child Guidance Clinic in 1973. At first her voice came to me mostly when I thought about Jay's work. But slowly, or not so slowly, her voice has become distinct to me, bringing a mood of playfulness, an understanding of children, and a capacity for fantasy that blends without clashing with highly disciplined thinking. Now I hear her voice whenever I work with young children.

When I think of Carl Whitaker it is with a certain warmth. We have been friends for the last 20 years. I don't remember when I first met him, but I have a feeling that it was at a meeting in St. Louis, where we were both invited by Washington University. I was offered twice the fee that he received, and I think the first family therapists' collective bargaining committee was formed at that moment.

Carl, who is one of the pioneers of family therapy, has insisted for the last 30 years that theory handicaps creativity and therapeutic freedom. Only in the last ten years or so, in the papers he has written with David Keith, has he elaborated his point of view about families and change. I have shared consultations with him with four or five families in a variety of circumstances, and I have incorporated in my work his benign pleasure in the absurd. I suppose that with aging there comes to all of us something that Carl discovered early in life—that human experience meanders and that a sense of direction is something that we impose on our existence only at our own peril. He challenges family members' ideas that there is one way of understanding their lives—that there is one reality and that they know what it is. He offers the flexibility of multiple perspectives. At the same time, there is a certain rigid demand that we accept the truth of our own deaths and of the existence of murderous and incestuous feelings in us all. In some way, while his techniques are marvelous, innovative and challenging, some of his ideas remain wedded to early psychodynamic thinking.

Like Murray Bowen, Carl insists on the need to encompass three generations in one's thinking about families and the transmission of family culture. But unlike Murray, he frequently insists on seeing three generations together in his practice. He is probably the family therapist who has done the most marathon sessions with large families, bringing with him a general acceptance of absurdity, human frailty and madness in his encounters with people, accepting their instinctual as well as their behavioral facets.

Four or five years ago, Carl spent two lengthy periods as a visiting professor at the Philadelphia Child Guidance Clinic. He found that his way of working was frequently ineffective with the poor families he was seeing there, and he began to play with some of the techniques we had developed which were more adapted to working with poor families. I hope that some of this has become part of his style, since I would like to think that he hears my voice as well.

I think the voices I hear lately are speaking in Italian. From the beginning I was attracted to the simplicity of the Milano approach. At the same time, I questioned that simplicity. If it was that easy, shouldn't we all merely connote positively, prescribe the symptom, and work in teams?

While we were using videotapes in America to analyze family therapy, their first use of videotape was to study the therapeutic team process. And there lies a most ingenious paradox. The study of the therapist team was to implement a theory in which the therapist introduces prescriptions from a distance. By becoming multiple, the team could become homogeneous, with idiosyncracies smoothed out in the therapeutic corporation. Their goal, like my early attempts, was to develop a simplified set of therapeutic interventions that could apply to a large number of circumstances. And Mara Selvini Palazzoli's latest thinking seems to be moving in the direction of a universal therapeutic strategy.

The roots of the old Milano team (Selvini, Boscolo, Ceccin, and Prata) touched a combination of the voices of Bateson and Erickson via Jay Haley. While following Bateson's theoretical lead, they developed systematic techniques in training and in therapy that are highly teachable and effective. I think the modification of their technique by Peggy Papp, Olga Silverstein, Peggy Penn, Gillian Walker, and the others at the Ackerman Institute— imploding the family with three alternative ways of being—is useful. So is Karl Tomm's exploration of the process *in* the session. These are valuable complexities in a therapeutic process that sometimes tends toward oversimplification. It is also interesting that in *Alla Conquista del Territorio*, the book by Mara's son for which she has written the introduction, the *new* Milano team states that their therapeutic techniques must be grossly modified to be effective in the public sector with poor families.

At the 1985 American Association for Marital and Family Therapy meeting, Mara's presentation brought confusion to hundreds of her followers. She emphasized family structures, the issues of power in families, and the importance of provocation and negative connotation, joining with many other schools of family therapy. In my turn, in spite of my tendency to confrontation, I find myself prescribing symptoms, scheduling sessions less frequently, and even, here and there, doing circular questioning.

Recently I was working with a family with three adult children whose mother committed suicide 20 years ago, when the oldest child was 12 years old. I asked them for memories of their childhood, but they could not describe their mother nor any other recollections. The father explained that he had tried to protect the children from their mother's death by never talking about her. I surprised myself by asking them to watch family movies and to mourn the mother's death. I thought Norman Paul might be proud of me.

Another day I was seeing a family with an anorectic child, where there is a possible history of an incestuous relationship between father and daughter. The girl was refusing to eat because she feared her food might be poisoned. I found myself remembering some of the writings of Hilde Bruch. I didn't know she was one of my voices, but so it seems.

Naturally pulling many voices together usefully demands an organizing frame. Briefly, the business of family therapy is change. Under this umbrella, I operate with a set of premises that are familiar to me. I look for distance and closeness within a family, and I map a family along those parameters. My experience as therapist, supervisor, and consultant continues to validate the perception that there are a limited number of organizational arrangements available to families, and that these are influenced by the social and historical context, by the family's own developmental stage, and by idiosyncratic factors. Each one of these possible family organizations makes certain demands on family members. A therapist therefore joins the family in a therapeutic system and tries to help the family actualize alternative ways of being. The therapeutic goal is to expand the family members' repertory of responses to the complexities of life.

Within this framework the possibilities are many and varied, as are the voices that speak to me. Today, they are the way I do therapy. Clearly the voices I hear do not mean that everything is the same or that eclecticism is beautiful. The demands of a situation, and one's own possibilities and limitations, still operate selectively. Perhaps this is like the harmonic context of a melody. Within that context, a theme appears, is taken up by other voices, and can reappear in counterpoint or in inversion. Within the possibilities open to us, the best in us always learns from the best of others. I am pleased to acknowledge that when I say to a man, "When did you divorce your wife and marry your office?", it is Carl's voice speaking. He might not recognize it in my accent, but it is there, as are all the others.

Discussion by Zerka T. Moreno

♦

Family therapists are to be considered as Daniel's entering into the lions' dens and should, therefore, be much commended for their work and courage. Dr. Minuchin's paper on historical perspectives dealing with his many voices has unfortunately, in my mind, left out a voice in the background. I hope I can bring it a little bit more into the foreground. But family therapists have in common, with psychodramatists, the fact that we do not emphasize insight, that we are more concerned with action and interaction and their nature, and with the here and now. Change is focused upon the future, upon integration and competence.

But I do have a question. Being naive by nature, I have a question about the anorectic child. I would like to know who she said poisoned the food and whether that was pursued. I would assume it was her mother, but I can't speak for the child. Her father? In other words, it had to do with incest.

But, as I read Dr. Minuchin's paper, I began to regret more and more that it had not been part of our mutual fortunes to have crossed paths earlier, and especially when J. L. Moreno was still alive. Certainly many streams are still forming the field of family therapy, but among the early family therapists was Jacob L. Moreno. He did not appear in print in this country until 1925, although he actually started working with entire families in Vienna in the second decade of the century.

In this country, largely because of his struggle to stay clear of the psychoanalytic fraternity, his work was not widely known. However, he crossed paths with, among others, Nathan Ackerman and Carl Whitaker in the 1940s. What is impressive about Moreno's work was that he systematically explored interactions and what these interactions were about—especially within the family—before anyone else in psychiatry. He described his treatment of a marital couple in Vienna in the early 1920s in a book that was published in this country in 1947 (*Psychodrama, Vol. I,* "Intermediate Treatment of a Matrimonial Triangle," Beacon House, Beacon, N.Y.). In 1937 he published his first paper on interpersonal therapy in marital conflict ("Inter-personal Therapy and the Psychopathology of Inter-personal Relations," in *Sociometry, Vol. I,* Beacon House, Beacon, N.Y.), involving also the husband's lover and using himself as a go-between while he constructed a systematic approach.

I myself took part in a weeklong treatment, with two sessions daily, of a newly combined family, each parent having brought some of their own children into the marriage. The situation was complicated by the fact that the father still had a child living with its biological mother so that we had, in fact, a triad of parents—father, mother and absent mother. We were unable to bring the latter into the treatment process; ideally, of course, we should have. This constitutes what Moreno called "The Family Social Atom."

We first worked with the entire family, hearing from each member how he or she perceived the family was working or not working. I am not going into all the details as to how we worked with this family the entire week, but I want to point out one aspect relating us to animals—the problem of a territorial imperative. It became clear during the week that some of the more immediate problems were due to the close living quarters of a number of the offspring. With the help of the biological siblings in the conflict, a schema of the house itself was drawn on the blackboard, showing where the bedrooms and bathrooms were. This was an upper middle-class professional family with six children living together—eight people in all, plus a housekeeper. With a seventh child coming to visit on weekends and holidays, that was quite a group.

First a tracing was made of the paths made in space by the young people. After it was made apparent in psychodrama how they bounced against one another, a new arrangement of the sleeping quarters was drawn up and different bedroom assignments made. These changes were part of the homework the family had to undertake upon returning home. They reported later that this successfully resolved one of the worse sources of daily irritation and arguments, namely, sharing time and space. By entering into the actual living space, we gained new perspectives and dimensions. Time and space are among the dynamic living categories in our world and cannot be overlooked since no two people live identically in these dimensions. Indeed, the question of whom we share time and space with—for instance, when we marry and start to join our lives with a partner—is of the essence.

Another problem arose with three sons of a family where the presenting problem was that two of the boys threw food at each other across the dining room table, three times a day. A sociometric reorganization according to their preferences as to whom they wanted to be close to at the table completely erased that particular problem.

I would like, therefore, in reviewing Dr. Minuchin's paper, to suggest that more attention be paid to the method of choices in the family, if possible, using the sociometric system.

My other recommendation would be for psychodrama to be used. I am, of course, dedicated to that approach when communication breaks down and the problems remain in some way incomprehensible and intangible.

One discovery we made in working with pregnant mothers was that there is a psychodramatic or fantasy child in the mind of parents. Mothers have this idealized child more often than fathers. They may find it painful to admit this to themselves or to family members, and denial is common. Nevertheless, the fantasy or ideal child can become a living reality in that its image and presence create an invisible but strong barrier between parent and live child. It may be that the live child is of the wrong sex, has come at the wrong time, or is not in some way the exact parallel of the ideal child. The parent will then clasp the fantasy mask over the real child and proceed to try to make the real child fit this image—not seeing or appreciating it in its own right. In this sense, then, positive transference is to the fantasy child and not to the biological child; the latter's is largely a negative transference.

The real child may never be informed overtly what is happening, but he or she will hear sentences such as, "How come you don't," "Why can't you," and "You can fit yourself into that scheme," and so on, implying the child's own worthlessness. Our approach to this is to let the parent play out this fantasy in psychodrama without the real child present, have that wished for child, and interact with it in a number of ways and scenes. Then the parent will be readier to give up the fantasy child, be able to perceive the real child somewhat differently—hopefully, more clearly—and may even begin to appreciate that the living child incorporates a number of features of the fantasy child. Thus, a new relationship can begin. We stress here the importance of completing unfinished business. We are concerned as much with the intrapersonal as with the interpersonal because often the latter can lead us to the former, and vice versa.

I might add that I have experienced this process myself. In my case, it was a fantasy daughter whom I never had. It was not that she interfered with my relationship to my son. Rather, I wished and yearned to have a daughter as well and wanted to complete my family. In two sessions, having had her with me on the psychodrama stage but especially in role reversing with her and becoming my own fantasy daughter, I was able to free myself from this involving need.

So here is another dimension indicated, that of the invisible fantasy world that may surround protagonists in the family drama and block their need for cooperation with other family members. Because

of this, I believe that psychodrama, with its action format, is able to deal more completely with the multiplicity of relationships inherent in families. And I haven't even touched on the multiplicity of cultures and socioeconomic levels in our country.

Role-playing has been found to be practical and useful in working with the poor, as Frank Riesman pointed out in his book *Mental Health of the Poor.* He found it to be the treatment of choice since their verbal skills are different from those of the middle class. Since action is their medium for living, action methods fit them better.

Family therapists think of themselves as action oriented, and they are. But psychodramatists go a little further into the action dimensions with family members, with the scenes completely embodied in front of them, both in time and space, in the rooms in which the events occurred, in the house in which they happened, in the garden, and so on. Within the context of a family at play, the drama soon turns into deadly earnest as the warming-up process takes hold.

Another important technique is that of role reversal. Ideally, family members who are stuck in their own role rigidity should learn to role reverse with the others, not merely to understand the others, but also to see themselves through the eyes of the others and thus possibly to start to change the relationship.

In the main, I want to say I learned a lot from Dr. Minuchin and other family therapists in terms of this wonderful sense of freedom to create absurdities, to introduce humor, and to work for change without having to constantly look at the past. We, too, bring in the past only where it reflects upon the present.

Therapy—A New Phenomenon

Jay Haley

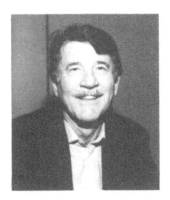

Jay Haley
Jay Haley (M.A., 1953, Stanford University) is Director of the Family Therapy Institute of Washington, D.C. He is one of the leading exponents of the strategic/interpersonal approach to family therapy. Haley served as Director of the Family Experiment Project at the Mental Research Institute and as Director of Family Therapy Research at the Philadelphia Child Guidance Clinic. He has authored seven books, co-authored two and edited five. Additionally, he has more than 40 contributions to professional journals and books. Haley is the former editor of Family Process *and the first recipient of the Lifetime Achievement Award of The Milton H. Erickson Foundation.*

Haley uses his provocative tongue-in-cheek style to provide an in-depth meta-analysis of the evolution of psychotherapy during the last three decades. He prods us to step aside and evaluate both our cherished theoretical formulations and our ideas about effective technique. Haley delineates seven guidelines for therapy, arguing that therapists must be agents on behalf of strategic change. Concepts prevalent 30 years ago are not only outdated, they are diametrically opposed to what is necessary for constructive psychotherapy.

Among the mysteries of human life, there are three special ones. What is the nature of schizophrenia? What is hypnosis? What is the nature of therapy? These mysteries share aspects in common. All of them involve paradoxical communication in a way that is exasperating to the theoretician who would like, as Gregory Bateson would say, to get them "to lie flat on the paper." All of them are controversial; each has groups arguing over its definition and nature. In each case there is a question raised whether it even exists.

Of these mysteries, therapy has become the most important issue. Vast sums of money are involved in the art and science of changing great numbers of people. In the scientific field and in the marketplace, enthusiasts contend about the many different kinds of therapy. I will discuss here my own adventures in the years I have taught and done research on this topic. I have been led to a certain way of thinking about and doing therapy. This came partly from my teachers, especially Milton H. Erickson, and partly from research. The research influences, which I will emphasize here, led me to uncertainties and confusion about this phenomenon over the years; and finally they led me to a logical position about therapy.

I began my research life in the 1950s inquiring into, among other things, the nature of schizophrenia, hypnosis, and therapy. In that decade, all three phenomena underwent a basic change from being regarded as an individual characteristic to being considered interpersonal in nature.

Schizophrenia, for the first time since the word was coined, was thought of as a behavioral response to a social situation. Families and hospital staffs were defined as part of the malady, leading to therapeutic milieus and family therapy.

Hypnosis, which had always been considered a one-person phenomenon, began to be defined as responsive behavior to another person. Instead of being the effect of magnets or a relaxation or sleep phenomenon, hypnosis was being examined as a peculiar response to the peculiar behavior of a hypnotist. The work of Erickson, with his emphasis on the interpersonal induction of trance, had its influence in that decade.

Erickson also had his influence on therapy which, for the first time in the 1950s, began to be thought of as an interpersonal phenomena. Prior to that time, one could read the literature of therapy and not find what a therapist did in an interview because he, or she, was really not there. The focus was on the patient and his hopes, dreams, past, and projections upon the therapist. In that decade it was discovered that what a patient said was a response to what the therapist was doing and was not merely a report on the patient's inner nature. As Bateson said, a message is both a report and a command, therefore it involves more than one person.

The first published interview of a therapy session, not just an anecdotal excerpt, was by John Rosen in 1948 (Rosen, 1951). He mimeographed interviews and also printed a verbatim therapy interview with a patient diagnosed schizophrenic. To read the dialogue of two people talking in therapy, rather than read just a case summary,

was a revelation about both schizophrenia and therapy.

It is curious that in the decade of the 1950s everyone began to think more socially. Animals were studied in their natural environments by ethologists, the organization of businesses became a focus, and all kinds of groups became popular. Families were actually observed in action; and, for the first time, the behavior of a therapist became part of the description of therapy as audiovisual recordings were used. Cybernetics, the science of self-corrective systems, provided a theoretical framework for the group processes being examined.

A major influence on those of us who were viewing therapy as interpersonal was Harry Stack Sullivan. I was supervised by Don D. Jackson, who had been personally supervised by Sullivan. To illustrate the change in thinking at that time: I was doing therapy with a hospitalized patient diagnosed schizophrenic and had been seeing him daily for a number of years. One day this gentleman began an interview with me by saying something like, "I was out on my submarine this morning, and we were to meet the refueling ship off Madagascar. Unfortunately the ship was struck by an atomic bomb and barely limped in late with its Chinese flags at half-mast." The routine therapeutic response would have been based on the idea that the patient, because he was locked up in a hospital and did not own a submarine, was expressing the fantasy of a disordered mind. The question might have been: Was he speaking randomly or was he expressing a symbolic meaning based on childhood experiences?

Because of Sullivan's influence, I had to face a different question: How was the patient's comment related to *me*? I realized I had been late to the interview that morning. The mention of a refueling ship being late could best be received as a courtesy comment on my lateness. By courtesy, I mean it offered me the opportunity to interpret to him what submarines really symbolized to him, or I could apologize for being late. Those were the days when schizophrenics were the great teachers in psychiatry—before it became the fashion to drug them.

DOES THERAPY EXIST?

As we look at these great mysteries today, it is the examination of the nature of therapy that has become the most explosive in producing new theories and innovations. It is also the most difficult to research. When we research a topic, we prefer a well-defined field where we can gather facts and make hypotheses. In studying therapy, we would like to know what the facts are, which theories explain them, and which techniques are the most successful in inducing changes that are well-defined.

When I began research on therapy, what to investigate and how to investigate it were not clear. In fact, the question being asked seriously for the first time was: Did therapy actually exist in the sense that it caused a change? Was there a correlation between a therapist's behavior and a desired change in the client, or was therapy an illusion? The fact that therapy was practiced by prominent people and had been for several generations did not necessarily mean that it was not illusory. There have been a number of scientific endeavors that proved to be delusions. One example is the science of phrenology, the study of character by the shape of the skull and the bumps on the head. That science was thought to be based on facts and had many enthusiasts among university scientists. There were national and international journals reporting research findings for many years. Today, we have dismissed it as an illusion; yet it remains a lesson for us all that many intelligent people can be misled for long periods of time.

Can we say that today there is much more evidence for the existence of therapy than there was in the 1950s? The number of clinicians has increased by the thousands, and the number of schools of therapy has multiplied. Yet there does not seem to be increased certainty about therapeutic theory and practice. We still face the unsettling question: Do therapists influence anyone at all?

When I began research in the 1950s, outcome research on therapy was beginning to indicate that therapy was not causing a change, and equally interesting was the investigation of spontaneous remission. One form this investigation took was research on the changes that occur when a client is on a waiting list anticipating therapy. Studies at the time seemed to indicate that 40 percent to 60 percent of the people on a waiting list recovered from their symptoms. Because of our observation of families at that time, it seemed possible that spontaneous change could actually be greater than that.

The merits of waiting list research were debated, but it was extremely important if a high percentage of people recovered from the problem without therapy. It meant that when a person happened to be in therapy at the time of spontaneous change, the therapy would get the credit. Assuming half of any therapist's clients recovered if the therapist just kept out of the way, the therapist who did nothing would be the most successful in achieving his 50 percent cure rate. Therefore, therapists would be encouraged to do nothing as a sound therapeutic approach. With half their patients getting better, the therapists would feel rather confident about their therapy approach. Believing that therapy is bringing about the change, the therapist would live in a financially stable illusion. Waiting list research seems to have been abandoned in recent years, perhaps fortunately.

It was not only the examination of waiting lists, but also the discovery of families and how they change that led to uncertainty about the effect of therapy. The following case illustrates the difficulty in defining what is a problem and raises the issue of spontaneous change.

A 19-year-old woman was referred to

me for a shaking right hand. It was an uncontrollable, intermittent shaking that had persisted through a year of therapy and a number of negative neurological tests. She was referred to me to cure the symptom with hypnosis, while her psychiatrist continued to work on the childhood roots of the symptom. I asked the young woman what would happen if her symptom became worse. She said she would lose her job because she was having increasing difficulty even holding a pencil to write. I asked what would happen if she lost her job. She said her husband would have to go to work. This helped me to think of the symptom as interpersonal, which I was trying to do at that time. I learned that she was recently married and that her husband was unable to decide whether to go to school or go to work. Meanwhile, she was supporting him. The symptom could be viewed as a marital issue.

Yet, in discussing her marriage, I found the issue could be defined as a larger unit. Her parents, not approving of the young man, had opposed the marriage and continued to do so. Each day her mother telephoned her to ask if she was coming home that day. She would point out to her mother that she was married and had her own apartment now. Her mother would say, "That won't last," and she continued to call, encouraging the young woman to give up her husband and return home. The shaking right hand and the husband's behavior could not be explained without a family view. The husband seemed to feel that he could not please his wife's parents, no matter what he did. If he went to work, it would not be a good enough job for their daughter's husband. If he went to school, she would be working to put him through school. So he was incapacitated.

I made a variety of skillful therapeutic interventions in this case, and the outcome was successful. The shaking hand was cured, the husband went to work, and the parents began to support the marriage. However, in my period of self-congratulation, I could not overlook another change

which had occurred during the therapy: The young woman became pregnant. Once pregnant, she was going to have to quit her job, and so her husband went to work to support her. Her parents, who wanted her back home, did not want her home with a baby. So they began to support the marriage. The symptom disappeared. Since she was in therapy at that time, the therapy got the credit, and I got more referrals. Yet, I think the change she went through might well have occurred if she had been on a waiting list.

This case and others helped us to give up the view that symptoms are deeply rooted in individuals and to consider symptoms as adaptive to a social system where they can come and go as the life situation of a person changes. Naturally, the longer someone is in therapy, the more chance a positive change will occur in their lives, independent of the therapeutic action.

It is not only possible that therapy has little effect, but it is equally possible that the confidence of the therapist in his theories will not be affected by the outcome. We would like to believe not only that we can determine what is therapy and what is not, but also when it is effective and when it is not. Our certainty that we are causing a therapeutic change is often taken as evidence that we are doing so. When I began to investigate therapy, I became acquainted with some unsettling research which made me cautious about having confidence in theories. Alex Bavelas, a social psychologist, was investigating the ways in which human beings construct theories. To summarize the particular experiment:

Bavelas gave subjects a panel with many buttons and a light. He told them the experiment was a timed test. The task was to find out which buttons to push to make the light go on. The subjects would begin to push buttons and watch the light. After awhile, they would be able to make the light go on by pushing the right series of buttons. They would explain, for example, that it was necessary to push the button in the top corner, the one in the lower corner, the one in the middle twice, and the third one from the end, and then the light would go on. They could demonstrate the proof of their theories by pushing the buttons and making the light go on again and again.

When they completed the task, Bavelas might or might not tell the subjects that in fact the light went on every 20 seconds no matter which buttons they pushed. They were living in an illusion that their acts precipitated an event which, in fact, was occurring independently of anything they did. Just as the therapist can have the illusion that he causes a change in therapy when it is actually the result of other actions, so did these subjects live in an illusion. Some of the subjects refused to believe it when they were told they were not turning on the light. The higher their academic status and scientific background, the more sure they were that they were turning on the light by pushing the right buttons. (Some of them would give up the delusion only when someone else was put through the experiment.) After that, I listened to clients and families with a more cautious concern about finding patterns. One of my first experiments was to test whether family members were actually behaving randomly with each other.

In my research on therapy, I tried to examine whether we were inducing the changes as we thought we were. The fact that several generations of therapists believed in the theories and the results did not mean the evidence was sound. A description of another experiment by Bavelas might portray the history of therapy. In this theory-building experiment, Bavelas would tell his subjects he wished them to develop a theory in an area where they had no knowledge. He would show them, for example, pictures of cells and tell them that some of these cells were sick cells and some were healthy cells. The task was to look at the cells and guess which were which. Since the subjects knew nothing about sick or healthy cells, they could only guess. Bavelas said he would tell them if they guessed correctly.

In actuality, the cells shown on the slides were randomly selected; none were particularly sick or healthy. In addition, Bavelas was following a program where the subject was told he was correct 60 percent of the time, no matter what he said. That is, when they guessed whether it was a sick or healthy cell, 60 percent of the time they were told they were correct in their guesses, and 40 percent of the time they were told they were wrong. The reinforcement was not contingent upon what they said but was independent of their responses.

The subjects would look at a cell and make a guess, then look at another cell and make a guess, and they would begin to build a theory. They would decide that a sick cell had a little shady area, and a healthy cell did not. Since they were told they were correct only 60 percent of the time, they would soon find that they were wrong when they said a cell with a shady area was sick. Therefore, they would decide something more was needed. They would add the idea that a sick cell needed both a shady area and a thing hanging down. Again, this would prove to be wrong since they were told they were right only 60 percent of the time. As they studied the cells, they had to increase the complexity of their theories of what makes a healthy cell and what makes a sick one.

When the experiment was completed, Bavelas would ask a subject to write down his theory of the difference between sick and healthy cells. He would offer a new subject this written explanation and tell him that the previous subject had worked out this theory on the basis of his guesses. The new subject was instructed to take this theory, use it if he wished, and correct it, if necessary.

The new subject would examine the theory and look at the slides. He, too, was told he was correct in only 60 percent of his guesses, and so he would find the theory he had been given was correct about half the time. Therefore, he would have to add his own complications as he made his guesses. In doing so, he created an even more complex theory, which he was asked to write down and pass on to a new subject, a third generation. This new subject would examine the theory and do the same task. The third generation subject would look at this more complex theoretical description and begin to apply it to his task of guessing sick or healthy cells. He, too, was rewarded as correct only 60 percent of the time. Naturally, he found the theory was not quite adequate, and he would add to it and make it even more complex.

When Bavelas approached the fourth subject and gave him the same instructions, the subject would look at the extraordinarily complex theory. He would say, "The hell with it," and discard the theory. Starting over, he would make his own guesses and build his own, more simple theory based on being correct 60 percent of the time. After constructing his theory, he would be asked to write it down and pass it on to the next generation of subjects, and so on.

Bavelas found a sine curve—theories would become increasingly complex over the generations until a revolution occurred and previous theories would be discarded. The person would start over again to build increasing complexity until someone discarded the theory again. I think this might be a description of the history of therapy, if not of all scientific endeavors. If we accept the idea that every therapist will have a 50 to 60 percent positive outcome rate when doing therapy, independent of the action in the therapy, he will make a hypothesis about how his therapy works. The hypothesis will increase in complexity as failures occur. He will pass it on to the next generation who will find the theory correct about 60 percent of the time. This generation will add complexities to the theory to improve it. They will pass it on to the next generation. At a certain point, young therapists will say, "Let's start over and think this business through in a new way." They will make a more simple theory, and so on.

I think it might be argued that behavior therapy began as a rejection of the theories of psychoanalysis which had become increasingly turgid and so complex that they were hardly understandable. Now behavior therapy is becoming increasingly complex with intricate learning and cognition theories. Similarly, many of us began family therapy as an attempt to make a more simple theory and discard the past complexities which were not relevant to the therapy task. At this point in family therapy, we have enthusiasts who are creating more turgid and complex theories with their circular, epistemological adventures.

In summary, we face the possibility that our theories of therapy are based upon processes of spontaneous change and not upon our actions. If so, we will have a reasonably good outcome, a high level of confidence that we know we are producing change, and the consensus of colleagues and teachers. As the number of generations continue, we will believe theories are improving, when in actuality they are only increasing in complexity to account for failures. All of this can happen without the outcome of our therapy being contingent upon our therapeutic interventions. That is the framework of uncertainty I faced when teaching and doing research into the nature and practice of therapy. It is still the situation today.

WHAT IS THERAPY?

Besides wondering whether therapy actually has an influence, those of us doing research need to determine what is therapy and what is not. Just as it is difficult to say what is schizophrenia and what is not, or what is hypnosis and what is not, therapy is difficult to separate out from other activities. Is good advice therapy? Is accidental, random influence that has a positive effect therapy? If a violent person is hospitalized and medicated, is that therapy? If so, what about the criminal placed for rehabilitation in the penitentiary?

We might define therapy as a client voluntarily seeking a therapist in order to change. Yet that is only one context, since therapists also work with involuntary clients, both in and out of institutions. We cannot examine therapy without examining its social context—and what is new in the world is the use of therapy to restrain people. Responding to public disorder, the government provided funds for mental health centers in poor neighborhoods where therapists had to deal with the question: was he or she an agent of social control, or was he or she a therapist helping a client? There are other questions about who the therapist serves. In society, is the therapist the agent of the state? In a family, is the therapist the agent of parents who want a child restrained? In a marriage, is the therapist who sees a wife for her anxiety the agent of a husband who would like to pay someone else to listen to his wife complain?

In the last few decades, we have seen the social impact of therapy developing everywhere within communities, and we can no longer think of therapy as simply the interchange between two people. It is a business, a calling, and the agent of many forces.

IS THERAPY THE SAME EVERYWHERE?

At one time, we could do research on therapy with the assumption that therapy was relatively independent of its context. However, today, therapy is done in so many different ways, in so many different places that such simplicity is not possible. Obviously, the practice of therapy is going to be different in different contexts; therefore, the theory appropriate to it will change with the context. For example, a therapist in private practice who has wealthy clients, or clients with insurance paying for the therapy, will have a certain theory and practice. In that situation, a therapist does long and leisurely therapy exploring the nature and origins of the client's discontent. The theory appropriate for that context would be one allowing the uncovering of subtle ideas in the person's psyche, anticipating the slow over-

coming of resistance, and assuming there is a long history of past influences which determine present thinking.

Such a theory and approach would seem bizarre in a mental health agency dealing with poor and working-class clients. Faced with a drunken husband, an erring wife, and a delinquent son, none of whom want to be in therapy but are required to by the court, how can the leisurely exploration of childhood fantasies be considered? In such a situation, a therapist must develop a theory that current influences are a consideration in therapy, redistributing power in a hierarchy and organization is important, and rapid change can be brought about by action and not by reflection. The goal must be a behavioral change rather than a shift in the content of a fantasy.

To researchers, these two extremes indicate that therapy must change its nature when it changes its context. In relation to the financial context alone, the private practice therapist paid by the hour and the agency therapist on salary are going to develop different theories about the pace and depth of therapy. To quote that great theoretician Mark Twain, "Tell me where a man gets his cornpone and I'll tell you what his opinions are."

It is possible that in the history of therapy the most important decision was the idea that it should be paid for by the hour. Suppose, in contrast, a therapist was paid a set amount for the successful outcome with a problem and was not paid hourly. Would theory and practice not change? We might see that day as insurance companies, who determine so much about the nature of therapy, consider orienting themselves to brief contracts for specially defined problems which can be successfully solved.

WHO SHOULD DO THERAPY?

In the period of time that I have studied therapy, not only has the nature of therapy come into question; but, inevitably, who is to do it and how they are to be trained have changed.

As therapists began to unionize by getting licensed, they needed to argue that their training was of such a nature that they had the right to tamper with people's lives, and other people without therapy training did not have that same right. Yet there is the curious problem that each profession requires different training. If psychiatrists agree that psychologists should do therapy, they admit their years of medical training are irrelevant. If psychologists say that psychiatrists or social workers should do therapy, they are saying their years of testing and research are irrelevant. If social workers say that psychiatrists and psychologists can do therapy, they are saying their courses in the history of social work are not essential to a therapist. While this issue was being debated in the established professions, there was an eruption of new people, who were outside the established professions, entering the field through family therapy and various forms of counseling. If they were allowed to do therapy, all that the professions had been teaching was not necessary.

I began to do therapy without proper training, whatever that might be, and I once trained others to do therapy who were not even college-educated. They were quite competent in doing therapy, even though they lacked not only graduate degrees but also what all the middle-class therapists had experienced, an undergraduate education.

In the 1960s, I left schizophrenia, whatever that is, and I set out to do good work with the poor and impoverished of society. At that time, the poor came into therapy, and we either had to teach the middle-class therapist to understand the poor, or we had to teach the poor to be therapists. We did both. Setting out to train people from the community to do therapy, we discovered that much of what was considered essential to be a therapist was not really necessary. The degree, the education in philosophy and psychology, the

courses on testing, all of it seemed inessential when people off the streets could be trained to be competent therapists, if properly taught and supervised. Obviously, whatever therapy is, therapists can be trained in many different ways and still do as well in their results, perhaps even better, than waiting lists.

THE USE OF METAPHOR

Besides all the social issues which arose during this period, a theoretical problem existed from the beginning of therapy investigations. The theoretical analogies, or metaphors, trapped everyone into a particular way of thinking. This helped prevent us from conceptualizing the new forms of therapy developing at that time. It would seem to be in the nature of a theory that it can restrict thinking. In this particular situation, the analogies were too limited to deal with the complexities and changes in the field.

I recall a learned and prominent psychoanalyst beginning a lecture by saying, "We all know what is strength and what is weakness. A muscle is strong or it is weak. It is the same with the ego. The ego is strong or it is weak." This kind of analogy was typical of the time. In actuality, the ego is a hypothetical entity, an abstraction created in an attempt to explain some behavioral phenomenon. To consider it strong or weak, like a muscle, and set out to strengthen it, presumably with therapeutic aerobics, is to take a metaphor literally in a most curious way.

Interestingly, in all three areas of mystery there is a confusion about the literal and the metaphoric. In schizophrenia, the person often says things like, "I have butterflies in my stomach when I get nervous, and they are blue and yellow." In hypnosis, metaphoric images are accepted as literal, as part of the nature of trance. In therapy, we use analogies, stories, and metaphors to influence clients who respond to them as to a literal message. Or, we create a metaphor as part of theory-building and take it literally.

When I began research, not only was the ego taken literally, but the entire intrapsychic structure was so real inside a person that it was as if it could be examined with a surgical operation. There was also the confining analogy of the steam engine. It was said that if a conflict did not burst out in one place from internal pressures, it would burst out in a symptom elsewhere. A much more sensible analogy might have been the idea of the "governor" of a steam engine which controlled the pressure. This was proposed by Maxwell in the 1870s. It did not become adopted as important until the cybernetic theoreticians made use of it, almost a century later, in their theory of systems.

There was another analogy, or metaphor, which handicapped us all and is still a source of confusion. Used to build theory, it was also used as a polemic against competing theories. It was suggested, as part of an old tradition, that the important entities for therapy within the human being were vertically spaced. That is, the conscious was up at the top, and the unconscious was down below. With that analogy one could speak of bringing something *up* into consciousness or putting something *down* into the unconscious. It was also possible to give *deep* interpretations because one knew that the important area was *down there* in the roots, not up here in the superficial surface. One could, as a polemic, say that the other person's therapy was *shallow*, while one's own therapy was *deep*. This was often said about those of us who did brief therapy by people who did endless therapy and called it deep.

I wonder how many hours of seminars and controversies have been devoted to that up and down metaphor? One can appreciate how limited it is by considering other alternatives. Suppose it had been agreed that the unconscious was to the left, not down below, and the conscious was to the right? One could say, "My therapy is more leftist than yours." One could also say, "I made a far right interpretation." An objection to brief therapy could be that it was *rightest* rather than shallow, with a whole new set of connotations.

A research difficulty for years was finding ways to measure a *deep* change in therapy in contrast to a *shallow* change. Now we can see the most serious problem in research is to escape from such analogies and, when we attempt to describe change, to recognize that we are talking about real people doing things in the real world.

Related to the existence of metaphors that are too confining for therapy is the difficulty we all face that theories were not created to change people but were created for other purposes. Psychodynamic theory is not about how to change someone but is about how a person is and how he or she got that way. Learning theory is not about change but is largely a description of what led people to their present ways of behaving. The systems theory of family therapy is not about change but is about how a governed system does not change. Not only do we lack theories focused upon change, but the only clinical language is one of diagnosis, which is irrelevant to therapy and, in fact, can inhibit a therapist's thinking.

GUIDELINES

Let me summarize some of our uncertainties about therapy and their relevance to current practice. We cannot be sure that therapy actually influences people, and the fact that previous generations were sure does not make it so. When we examine therapy, assuming it exists, we have trouble saying what it is and what it is not. Not only is it difficult to differentiate it from social control activities and educational processes, but therapy also seems to differ in different social contexts and is not a single type of behavior. When we try to think about therapy, we are confined and restricted by clinical metaphors.

Given all these uncertainties and doubts, how should a responsible therapist and teacher act today? How should we proceed if we are not to delude the public paying for our services?

To a great extent, it is these uncertainties from observation and research that have led me to the particular kind of therapy I developed and teach. At the risk of being accused of being simplistic and shallow by people who were sure their therapy was deep, I developed certain guidelines for a therapy which seemed to me to be the most trustworthy. Let me outline these guidelines:

1) If it is possible that change occurs independently of therapy, with a risk that the therapist is taking the credit when he should not, it follows logically that therapy should be brief. If clients are seen for years, they graduate from school, get married, have children, get divorced, and go through all kinds of life's changes which can, in error, be attributed to therapy. Short-term interventions can better reveal whether it is the therapy or outside forces which are inducing change.

2) When there is uncertainty about change, it would seem better to focus upon the most observable situation and not to dwell upon what cannot be seen. It follows logically that one should be concerned with the current, real-life situation of a client, which can be examined, rather than the past, for which there is no evidence or fantasies, and for which there can be none.

If one believes that a person's past will program his or her present, it becomes part of the goal of therapy to change the past. With today's skillful reframing techniques and with the careful use of amnesia, it is possible to keep people from having the awful pasts they once had. The use of amnesia is particularly valuable. We can get along with each other, if we forget today what we did to each other yesterday. To reframe the past with psychodynamic ideology, bringing out all its worst traumatic aspects, seems less helpful than to reframe the past in a more

positive way and give amnesia for the worst of it.

3) If there is uncertainty about how to verify the outcome of therapy, it would seem logical for therapists to focus on a particular problem. In that way, one can determine whether the problem is still there or not. To accept for therapy ambiguous character problems or system relationship problems, when one can never determine if they were successfully changed, does not seem reasonable.

4) To gather evidence about what is happening in the life of a client and to determine if therapy is inducing a change, it would seem best to bring in the family. Not only can the family contribution make therapy more successful, since relatives inspire changes that a therapist alone cannot, but it also helps the therapist stay in the real world where change can be observed. A wife who offers only fantasies about her husband is not providing the information that one gets when she provides her husband. What a handicap it now seems that therapists in the old days declined to see relatives or even speak to them on the telephone because it would have interfered with the therapist's fantasies about the family.

5) If one wants to be more certain whether the therapist has an influence or not, it seems sensible for the therapist to focus on behavior and give directives for change, instead of only talking about ideas. To discuss issues insightfully leads only to a change in the client's ability to discuss insightfully. A behavioral change can be observed. This issue is separate from the fact that people are more cooperative and less resistant to change if one does not make interpretations or give insight.

6) If one wishes to influence a client to change, it logically follows that a therapist should organize the therapy so that happens. To sit back and listen and say, "Tell me more about that"—this produces a therapy without destination. If therapy is to achieve a goal, the therapist must set one. To get there, the therapist must, as much as possible, arrange what hap-

pens. To let a client initiate all conversation, behavior, and ideas, when the client has come to the therapist because he does not know how to change, seems naive.

7) If we wish to be sure that we are not taking money under false pretenses and that our therapy is changing someone, it would seem logical to train therapists in skillful therapy techniques. Just as therapy should focus on the observable present, training should focus on the observable actions of a therapist, preferably on videotape or in a one-way mirror room. To depend upon personal therapy of the therapist as a way of teaching how to change a client is to wonder if the therapist has learned how to change anyone at all.

Perhaps most important, it is reasonable that a therapist should have confidence in his or her ideas and actions in therapy. The past emphasis on personal therapy produced therapists who were uneasy about their unconscious conflicts and hostile, aggressive, internal impulses. It now seems naive to teach therapists self-distrust and then expect them to confidently offer hope and help to the helpless and unfortunate.

These guidelines are based upon a rather obvious idea about therapy, and what becomes evident is a curious finding. It seems apparent that the procedures I am recommending for therapy are precisely the opposite of what was done 30 years ago when I began my therapy investigations. At that time, and still held occasionally in the large cities, there were some assumptions: It was assumed that therapy should be long term; it should deal with the past and not the present; it should not focus on a problem but on vague character issues; all relatives of a client were avoided; insight and interpretation were the therapeutic focus instead of action; a person was helped to remember every miserable moment of the past; and training consisted of personal therapy for the therapist.

There was another issue which shows a difference from the present focus of therapy. In those days, a therapist did not take responsibility for change. If someone asked an analyst, "Is it your job to change people?", the analyst would say it was not. The task was to help people understand themselves—whether they changed or not was up to them. The opposite posture seems more reasonable today in terms of accountability. The therapist is no longer a consultant but a people changer who fails if the case fails. As Erickson would put it, a therapist must learn many different ways to change many different kinds of people, or he should take up some other profession.

In summary, the kind of therapy we have today as the mainstream is the opposite of what was done in the beginning. Some people have changed because of the influence of teachers, others out of trial and error, and others after examining therapy research. Today there is a generation of people who have seriously taken up the career of changing people. They are not advisors, consultants, objective observers, or diagnosticians. They are people whose task is to be expert at influencing another person. They are skilled at getting people to follow their suggestions, including suggestions the person is not aware of receiving.

We have arrived at a revolutionary time in the therapy field. Rather than being pessimistic about whether therapists influence people at all, as I suggested was the beginning of therapy, we are now concerned that therapists will become so skillful at influencing people that we must worry about how to govern therapists.

Although therapists are not extraordinarily skillful today, let us project into the future and see what it might be like if present trends continue. There will be a group of skillful people who have spent years of training and practice influencing people. They will know how to give directives that are followed and will know how to influence people outside their awareness. They will be able to marshal the forces in the family and in the community to bring about the changes they wish. Groups of such therapists will combine their thinking in planning strategies to produce change. With therapists and their teachers becoming increasingly skillful in their craft, therapists will use power over other people to benefit them. What about limits on that power?

When we look at the three mysteries of human life, people have always been afraid of schizophrenia and they have been afraid of hypnosis. The time is approaching when therapy could raise fears; and, in fact, it already has. As we train therapists to be experts at influencing people, their skills must be confined to positive goals. It is the same problem that teachers in the martial arts faced when they taught the most scientific ways to use physical force in combat. It is not helpful to say that therapists should not be interested in power, when skill in achieving power over others is often necessary in helping people. It also does not seem reasonable to teach therapists to be inept as a way of preventing their influence. Obviously we want therapists who can help people in distress because they are skillful and know their business. But how will we control these people who are becoming expert at controlling others?

Logically it follows that training therapists in technical skills must be within a framework of ethics and self-discipline. Our problem becomes more complicated as so many different kinds of therapists enter the field, and as therapy becomes more of a business and less of a calling. Technical skills can be used to turn people into patients for financial gains, as well as to change them. Possibly the model to turn to is one developed by others who needed to control people trained in the skillful use of strength and power. We might ultimately adopt a model from the martial arts and Eastern religion, where people are taught ways to achieve power within a framework of harmony and restraint. An adaptation of the aikido philosophy might be appropriate. We could define therapy as, "The art of defending oneself and society without taking advantage of, or harming, other people."

REFERENCE

Rosen, J. (1951). *Direct analysis.* New York: Grune & Stratton.

Discussion by Salvador Minuchin, M.D.

◆

The previous panels at this conference joined psychoanalytic and behavioral therapy, family therapy, Zulus, and Eskimos, presenting questions about life, therapy, and the process of change. This panel, where Cloé is being discussed by Watzlawick, and Jay discussed by me, is different. It's all in the family. So it's natural to expect a few family quarrels.

First, as always, there is style. Jay aims to challenge. This is a stance that really fit the younger Haley, the iconoclast, better than the present Haley, director of a prestigious institute. But of course we are prisoners of our pathways. Just as I must always carry my early Talmudic upbringing, Jay must remain wedded to his iconoclastic leanings.

Then, there is the question of how his paper is organized. Here I want to borrow from literary criticism to question whether this paper was written from the beginning to the end as one piece, or whether it is a quilt pieced together from different periods of his thinking. I am inclined to think it is a quilt. The first part of the presentation is vintage Haley. It uses simple declarative sentences and the peculiar mixture of facts imbedded in opinion with which Jay surprises readers and shocks them into accepting his assertions. This part is Jay the pioneer, reminiscing on his earlier challenges to the field, his skepticism, his research on therapy, his challenges to psychoanalytic thinking, his evolution as a trainer, his training of paraprofessionals, and his integration of Bateson's and Erickson's theoretical trends, continuously warring inside him as his ideas evolved toward the strategic approach—the particular brand of therapy the Washington institute teaches. I would guess that this part of his presentation was gleaned from Jay's early writings to substantiate the second part of his paper, the guidelines: the description of what he thinks therapy and training should be—the Magna Carta of his institute.

If this is the progression, I would say the results are not entirely successful. The guidelines would stand alone. But they are not the product of 30 years of reasoned inquiry and research into the field of therapy. They are the product of the last ten years (and it is not a coincidence that the institute is celebrating its tenth anniversary). The attempt at melding does not really do justice to the complexity, or to the meandering, of those 30 years.

The summary is relatively unrelated to the other two parts. As a matter of fact, it conflicts strongly with the first part. Where the first part questions whether we can be certain that therapy influences people, the summary warns us to beware of the therapist's power. The summary arises from Jay's current explorations. But it also states a basic theme. Regardless of his attempts to hide it, Jay Haley is a moralist. In the Socratic tradition, he is concerned with the consequences of our success in creating the delusion that our knowledge is complete and that the power

springing from this knowledge will be basically benign.

For the rest of this discussion I will focus on what I think is Jay's moral intent: his cautionary tale about the consequences of knowledge misused.

The paper starts with a simple question: Is there such a thing as therapy? Presumably, the 7,000 participants of this conference would answer with a resounding yes. "Not so fast," says Jay. "How do you know that therapy actually exists, in the sense that it is causing change?" In reply, we can posit a simple description of therapy. It is an encounter between two parties, one defines himself as needing help, cure or change, and the other claims a body of knowledge that can do the trick. The process of therapy occurs in a field of verbal exchanges. Though it may be individual, familial, psychodynamic, behavioral, hypnotic, systemic, voluntary or involuntary, out- or inpatient, and so on, the therapeutic encounter clearly partakes of the above elements. But the problem that concerns Jay is not whether the therapeutic encounter occurs; we know it does. But how do we know that it has produced the change we want to produce? And, of course, here we step into a mare's nest, because change is measured only against one body of meaning: the therapist's.

To support his pessimism, Jay highlights his early research in the 50s on the waiting list. "Not so fast," say Smith, Glass and Miller, prestigious investigators of the therapeutic process, who reported, in 1980, a meta-analysis of over 500 studies comparing some form of psychological therapy with a control condition. When averaged over all dependent measures of outcome, they report, psychological therapy is .85 standard deviations better than the control treatment. "Not so fast," say Prioleau, Murdock and Brody ("An Analysis of Psychotherapy versus Placebo Studies," *The Behavioral and Brain Sciences*, 1983, 6, 275–310), who reported that when they examined a subset of 32 of these studies dealing with psychotherapy versus a placebo treatment, they found no significant differences. Dozens of other prestigious names, among them Jerome Frank, Hans Eysenck, and Sol Garfield, join the debate in a seesaw of opinions that depend on the perspective of the investigator. The field remains ambiguous and confusing; it would be useless to assert that we even have a definitive study.

Just to complicate matters, what are the criteria by which we measure change? Our research with psychosomatic patients (anorectics, asthmatics, and brittle diabetics) showed an 85 percent cure of the identified patients' symptoms, lasting over a follow-up period ranging from seven to 12 years. By Jay's guidelines, we passed with flying colors. There were behavioral changes in the predicted direction in the identified patients after our intervention. And criteria for change were simple and clear: reduction of the number of days in the hospital, reduction or disappearance of medically inexplicable difficulties in our diabetic patients, weaning of asthmatic patients from cortisone dependency, increase of body weight in anorectics. Clearly we produced change, in the desired direction. But we had a much more difficult time measuring what we thought was the real breakthrough in our study, namely, that the changes in the identified patients' symptoms were due to our interventions in the body of the family.

So I would like to add the variable of measurement to Jay's concern about the meaning of change. Might we be measuring certain things simply because they are measurable, like the drunk looking for his lost key under the streetlamp because that's where the light is? In any case, I have never seen any evidence that convinces me that changes in the theory and practice of therapy are guided by research on therapeutic outcome. It seems much more likely as Bavela's parable suggests, that, in social science at least, paradigmatic change does not follow scientific evidence. It may well be that in our field, a field of persuasion, after all, what new paradigms really follow is cultural trends—the ethos of our era.

For example, Freudian metapsychology held sway for about a generation. But by the 50s, that theory, based on the cultural and scientific ethos of the nineteenth century, had already been subjected to multiple schisms and deviationist detours within its own advocates. Challenges were posed by the neo-Freudian psychoanalytic schools. Kardiner, Horney, Fromm, and Sullivan were some of the challengers who introduced cultural dimensions to a theory that belonged to a period grounded in unending expansion and unlimited resources.

When family therapy came into the field, it entered upon the cultural and scientific changes of the late 50s. When it encountered cybernetics through Bateson, his ideas became enormously significant simply because it was time to accept the idea that people are interconnected participants in a larger context, in a world increasingly aware of the dwindling of resources and our own wastefulness. We could not have avoided that paradigmatic change because, like Freud, Bateson and the early family therapists were people of their time, using the scientific metaphors that governed the period.

As we developed the theory and practice of family therapy, we followed the steps that paradigmatic expansion necessarily follows. The increased complexity of our theory-building is the result, but as Bavela's experiment demonstrates, increased complexity does not necessarily denote increased knowledge. We often tend to equate the two, as in the current effort to marry family therapy to Maturana's closed systems biology. Or perhaps, following the conservative trends of our time, family therapy is searching for a conservative theory.

At any rate, as every fable ends with a moral, we must search for the moral of Jay's paper. Since so much of it is devoted to questioning our certainty, one would expect that at some point Jay would turn to questioning his own. But he doesn't do that. As a family therapist who worked with Jay for ten years, I share many of his ideas of therapy and training. But I would not be so certain that my body of knowledge encompasses all situations. I would not feel so certain that change can be measured only behaviorally, or that therapy should be only brief, or that the past should be dismissed, or that relationship problems can never be determined, or that directives for change are always better than talking about ideas. This paper may answer a myriad of questions in the field, but it doesn't answer them all. And it occurs to me that, here and there, there may be a question that even Jay has not asked.

It seems to me that this meeting was designed by the Erickson Foundation not as a Tower of Babel, but as a congress of people exploring the field of mental health from different perspectives. In this context, perhaps family therapists could learn something about respect for the individual's resources from the followers of Milton Erickson and reencounter the individual in the system through that learning. Perhaps object relations analysts could expand their theory and practice by realizing that there are external objects in continuous transaction with the internalized familial object. Perhaps group therapists could unearth the 1950s question about the differences between artificial and natural groups. Perhaps behavior therapists could begin to reconsider a theory that encompasses only two people. Maybe RET people could gain uncertainty. . . .

I am not naive enough to think that this change could be achieved in 27 speakers. Our pathways are too well-worn for that. But our parallel monologues have been heard by 7,000 participants who, I hope, will expand our present theories. I want to thank Jay for articulating, as always, such a clear map of where he stands and allowing me to dance around him, trying to tip his balance.

Psychotherapy—Past, Present, and Future

Murray Bowen, M.D.

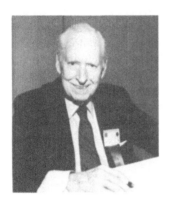

Murray Bowen, M.D.
Murray Bowen is one of the pioneering figures in the history of family therapy. His medical degree was awarded from the University of Tennessee in 1937. Currently, he is Clinical Professor and Director of the Georgetown Family Center of the Georgetown University Medical Center, and conducts a part-time private practice of family psychotherapy. He has published approximately 50 papers, book chapters and monographs, mostly on family psychotherapy and family systems theory. Among these is his landmark paper, presented in 1967 and published in 1972, which started a trend toward defining oneself in one's family of origin in lieu of more conventional therapies.

Bowen describes the evolution of psychotherapy by outlining its antecedents and describing major events that shaped contemporary psychotherapy. He calls for therapists to take the responsibility to fill gaps in academic and theoretical knowledge.

Some form of talking therapy has been present since the human sought help with personal problems. Talking therapy has gone through many stages, and its antecedents are deep in human history. Change was slow until psychotherapy was formalized a century ago. The greatest change came in the last half of the twentieth century. This chapter will review some of the important changes that have marked the development of psychotherapy, and the last section will contain some educated guesses about the future direction of this profession.

PSYCHOTHERAPY IN THE PAST

ANTECEDENTS TO PSYCHOTHERAPY

Antecedents to psychotherapy date back millions of years into evolutionary history when egg-laying reptilian mothers protected their young. As evolution proceeded to mammalian life, it was routine for mothers and/or fathers to feed and protect their young until they were physically viable, for adults to live in groups that could be called families, and for multiple families to live in conglomerates with others of their kind. The family has been around a long time. It contained the basic instinctual pattern of the relationships between parents and their young. Evolution contradicts the notion that family relationships were developed by the human family. The comments in this chapter are presented for comparative purposes rather than to provide detail about evolution. Serious authors have detailed considerable knowledge about this subject in recent years (Sagan, 1980; MacLean, 1973; Wilson, 1975). Wilson is among sociobiologists with evidence that altruism is present in lower forms of life. He believes that automatic helping of others is an instinctual way to ensure survival.

The most rapid change in man, as he has evolved to his present human state, has been the development of his brain. A simple description would say he began with a hindbrain and midbrain that governed his automatic, protoplasmic, and instinctual life. Comparatively late in evolution he began to develop a prefrontal cortex or forebrain, which enabled the human to think, reason, and reflect. MacLean has spent his life studying brain development. He used the term *the triune brain* to describe the amalgamation of the three brains into a single organ. While retaining the basic function of his early brain formation, the human developed an intellect, tools and agriculture, languages, the ability to read and write, and all the other functions that went with his developing culture.

The time span of events in the universe is beyond ordinary comprehension. It is estimated that the earth began some 4,000 million years ago; that the earth remained inert about 3,500 million years; that living cells developed about 500 million years ago from the interaction of the earth's chemical elements, water, and the sun's heat; and that all animal and plant life on earth evolved from that beginning about 500 million years ago. This is a graphic representation of evolution. From ordinary comprehension, it is microscopically slow. With a broader comprehension, it is

a process that begins slowly and gains momentum. Living things reproduce themselves almost exactly, but not quite. Over a long period of time, the slight changes between the generations add up to the major change known as evolution.

It is a fact that the human brain, skeleton, muscles, lungs, digestive tracts, and internal organs (such as the reproductive organs) are similar to those that existed in earlier subhuman life forms. Paleontologists and archeologists proliferate. The human emerged from a subhuman state less than a million years ago. Most current ideas about primitive civilization go back less than 30,000 years, and the sparse recordings of history go back less than 10,000 years. Our current calendar goes back to the birth of Christ less than 2,000 years ago. The human, with his developing brain, has been able to comprehend the rhythm of the universe, the solar system, the earth, the seasons, day and night, the tides, and the weather. It is a giant explainable and predictable natural system that interlinks with numerous variables that are also part of the natural system.

The integration of the parts of the human brain will probably continue to pose problems. With the cerebral cortex the human has worked to define the nature of the universe, the nonliving world, and items of life other than his own. This area includes the accepted sciences which can be proven, measured, validated, and predicted, such as astronomy, chemistry, physics and other disciplines from the sciences. At the opposite end of the spectrum are the arts, made up of feelings, subjectivity, impressions, imagination, and ideas that can be neither validated nor proven. These include art, music, dance, theatre, literature, religion, and other disciplines based on human subjectivity and experience.

In the middle ground are numerous disciplines. Biology is one that is almost a science, but not quite. There are those who say biology is based on certain concepts that do not meet the criteria of sciences. Medicine contains elements of science and the arts. Psychoanalysis was governed by the *scientific method*, which indicated it was not really a science, but that it might eventually become a real science if research people handled subjective data with scientific rigor. Psychiatry, psychology, anthropology, and sociology were clearly in the arena with the nonsciences. The same could be said for the "social sciences"—a term used to convey the notion that they aspired to a scientific status.

I became interested in psychoanalytic research shortly after World War II, wondering what it would take to elevate theory to a scientific level. This interest has continued for 40 years. Psychoanalysis was filled with nonscientific *feeling* concepts and concepts based on Greek plays. My curiosity about theory remained latent for almost a decade until family research began in the 1950s. The family seemed to contain variables for theory that were missing in individual theory. The family research, plus the previous thinking about theory, plus ideas from evolution, all led to the effort to conceptualize human behavior into the same natural systems ideas that governed evolution. This was quite different from general systems ideas that were developed by von Bertalanffy. An effort was made to integrate family relationships into the systems concepts of evolution. The concepts of family systems theory and therapy were presented in *Family Therapy in Clinical Practice* (Bowen, 1978). More detail about theory is beyond the content of this chapter on psychotherapy. On a practical level, theory governs the way the human thinks about human affairs.

The human uses some kind of theoretical notion to govern thinking and action. Through the centuries, the acceptance of a new way of thinking has been uneven. Overall, there has been a lag time between the introduction of a new idea and its general acceptance. There have been situations in which the old idea persists, and other situations in which the old idea breaks out in pockets. Continuation of the old appears related to an increase in societal feelings, reactivity, or religious ideas. Through theory man knew the earth was round as much as 2,000 years ago, but the notion of a flat earth persisted for centuries. The idea that the earth was created in its present state persisted long after the idea of constant change and evolution was established.

Distortions about good and evil spirits have been common. Primitive man believed that favorable times were controlled by approving spirits and bad times by angry spirits. He also believed his own goodness or wickedness governed the spirits. He devised rituals to get himself in harmony with the spiritual world. Primitive medicine men believed an illness resulted from evil spirits, and good treatment was a ritual to drive out the evil spirits. Witch doctors devised a variety of rituals to drive away the same misassumption about an evil spirit. Witchcraft came to be centered in England about two centuries after its beginnings in 1500. This era included the Salem witch burnings in colonial New England. Witches were assumed to be living devils and, after public trials, they were burned alive to kill the devil. This was a brief period when religious zealots put superstition into action. One can hope such actions are behind us, but they can surface even now when frenzied feelings overcome calm knowledge. Even in recent centuries, medicine has included numerous superstitious notions about the cause of physical illness.

The human has the ability to think for himself if psychotherapists and professional people can convey a calm notion of the problem and permit the patients to work it out for themselves.

THE ROOTS OF PSYCHOTHERAPY

A version of psychotherapy began in prehuman evolution when mothers protected their young and individuals became aware of the importance of others. In each evolutionary period the awareness has been deepened and broadened. There are birds who choose a mate for life and who go into mourning and die when the mate is killed or lost. There are 17 species of mammals more monogamous than the human. Their entire lives are spent relating to each other, raising their families, and living in groups of other pairs who do the same. This behavior is instinctual. The early instinctual behavior continued as the primitive human developed a forebrain.

As culture proceeded through the centuries, the roles of clan members became more formalized. There was always a clan member, a senior person, or an elder to whom the individual could turn for knowledge, guidance, and support when it was needed. As far as we know, the human sought counsel from others besides his parents for certain crises that developed in his own life. As time passed, the settlements grew and the roles of males and females became specialized. There were humans with knowledge, experience, technical expertise, and personal characteristics who served as resources for advice and counsel. As the villages became more complex, the roles of various clan members became more professionalized. There were the early physicians, ministers, teachers, and experts in human relationships to whom people could turn for advice and guidance. There is evidence that some form of psychotherapy was being practiced long before the profession was identified.

THE MODERN ERA OF PSYCHOTHERAPY

Psychotherapy attained a new level of excellence with the work of Freud (1949) about a century ago. Through most of the nineteenth century, people with psychotic problems were housed in institutions under the care of psychiatrists, often known as "alienists." The term alienist described the alienation that involved the patients. Neurotic problems were treated by psy-

chiatrists who were also neurologists. Treatment involved symptomatic support or rest cures in sanataria.

Freud was trained as a neurologist. He developed a completely different theory and a method of *talking* therapy that gave birth to psychoanalysis and, ultimately, revolutionized psychiatry and psychotherapy. Freud's theory conceived of an unconscious which included unacceptable sexual and social thoughts and impulses. It remained out of conscious memory by repression and the mechanisms of defense. The intensity of the unconscious determined an unexplained life course and unforeseen symptoms. Through a process of free association in the presence of a nonjudgmental analyst, the person slowly remembered items from his own unconscious. The analyst was always there to help integrate the unconscious items.

Freud was the first to do a detailed study of two-person relationship patterns. In the presence of a nonreactive analyst, the patient's fantasied relationship with the analyst was an exact replica of early life relationships to parents, spouse, and all other people. This transfer of emotional patterns to the analyst was known as *transference*. It could be analyzed if the analyst *knew* his own unconscious. It was common for an inept analyst to respond to the patient with his own unconscious processes. This was called *countertransference*. The analyst was an unwitting pawn in the whole process. The countertransference could block further analysis and change the entire therapeutic relationship into another acted-out relationship.

The finding about the replication of early life relationships with other people was one of Freud's important contributions. The replication extends into marriages and all other significant relationships. It is a situation in which one unconscious responds automatically to another. Freud dealt with this by requiring new analysts to undergo their own personal psychoanalysis. This has been fairly successful when analysts accept full responsibility for their unconscious processes. This procedure stills holds in psychoanalytic training centers. The whole process tends to become lost in the recent surge in psychotherapy when therapists believe the situation can be handled by yet another technical maneuver.

The principles of psychoanalysis have been a major force in the development of the entire field. Freud was a physician and he tried to develop his theory as an extension of medicine. The distance between physical and emotional illness was too great for the concepts of the time. Because psychoanalysis did not require detailed medical training, he began to admit students from related disciplines to psychoanalytic training.

Important changes occurred during the first half of the twentieth century. Psychoanalysis was effective with neurotic problems but not with the more severe forms of illness. Therapy required more activity from the analyst and this involved countertransference. Psychoanalytic technique was modified to "psychoanalytically oriented psychotherapy," which permitted more activity from the therapist and less fantasy from the patient. The best therapists were still those who knew and respected the countertransference phenomenon.

Another change involved the "team concept." Psychiatric hospitals and clinics began using psychologists, social workers, and experts from other professional disciplines as part of the diagnostic-treatment teams. In the 1920s, this trend led to the establishment of the American Orthopsychiatric Association, a national organization for members of the mental health disciplines.

A series of changes in the 1950s and 1960s influenced the direction of psychiatry and psychotherapy. They are (1) the introduction of the major tranquilizers in 1954; (2) the beginning of family therapy in 1957; and (3) the National Mental Health Act in 1963. Each of these changes will be discussed separately.

The Introduction of Tranquilizers

The use of tranquilizers increased rapidly. The serious forms of mental illness became more symptom free, state hospital populations decreased, and more patients could be managed as outpatients or in halfway facilities. Tranquilizers have done more than anything else to change the practice of psychiatry in this century. They are also used for the less severe forms of mental illness. An increased percentage of tranquilizers is prescribed by internists and general practitioners for all kinds of mild anxiety symptoms.

Family Therapy

Family therapy illustrates principles that have involved the helping disciplines for several decades. It burst into professional awareness when it was discussed at a national meeting in March 1957. The theoretical jump from an individual to a family orientation had been slow and difficult. It violated important principles of theory, such as transference. For several decades the profession knew that the family was important in all forms of mental illness. The transference situation required that each family member be treated in individual psychotherapy with a separate therapist. There were all kinds of theoretical principles involved in whether, or how much, the separate therapists could meet, either socially or professionally. If they met to discuss the family issue, there was one kind of problem. If they did not, there was another kind of problem. If a nonsymptomatic family member was in individual therapy, there were questions whether it was to help the identified patient or the other family member him or herself. There were no easy answers.

The average professional was not aware of the years of work on theory, emotional connectedness, and transference that had gone into the creation of family therapy. Most responded as if it was no more than a simple shift in technique, and that anyone could do family therapy if they found the correct technique. The field proliferated with professional people from divergent backgrounds. In the rush to do therapy, theory was bypassed. Group therapists became involved in large numbers. Formerly they had put family members into separate groups; now they began to put multiple family members into the same group.

I was involved in the development of family therapy and in most of the meetings that followed. Most of the people who developed family therapy had mastered the countertransference phenomenon in their former training. I believed the rush into family therapy would subside when therapists encountered countertransference snarls. However, that did not occur. The countertransference was less operative as long as two or more family members were present in the therapy sessions, or if the therapy was kept brief.

The number of family therapists increased at an unprecedented rate. When someone learns a technique, they teach others. The proponents of one technique are quick to challenge the proponents of another. It resembles the multitude of different sects in the great religions. By the late 1970s a few professionals became interested in theory, but most of the interest dealt with old issues from individual theory. The rapid evolution of family therapy has been an interesting phenomenon.

The Mental Health Act

The Mental Health Act of 1963 was a government action to establish a network of centers and "storefronts" which made services available to the masses. Psychiatry had become more socially acceptable. A segment of the population had long associated psychiatry with "crazy" people. For example, people were hesitant to mention psychiatric treatment on employment applications lest they be permanently categorized as deranged. Along with the other changes, the Mental Health Act helped change the public image from the treatment of chronic sickness to a more positive orientation that ensured good health.

The focus was on brief therapy and the termination of the therapeutic relationship after a few interviews. Brief therapy and crisis intervention became catchwords as if the process had been invented by this different orientation. Staffing the centers provided employment for hundreds of newly trained therapists who never had time to learn some of the important fundamentals of theory, transference, and the important function of the therapist in mental health situations. The brief orientation invaded the various teachers and training centers. This helped foster the notion that theory is superfluous and techniques can be learned quickly. From an evolutionary standpoint, the Mental Health Act created a positive public image for mental health and psychotherapy. The negative side of the extremely rapid growth will probably fall to those therapists who accept the responsibility to keep knowledge abreast of the rapid change.

PSYCHOTHERAPY IN THE PRESENT

The goal of this section is to present a few systems ideas about forces in medicine, in psychiatry and in associated professional disciplines that have governed the present development of psychotherapy.

There have been profound changes in psychotherapy in the past 60 or 70 years. Most of the change occurred as psychoanalytic therapy related itself to medicine and mental health. Freud developed "a new psychiatry." His ideas attracted a number of physicians from other countries who were eager to learn and to be psychoanalyzed. Central Europe was the center for the new ideas. There was a premium on being analyzed by Freud, or by someone who had been analyzed by Freud. The new ideas were brought to the United States by progressive young psychiatrists who were immediately in demand by other psychiatrists for psychoanalysis and training. A few who were already connected with medical schools aspired to have this analysis and training connected with medical schools. A series of theoretical and practical reasons prevented that union.

The more experienced psychoanalysts formed freestanding psychoanalytic institutes in some of the larger cities. These institutes had no direct affiliation with medicine. The psychoanalysts did their psychoanalyses in private offices and met regularly in the institute buildings with all the analytic candidates for the long period of supervision and training that was necessary for final membership in the American Psychoanalytic Association. It was common for training analysts to have long waiting lists of prospective candidates. The institutes were careful to see that candidates were qualified before graduation. The more promising young psychiatrists found reason to be psychoanalyzed for their own personal problems and to complete the long training and supervision before practicing on their own.

Psychoanalytic theory spread very fast. No one else had a theory to compare with psychoanalysis. In addition to teaching, the new analysts psychoanalyzed a few patients and members of the other psychiatric disciplines. The actual number of analysts was small, but they held important positions and they were active in psychiatry. Psychoanalytic theory was dominant in psychiatry and the mental health professions.

World War II changed psychiatric practice. Most of the psychiatric leaders in the armed forces were also psychoanalysts. Psychiatry was finally becoming popular as a private practice specialty. Numerous young psychiatrists sought psychoanalytic training after the war. By midcentury, more and more vacancies in chairs of psychiatry in medical schools were being filled by psychiatrists who were also psychoanalysts. In this period psychoanalysis was closest to medicine. The psychoana-

lysts of that time were idealistic. There was evidence of the extent of the mental health problems in the population. They believed that psychoanalytic ideas could conceptualize world problems, and the ideas could be taught as a way to prevent mental illness.

The previous section outlined three forces that appeared to operate after midcentury. In addition, there was another force that began in the 1960s and gradually became more operative over the following decades.

Freud had never been able to integrate psychoanalytic theory with medicine. Psychoanalytic theory functioned as a theory that described the underlying problem, but he used the analogy of psychopathology to say it was similar to pathology in physical illness. In the field of science, a similarity between bodies of knowledge does not make a theoretical connection between the two. His theoretical concepts included speculation, feelings, and ideas from literature that could not be validated, measured or proven by scientific methodology.

By the mid-1960s, there were growing rumblings that psychoanalytic theory was not really scientific, and this sentiment increased gradually for a decade or more. Part of this appeared to be the interplay between medicine and psychiatry. The scientific side of medicine is based on factors that are called *biological.* It bases theory on a premise in use for centuries. It maintains that functioning in an individual is determined by the physical beginning, including hereditary, genetic, pathological, and other factors; that the cause of illness can be determined in medical research; and that treatment involves physical factors and the discovery and use of chemical substances. Psychiatry is said to involve biological, psychological, and sociological factors. This division is simplistic according to present knowledge, but it will do for the purpose of this chapter. Psychological and sociological factors are not quite scientific.

The theoretical distance between medicine and psychiatry has always been there, even when they appeared harmonious on the surface. Before World War II, psychiatry usually operated as part of the department of medicine. Psychiatrists complained about lack of representation in medical school decisions. Some states went to the point of building psychiatric institutes physically removed from the departments of medicine and surgery, which are the most powerful departments in running a medical establishment. The new institute buildings removed psychiatry physically. The distance was perpetuated. Some medical schools attempted to solve the distance problem by putting department offices near each other in the medical complex. The theoretical distance still prevailed, despite the efforts of the chairmen of psychiatry to be good friends with the other chairmen.

Another factor operated in medical schools that illustrates the theoretical posture between psychiatry and medicine. Immediately after World War II, it was unusual to hear the term *eclectic* except in rare instances to refer to some different theoretical approach. In the 1960s when psychoanalysis was being discredited, it was common for departments of psychiatry to be called *eclectic* which meant they taught and used all kinds of different approaches, even though the chairman was basically psychoanalytic. The term *eclectic* referred to a broad spectrum of different approaches, methods of psychotherapy, electroshock therapy, drug therapy, and others. The use of the term increased in the 1970s until the department appointed a chairman who emphasized drug therapy as a cure for mental problems. When the chairman was finally known as a "biological" psychiatrist, the use of the term eclectic was dropped.

The biggest change came during the 1970s. More and more department chairmen were biological psychiatrists who taught drug therapy and little else. At the extreme there were a few whose total time of psychiatric residency was devoted to drug therapy. The psychiatric residents received no training in psychotherapy, except for a brief lecture course in a family therapy section run by professionals in social work or psychology who had Ph.D. degrees. Family therapy and psychotherapy were relegated to nonpsychiatric members of the mental health professions. These situations are an absolute ultimate in a 30-year trend in which physicians are trained in the biological sciences and psychotherapy is referred to nonphysicians.

In summary, although there are a number of different ways to understand this development, the theoretical is the most important. Psychological factors are present in every human illness, whether that illness is acute or chronic, or whether it is manifested in a psychological, physical, or social problem. When the human is divided according to symptom manifestation, the diagnosis misses an important cause that may underlie dozens of medical and surgical conditions. There is strong evidence that schizophrenia, manic depressive psychosis, neurosis, and all the other psychological states are not separate entities, but are qualitatively the same. When the clinician is assigned to one small area, it is easy to miss the overall picture. There are both positive and negative factors when an evolutionary process goes to specialization. There are positive aspects about focusing on detail. But when broad aspects are poorly defined, the focus on detail tends to be more negative.

The broad configuration is one in which psychiatry, mental health, and psychotherapy have separated themselves from medicine. It appears that medicine may have played a major role in that. For some years medicine has been moving to bring psychiatry into better theoretical harmony with its body of knowledge. The choice of *biological* psychiatry may eventually prove to be a bad choice; but when medicine applied insidious pressure, there is some evidence to support the thesis that psychiatry was given a choice to either go *biological* or else. If psychiatry goes biological, as is the trend these years, it would be necessary to give up its association with psychotherapy and family therapy. The other side of the broad configuration would say that both psychiatry and psychotherapy, including family therapy, have played equal roles in this. Psychiatry has already decided to go *biological* in preference to relationship therapy. In 1977 a national family therapy organization received official government approval to call *family therapy* an autonomous and separate discipline. This approval was the response to the organization's promise to do regular inspections of family therapy training centers. In return, the organization received permission to accredit family therapists for practice. By this action, initiated from within family therapy, the fields of family therapy and psychotherapy were officially approved as separate and autonomous disciplines.

To summarize this point, family therapy, with its right to do "individual, marital, and family therapy," has been declared an autonomous discipline that is not related to any other existing discipline. By this action the discipline achieves some remarkable freedom to determine its own course, but it also assumes tremendous responsibility to go it alone. The field of psychotherapy now includes hundreds of people who seek more knowledge than was possible in their training.

PSYCHOTHERAPY IN THE FUTURE

This chapter has presented variables that appear to have been important in the overall evolution of psychotherapy. On a very broad level, for centuries into the future, human beings will continue to need people who function as psychotherapists. During the next few years, the practice of psychotherapy should continue much as it is today. Practice is far less secure for ten to twenty years from now. This is based on marked changes within the profession in the past ten years.

Changes in the mental health disciplines have made psychotherapy the primary responsibility of psychotherapists. This arrangement may continue into the future if psychotherapy addresses itself to knowledge and serious deficits in theory. If it does not deal with theory and academic knowledge, it is likely that one of the interlocking disciplines will fill the gap, and there will be another shift in the complex of disciplines. The current shift of practice responsibility to psychotherapy may facilitate practice for psychotherapists, who make a living from it, but it is not seen as healthy for the total benefit of mankind.

REFERENCES

Bowen, M. (1978). *Family therapy in clinical practice.* New York: Jason Aronson, Inc.

Freud, S. (1949). *Collected papers.* London: Hogarth Press.

MacLean, P. (1973). A triune concept of the brain and behavior. In T. Boag & D. Campbell (Eds.), *The Hincks memorial lectures* (pp. 6-66). Toronto: University of Toronto Press.

Sagan, C. (1980). *Cosmos.* New York: Random House.

Wilson, E.O. (1975). *Sociobiology.* Cambridge, MA: Harvard University Press.

Discussion by James F. Masterson, M.D.

Last night, it took us approximately five hours to fly from New York City to Phoenix. This morning, in 50 minutes, Dr. Bowen has taken us on a journey of four thousand million years, to the present. No mean feat. In doing so, he has condensed a number of ideas, as well, as I'm sure, a good deal of time and thought, into a succinct presentation of one man's view of the evolution of psychotherapy.

He begins by reminding us that we are descended from the animals and bring with us physical structures from that time, such as the hindbrain and midbrain that continue to function. What uniquely characterizes us, however, are the forebrain and the cortex, which enable us to think, to plan, and to study. He reminds us that we are newcomers in this long saga of evolution, only about 30,000 years out of four thousand million. He also stresses that the animal kingdom had family relationships long before humans developed.

I've always been fascinated to watch on our public TV channel a nature series which shows fascinating evidence of all these factors about family life of animals that Dr. Bowen mentions. I also was fortunate to attend a lecture on the triune brain which traced the evolution of the capacity for vocalization in the development of animals, describing it as an evolutionary way of trying to deal with separation stress.

I was impressed in Dr. Bowen's paper by the nice sequence of ideas as they emerged and the intellectual discipline of his presentation. He underlines that there was a disappointment in the results of psychoanalytic work that led to the development of family systems theory and therapy in the 50s. I'd like to come back to that a little bit later in my discussion. He then goes on to make some comments about theory, and about how theories govern the way we think about human affairs. Of course, we all have theories—personal theories. The paranoid patient's theory is, "Everybody's out to get me." This is a theory that is necessary for him to manage his internal and external life. I think theories are our way of organizing our perceptions of ourself and the world. On the one hand, they provide interpsychic equilibrium and a sense of comfort and confidence in dealing with out inner and outer world. Hopefully, our theories also say something about the truth. Perhaps whether your own personal theories lean more towards comfort or towards truth will depend a great deal on your own development—or how far you have come.

Dr. Bowen mentions that new ideas are not readily accepted. I think one of the reasons they are not is that our own theories provide us with comfort. And we have to forego that comfort to accept new ideas. This will often lead to ignoring new ideas and reinventing the wheel. I have experience along this line myself. I published a book in 1967 called *The Psychiatric Dilemma of Adolescence* (Boston: Little Brown; reprinted New York: Brunner/Mazel, 1984) in which we presented follow-up evidence about adolescents who were symptomatic. The theory at the time was that this was due to adolescent turmoil and they would grow out of it. Our evidence showed clearly that they did not grow out of it and required treatment. About two years ago, I was in one of our better departments of psychiatry in the United States and a speaker presented a paper on adolescent turmoil saying that most likely they would grow out of it, referring not at all to this prior work. So, we are always reinventing the wheel.

In his thoughts about the effect of theories on mankind, Dr. Bowen referred to the brief period when religious zealots put superstition into action. And he hopes, I think somewhat wistfully, that that is a part of the past. I wonder, myself, how much a part of the past it is when we consider the phenomenon of Jonestown, of the Bhagwan Shree Rajneesh and of the Maharishi.

In turning to the roots of psychotherapy, Dr. Bowen emphasizes that there were always senior people available for help. As a therapist who works mostly with personality disorders, borderline and narcissistic disorders, I couldn't help thinking that this is exactly what was missing in early development for these patients and their families. There were no people available to provide appropriate and adequate help. Then he turns to the modern era of psychotherapy and outlines some of Freud's discoveries. It has always been a matter of interest to me that you constantly hear how Freud is dead and Freudianism is dead. I think one of the reasons this thought arises is that most of his discoveries have been coopted by other disciplines. Therefore, we can say that Freud is dead, while we use his discoveries for other purposes.

Dr. Bowen emphasizes the great importance in the modern era of countertransference in doing psychotherapy. If the therapist is not aware of his countertransference, he ends up providing just another acted-out relationship for the patient. An interesting historical point on countertransference is the difference in the way Freud and Breuer handled countertransference. You will remember that Breuer worked with Anna O. She was bedridden, paralyzed from the waist down. Breuer, at the end of the day, used to come and sit by her bedside, put his hand on her forehead, and have her free associate endlessly to thoughts that came to her mind. And he would sit there sometimes the whole night, eight or nine hours, with his hand on her forehead. Over a period of time, as her symptoms remitted and others returned, he became extremely

involved with her. He was a very conscientious physician. Finally Anna O. developed a false pregnancy, pseudocyesis, based on her erotic transference to Dr. Breuer. And when he saw this, he was so appalled that he dropped the case like a hot potato; he never contacted her, never had anything to do with her. Since he was such a conscientious physician, you can imagine the kind of power that kind of transference must have had.

A little more than ten years later, Freud had a similar experience. Rather than react to it with the kind of transference Breuer had, he took a step back and reflected on what the patient was presenting and feeling. Thereby, he discovered the concept of transference.

Dr. Bowen mentions the changes that occurred in the 50s. One of the changes is one in which I myself was involved. At that time, psychoanalytic thinking was widely emphasized, but it became clearer and clearer that as practiced by classical psychoanalysts it did not work with patients with personality disorders. We struggled for many years to use classical, instinctual theory to try to understand the various personality disorders, but it didn't work. And it wasn't until we changed to a developmental and object relations theory that the door was opened to therapeutic techniques which would make the treatment of these patients possible. One could see this as an offshoot from that early pool of psychoanalytic thinking, as perhaps family systems theory is also.

Dr. Bowen mentions the introduction of tranquilizers in family therapy and the Mental Health Act in recent years. There is no question about the fact that the introduction of antipsychotic, antidepressant drugs has had a profound effect on the practice of psychotherapy. I think we have to accept the fact that the talking cure, as it used to be called, doesn't work with everybody. So the drugs have been a great help for many people. One of the problems, however, is that large categories of patients are removed from the hands of psychotherapists and probably treated mostly by internists or general physicians. Another offshoot is that psychiatry itself, as Dr. Bowen mentioned, has become more and more "biologicized," as I call it. We are becoming more and more biologic and less and less psychodynamic. One of the great agents for this has been lithium and its effectiveness with the affective disorders.

I had one experience which dramatizes this point. I have long been interested in the psychotherapy of anorexia nervosa and closely followed the literature and results reported. At an American Psychiatric Association meeting I had to discuss a paper on treatment of anorexia nervosa. Thirty adolescent girls who had had every kind of treatment known to man, without success, were given antidepressants, I think for a period of 18 months. They were all cured. In discussing this paper, I said I was delighted and astonished to see such a cure rate; I had never seen more than 20 percent before. But, there was not a single reference in this paper to the personality structure of the patients before they had the drug or after they had the drug. In the audience of several hundred psychiatrists, there were only two questions raised when I finished my discussion: Question #1: the dose of the drug; Question #2: the side effects.

Dr. Bowen mentions the explosion of family therapy and raises crucial issues about the importance of thorough training. I often wonder what are the consequences for individual psychoanalytic psychotherapy of the explosion of family therapy. Now he mentions that the Mental Health Act was positive in that it made psychiatry and psychotherapy more acceptable, which is probably the case. But it had an equally large handicap in its emphasis on short-term therapy. As a matter of fact, you're looking at one of the victims, because at the time it was passed, I was in charge of an inpatient unit for long-term treatment. After the Mental Health Act was passed, the funds for this unit were cancelled, as they were for all such units, and they were not able to

function. I can't help but wonder, because of the mental health center's focus on brief psychotherapy and crisis psychotherapy, if perhaps a cruel illusion is not being foisted on the American people—that their basic problem has to do with crisis. And I wonder how many times you have to go to a mental health center with a crisis before beginning to wonder if there is something more fundamental involved than what is seen in the crisis.

As he turns to emphasize the changes from the 50s to the present, which have been many and dramatic, Dr. Bowen emphasizes, for example, that the chairman's point of view has changed from psychoanalytic through eclectic to biological. There has been a devaluation of psychotherapy and an enhancement of biological approaches. There are a number of forces that he has not mentioned which I would like to add. There has been a dramatic increase in the number of psychologists and social workers in the last ten years. There was an article in The New York Times which noted that psychiatrists in the last ten years had remained more or less the same number, psychologists had doubled, and social workers had tripled.

Another dramatic change is the brain-biological research that is going on. Just to give one example in regard to our concept of anxiety, you may recall that Freud initiated the concept that anxiety was due to overflow of neuronal excitation. In other words, there was no psychological content to it. That was his first theory. Then, of course, his second theory was that anxiety is due to conflict. Recent biological brain research is demonstrating that there is, perhaps, a center for the control of anxiety level in midbrain. This center probably evolved to deal with separation stress, to warn the organism. The center itself can become deregulated and can fire off at times other than separation stress; secondly, it can maintain too low a threshold of separation anxiety. So if a patient comes to you with symptoms, rather than being due to conflict, they are due to deregulation of center. Rather than providing psychotherapy, what you would provide is drug treatment. If it's the center firing off irregularly, the benzadiazapenes are supposed to be quite effective; if it's low threshold, the antidepressants are used. So the biological brain research is causing us to think more broadly and widely about the possible etiology of the problems our patients bring us.

There has been in the field of the personality disorders as large an explosion of knowledge as there has been in the area of family therapy. This knowledge continues to expand at an ever-increasing rate, and new therapeutic techniques have been developed which are effective with patients who used to be thought not to be treatable. Some more recent influences are less positive. First, we have the commercialization of medicine, which will inevitably lead to placing greatest emphasis on cost effectiveness for psychotherapy. And, finally, we have the introduction of Health Medical Organizations and Employee Assistance Plans. Now what these two, it seems to me, suggest for the future, as Dr. Bowen indicates, is that private practice is going to be less and less common; psychotherapists, if they will be working for Health Medical Organizations or Employee Assistance Plans, they will probably be doing mostly brief therapy. My hope is, that in this tidal wave towards brief therapy, the therapeutic needs of patients for more longer-term and intensive psychotherapy are not going to be overlooked.

I'd like to thank Dr. Bowen for this four-thousand-million-year journey where he has presented a number of ideas which, hopefully, have jogged some of our own personal theories and opened us up to a pursuit of more ultimate truth.

QUESTIONS AND ANSWERS

Question: Dr. Bowen, I was somewhat surprised at what I perceived to be a hoped-for isolation of family therapy and psychotherapy from medicine and the sci-

ences. I was surprised by that because of the current excitement and promise of the marriage of the two through the expressed-emotion research which shows such promise for devastating disorders. At the same time people are evaluating serious, emotional psychiatric illnesses using recombinant DNA research, trying to find causes and patterns. It would seem to me that the marriage of widely disparate studies and disciplines, all looking for the same closing of the gap between theory and what the theory is trying to explain, would be a very helpful way to study the human being and the human species. I think this conference itself shows promise in trying to get people from widely different areas and theories and beliefs together to discuss the problems that we all face in treatment.

Bowen: I'm in favor of everything. Anytime you isolate one way of thinking from another discipline, you are increasing the time it takes for resolution of the problem. So I'm very much opposed to separating mental health from psychiatry, or psychiatry from chemistry or evolution or anything else. The more that all the disciplines are brought together, the better. Bringing the disciplines together is a lot more complex than bringing them together in something called multidisciplinary research where several disciplines meet together in a room and accomplish nothing. It takes more than physical contact between them. It takes a thinking contact and the more we separate one from another from another, the longer we extend the time before they will eventually be connected. I think right now we have a big split between psychotherapy and medicine. All kinds of people in medical school can get jobs, but the medical school will still distance you.

Question: Dr. Bowen, can you comment a little bit about your own thoughts on the future of family therapy?

Bowen: I think family therapy in the long

run will bridge the gap between individual and human behavior. Mankind has tended to ignore that. But I think the difference between the family and the individual is going to be a gap that makes theory about human behavior possible. I think it will eventually make human behavior into a science. But I think we are far from understanding the implications of one's own family. I could go on at length about that but not in a short session.

Question: I was wondering if both speakers could comment on what influence you think the modern feminist movement has had on psychotherapy?

Bowen: I don't know how you figure that one out. I don't know whether psychotherapy influenced the feminist movement or the feminist movement was influenced by something else. I believe that in this current trend mankind is in favor of compartmentalization.

Masterson: I think it has had quite a strong influence in several directions. One, I think it has made all psychotherapists, particularly male psychotherapists, much more aware of these issues which they may not have dealt with adequately in the past. On the other hand, I think it's had some other practical effects. I haven't seen a female homosexual as a patient in the last ten years, yet I used to see female homosexuals as well as males as patients. So I suspect that female homosexuals are going to female therapists.

Question: Dr. Bowen, could you comment on the future of psychotherapy in the childhood area?

Bowen: I don't think really that you can separate child psychiatry from the rest of psychiatry. Child psychiatry, as it was originally described, was psychotherapy with a child. When you approach the family instead of the child, I don't think that psychotherapy with the child is necessary. That is simply a viewpoint. In other words,

I think child psychiatry is a very good training area. But technically, I don't think it's essential.

Masterson: I think child psychiatry is in for dramatic changes because one of the greatest contributors to knowledge in the past 30 years in the area that I worked has been direct child observation research. The work of people like Margaret Mahler, M.D., and John Bowlby, M.D., has taught us so much about normal development. These studies are now being carried even further and in more technologically sophisticated ways by Virginia Demos, D.Ed., at Harvard and Daniel Stern, M.D., at Cornell and the changes in what we're learning are phenomenal. For example, that child who we used to think did not have a full perceptual apparatus till three months of age or more, is now seen as a fully articulated perceptual apparatus by the age of three or four weeks. In addition, we used to think that the child was a kind of passive agent of the mother's, but it's been demonstrated again and again in films that practically from the first week of birth the child is a very active agent in interaction with the mother and his own development. I think infant psychiatry has become a new specialty in the past few years. I think there will be dramatic and important changes in knowledge and therapeutic technique.

Question: Dr. Bowen, I have a question about your prediction for the future. You said that you thought that knowledge would be the most important thing and that technique would be less important. In light of the trend toward technique in medicine and the lack of philosophy in our educational programs, is it your *hope* that knowledge will become the paramount focus or is it what you *expect* to happen?

Bowen: I think one of the problems with medicine is that it is fairly fixed. There has been no force to cause medicine to change its orientation. When systems ideas came into medicine, this was sort of foreign to medicine. I think this applies to everything that medicine does. I think medicine has to change eventually. Psychotherapy can do much to try to help medicine; there's a big future for you in that area. If you permit yourself to be externalized by medicine, the future for mankind is less hopeful. I think all of the sciences have to join with medicine. Medicine has moved forward in many ways. A week ago I went to a symposium on organ transplants. You wouldn't believe some of the things that go on there. If your liver runs out in middle age, you can check in to get a new liver. That is how far organ transplants have gone—livers and hearts and kidneys and eyes. So medicine has come a long way technically, but theoretically, it hasn't come so far. In that session on organ transplants, they were talking about the response of the individual, not about the family. The family is what makes it go. So everybody is a part of medicine. Medicine has to do with the human being and you have to work with the human being. I don't think you can separate yourself from medicine.

Advances in Strategic Family Therapy

Cloé Madanes

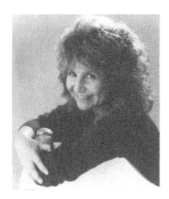

Cloé Madanes
Cloé Madanes is Co-Director at the Family Therapy Institute of Washington, D.C. The author of two books on family therapy, she is renowned for her innovative directive approaches to psychotherapy and supervision.

During the decades of the 1960s and the 1970s, new explanations of human motivation were found in the social context of the individual. The clinical focus shifted from the individual to the nuclear family and the extended kin. Family structures were described and the importance of maintaining generational boundaries was emphasized, as was the fact that all organizations have hierarchies. It was observed that people with symptoms are involved in incorrect hierarchies, such as when a problem child determines what happens in a family. The issue was how to describe problem hierarchies and how

to think about changing them. It became obvious that symptomatic behavior is adaptive and that a person behaves in abnormal ways when in an abnormal context. The problem was how to describe the family as a social context and how to change the behavior of its members.

Bateson, Jackson, Haley and Weakland (1956) proposed that there is a human dilemma when dual levels of message are incongruent. Similarly, there is an organizational dilemma when the organization has incongruent hierarchies. Thus, an organization with an incongruent hierarchy requires conflicting levels of communication, or symptomatic behavior (Madanes, 1981).

The Bateson project described conflicting levels of message in context and coined the term *double bind* to describe dual mes-

The ideas expressed in this paper have been published in slightly different form in Madanes (1981), *Strategic Family Therapy*, and (1984), *Behind the One-Way Mirror: Advances in the Practice of Strategic Therapy*. San Francisco, CA: Jossey-Bass.

sages that conflict paradoxically. They made the shift from describing madness and other symptoms as individual phenomena to describing them as communicative behavior between people. However, the organizational context in which communication takes place remained largely undescribed. A mother would say to her child in some form, "I want you to spontaneously do as I say." The child would respond in a peculiar way to this peculiar set of messages. Why the mother communicated in this conflicting way could be explained only by references to her nature or to her need to respond to a child who was communicating strangely. Whether it was a problem child or a symptom of a marital couple that was described, a way to conceptualize the larger social context to which family members were adapting was lacking.

One way of understanding the context of conflicting levels of message is the conflicting hierarchies in the organizations where people communicate. A mother who asks her child to obey her spontaneously can be in an organization where (1) she is in charge of the child by the fact of being a parent but (2) the child is also in charge of the mother because of the power of symptomatic behavior or because of the power given by coalitions with family members of high status. Therefore, the mother must give directives because of the nature of her position, but she can only express helplessly the wish that the child might do as she says (Haley, 1981).

In any organization, there is hierarchy in the sense that one person has more power and responsibility than another person in determining what happens. Parents have legal responsibility to provide for and take care of their children. As children grow into adolescence, parents are expected to relinquish some of this power, so that children gradually take increasing responsibility for their own lives. When adolescents become young adults, the relationship shifts to one of increasing equality between parents and children, and eventually children take care of their parents in their old age.

In a marriage, spouses usually deal with hierarchical issues by dividing areas of power and responsibility. For example, one spouse might make all the decisions having to do with money, while the other spouse makes all the decisions involving relatives. One spouse is superior to the other in certain areas and inferior in other areas.

The hierarchical organization of a family includes certain members dominating, taking responsibility, and making decisions for others. It also includes helping, protecting, comforting, reforming, and taking care of others. By the nature of their position in the hierarchy, parents help and protect their children more frequently than children help and protect their parents. In this sense, parents have more power than their children. In a marriage, spouses help and protect each other at different times in different situations.

When a child presents symptomatic or problem behavior, the parents express their concern in protective or punitive ways. The disturbed behavior of the child gives him power over the parents, who focus their concern on him and yet fail to help and to change him. In this sense, the child has power over the parents, often determining what the family can do, what they will talk about, how time will be spent, and so forth. Yet, because the child is disturbed or symptomatic, the parents have to take care of him even more. In this sense, there are two conflicting hierarchical arrangements in the family. Both parents and child are simultaneously in a superior and an inferior position in relation to each other. The hierarchical incongruity may become a hierarchical reversal if the parents lose all power over an adolescent or young adult who dominates them by terrorizing them through violent, delinquent, or bizarre behavior.

When it is a spouse who develops symptomatic or problem behavior, two incongruous hierarchies are simultaneously defined in the marriage. In one, the symptomatic person is in an inferior position because of helpless and disturbed behavior, and the other spouse is in the superior position of helper. Yet at the same time, the symptomatic spouse is in a superior position by not being influenced and helped, while the nonsymptomatic spouse is in the inferior position of being an unsuccessful helper whose efforts fail and whose life can be organized around the symptomatic spouse's needs and problems. Such symptoms as depression, alcoholism, fears, anxiety, and psychosomatic complaints may serve this purpose, organizing the nonsymptomatic spouse's behavior in many different ways. Several examples of areas that can be dominated by the helplessness of the symptomatic spouse are: how free time will be spent, how money should be used, how to relate to the extended family. Even the way the nonsymptomatic spouse should be helpful, and the fact that he or she should keep trying to help even though he or she always fails, are often engineered by the symptomatic spouse. The couple is caught in an interaction that simultaneously defines their power and their weakness in relation to each other.

A symptom is an incongruent message in the sense that the symptomatic person behaves in unfortunate or inappropriate ways and denies that he has control over his behavior because it is involuntary. In a wider context a symptom can be seen as appropriate to an incongruous position. Defined spontaneously as powerful and helpless, a person will behave in symptomatic ways.

INTERACTIONAL METAPHORS

One of the reasons that professionals get into clinical work is because they are interested in the reasons why people do the things that they do. It is a mystery why people behave the way they do, as well as what to do about it. One of these mysteries is in the area of metaphorical communication.

People communicate in analogical ways; their messages can be assigned meaning only in a context of other messages. An analogical message usually has a second

referent different from the one explicitly expressed, and it also carries an implicit request or command. For example, when a wife says to her husband, "I have a headache," she is explicitly making a statement about an internal state, but she may also be analogically expressing her dissatisfaction with her situation. Or she may be requesting that the husband help her with the children.

All human behavior can be thought of as analogical and metaphorical in different ways and at various levels of abstraction. A behavior is analogical to another behavior when there is a resemblance between them in some particular way, even though they may be otherwise unlike. A behavior is metaphorical for another behavior when it symbolizes or is used in place of another behavior. Symptomatic behavior has been considered analogical and metaphorical in certain specific ways:

1) A symptom may be a report on an internal state and also a metaphor for another internal state. For example, a child's headache may be expressing more than one kind of pain.

2) A symptom may be a report on an internal state and also an analogy and a metaphor for another person's symptoms or internal states. For example, a child who refuses to go to school may be expressing his own fears and also his mother's fears. The child's fear is analogical to the mother's fear (in that the fears are similar) and also metaphorical (in that the child's fear symbolizes or represents the mother's fear).

Building on these ideas about metaphor, the next step is that not only can an individual person's messages be assigned meaning only in the context of other messages, but also the interaction between people is analogical and can be assigned meaning only in a context of other interactions. That is, a sequence of interaction usually has a second referent different from the sequence explicitly expressed.

The interaction between two people in a family can be an analogy and a metaphor, replacing the interaction of another dyad in the family. For example, a mother may be upset and worried, and her husband may try to reassure and comfort her. If a child develops a recurrent pain, the mother may become preoccupied with reassuring and comforting the child in the same way that the father was previously reassuring and comforting her. The mother's involvement with the son in a helpful way will preclude her involvement with the husband in a helpless way, at least during the time in which the mother is involved with the son. The interaction between mother and son will have replaced the interaction between wife and husband.

The system of interaction around a symptom in one family member can be a metaphor for and replace another system of interaction around another issue in the family. Mother, father, and siblings may helpfully focus on a child's problem in a way that is analogical to the way they focused on the mother's problem before the child's problem developed. The focus on the child's problem precludes the interaction centered around the mother's problem.

The distinction between the literal and the metaphorical levels of messages is an issue of contemporary psychopathology. A concern with metaphor has characterized the development of psychoanalysis, the theories of schizophrenia, and Gestalt psychology. These theories have been plagued by confusions between what is communication and what is thinking about communication. Korzybski (1941) and the movement of general semantics offered some clarification when emphasizing that the map is not the territory. The whole of psychoanalysis is a theory of metaphor that confuses map and territory, where the oedipal drama, for example, is not thought of as a metaphor or a map but is taken as a literal event.

Schizophrenia has been described as a difficulty in discriminating between the literal and the metaphorical level of messages, and generations of therapists have struggled to understand the metaphors of the schizophrenic in the belief that that understanding would lead to a solution to the mystery of psychosis. All the psychodynamic and experiential therapies are based on understanding the metaphor of adult language and of children's play.

Within this tradition of interest in metaphors, new complexities are introduced when describing metaphorical sequences of interaction. A system's metaphor and a metaphor in a dream are not of the same order. To focus on the metaphor expressed by a sequence of interaction is of a different order than focusing on the metaphor expressed in a message or an act. There is a shift to a different level of analysis when metaphorical communication is thought of as expressed not only by individual messages but also by relationships and by systems of interaction (Madanes, 1984).

The description of metaphorical sequences of interaction provides a bridge between the individual psychodynamic and experiential therapies that focus on understanding the metaphor and the family therapies that are concerned with the organization of the family.

POWER AND INTERPERSONAL INFLUENCE

Family members influence each other in helpful ways that are often unfortunate— instead of resolving a problem, they only distract from it, preventing a resolution and creating a new problem.

A child's disturbed behavior, for example, helps the parents by focusing their concern on him, providing a respite from the parents' own troubles and a reason to overcome their own difficulties. For example, a mother may become involved with her problem child instead of being concerned about improving her husband's shortcomings or instead of being involved in her career in a way that the husband might find upsetting. A child's difficulties can make a father feel needed at those times when he feels rejected by his wife.

These ways in which the child protects the parents make the child appear to be helpless because of his disturbed behavior, yet he is powerful as a helper to the family.

The question arises as to whether the child really plans to be helpful or whether it is the parents who elicit this kind of behavior from the child. Does the father, for example, elicit the behavior in the child so he can be free from having to support his wife in her difficulties? Or does the mother elicit the behavior in the child to free the husband from supporting her? What is the truth is really not the question. The important consideration is what kind of punctuation of the events will best lead to designing a strategy for change.

PLAYFULNESS AND HUMOR

My therapeutic strategies have been characterized by the use of playfulness and humor. When people are irrationally grim, the introduction of playfulness can elicit new behavior and bring about new alternatives. A humorous redefinition, explanation, or directive takes the family by surprise in a way that gives strength, drama, and impact to the intervention. This allows the therapist's creativity to match the creativity of the symptom. What makes change possible is the therapist's ability to be optimistic and to see what is funny or appealing in a grim situation.

Humor involves the ability to think at multiple levels and in this way is similar to metaphorical communication. When a therapist talks about a meal or a tennis game in ways that are metaphorical of a sexual relationship, the humorous aspect of the communication becomes apparent as soon as the connection is made between the two levels. Thinking at multiple levels also involves the ability to be inconsistent, to be illogical, and to communicate in non sequiturs, jumping from one subject to another, associating what seems to be unrelated in ways that appear humorous and are therapeutic.

To give an example of a humorous therapy, a young man's family consulted about his compulsive gambling. It had ruined his career and was threatening his life because of his connections with mafia types to whom he owed large sums of money. The father was a busy physician; the siblings were successful and irate because the mother and aunt were always giving the young man money to bail him out or to allegedly support him, when in fact he spent the money at the race track.

The therapist explained to the mother and aunt that the young man needed their guidance and instruction in the one area of his life that was most important to him: gambling. Once a week, mother and aunt were to take the young man to the race track and, standing on each side of him, examine the horses and the jockeys before the bets were placed, while making loud comments such as "I want you to bet on the black one, he's so cute!" or "I will only let you bet on the jockey with the red shirt, he has a kind face." These types of comments and instructions would be given by the two little old ladies no matter what friends of the young man were present. Then they would stand in line on each side of the young man as they waited to place their bet and would protect him and interfere with any old friends who might try to approach him, pushing them away and saying, "You are not allowed to talk to my son," or "You are not allowed to talk to my nephew." They would instruct the young man on what horse to bet on, give him the money, and he could bet only on that horse.

In addition, every evening, mother and aunt would gather as much of the family as they could for a game of poker or blackjack. During the game and as often as possible, mother and aunt would criticize the way the young man played and instruct him on how to gamble more intelligently.

The family was puzzled by these instructions because the mother and aunt had never been to the race track and did not know how to play blackjack or poker, but they promised to learn right away so they could be adequately instructive and critical. The young man was exasperated, particularly during the two sessions that were spent rehearsing the scene with the mother and aunt at the race track and pretending to play poker and blackjack during the session. The sister and brother were happy to collaborate since they were interested in stopping the flow of the family's money to their gambling brother. The father, who was a secretive person, collaborated when the therapist insinuated that if this did not solve the problem of the young man's compulsive gambling, perhaps the vices of other family members would have to be disclosed. The young man complained that the therapist did not understand anything about gambling and said that anyhow he had decided to get a job, pay his debts, and start a new life, which he did.

PARADOXICAL STRATEGIES

Most people who come to therapy cannot follow good advice. Most therapists work from a position of weakness with people who are not particularly eager to follow their suggestions. Usually, clients and families need to be influenced indirectly in order to change. In my therapy, family members can be asked to do, in playful cooperation with the therapist, what may appear to be absurd and unrelated to the therapy but is therapeutic. Here are two of several strategies that I have developed.

PRESCRIBING THE PRETENDING OF THE FUNCTION OF THE SYMPTOM

This is a strategy where family members perform, in a playful way, actions that represent what the therapist believes to be the function of the symptom. These actions do not literally represent the function of the symptom but are a condensed, abbreviated, somewhat symbolic, and

somewhat humorous version of the family drama. A special characteristic of this type of paradox is that it reverses the positions of family members with respect to who needs help and who is helpful. For example, if a daughter is suicidal, the mother is asked to pretend to be depressed and the daughter to help the mother; if a child has fears, a parent may be asked to pretend to be afraid and the child to protect the parent. The therapist conceptualizes the function of the symptom as a parent covertly asking for help and a child covertly helping the parent through symptomatic behavior. In the playful prescription of the paradox, the parent overtly asks for help, and the child overtly helps the parent.

An example will clarify the approach. The mother of a boy with nightmares and night terrors recently remarried. Her new husband was an older man who was reluctant to become involved with her children—to the point of actually saying in front of them in a session that he was not and did not want to be their father. He was kind to them and they found him appealing because he was an interesting man, but he insisted on keeping them at a certain distance. The biological father lived far away. The mother was struggling to develop a career and had a tendency to be obsessive in her doubts about the well-being of her children and about the decisions she had made in her life. She described herself as an anxious and fearful person.

The fears of the child were approached by asking the mother in the session to pretend that she was very afraid because she had seen a cockroach (the mother had previously expressed her fear of bugs). The stepfather was then to call the boy, "Jimmy, to the rescue!" Together, hand in hand, they would run to the mother and the boy would stomp on the cockroach. Then they would play another scene in which, instead of being afraid of a cockroach, the mother was afraid of a thief breaking into the house. Once more the stepfather would call, "Jimmy to the rescue! We must save your mother!" Together, they would repel the intruder. The family was asked to repeat these performances several times in the session and to act them out every evening at home.

The idea behind the directive was that the child's fears were a metaphor for the mother's fears and that the mother was covertly asking the child to help her to integrate the stepfather into the family and to elicit from the stepfather the kind of concern that she wanted. The child was covertly helping the mother by developing a symptom that engaged the father.

In the dramatization that was prescribed, not only was the mother overtly requesting the child's help and the child overtly helping her, but the child was doing so in collaboration with the stepfather, holding his hand and participating in an action initiated by the stepfather. This togetherness between the stepfather and son was what the mother wanted. Her fears centered around the distance between her son and her husband. In the next session, the stepfather told the therapist that he understood the intervention and that the dramatization was no longer necessary. He and the boy would find more interesting things to do together. The night terrors did not recur (Madanes, 1984).

Another example is the case of two adolescent sisters who repeatedly attempted suicide. In this family, the father, by appearing extremely depressed, was covertly requesting his daughters' help in preventing his wife from leaving him; the girls, by attempting suicide so that the mother could not leave, were covertly helping the father who loved his wife and wanted to keep her. A playful dramatization made evident the father's depression and the daughters' concern and enabled the father to spontaneously correct his relationship both with his daughters and with his wife (Madanes, 1984).

This kind of paradoxical intervention is appropriate when the therapist understands that the gain the child derives from the symptom is being helpful to someone else (usually one or both parents), even though this helpfulness is unfortunate. If the therapist understands not only the child's gain but also the covert request made by others for the child's help, then the strategy is simply to elicit an overt, rather than covert, request from those others and to have the child help overtly rather than through symptomatic behavior. Pretending to help parents in other absurd ways (through dramatizations in and out of the sessions), rather than in the absurd way in which the symptomatic behavior is helpful, serves this purpose and matches in playful ways the creativity of the symptom. This intervention is indicated when the therapist can see that the child is motivated mainly by love and concern, but it should not be used when all the therapist can see is rebelliousness and hostility (not because the intervention could cause harm, but because the family will refuse to collaborate).

PRESCRIBING A REVERSAL IN THE FAMILY HIERARCHY

This strategy consists of putting the children in charge of the parents. All the children (or one particular child) are asked to take charge of some aspect of the parents' lives, such as their happiness. Sometimes the therapist gives the children authority by putting them in charge of each other, in this way replacing the parents. This approach is appropriate when the parents present themselves as incompetent, helpless, and unable to take charge of their children, while complaining that the children are out of control. It is also appropriate when a parent presents disturbing behavior, such as delinquency, alcoholism, or drug addiction, that disqualifies him or her from a parenting position.

As the children are put in charge (in practice or in fantasy), the parent responds by becoming more caring and effective. The intervention is paradoxical because the parent typically complains that the children are "out of control," meaning out of the control of the parent, and the therapist responds by putting the children in control of the parent rather than under the control of the parent. The therapist prescribes a reversal of the hierarchy, which leads the parents to take charge and correct the hierarchy by taking more responsibility for themselves and for their children.

This approach is useful when a parent is ineffective, although it is not necessary to understand *why* the parent is ineffective. It is necessary, however, to give the family some rationale for putting the children in charge. The rationale might be, for example, that the parents are unhappy and need to be taught how to be happy or that a parent is tired and needs to be relieved of responsibilities. Whatever the rationale, the children need to be given concrete tasks and concrete topics to discuss in the sessions in relation to the parents.

Most of the content of the therapy interviews is centered on the children taking charge and on how they are going to do this. The approach is particularly useful when the parent does not provide appropriate caring behavior, when child abuse or neglect has occurred, or when the parent is the presenting problem. It is particularly indicated when the children are seen as being concerned about and caring for the parent but rejected in their affection. Whether the children are asked to take charge in realistic or fantasized ways the tone of the sessions should be light, benevolent, and humorous.

As the children give love to the parents (by actually giving them directives, by taking care of them, or by fantasizing about how they would take care of them if they could), the parents not only become more responsible and caring toward the children but they also resolve their own problems. Children are often surprisingly wise in their directives and advice and, with the therapist's encouragement, they can be very helpful.

When the children are put in a position of authority, it is important to allow them to make positive suggestions and to forbid all criticism of the parents. In this way, cross-generational coalitions that divide the parents and support their disturbing behavior are blocked, and a child cannot express overtly a parent's covert criticism of the other parent. At the same time, an alliance between the children is encouraged so that they can support each other and need not seek coalitions with the parents. This, in turn, gives the parents the satisfaction of seeing that their children are strong, united, and benevolently concerned about each other and about the parents—all factors that contribute to the improvement of the parents' situation. As the parents improve, the children are happy to see that their efforts have succeeded and that they have helped their parents. With increased self-esteem and competence, the children, who characteristically have serious problems of their own, often spontaneously resolve their own problems.

This approach is appropriate both with shy, withdrawn children and with rebellious, misbehaving ones. It can be used with young children, adolescents, or young adults. No matter how withdrawn the child or how disruptive his behavior, the approach can succeed if the therapist is able to appeal to the child's sense of humor or to touch the chord of love that can always be found between parents and children. The strategy is especially useful when parents are very rejecting, because little or nothing is expected from them and all demonstrations of love and concern are initiated by the children.

The approach of prescribing that the children take charge of the parents is paradoxical when used in situations in which the parents are covertly encouraging the children to be in charge because of the parents' incompetence, symptomatic behavior, or neglect, or because one parent is siding with the children against the other parent. The therapist encourages the children to take charge in an effective, benevolent way—quite differently from the way in which the parents were covertly requesting that the children take charge. As the therapist's prescription makes the covert request by the parents overt, the parents react against the therapist's prescription and take charge of themselves and of their children. The therapist appeals to the love between parents and children, to the children's altruism, and to their ability to communicate in metaphor (Madanes, 1984).

CONCLUSION

To conclude, I want to point out that the techniques of strategic therapy are deceptively simple but also complex: Simple in that they are often playful and appeal to the child in all of us; complex in that they involve metalevels, paradox, and metaphor. Picasso (1973) said "Art is a lie that makes us realize the truth," and

"Through art we express our conception of what nature is not." Similarly, the therapy I have described is make-believe that makes us realize the truth. By expressing what real life is not, it clarifies what real life is.

REFERENCES

Bateson, G., Jackson, D.D., Haley, J., & Weakland, J. (1956). Toward a theory of schizophrenia. *Behavioral Science, 1* (4), 251–264.

Haley, J. (1981). Foreword. In C. Madanes, *Strategic family therapy.* San Francisco: Jossey-Bass.

Korzybski, A. (1941). *Science and sanity.* New York: Science Press.

Madanes, C. (1981). *Strategic family therapy.* San Francisco: Jossey-Bass.

Madanes, C. (1984). *Behind the one-way mirror: Advances in the practice of strategic therapy.* San Francisco: Jossey-Bass.

Picasso, P. (1973). Quoted in *The Arts*, 1923, reprinted in *The New York Times*, obituary.

Discussion by Paul Watzlawick, Ph.D.

I would like to point out that since what Cloé has presented is similar to the way we at MRI think and work, it becomes difficult for me to maintain at least a semblance of objectivity. Therefore, all I can do is to take the role of the devil's advocate and level at her those objections that are most frequently made against this type of therapy. So let me pitilessly pluck her paper to pieces.

Madanes implies that the responsibility of therapy lies on the therapist. Some would immediately reply that this makes our clients even more helpless. It encourages dependence. Both Madanes and I would disagree. As I tried to show earlier, whenever success or change for the better occurs, we seem stupid. We do not know

how the change came about. We need to have this explained to us. We must have done something differently. What could it have been? And we get the client to explain to us the reasons for the change. We think there is no better way of getting people acquainted with their own resources.

Much more important, I think, is the charge that this approach is insincere, that Madanes doesn't say what she really feels and thinks. This is a charge leveled by those therapists who believe that only what wells up from the depth of their innermost being is the real truth and therefore this is what matters. I think Cloé would have an answer to that charge. She also seems to imply that the therapist is constructing a different approach or a different technique for every specific problem. Now this can very well be taken as an outrageous statement because it seems as if we are supposed to give up our entire diagnostic vocabulary, along with the dignity and the hermetic qualities that go with these words. Where would we get if the terms contained in DSM-III were only used on insurance forms. We need names, especially names of Greek origin, because this impresses our clients. And it is also well known that the moment there exists a name, the thing that is named must exist. As I have already pointed out, it is inconceivable to ask that in our intellectual universe, there should be those little angels you see on Baroque paintings that consist only of a head and a pair of wings, with no body. They should flutter around in our intellectual universe.

Then there are those "enfants terribles" like Szasz and David Rosenhan who point in a very different direction. In any case, I think that Cloé would probably say that the system theorists have the answer to the question that I just raised when they say that every system is its own best explanation and therefore categorizations are semantic traps. She thinks of symptoms as contracts between people and the only conclusion that one must draw from it, with horror, is that pathology resides not in but *between* people. Then the biologists, for instance, tell us that they have long since given up the idea that you can study one entity in isolation, that the only thing you can study is the interaction between such entities, no matter what these entities are, from the atom in the case of the physicist all the way up to nations. We have to realize that a relationship is more and different from the ingredients that people bring into the relationship. Therefore, any attempt to decompose a relationship into its elements can lead only to absurd reifications.

She also seems to be saying that diagnostic categories can better be seen as specific difficulties in a family's progress from one stage to the next, from one life cycle to the next. She again attacks the dogma of linear causality. I asked myself, "How did the evolutionists get over this problem?" I saw that in time this slight gradual increase in behavior vis à vis changed environmental conditions made less and less adaptive the behavior maintaining adaptations that at one point were perfectly valid. How can this change be incorporated into a theory of linear causality? As we watch families, we begin to understand, or think that we begin to understand, the difficulties. We can see that these families are clinging, as we all do, to adaptive behaviors that at one time were evidently quite appropriate, useful and effective, except that by doing more of the same as the environmental conditions changed, people then get into very serious problems.

She implies that families that come to us offer resistance to change. Anybody who comes into therapy is really saying that they expect just one thing from therapy: to be taken back in time to the point before the problem arose because then everything was nice, everything was well. They had no problems. This clearly is one thing the therapist can under no circumstances accomplish. But apparently Cloé ignores the fact that resistance "should be interpreted." It has to be shown how it has originated in the past of the person. What she suggests apparently cannot have any lasting effect. But I cannot overlook the fact that there was a man, I think in a place called Phoenix, who had very different ideas about how we can deal with resistance. I think his name was Erickson.

Cloé says symptoms such as depression, alcoholism, fears, anxiety, and psychosomatic complaints may organize a non-symptomatic spouse's behavior in many different ways. Some would say that what she is really talking about here is the secondary gain. Using this explanation has the advantage that it saves and maintains the intrapsychic and introspective dogma. She tries to talk about "what for." She tries to talk about the function of the symptom and somehow she seems to have success by looking at where this particular so-called symptom fits into the wholeness of that particular human relationship system. She says that people communicate in analogic ways. I would prefer that she say that they behave by way of stimulus or something similar, because analogic, unfortunately, has a well-defined place in human communications theory. It refers largely to nonverbal behavior. I know that she means behavior that is based on some analogy of the meaning that is supposed to be conveyed or it is supposed to have.

I very much like her insistence on the fact that the therapist is trying to look at patterns. I probably would have preferred a stronger accent on the fact that these patterns, redundancies or repetitive occurrences, and the meaning attributed to them, are read by us into the system. It is the observer who leads them into the functioning of the system. As far as we know, they are not necessarily there, in a real sense. Towards the end of her paper, things go from bad to worse. She begins to undermine terms like "real," "truth," etc. I think this leads to an outrageous nihilism. Long before her, the Nobel prizewinner Julian Schwinger, in his book *Mind and Matter*, said that every man's world picture is and always remains a construct of his mind and cannot be proved to have any other existence. So maybe she is right when she talks about the therapist "rearranging realities," which is her expression.

I like to remark about humor. I would prefer if she had added that the use of humor at times is very dangerous, especially with people who don't have humor or with people who are very seriously suicidal or depressed. I think they would resent humor. But the use of humor with so called schizophrenics is an excellent way of somehow communicating to the patient, "I can see your point of view."

When Cloé talks about paradoxical strategies, I again have a purely linguistic objection to what she is saying. Paradoxical, I think, ought to be reserved for the very definitive definition or definitive meaning that this term has in formal logic. I see a danger there, and Cloé points to this danger when she talks about these strategies seeming to be deceptively simple. The danger I see is that people have come to consider as paradoxical any kind of outrageous, outlandish, weird behavior on the part of the therapist. This is not at all the case. When we talk about paradox, we ought to stay within the bounds of the classic definition that has been given to this particular pattern, to this particular structure in formal logic. Otherwise, we get to the point where our work is being discredited by people who just do weird things and think that, just because they are weird, they are paradoxical and, therefore, they are good.

At the end, there is a mistake I would like to point out. Cloé says that by expressing what real life is not, one clarifies what real life is. My position there stops at the comma; we can find out only what real life is not. That is all we can ever know about reality and I am willing to defend this point of view.

But let me draw my conclusions. I believe I am speaking for all of you when I say that I think this young lady's license to do therapy should be revoked before she can do any more harm to theories and any more good to her clients.

Going Behind the Obvious:
The Psychotherapeutic Journey

◆

Virginia M. Satir, M.A., A.C.S.W.

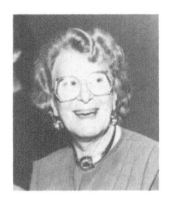

Virginia M. Satir, M.A., A.C.S.W.

For almost forty years, Virginia Satir has practiced and taught psychotherapy. One of the founders of family therapy, she has co-authored four books and authored five. Additionally, there are a number of books about her approach. She is recipient of the Distinguished Family Therapy Award from the American Association of Marriage and Family Therapy.

Satir is cofounder of the Mental Research Institute. She is past president of the Association of Humanistic Psychology and has a number of honorary doctorates. Her master's degree was granted in 1948 from the University of Chicago School of Social Service Administration.

Using World War II as a turning point, Satir makes a personal statement and discusses how psychotherapy has evolved in a broader social matrix to the point where healthful human values can be emphasized as a basic foundation. It is important to understand and utilize systems. Positive parts can be developed rather than focusing on pathology. Also described is her personal evolution as a therapist in terms of perception and procedure.

I want to take a journey with you and ask you to take one with me. I am going back to the year 1900. I want to look at today in relation to what has happened since that time. In 1900 we would have seen more horses than cars, more fields than cement. Our pace would have been slower. Our clothes looked different. Many people were immigrants from Europe, bringing with them all of the cultural and national gifts of their heritage. At the same time, they were bringing all the anxieties of living in a new land. Cities were small. Most people lived on farms doing agricultural work.

Today the context in which we live is quite different. The average life span of individuals in 1900 was not more than 55 years, slightly more for women than for men. Today the average life span is closer to 75 years. However, people were born, lived, mated, parented, and died then as they do today. People today have the same number of bones and are structurally the same as they were at that time.

What is different now is the way that

human beings view themselves. In 1900 there was very little awareness that human beings had an unconscious, a place within from which they were motivated without their conscious attention. Since that time we have unearthed some of the secrets of the unconscious; we also know more fully how the body operates. There have been breakthroughs that have helped us to understand the relationship between mind, body, and emotions. We understand more about how this triad cooperates to create illness as well as health. Today we call this concept—the interconnections between these three components—holistic health.

In 1900, rules for how people were to view themselves and their behavior were rigidly defined. Everyone was clear about the idea that the man was supposed to be treated as the head of the family, that is, as an intellectual giant and a wise decision-maker. His wife and children were considered to be his chattel. Under the best of circumstances he was a benign dictator. Under the worst of circumstances he was a tyrant. This was how it had been for hundreds of years. The fate of women was held entirely in the hands of men. No woman could own property or handle her own money without the support or permission of her husband or father. A woman's role was primarily that of serving men and being the bearer and the caretaker of children. Even in today's society, many people behave as though the woman is still the primary parent. The idea that men are part of the emotional and psychological life of the family is a recent awareness. Today, for the most part, women can work ouside the home, earn their own money, own property and be part of the business world. More and more, men are willing to be a part of family life and recognize that they have a most important role in helping children become whole beings.

Around 1900 we were seeing the beginning of the industrial age. Children were looked upon as a source of labor and money for the family. It was also a period that marked the beginning of the change from agricultural to urban life. Children as young as the ages of four and six worked in factories, coal mines and textile mills, often working ten hours a day, six days a week. There were no mandatory provisions for education. Many children were neglected, abused and dependent. At this time socially conscious women started a movement to assure more rights and better care and protection for children. One very important outcome of this was the development of the child guidance movement, and along with it came the formation of the juvenile court in 1899. This movement operated on the premise that when parents failed or were unable through death or otherwise to care for their children, the state had an obligation to act in loco parentis (as a parent to the child). This principle is still in effect today.

This was the first legal intrusion into the family by authorities. It provided a base from which to examine and frame the behavior of parents toward their children. The absolute power of the father had been challenged and was diminished. Orphan asylums for dependent children sprung up. These were largely for children whose parents had died, and for children who had been deserted or born "out of wedlock." The care and guidance were taken over by the staffs of the asylums. These staffs became the substitute parents for the children. It is only within the last 35 years that foster home care and small group homes have largely replaced these institutions.

During this period of the 1900s, children were still seen as non-people. They were beings to be manipulated, to be trained to be conforming and obedient. There was more in common between rearing children and training animals. I think many animals fared better than many children. Few people seemed to notice that children were people from birth, and that their treatment as children framed their behavior in adulthood.

In 1900, women did not have voting

rights. The constitution granted freedom to all men. "Men" were interpreted to exclude women and black people. As a result neither women nor minorities had the vote. Then, as now, there were people who rose up against these indignities and inequities. Women succeeded in getting the right to vote in 1920. Black people won their right to vote in 1953. This meant that women and blacks now had a way of influencing their lives through legal channels. Although women got the vote in 1920, it was nearly 40 years later before they actively took up the cudgels of becoming equal to men, persons in their own right. This effort began with the appearance of the women's movement which is still going on today.

As the status of women changed, it was inevitable that the relationship between men and women would also change significantly. Women are no longer subject to men in the way they once were. Progress has been made. However, because of laws and outmoded attitudes, the realization of equality for women is far from complete.

People often ask me if I think the family is falling apart, disappearing or being destroyed. My answer is that what is happening is that we are going through a much needed evolution that has had revolutionary aspects. Women are rising from positions of victimization to standing on their own feet. They are discovering their possibilities.

For eons family structure had remained the same, with a person's identity being invested in a role; the male dominated family structure was firmly entrenched. When a change occurs that is as profound as the change in women and their relationship to their role in society and to themselves, there is bound to be an upheaval in the ongoing system. That is what is happening in families today. Changes are always connected with chaos and that's what we are seeing right now. The family structure will have a much needed facelift when we reshape our attitudes and expectations about the equality and value of human beings.

There also will be a change in how power is used. When people are viewed as equals, power can be used to empower individuals instead of controlling others. The most prevalent use of power among individuals is to control others because of their age, status, relative wealth, sex, or race. The difference here is between seed power, which is based on growth and cooperation, and gun power, which is based on threat. We have never had a time when the choices of our use of power were as clear and so available.

At the end of World War II, we all heaved a sigh of relief and had hope of building a more just world. The U.N. was a manifestation of that dream. These hopes were also translated into a new psychological construct—the human potential movement. In 1946 we heard the voices of Abraham Maslow, Rollo May, Carl Rogers and others who believed that human beings are and can be more than what their behavior led us to believe. We set on a journey to find out what else there was in the human being that had not yet been discovered and accessed. Major outcomes of this thrust were the possibility that individuals could exercise more control over their health; they could have more satisfaction and happiness in their lives; they could have rewarding and nurturing relationships with one another. They did not have to settle as Hans Selye, M.D. suggested, settling for being "only a little bit sick."

I believe that the development of family therapy was an outcome of this search for human potential. For the therapist, this suggested a change from concentrating on the elimination of pathology to the promotion of health. The trend is obvious in those institutions and persons who are on the cutting edge of today's world. That is, that people work together on the basis of cooperation rather than authoritarian means. The family is the place where human beings start their journey toward becoming adults.

Over time, many theories and techniques have been advanced to guide thinking in new directions. These change according to the beliefs we have about the nature of human beings and what we want them to become. For example, if our goal is to eliminate pathology, we behave differently than if we aim toward developing health. Previously, therapy was generally directed at helping people adjust to their environment; it did not include giving them tools to reshape their environment. This necessarily brought them in line with what was expected and what was acceptable, often at the expense of whatever new might be emerging. In short, therapy played the role of a universal super parent who knew what was good for people. This role changed radically after World War II with the inception of the holistic health focus.

Since 1946, almost every sacred cow has been scrutinized—for example, rights of minorities, women, and sexual behavior. In 1930, it would have been unthinkable for a professor at a university to openly live with someone without being married. Today, there are many places where this would hardly cause a raised eyebrow. Having babies without the benefit of marriage once was a source of disgrace. Today some women actively seek to become mothers without being married. Many of these changes have brought considerable pain, anguish, and often destructive behavior. They were indeed a challenge to the status quo. These changes came about as responses to the chains of conformity, in an atmosphere of freedom where it seemed possible to break the chains. As I mentioned before, whenever change occurs there is always chaos. As the chaos manifests itself, new directions emerge which can be seen clearly when the chaff falls away. Not everything that gets stirred up in a period of crisis indicates a new healthy direction. There needs to be a time of settling and sorting. I think as far as the human condition is concerned, we are at this point now. We have some new directions that are forming. We also have a lot of chaff to wade through. I hope that we will give ourselves per-

mission to change course if we find out that we are on the wrong track.

Therapists are a product of their own time. Now we have much new knowledge and information, and we know more about how the body and brain work. We have developed therapies to match our understandings. For example, bioenergetics and rolfing use the body as an entry point. "Super-learning" speaks to integrating cognitive and intuitive learning. Our knowledge about communication has deepened and broadened, especially through cybernetics and general systems theory. Family system therapy is an application of this knowledge.

Before 1946, a good therapist was one who kept the therapeutic intervention rigidly within the frame of a single theory. Being eclectic was considered unprofessional. When I was in graduate school, I was asked to declare whether I was Jungian, Freudian or Adlerian. The implication was that I had to choose one and put on blinders for the others. The goal for this limiting decision was to give focus and a sense of confidence, thus preparing me to fulfill professional expectations. I think this goal resulted in a cookie cutter approach, wherein the patient had to fit a mold. Those patients who were unwilling to be molded were considered resistant. I wonder how much farther we would be now if we had used an approach which allowed us to check our techniques for fit and then to give up our rigidities to create something that fit better. Today we are less rigid on this point. We are less likely to feel there is one right way. Many more people are open to new learning.

Let us consider another aspect of life since 1900. From 1900 to 1914 industrialization was occurring rapidly. From 1914 to 1918 we were involved in World War I. Usually a crisis such as war, along with its devastation, also brings some new possibilities. This was true for World War I. From 1918 to 1929 we saw a phenomenon that had never existed before. It was referred to as the "flapper age." This was a period of discarding values, with the result that personal behavior excesses flourished. It was as if the back of the work ethic had bent and people were ready to experience some hedonism. Even though there were prohibition laws, this did not stop people from drinking. They just got more creative and more resourceful. There were many illegal sources from which liquor could be obtained. There are many stories about moonshine stills and the ways the moonshiners could outwit the "Feds." There was an upsurge of criminal behavior. Al Capone was king of the underground and Chicago was the home of his mobsters. Al Capone never was punished for direct criminal behavior. He was caught on income tax evasion.

From 1929 to 1941 we were in the worst depression in our history. In Chicago in 1932, I remember seeing the streets lined with unemployed men. It was a time when many people committed suicide, when they lost their money and saw no prospects for jobs. Many people became prematurely old. It was a time of great despair and hopelessness, anguish and pain. There was no protection against this awful turn of events. People had been thoroughly indoctrinated with the idea that they should take care of themselves. The Great Depression highlighted the fact that people could not control all the forces that acted upon them. Society was much more complicated.

New laws changing banking and investment policies grew out of this dreadful situation to protect people against loss of their savings. In the Depression, many people who had diligently saved lost their life savings and faced the rest of their lives as paupers. "Bums" and "spendthrifts" had always been around; they were taken as a matter of course. But, when respectable, hard-working thrifty people lost their money, changes were made.

The calamity of the Depression also painfully brought to the fore the plight of many disadvantaged people. There were no federal programs for assistance. Some forward-looking states had programs for the "disadvantaged deserving" people.

The Social Security Act of 1935, was a law that embraced the idea that the federal government had a place in augmenting and extending resources related to earned work credits for all citizens who needed those services. And, it was a matter of right, not charity. This dignified the human being who worked. It also recognized that human beings were mutually dependent within a complex society.

World War II started in 1941 and continued until 1945. The horrors of this war demanded that we work to avoid the repetition of such a holocaust. Hitler and his colleagues represented the extreme in the phenomenon of one person deciding who was right, who was wrong, who should live, and who should die. This is a natural outcome of relationships based on submission and domination. In general, this was the way Western society operated and was linked. Those who had power decided what was best for others and then proceeded to enforce their decisions. Fear, threat, and enticement were the chief means by which this was accomplished. There was little room for autonomy or self-responsibility.

As the voices of humanistic approaches became stronger, it seemed clear that empowering persons to become their own decision-makers and to learn how to create a value of equality between and among people held the greatest promise for human beings to live and manage their human affairs. There is increasing evidence to show that persons who give their decision-making power to others are more vulnerable to illness and other human dysfunction. My challenge is: Can the therapist assist clients to develop their capacities to cope with what is needed, or do therapists decide what should happen and then use their power to try to make it happen?

I am on the side of using myself to help my patients or clients find their own resources to cope differently, and then to decide what it is they want. I look back at World War II and Hitler's involvement. It is frightening to experience the phenomenon where one person could be the catalyst to so many people losing their minds and hearts, allowing themselves and others to deliberately behave in the most inhuman ways imagineable, as many of the Nazis did to the Jewish people.

Whenever there are people not standing on their own feet, and whenever they give their power over to someone else, they essentially have to lose their minds to make it work. This is fertile ground for cultism. There is a crying need for us to use our energies so that everybody should be so informed and therefore able to stand on their own feet, so that they do not have to give their power over to someone else. For me, that is the core of my therapeutic endeavor. Taking and managing one's own power is not something most of us were brought up with. It is 180 degrees different from practicing obedience and conformity, which is what most of us were taught as children.

At the end of World War II came the next development of the seeds that had been set in the early 1900s. Now there were new possibilities for all people in the world to responsibly pursue their humanness and freedom. We are still at the edge of this process. We are moving from a time and place where the pairing relationship characterized by "who's on top and who's on the bottom," who is dominant and who is submissive, is changing to who is across from us.

At this point we are beginning to sense that a healthy relationship must be between equals. This has very important implications for therapy. We are only beginning to develop models of what relationships of equality between people look like. We have to redefine what "equal" means. Generally speaking equality has meant "the same as." Actually human beings are unique. There are no exact duplicates. Within that fact, equality has to mean the equality of value and worth in the eyes of each toward the other. Neither being is dominant nor submissive to the other. What kind of therapeutic interventions will therapists have to learn to cre-

ate that kind of equality? How can equality be modelled between therapist and patient? If that modelling is not apparent, the words will have little meaning. "Do as I say, not as I do" gets few followers.

When the human potential movement was sufficiently developed to have a form, the nucleus of that form was how to make contact with one's self as well as others— how to look, how to listen, how to touch both self and others. For many people these three skills are tied up with prohibitions from childhood. All three often are triggers that have sexual and negatively aggressive connotations. Today there are few people who know how to look, to listen, to touch someone comfortably, in a way that is free from implications of aggression or sex. Touch has been singled out for more fear and censorship than looking or listening. There have been some unfortunate results related to touch contact. Unfortunate results have come about from the way that people have looked or talked to each other as well.

It is interesting to me that nobody suggests that one stops looking, gouging out one's eyes, or closing them because they have been misused. They look to reshaping the use. Nor does anyone suggest cutting off ears because one has heard the unhearable. Yet people suggest stopping touching because it is sometimes misused. What we need to do is to learn how to use touch creatively and safely and to learn that it is a major means of contact. Senses are a source of communication, a vehicle for sending information, and a means of connecting personal energy. Senses are the real basis of contact. Contact is the basis of trust. When trust has been established, real and relevant work can go on.

Another important goal of the human potential movement (holistic health) was an emphasis on what was already growing and positive within the self. A primary idea was to help individuals further develop their positive parts. In so doing, they would create the energy and strength to cope more effectively with their barriers. There are some of us that feel that if one works only on pathology, it's like beating a dead horse. It's not going to go anywhere.

Before World War II, the usual unit of treatment was the individual. People behaved as though they believed that the individual became pathological by him or herself and would have to get well by him or herself. There was one exception to this. Child guidance clinics were functioning on the premise that mothers affected their children. Thus both the mother and child were seen, but separately and by different therapists. The therapists often developed adversary positions toward each other, resulting in negative system therapy at the level of the therapists seeing the relationship between the child's behavior and the impact of the mother's behavior. This was a step philosophically toward the idea that individuals impact each other. If the mother affected the child, the child was also affecting the mother.

Once that idea was established, then other relationships could be viewed from a similar perspective. Dr. Harry Stack Sullivan in the 1930s advanced the theory that the behavior of any person included the effects of the impact of the behavior of others. However, the idea was not translated into using the physical presence of anyone other than the one who was exhibiting symptoms.

The atmosphere of the 1950s and 1960s was such that there was freedom to discover new paths to change. During this time there was encouragement to confront and reevaluate the "accepted truths" about human behavior and treatment.

In the last 40 years, researchers and clinicians have proposed new views about the nature of human beings, their behavior, and how to change behavior. In a way, we were now a little like the proverbial story of the six blind men and the elephant. Each one viewed the elephant from his own place. They quarreled about who was right. Perhaps we need to take a lesson from that story. Instead of quarreling about who is right, we can contribute and share with each other about what we have seen. Actually, this period brought us a rich smorgasbord of fresh ideas. I think it behooves all of us to become familiar with these new approaches.

One such idea stands out among the rest. This is the concept of systems. As we became more fully acquainted with the phenomenon of how persons impact one another, we were at the beginning of understanding the concept of systems. Briefly defined, a system is an action, a reaction, and an interaction. Out of this series of connections, people enforce, support, and reinforce the status quo. By engaging in a new set of interactions, something new follows. When we add this system awareness to the new vista that Freud opened up for us, namely, that we had within us the seeds of our destructiveness as well as our constructiveness, we essentially have a new basis for psychotherapy.

I have been delighted that at this conference more sharing with a sense of contribution has gone on than at any other gathering I remember. Perhaps this speaks to our maturity and that we are learning the lessons of the "elephant story."

We are only 14 years away from the year 2000. I feel that much anticipation and preparation are going on in relation to that event. Most of us in this room will probably see the year 2000. Many futurists are writing about what the year 2000 will be like. I think that we are preparing to develop ways to be in touch with the broader, deeper, and higher consciousness of what it means to be more fully human. I think there are many places on our planet where people are already deliberately and consciously working on developing this new consciousness. We are in the throes of an evolutionary leap concerning humankind. These leaps are accompanied by struggle. Until now, human beings, as such, have not been valued simply because they are human. We are apparently just beginning to notice that human beings are miracles of creation. Have we yet been able to develop a sperm and egg that can reproduce itself?

We know that each human being is unique and has no exact duplicate anywhere. Within this reality, it is hard to understand torture, racism, sexism, and war. The only way it can make any sense at all is that some people are not considered humans, such as slaves, women, and children.

As we move toward the twenty-first century we are bringing a growing awareness that each human being is of value and a source of powerful energy. The challenge is to access that energy and convert it to constructive ends. We have already begun to develop therapies and educational approaches that reflect our growing knowledge about how to do this. The seeds were set in motion at the beginning of this century.

Now I would like to put myself into the background that I have described. I was born on a farm in Wisconsin in 1916. I lived in a family where I was free to search for whatever I needed to find out. I was ill a great deal as a child which, I think now, was partially a reflection of the negative parts of my parents' relationship to each other. I had no question about my parents caring for me. However, I didn't really understand why they treated each other the way they did. As a result, I made a resolve that when I grew up I was going to become a children's detective on parents. The first breakthrough on that route came when I found out that parents were only children grown big, carrying with them whatever they had learned as children. If they had not learned anything new since their childhood, they simply found a new form for that old learning. People have always fascinated me and they still do. Life fascinates me.

To start my professional career I went into teaching. I felt delight with each new piece of information that could help me to understand the giant jigsaw puzzle of how "people worked" and how the pieces fit together.

I did not want to be an armchair expert. I wanted to have "hands on" experience to extend my learning. I arranged my teaching jobs so that in the six years that I taught school, I had five different teaching experiences. This allowed me to be in touch with white children, black children, rich and poor, immigrant children, urban and farm children. My goal was to help the children find learning to be a wonderful experience and thereby get all the benefits they could from it. I had revered my own learning experiences. I wanted the children to feel that school was a wonderful place to be and learning was exciting.

As a step toward providing this context, I became acquainted with each child's family. Every night after school I went home with a child to meet his or her parents. I hoped to interest the parents in becoming part of my school family. Most of the families accepted. Retrospectively, I know that this helped with discipline because I had few discipline problems. My students responded with excitement and performed well academically. Visiting the homes also gave me a chance to learn how different families operated. One day one little boy fell asleep soon after class started. When I asked him why, he told me that his father had been drunk the night before and had locked him out. I went home with him that night. In a very straight and innocent way I told the father that little boys can't learn in school if they don't get any sleep. Therefore he needed to see that his son got a good night's sleep. He agreed to do that. He kept his promise. Later I learned that he had stopped his drinking. This experience triggered my inquiring self to search out more about adult behavior. I began to see that I needed to know much more about behavior than what I knew at that time.

My next step was to go to graduate school, where I enrolled in a social work program. I was a good student and learned well. I also followed the principle of relating whatever I had been taught to its applicability to human beings and their behavior. Sometimes the theory and its application seemed in conflict. The theory base was psychoanalytic. All of the pathology seemed exciting to me and very new. Sometimes, I couldn't tell whether the concepts applied or not. However, since I had faith in my teachers, I accepted their teachings even when I was in doubt. I have found since that I have discarded many, reshaped others, and built on still others.

In the institution and agency settings where I worked, I discovered that I had a special ability to work with seriously disturbed and high-risk people. Little in my training helped me to understand how I got such good results. Later, I went into private practice in Chicago. Being a nonmedical person, I did not have access to the so-called cream of the psychiatric crop. Therefore, I saw the people no one else wanted. Among these people were alcoholic men who had been taken out of the gutters on West Madison Street in Chicago, children who had been moved from pillar to post and were considered impossible, and others who had moved from therapist to therapist. Since I was nonmedical, I was unable to get liability insurance. I needed to work and have no casualties. I had to develop reliable ways of protecting myself and, at the same time, take the risks necessary for people to grow. If I wasn't successful in helping people, I would not have a livelihood. I had little room for error. If I did err, there would be serious consequences. I was with high-risk people and I was taking high risks myself. This was a tough, but good context in which to learn some basic lessons.

My early educational training and experiences stood me in good stead. I automatically looked at these people in terms of finding their strengths, making contact with them, listening to what they thought and felt. I believe now that the above factors were largely responsible for the positive changes that took place. I have since learned how to make conscious use of these awarenesses to engage people by looking at them, by listening to them, and by touching them. To do this, I need to be centered and live the values I espouse.

One of the valuable things about working with people that no one else wants is that they have already been discarded. Therefore, one is under no threat of failure. One is free to do all the experimenting necessary. To my surprise, my way of working with so-called "impossible people" was beginning to pay off. I really didn't know too much about what I was doing, except that I was applying things that weren't supposed to be applied—looking at people from a positive point of view, connecting with them as people, and minimizing emphasis on pathology in order to work for their growth. Word got around, and I soon had a very large practice. In time, people came who weren't the "impossible people." What I began to see was that the same approaches worked with everyone regardless of their symptoms.

I will describe briefly the first situation when a lot of things came together for me. Actually, the learnings in this case formed a basis of what I do today. It was the spring of 1951. A 28-year-old woman came to see me. She was labeled "ambulatory schizophrenia." She had gone to many different therapists without particularly good results. We worked together for about six months. Things were beginning to change. One day I had a phone call from her mother who threatened to sue me for alienation of affections. That day I heard two messages, something I had never before been conscious of. One was a threat in her words, and the other was a plea in her voice tone. I ignored her threat and responded to her plea and invited her to join her daughter. She accepted. When the mother came in, my patient behaved as she had the first day I saw her.

When peculiar things like this happen to me I stand back and observe. I don't act. I realize that I don't know what is going on and I must take time to understand. Within six months, we, mother, daughter and myself had developed a new relationship. I realized that what I saw here were the bare bones of the beginning of my communication theory. That is, whenever one speaks, there are always two messages: a verbal message and an affective message. I had also begun to see that between these two people there was a cluing system that seemed to be operating. I noticed the tilting of a head, or an arm moving, or a voice drop, and then I would see a reaction. It didn't seem to have anything to do with the words. The words could be "I love you" but all the rest of it was something else. I began to look more closely at this system of cluing. As I learned about this phenomenon with my patient and her mother, I used this knowledge with other people.

This cluing system was the beginning of what I came to know as the family system, made up of overt and covert emotional rules. As I studied this cluing system together with the verbal and nonverbal message, I realized that the two messages in the communication came from two quite different places. The verbal message came from the cognitive part of the self, whereas the affective one, manifested in voice tone, breathing and the posture, was a message from the body itself about what was currently going on. It was perfectly possible for somebody to say "I love you," while at the same time turn the head in such a way indicating "no." Later, I became aware that when the affective and verbal parts of the message are discrepant, the affective message is most impactful.

In another six months, I suddenly had the idea that maybe there was a man in this family, that the woman had a husband, and the daughter had a father. I remind you that at this time men were not considered part of the emotional life of a family. When I asked, I discovered that there was a man and that he lived in the home. I asked if they would ask him to come in. They agreed. Actually, the father was not supposed to do this, according to what I had been taught. I had been taught that family members are natural enemies of each other. When the husband/father appeared, the relationship between the mother and daughter became

chaotic. This was much like the change that occurred when the mother first joined the session. As I watched this interaction, I saw the effect of a third person on a pair. For example, I saw how the third person was used as a bridge between the two. I also noticed how the third person was invited to take sides and how the third person was blamed for whatever was going on whenever the other two were at odds. I worked with these three people until we got it righted.

One day I had another thought that maybe there was another child in the family. I asked and the response was "Yes." We were so individually oriented at that time that one did not think in terms of other children. I invited that person to come in. When he did, he turned out to be an absolutely fantastic-looking male, two years older than his sister, big, juicy, luscious looking. It was immediately apparent he was the worshipped one. He was the wonderful, smart one in the family and his sister was the bad, crazy one.

I have since seen this phenomenon many times in troubled families. Each child has a stereotype. One child is the bad one, another, the good one, the smart one, or the dumb one. These labels are powerful sources for reinforcing the behavior the stereotype implies. These are and become a part of making a system balance. I see two kinds of balances. One is a balance in which each part gets as much as it gives. This is healthy. The other is where one part pays a lot more than it gets. The latter balance is apt to have an identified patient who is a person wearing the symptom. With the appearance of the son, I had access to the whole family.

Since I am very visually minded, I saw these people in exaggerated stances to themselves and to each other. That was the beginning of my sculpting technique. In this family I saw the son standing up on a chair with the other three below worshipping him, hands outstretched. My patient was obscured from contact with the parents because she was pushed behind them. This was my initial attempt to manifest communication through body postures. I later completed these tools and called them *blaming, placating, super-reasonable, and irrelevant* stances.

I learned that if I put people in physical stances, they were likely to experience the feelings that went with that stance. For example, if I put someone in a placating stance he or she would begin to feel helplessness and also, often, rage. Putting people in the stances also allowed me to circumvent the threat that went with a sense of becoming aware. It bypassed negative confrontation and accessed information instead. It was also a means of stimulating interest. When used with the proper timing, this tool is almost always successful. It is a quick, reliable, and interesting way to get to the feelings. This tool also allows for the use of humor which in itself is healing. We can get to a sense of the ridiculous without developing threat.

As I became aware of the new factors I learned with this family, I applied them to other families. I began to see similar results. It was at this point that I was keenly aware of the relationship of communication to the behavior of individuals in the family. I had the beginning notions of how family systems are built and how in turn that system reinforces the behavior of individuals in the family. I defined, redefined, broadened, and deepened my understanding as I went along.

I obviously did not stop here. I discovered what appeared to be important truths. Following these truths took me in directions quite different from what I had learned in graduate school. This was happening not only for me. I am grateful to have been a part of an exciting period when the rigidities imposed by professional constraints were giving way to an air of inquiry and experimentation without losing professional respectability. I should like to see that spirit continue.

In this century, we have made breathtaking changes in our outer world. For example, we have gone from transportation by horses to airplanes, from the party-line telephone to satellite communication, from science fiction to drawing board plans for actual cities to be built in outer space.

Changes in human consciousness have proceeded at a much slower pace. We still see war and other forms of threat as viable means of handling conflict. We still categorize and stereotype people, substituting role for identity. We still do not behave as though all human beings have value. Our tendency has been to see behavior and the person as one.

I see the person as an outcome of the manager of his/her behavior. I therefore put emphasis on the preparation and development of the manager. It is hard to play beautiful music on an untuned violin, no matter how great the skill is.

I equate the evolving, healthy person with a beautifully made and finely tuned instrument. Our instrument is finely made. We need to learn how to tune it better. That means developing a philosophy and an approach that are centered in human value and use the power of the seed which is based on growth and cooperation with others.

This conference is affording all of us the opportunity to look in depth at where we have come in the last 80 years, where we are now, and where we are going.

Discussion by Erving Polster, Ph.D.

One of the major things about Virginia, which is even more evident this time, not actually working with people but giving this lecture, is that she is a magnificent storyteller. This happens to fit in with what I'm concerned about these days, which is how we include storytelling in psychotherapy, how we include it in our lives, and the sense in which stories confirm our existence. And she of course, with her stories, confirms the existence of a process that has been going on since 1900, which has certain culminating characteristics at this conference in terms of the coming together of people from diverse points of view in an atmosphere of mutual recognition. Virginia gets that across very beautifully. She lives that and so there is in that living of it the support for being able to tell us her story as it relates to our story and as that relates to the story of our culture since 1900.

Virginia said something toward the end of her talk which accentuated one of the things that comes across to me in what she does. She said that she accesses what people don't know they have and then makes it clear that they have it. I would put that in somewhat different words, but I think it would amount to something very similar, and that is that when we work with people in therapy, it's their business in working with us to be uninteresting. And it's our business, in being their therapist, not to be fooled by that and to realize that in spite of everything they do to the contrary, our patients are fundamentally hugely interesting. The trouble is they haven't noticed it, or they've noticed other things about themselves that stand in the foreground which becloud the fact that they are indeed interesting. Or they pretend to be interesting about things which they actually are interesting about if they only wouldn't be pretending it.

So, I see Virginia as a person who has such great fascination in whomever she's dealing with that there is no way that that person can't wind up feeling that fascination, and thus feeling fascinating, and feeling, thereby, confirmed in being enabled to go further with the liveliness in their spirit.

Another thing Virginia does is seen when she talked about the various levels of human experience, going from the large dichotomy of mind and body to the rather smaller diversities which she described so beautifully in the many things that people do. She would be interested, though she didn't say this, in what they had for lunch or who their best friends are, or when they like to sit alone, when they like to be with people, what book they're reading. In other words, she gets a sense of the variety that exists within each person. And so when you get that variety working and start to coordinate it, you could say that Virginia is, in a sense, doing group therapy when she is working with an individual. She is trying to coordinate all the varied aspects of a person and make one whole person out of that diversity.

This is Virginia's way of getting to depth, to the obvious and the not so obvious. Her sense of the reaching of depth is what I think of as a horizontal relationship of experience to meaning, rather than a vertical one. When you get a vertical relationship of event and meaning, what you have is an interpretation or a symbolic structure—some immediate reaching into the depths of what's happening with a person. But when you have the horizontal experience, you have a process in which the meaning evolves and at one point becomes clear, even though you haven't delved into the depths of each particular event. By doing that, she is enabled—and all of us could be, too—to take events seriously for their own sake, without having to be concerned with what do they really mean at each moment.

QUESTIONS AND ANSWERS

Question: You've mentioned several times the issue of different cultural roles. Could you say something about how you work with people who don't share your cultural beliefs or your beliefs about appropriate roles for people to play with each other?

Satir: If while I address everybody around me we all sit in a Turkish bath and we're free enough to look at each other, I think we would all come up with similar observations. Now, in a funny way that's a metaphor for your question. I know that every human being breathes, for example, and that surgeons can be successful because they don't have to learn how to operate on an Irish person or a Swedish one or whatever. They know how to operate and I think that's the way I work. Now how do you find a way to have meaning? How do you work out a way to understand each other?

I have done a lot of work with the Sioux Indian people in the past ten years. One of the first persons I saw was an old Indian chief, about 80-years-old with no teeth and gnarled hands, who lived in a hogan. He brought eight children, two of whom had been labeled schizophrenic. I had never worked with an Indian man before. I knew that I could talk to him even though I didn't know if he would understand me or if I would understand him. I said to him, "I have never worked with an Indian man before and I would like you to teach me what I need to know in order to understand you, and I will do the same with you."

So even though I can't go in just anywhere and know that I know the meaning

of things, I have a means by which I can ask people to help me to understand them so that I can better work with them. What I work on is the process of things and I have worked with many families around the world whose language I didn't know. We always work successfully because it was working on a process. Everywhere I go, I find I can reach out a hand and somebody will take it. The messages I get from that hand are not cultural, they are human.

This is what I do with all my students: I teach them how to understand not by figuring out ahead of time to be able to understand but by asking people to teach them how to understand them. They will do the same themselves and then they can have something together. I don't know if that helps you out but that's the way I work it. That's how I can work with people everywhere in the world.

Question: To what extent have you been able to work with people from the Soviet Union?

Satir: I have not worked at all with people from the Soviet Union. I have, however, worked with people from the Eastern bloc countries. I was invited officially to one of the countries for two weeks and found, of course, that the problems are the same even though people have different ways of coping. Since there is an extra environmental factor there, I worked out a way to work only in process without practically any content. Thus, I'm always mindful of the context. I had in my group a writer who had made some human rights statements. He was doing some menial work and his typewriter and car had been taken away. He was there with his wife and they were having terrible problems. What I did was to use just process terms such as, "Take your wife's hand and say to yourself what you're feeling." I let most of the work go on in hands. If there was something I knew he was angry about, I asked him to fantasy it inside. Then I gave him help with how he could have an internal temper tantrum so that he wouldn't get into further jeopardy.

Question: I came into psychotherapy through the child guidance movement. Many classical analysts at that time were against family therapy and didn't see relatives or parents. In this agency they had the most wonderful classical analyst, but still they saw families and parents. There was an evolution from individual psychoanalysis to family work. I wondered why you didn't mention the work with the child guidance movement as part of the evolution of psychotherapy?

Satir: I'm glad you brought that up because the Juvenile Court Act of 1899 was the precursor of the child guidance movement. That was the first time that the state took an interest in what was happening to children and a court was established to protect them. Out of this the child guidance movement was formed based upon the fact that children sometimes needed to be protected from their parents. Many of the child guidance clinics later, in spite of their sophisticated development, kept that model—the parents were seen separately from the child. But there were others who did see them together. I'm so glad you brought that up because it was a significant development.

Question: How did you know the disguised cry for help behind the threat that "I'm going to sue you because you've alienated my schizophrenic child"?

Satir: That's a wonderful question and the best I can do is to answer it retrospectively. There have been times in my life when I was able to hear in ways I wasn't able to hear before. I can't give you a better answer than that because I certainly wasn't saying to myself that there was a double-level message. I didn't know the question to ask but I had a good relationship with this woman and in my mind there was a certain absurdity to a woman not wanting her daughter helped.

What was going through my mind was an awareness that if the daughter was so badly off, the mother must be badly off too. That wasn't in the forefront, but one of the other things I did to help young students and people who studied with me was to develop cuddle zones for parents because so often parents are asked to do things and to give things that they themselves never had. I think it was some awareness on that level. Also, I wasn't going to let this young woman down and I certainly wasn't about to be sued. So those were kind of bottom lines, but it didn't feel that way to me. It felt like an awareness that I just picked up.

Question: You spoke of the process of evolving. What is your perception as to where we as human beings are evolving?

Satir: I think we are evolving toward a state of becoming more fully conscious and human. We have always had individuals who were in that space, but more and more people can see themselves doing this. Usually, that was left to religious figures in the past. Now I think we have never had a world in which people were evolving so fully.

I think we're going to have to do a lot of different things as this happens. I can see, for instance, that the adversary system will change so there is more justice involved. I can see that family relationships will change. Just think what it would be like if we succeed in our model of a pair getting together, where two people are standing on their own feet and are able to move the team, to support each other but never in any way substitute for one another, to make a model of the union of uniqueness and differentness, what in some places might be called a union of sameness and diversity. What fantastic things can happen if we do that! I have a hunch that human beings, once they don't have to put so much energy into figuring out who loves them and under what conditions, can create an immensely positive and effective world.

I want to say one other thing. I don't think that passivity and peace is the same as passivity and fun. I don't think that aggression in and of itself is a bad thing. You like to stretch your muscles and do things. It's the meanness about this that makes it so bad. I don't know how the world will look like when we have fully evolved people. For example, China is doing a wonderful experiment, but I don't know what it's going to be like if they succeed in their goal of all families having only one child. We've never had a world like that. We have new things. Everytime you change, you have to change something around you. I hope we all have the courage to do the changing that we need to do. I'm looking forward to it.

Question: I don't have the courage you were expressing. I am a therapist treating young children and have been a therapist for 20 years after years of teaching young children in New York City. I am very concerned that while we are in this evolution, I am seeing more and more children. I come from the Philadelphia area. I work with the poor and the rich and the black and the white and the plaids. I am tired of hearing about families that, in my own terms, I am trying to find. I'm talking about children in trouble, who are hurting and abandoned not because their parents are cruel or sick, but because they must work or are unknown. I'm talking about children who are not receiving nurturing, neither from their birth families nor from their surrogate families. I have no one to appeal to in those cases. I cannot find the fathers—often not because they aren't present, but because they're busy working 14-hour days to keep up with their obligations. While this evolution is taking place, what do people who work with young children do?

Satir: That's where I was many years ago and that's where I learned how to do some things because of my strong feeling that the experiences we have as children are going to be reflected in us as adults. I

know that there are plenty of people who give birth to children but who are not much more than children themselves, and many of them are very deprived. It is similar to what a friend of mine who was in the Battle of the Bulge told me: There were so many wounded who were going to die and he could only work with a certain number of them.

Question: It used to be called triage. We used it when I was working in New York City right after World War II, but here we are in 1985.

Satir: I know, but we have to be as creative as possible. Many things happen and can happen. Do you have a support for yourself?

Question: Yes, beautiful support of family, of grandchildren. I am well respected, a clinical professor in a medical university. I have not had the chance to write some of my thoughts because I've worked so ridiculously hard in trying to prevent psychopathology in young children in our city. I haven't once heard this subject addressed in this conference. I feel great respect for the people who are here, but I am seeking not the answer but some awareness that all of us are working hard to try to help, to create that future that you were speaking of. Certainly, I want to participate. I need to find some new approaches for these children. I've tried politics, I've gotten nowhere in my writing, in my speeches, in so many meetings. I am so tired of these movements.

Satir: I hear what you say and I can share it. You want to know if you're alone in this or if there is any kind of support because after awhile the need gets overwhelming. I, too, had the people no one else wanted. When I told others how relieving it was to find somebody who could even talk about the same thing, at least it made me feel I was not alone out in left field. I hear you at this point saying something like that. I for one would like to tell you that I know what that's like and I also know that I'm not going to be able to do everything all at once. I will try. When I was in a girls' home in the early 40s, I used to go to cemeteries, to all kinds of places because I was convinced that people needed to know what happened to their parents. When I made contact, I found that it wasn't that the parents were working so hard that kept them away; it was their feeling that they weren't going to be valued and there wasn't any point to it. How many times did I find men who had "abandoned their children," that's what it said in the records, who said they didn't think they were of any value.

I could give a whole talk on this subject just from my experience. I would encourage you to talk more about this and get more people interested because often you live in a certain place and don't know what's going on in another part of town. For example, now there are a lot of people, rapes have been going on for a long time, molestation and sexual abuse of children have been going on for a long time, but until relatively recently people didn't talk much about it. Now it's very open. I often wish I had a magic wand with which I could change things. I suggest that you get yourself on programs and talk about this kind of thing. . . .

Question: I've done that for 20 years. I've been on programs, on T.V., I've been in Washington. . . .

Satir: Has something happened for you?

Question: No, it isn't me, it is a public policy, a social policy. We are not political enough, we are a huge body of human behavior scientists. I am not naive about this and know I'm not alone. Don't answer it in that sense. I would say I am appropriately depressed at what I see. If I were not, I would not be in touch with reality. But it's not me that I'm asking about. You are in the forefront. You and your colleagues have written beautiful and mean-

ingful books that I read. You have a chance to make a push for reason, to get together and say we need policies for children. We need help for single parents, whether male or female. We can't change what's happening. We can't put mama back in the kitchen. We must go out there and do something about this.

Satir: I appreciate what you're saying. I could tell you, for instance, that I am on the task force of the California legislature to do something about battered women. That's my way of helping. It didn't come up and I think maybe it's important that we do talk about this sometime. I'm glad you brought that up because we need to have it brought to our attention. So thank you.

Question: Would you be willing to share what "spiritual" means to you as you talk about body/mind and spirit?

Satir: When I was a child, there was much religious controversy in my home. My mother was a Christian Scientist and my father was a Missouri senator. While I know today that that wasn't really the issue, it took that form. As a result, I became ill and nearly died because my mother couldn't let me go for medical care. My father finally took me when I was virtually dead, but they revived me. As far as I was concerned as a child, religion and spirituality were the same thing and religion was bad because it nearly killed me. I later had terrible experiences with people in certain religions who said to me, "If that person isn't of this faith, I won't help them." That was when I was working with the people you are talking about and it made me very sad and upset. For me, religion didn't have much in common with spirituality.

However, I was raised on a farm where life was showing itself all over, the new plants and the animals and all of that. There was a reverence for life there. That was also true in my family. As I moved and looked at life within human beings, the spirituality part was for me first of all the manifestation of life, the sperm and the egg. The spirituality is a relationship to life, which I know now also exists in many religions and in many religious people. But the spirituality is that piece of manifestation of life. When the body lies in the casket, everything is there but the spirituality which makes for life. What happens to that, I'm not sure. I was feeling sad when the last woman was talking because I could feel her pain and I know that pain myself. Part of that pain translated into what I heard her trying to do. I certainly would love for all of us to know that kind of pain as well as the joy which is also a part of the spiritual. I see every human being as being a part of me in some respects. I do a lot of work with accessing intuitional things, which I think is part of a universal intelligence.

Buckminster Fuller said once, "I learn things that I was not taught. It's in the atmosphere and the intelligence is all around." That's a whole piece of it as well.

The Dynamics of the American Family as Deduced from 20 Years of Family Therapy: The Family Unconscious

◆

Carl A. Whitaker, M.D.

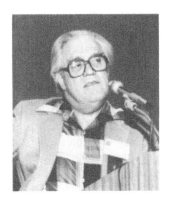

Carl A. Whitaker, M.D.

Carl Whitaker (M.D., Syracuse University, 1936) has practiced psychotherapy for more than 40 years. For nine years, he was Professor and Chairman of the Department of Psychiatry at Emory University College of Medicine. For almost 20 years, he was Professor of Psychiatry at the University of Wisconsin Medical School. Whitaker is one of the founding fathers of family therapy. He received the Distinguished Family Therapy Award from the American Association of Marriage and Family Therapy. His approach has been named the "experiential school."

Whitaker has co-authored two books, edited one, and there is an edited volume about his approach. He has almost 60 contributions to books, including introductions, chapters, and forewords. Additionally, he has published more than 70 papers. Whitaker is former president of the American Academy of Psychotherapy.

This chapter consists of two sections: roughly, diagnosis and treatment. In the first section, Whitaker proposes a schema for understanding family dynamics by discussing three types of families. In the next section, he outlines his method of therapy, underlining the inherent power of the family to serve as its own best therapist.

Let me set the stage for a very personal essay on our topic, "Growing up as a social isolate on a dairy farm in the Adirondacks." I went to high school, college and medical school in Syracuse, took a residency in obstetrics and gynecology, and then got waylaid into psychiatry by becoming fascinated with schizophrenia. I spent 1940 to 1945 doing play therapy and working with delinquents. From 1946 to 1956, I did intensive clinical work with individual schizophrenics, utilizing a cotherapy, foster-parent model. In a rented house, supervised by full-time nonprofessional caretakers, I saw one patient at a time, for four interviews a week, lasting from one-half to three or four years. From 1956 to 1965, the same small clinical treatment team used cotherapy in general private practice of psychotherapy with individuals, couples, groups and families. From 1965 to 1985, I have devoted myself exclusively to the treatment of families, defining family as a two-or-more generation unit.

THREE-GENERATION FAMILY STRUCTURE

I intend to present a series of observations and assumptions that are part of my personal belief system which has evolved out of 45 years of clinical work, made possible by the cooperation of two very generous university settings that allowed time for study and the opportunity for private practice, as well as the privilege of utilizing training residents and colleagues as cotherapists. Most of the therapy was with the *team as therapist* rather than an individual or even two individuals. My observations are those of the garage mechanic with no specialized training in wind dynamics, fuel dynamics or the dynamics of metal stress; and, for the last 20 years, my work has been restricted to medium-sized cars. The previous ten years in the ghetto of Atlanta are relevant but not being reported.

Perhaps it would be easier to understand my framework if I explain that I am not a research thinker, and probably it would be easier to think of me as a family anthropologist observing families in their struggles with the stresses of life and change, I am now trying to put some of that change into words. I hope to maintain my own specific observation site, making no effort to summarize nor incorporate into my thinking the observations and presentations of others who work in the field. I make no apology for this naive approach.

In general, I am convinced that the family is not only a product of social roles and social rules and a biocultural dynamic force, but also the family is an organism. The family is essentially a subject or a territory composed, as in the individual, of a physical territory plus a set of physiological and psychological forces. It is clear that the physical or, if you will, the

anatomic factors have an influence on the physiological factors, and the physiological factors have an effect on the psychological. And, of course, the dynamic forces of each of these three territories are an influence on each of the other two.

TYPES OF FAMILIES

In a broad sense there are three types of families: the biopsychosocial families, the psychosocial families, and the social families.

The so-called natural family—two sets of grandparents, two parents and their children—constitutes a biopsychosocial family. It is 220 volts—dangerous, powerful currents. It has a biological, sometimes called a genetic, identification. The members are part of a family unconscious and, as is said by the comics, they are stuck with each other. The 220-volt power of this unit can be effective in generating either short circuits within the family or concentrated shocking effects on the world around it. The identification between the grandparents, parents and children of this three-generation unit is powerful and inevitable. It includes the unique factor that when any one looks in the face of another, he sees some physical and symbolical component of his own personhood, and he experiences the profound power.

In the process of family therapy, when the grandparent generation is part of the interview, it is very easy to move from three generations to five generations when the grandparents talk about *their* grandparents, with the same kind of intensity that they talk about their grandchildren. Although the in-law grandparent couples and the parent couple are really only psychosocial relationships with characteristics of the in-law dynamic, each generation produces an increase in the investment and reverberations that come from the identification that takes place down the hierarchy and that reverberates across the *family marital contract dynamics.*

It is clear that the *family unconscious*

is transmitted down this family tree for a series of generations, either augmented or weakened by the experience of each generation, but nevertheless it carries its own power vector. The power of this unit is indicated by the force of what happens with the negative vectors. The war between husband/wife, parent/grandparent and grandparent/in-law has the character of psychological suicide or civil war and is *never* low-voltage *in character,* even though it *may be* low-voltage *in expression.*

The *psychosocial marriage* is a term utilized to describe any marriage or any two-person relationship. It is probably 110 volts, a semidangerous teaming. It consists of a psychological choice plus an ongoing, more or less profound series of investments in each other and in the *team.* The simplest way of illustrating this is to say that since Muriel and I met and courted in 1935, married in 1937, had six children and now have ten grandchildren, the 50 years have been a massive investment. *Note that* the investment in any teaming relationship is dependent upon the clarity of the decision for continuity. One can describe marriage as a decision to relate whole person to whole person with a guaranteed continuity which, of course, is always available for rupture. But if it is repaired, it, like a broken bone, is stronger and becomes not only the base for a lifetime of psychotherapy with each other but also for a lifetime of détente. The investment is irreversible, like an irrevocable trust. The principal is not available to either of the members, only the interest is available; and it may be reinvested or moved into a separate account.

The *psychosocial family* has many variants. The second marriage and the third marriage, the presence of children from his first marriage and her first marriage, and the arrival of children to this second or third marriage, for example, all create a very complex dynamic understructure of stress. The understructure may be hidden by the same kind of complex dynamics that individuals use, as well as by the

many dynamic maneuvers that are characteristic of psychological unions and social teaming. If one presupposes that all families have essentially the same undercover dynamics (just as all individuals have the same undercover dynamics), it becomes increasingly clear that the dynamics of a psychosocial marriage or of a psychosocial family structure are very complex.

Take the example of the second wife who, even though she may have had a serious defect in the first marriage, retains that psychological investment, both the positive and negative, or a mixture of the two. In essence, she lives in the paranoid assumption that the second marriage will be just like the first one. Or if she has children from the first marriage, the wife could assume that the second husband will be a father to those children. This delusion is just as distorting as her assumption that she has turned her back on or grown past her love for and bitterness about the first man. Part of the undercurrent dynamics is the assumption that the second man will be the *hit man* to control the children from the first marriage; another part is the way that the new husband has the delusion that his wife is turning her back on the first marriage and that the joy of their current courtship is a process that will continue and grow indefinitely.

Simultaneously, the same kind of process occurs on the second husband's part, much of it unknown to him. He retains his investment in his first wife, and he holds the usually covert assumption that the second wife will be a good mother to *his* children, who had a bad mother during the first marriage. The second wife, of course, is not able to carry out this delusion except in a socially adroit, maneuvering manner. The second husband discovers quickly that although he is expected to be and would like to be the new father, he is, in essence, a part of a triangle. As soon as he exerts his own authority on her children, he finds that the bond between mother and children is much more powerful than the one between second husband and second wife; thus, he is end-lessly defeated.

Meanwhile, her children and his children, in an effort to be loyal to their own mother and their own father, are at war trying to destroy the new union. They not only refuse the role efforts of the step-parents, but also they utilize their power to split the couple so that they themselves can maintain the oedipal gains that accrued to them through the process of divorce and remarriage. The arrival of a new baby to the second marriage couple precipitates a whole new set of covert dynamics, the most prominent of which are bitterness and jealousy on the part of the children from both previous marriages. The children of the first marriages become more aware of what they are missing by not having a team of genetically identified parents; and the triangles of mother, children and stepfather, and father, children and stepmother, are augmented by the reality of the new *biological* triangle.

At the same time, the power of the parent and stepparents is reinforced and often made into a caricature by the four sets of grandparents. The eight people who have psychological and biological connections with the two parents of the second marriage also have biological connections with the ex-spouses. This makes a three-generation salad that resembles the dynamics of the Middle East political arena. However, it should be clear that history is not something that disappears and the fact of social adaptation, psychological maneuvering and compensatory dynamics does not change the underlying dynamics of this United Nations-type war. No parent should tolerate the son-in-law or daughter-in-law who has stolen his or her biological offspring. Therefore, the grandparents live in an atmosphere of bilateral paranoia. The situation is much more complex with divorce and remarriage and it becomes clear how the relationship between the grandparents and the ex-spouses adds to the complexity of the dynamics in the second marriage family.

All of these undercurrent dynamics of the family unconscious are usually fairly well-hidden. Actually, most families live in relative blindness to the facts of this atmosphere and make social adaptations of such complexity and in such multi-colored shadows that, unless one assumes the family as a universal, it would be easy to pretend that everything was peaceful and creative. Even the U.N. building looks peaceful to the people on a *guided tour*.

Parenthetically, it is important to bear in mind that the voltage of the biological unions is always stronger than the voltage of the psychological or social bonding. Metaphorically, the situation has similarities to Jewish people settling on the West Bank or immigrants from Mexico or the Caribbean establishing their families in the United States.

THE SOCIAL FAMILY

It should be clear that the biopsychosocial family and the psychosocial family are two distinct classes, and it doesn't necessitate bifocal glasses to think about the social family as a variant of this process. The most obvious examples are the fraternity house, the football team or the tennis team. Calling this a social family does not weaken the fact that there are psychological dynamics which reinforce the organizational process. The voltage in this type of unit is closer to six volts than to 110 or 220. The establishment of a whole by 11 men or two tennis partners is good evidence that the whole is greater than the sum of its parts and that each individual contributes to and benefits by their union. However, the experience leaves only minor residuals in comparison with divorce in the biological or the psychosocial family unit.

To stay with our metaphor about investment, the principal of the social investment between the acquaintances can be reinvested, and it is assumed that these family or teaming relationships have a definitive ending, jointly agreed upon and available within the social regulations of this situation. It resembles a foster family. The psychosocial marriage includes a war of two sides or four sides, each with allies and each involving psychosocial and economic components. The social family may have negative dynamics but usually it's not a war; it's a cooperative process and a time-limited investment. Although it may be augmented by transference factors from the intimate families of the members, cooperation is the bottom line of this kind of family.

The adoptive child in a biological or psychosocial family is covertly a social relationship. Except for the transference factors, it is temporary and the relationship makes for limited investment because of the tentative and conditional attitude about the future of the relationship. Continuity is not guaranteed. The foster parent and foster children belong in this same social family group, and the same dynamics apply as in the business partnership or the athletic team.

Talking about the factual base for family relationships raises many fascinating metaphorical issues and questions. For example, I assume that marriage is not the union of two people but the contracts of two families, each of whom sends out a scapegoat to reproduce itself. This helps to clarify the covert dynamics of family history, since the battle over whose family is going to be reproduced never ends, even though it may be carefully covered and artfully designed.

THE DYNAMICS OF THE THREE-GENERATION FAMILY

Assuming that all families are covertly and dynamically identical, as are the human psyche and the human body, we can talk about the schema and its distortions. Metaphorically, the family is like a wheel. Mother is the center hub, the core of intimacy. The children represent the spokes connecting mother and father. The father is the rim of the wheel, intermediate be-

tween the intimacy of the family and the realities of the community and the outside world. The family as a multigeneration culture is basically controlled on an unconscious level, carrying massive vectors from past decisions. Control options reflect the total dynamics of the family as a whole expressed through the subgroups of parents and children, males and females, two- and three-generation or more triangles, influenced by genetic, experiential and environmental pressures.

Beginning with the grandparent generation, there is, of course, a covert tribal war. Marriage of the children—the second generation—is, in one sense, a bilateral adoption by the grandparents, with overtones of a psychological affair between the families. The second generation originates many times with the failure of the husband and wife in their divorce from their parents and without the preliminary evolution of personhood by the individuals or the critical puberty ceremony that readies entrance into adulthood. Marriage can then be defined as two 16-year-olds who adopt each other or become symbiotic in order to create one 32-year-old as a way of graduation into adulthood. Marriage can also be thought of as a bilateral, pseudotherapeutic plot. He's just the man for her as soon as she gets his alcoholism straightened out. And she's just the woman for him as soon as he gets her over her compulsiveness. Their contract, covert though it is, establishes a relationship for the years to come. Years ago, in *The Devil's Dictionary*, Ambrose Bierce defined marriage as a community consisting of a master, a mistress and two slaves, making in all two.

Many symbolic complications involved in the marriage are also covert. One of the most powerful is the fact that each partner expects the other to replace mother and the security received from her. The loving investment in each other tends to produce the praxis that makes for a concretization of this phenomenon. There are also present, of course, the oedipal reverberations of the wife fulfilling the husband's fantasy reverberations of his mother romance and the wife's attachment to her husband reflecting her sensual fantasies about her father. It is valuable for a professional therapist to realize the understructures of this kind of bilateral psychological incest and the triangular jealousies that shadow it.

To a lesser degree, the sibling relationships of his childhood and her childhood are also replayed in the experience of the adult marriage. First, the *concretized orgasm* of the first child has many implications—one of these is that the child is the realized projection of the four-year-old girl's fantasy of pregnancy by her father. Second, by covert common agreement, father and mother accept the first child to be symbolically mother's mother, so that this new two-generation family unit will have the security that the mother had in her family of origin. The second child becomes symbolically mother to the father so that he too can have reverberations from his family of origin and the security and freedom to model his new lifestyle.

The arrival of the third child usually coincides with mother's "thought" control of the children by virtue of father being, as Margaret Mead says, a social accident and deeply invested in tools and the reality of the outside world. So, this third child is, by common consent, the father's partner or playmate to prevent him from, at least psychologically, mating with another female, even if she's a tractor or a Ph.D. thesis. To carry on this schema, there is the possibility that the fourth child can be nonsymbolic and less a victim of the family dynamic system.

Parenthetically, the character structure and family role process are massively influenced by the family experience before, during and after the pregnancy, by the death of mother's mother or father's mother, or even by some sudden success or failure in the family's relation to the outside world. These factors can have a great effect on the significance of the baby's arrival. One of the basic distortions

in this second generation is the breakup of the marriage and the development of a second marriage. The amount of investment on each side of the mating changes the dynamics, and the second marriage is reverberating with projections and paranoia and the tendency to repetition compulsion characteristic of all human organization.

The children as individuals and as relationship systems also become reincarnations of past roles: mother's ex-boyfriend, father's ex-girlfriend, a relationship between mother's brothers and sisters and father's brothers and sisters. These are all reflected with great accuracy and with greater or lesser power in the dynamics of this new family lifestyle. The children also carry out counterculture models of the parents' lifestyles, either in terms of social conformity, rebellion, or liaison roles with society or with God—for example, the schizophrenic endeavoring to hold open mother's childhood delusion of virginity or the son stealing cars to prevent father from cheating on the income tax.

THE THERAPIST IS AN OUTSIDER

The initial establishment of the therapeutic relationship entails what sometimes is called *diagnosis* but should be called *the formulation of a therapeutic alliance*. This involves development of a process by which the therapist becomes identified with the pain of the family. His caring for them becomes the anesthesia for confrontation and the alliance that may bring about change. The therapist should lead in this formulation and try to establish within himself a sense of relationship to the family. This process should not be an effort to change the character of any person or even the character of the family. A static diagnostic process, expressed as "Is he depressed?" or "Is she overactive?", becomes a denial of the person and, more important, a denial of the relationships. The best process is to deny all diagnoses of individuals by any member of the family and, even more critically, to deny any individual's effort to characterize himself.

The effort to establish a therapeutic alliance is best brought about by getting *each member of the family to characterize the relationship between two or more significant others not including himself.* This may include, of course, characterizations of dyads or triads, but essentially it is a description of the relationship of the whole and its operation. Fred Ford (Ford & Herrick, 1974) established the idea that some families are "two against the world"; others are "everybody for himself"; and still others are "the children come first." This kind of understanding makes the family alive for him and for the family.

A good example of how graphic this can be is the request for an evaluation of the relationship between the in-laws. Father can say important things about the relationship between his mother-in-law and father-in-law and their family operation. As the therapist listens, he begins to accumulate a set of multiple perceptions of how the family achieves morale and how the subgroup morale is operating. As his perceptions become more established, the therapist can move to assume that all pathology and all relationship variations in any family are characteristically available in every family. This makes it easier to help the family see some of the covert components that are covered by or hidden behind the overt relationships. This generalization, of course, is of the same character as the concept that all individuals have the same kinds of defense systems in varying proportions and in varying combinations.

The therapist may carefully begin to interpret the process as he sees it operating, although he must be careful that his caring, like any anesthesia, precedes the use of confrontation. This parallel play process has more value if it takes place while the therapist talks through one person to another. The infiltration quality is even more useful if the therapist uses himself as a metamodel for reformulating what he's seeing take place within the family's description of itself. It is most valuable if you begin with the individual farthest outside the family, then move to father's father, mother's father, father's mother, mother's mother, father, children and, finally, mother, whose understanding of the intimacy in relationships is more profound and should be protected. It is helpful for the therapist to be wide-ranging and to talk way-out. He can assume universal paranoia and universal identification. Having presented his infiltrative ideas, the therapist can deny their validity and share his doubts about all wisdom or insightfulness. He can open the relationship even further by sharing some of his own pathology or suspicions of himself.

This freedom to flip into the patient role helps the therapist break down his own delusional grandeur and sets the pattern for the family to expose itself. It may help the family break its delusion that there is a magician somewhere who can fix everything. It is valuable for the therapist to share his anxiety and to use his sense of absurdity. The family, thereby, gets an awareness that reality is a multifaceted projection of the therapist, his world, and his experience. The family's world becomes merely a backdrop or another variant of the human condition. The therapist should share fragments of his own past history in a free associative manner, even if it has no relevance to the issue at hand. It is, however, important to limit and/or deny any bridge between the family and the therapist's current personal life. Members of his family have the right to their anonymity. The therapist's free association is his privilege and his family's right to privacy should be respected.

It is important to maintain the therapist's conviction that each appointment is both the first interview and the last interview. The first interview is, in essence, a blind date; and every subsequent interview opens the possibility of divorce or at least the separation between the family as foster child and the therapist as foster parent.

It is critical also for the therapist to be clear in his own belief system so that he separates the talking about, or the microcosm of psychotherapy, and the family's unique and multigenerational lifestyle and belief system. The therapeutic job is to help family members struggle with their yen to change their own lifestyle while maintaining the sacredness of family nationalism. The family lifestyle and family pattern are not up for reorganization except by them. The therapist should protect their right to secrecy and reinforce for them the fact that their living is beyond anyone's seeing or knowing and certainly beyond any verbalization.

Family change is a long-term, mostly unknowable and unexposed process in living. Portraits, caricatures, dreams and horrors are the jewels that enrich it. The voltage change of the therapy may, at the time or in later times, help deprogram and set the stage for gradual reprogramming of the family as an organism. Ninety percent of the family's dynamics should stay unknowable. It may be, however, that the evolution of the joint therapeutic dream will, at moments during and subsequent to the therapy, help to alter the family's lifestyle into a more satisfactory evolution.

Parenthetically, it is important for the therapist to be aware of and frightened of his own temptation to become a peeping tom. This belongs to his personal lifestyle and is best restricted to adult bookstores, X-rated movies, and his own psychotherapy. He may neutralize some of this by helping the family learn how to peep at him. The therapist needs to be aware and protect himself from teaming with subgroups in the family. He must be careful to protect the sacredness of the family as a whole, even though they may try to resolve some of the stress by fragmenting, increasing the entanglement or distorting the family's wholeness by phobic and protective acting out or acting in. All the dynamics of the individuals described by researchers are also present in family dynamics, except with much superior coloration based on the alliances and exposed by the cold-war qualities of the family itself and its subgroup.

It is valuable to recognize that the extended family is the United Nations within which the family deals in the politics of the in-law struggle. As previously mentioned, we find here the quaint process of the two or more older generations sending out one of their children as the family scapegoat to marry and reproduce their kind. Here begins the struggle of whose family will be reproduced in the child.

The therapist in a quaint way is the president of the United Nations, elected for a brief time with little power; his personhood is his only strength. Identification with the family is his gavel. It is critical that the therapist stay aware that his own introject is the family he's dealing with, not the one in front of him, and that his capacity to care is the anesthesia for confrontation. Thirdly, he must endlessly struggle with the movement into the family and the critically important movement out of the family. He thus models for the family members and subgroups an increasing freedom to separate, which then creates an increasing freedom to belong more intimately.

THE THERAPIST VIS-À-VIS THE FAMILY SYSTEM

The application of beliefs and the understandings of the family dynamics in a therapeutic process are essentially centered around the therapist's belief system. His capacity as an individual and his capacity to team with a cotherapist make the process of therapy one system operating on another system rather than a subsystem trying to alter a system farther up the hierarchy. His belief system consists of the *known components*, those things which he's aware of, the *knowable components*, those things which he has become aware of with experience and evaluation, and the *unknowable*, those parts of the belief system which are beyond intellectual understanding. Secondary factors in his personhood and his belief system are the rational component (either intellectual and technical or political) and the irrational (those components that are a covert part of his experience, his evaluation and his symbolization of that experience). They also include the cultural and personal delusional components in his own living process, whether they are systematized or nonsystematized and whether they belong in the typical four stylistic character patterns of paranoid, simple, catatonic or hebephrenic.

Components in the interaction of his personhood and the family system are the context of their meeting, their motivation and the interlocking of their two lifetime experiences. The therapist's operational adequacy is the result of his own integration and his own growth, his freedom to expand the belongingness of his family of origin and his nuclear family. They result in the dialectic balance between belonging and individuating. Professional application of this dialectical balance between individuating and belonging we call *the therapeutic alliance*, resting on the freedom of the therapist to separate his functional role from his personal living.

THE THERAPIST'S RESPONSE TO THE TRAPS AND MAZES OF THE THERAPEUTIC PROCESS

It is important to list the traps that threaten the therapeutic process. The most obvious ones are the tales of the past, the pain of the present, the phobia of the future, the fun of seduction and the myth of magic. The mazes include the game of rude excavation, the excitement of identification, the replay of the therapist's own therapy, the therapist's escape from his own reality, the construction of a joint delusional system and the temptation to a lifetime symbiosis.

A series of therapeutic moves is possible; although these moves are not technical, they may be lifesaving. The most critical is the process of joining, individuating, rejoining and reseparating from the therapeutic alliance. It is valuable to change roles within the transference projections by way of open boredom, therapeutic manipulation of the transference or explosive denial of it. It is possible also to fragment the family's projections and fantasies by direct invasion of their covert inferences and a parallel play in the therapist's own fantasy world. The therapist can share the "shards" of his own pathology. Bits and pieces of those residual patient components make the family's experience less a self-exposure and more a participant experience.

The therapist should make deliberate efforts to deny the presumed projections by the family—whether they are true or not is not important. It is useful to steal the patient role and force the context in which the family becomes the therapist and the therapist becomes the patient. These efforts make for less stress and more freedom to negotiate change.

It is also valuable for the therapist to invoke the consultant and thus widen the generation gap. This may be done either in the context of the cotherapy setting or with a deliberate introduction of another person into the therapeutic interview.

There is also value for the therapist to expose his impotence. The family needs to be *endlessly made aware of* its own power and of its capacity to destroy the therapeutic process. Finally, the therapist needs to make endless efforts to accumulate evidence of the need to end the relationship so that therapy is seen as a time-bound alliance which can only succeed by failing.

REFERENCE

Ford, F. & Herrick, J. (1974, January). Family rules—family lifestyle. *Amer. Jnl. Orthopsych. 44*, 1.

Discussion by Albert Ellis, Ph.D.

━━━━━━━━━◆━━━━━━━━━

Let me comment first of all on the notable points of agreement that I have with Carl's paper and presentation. Carl and I have been differing for the last 30 years or so, but we do see eye to eye on a good many things and he nicely brought out some of them.

First of all, he said, to my gratification, that everybody has a belief system. Of course, that is one of the things I have been beating the drums for during the last 30 years or so. I am glad he finally got around to acknowledging the belief system. I want to add that not only does everybody have a belief system, including therapists, which I think he really meant too, but also that is why therapy works, no matter what kind of therapist you are. What you do or what you say to the client is just one of the things that help the client create basic personality change. Really, it is their belief in what you do or say. If you did or said the same thing and they had a different belief and you didn't induce them somehow to change their belief, then you could be the best therapist in the world and it wouldn't work. Similarly, you might be the worst therapist and it would still work because of the clients' beliefs in some of the things you say.

Carl then said that you are an instrument of change. I would heartily agree with that. You bring yourself, your personality and your ideas and theories of psychotherapy, not to mention the practice, into what goes on and therefore you are an instrument of change. I would add, as I am not sure he clearly added, that the clients are the changers. You do not really change them. You help families or individuals or groups change, but they really change themselves and you are an instrument in helping them.

Then Carl said the therapist had better

have enough strength so that the clients, the families, can trust him or her. That is correct. Recent research has shown that one of the main ways therapists build rapport is not simply by being warm and responsive to their clients, as Carl Rogers has said for many many years, but also by showing clients that they, the therapists, do have strength and confidence in their own ways of acting and feeling and teaching. They show clients confidence in themselves and that is frequently taken by clients, and by the families if the family is the client, as assuring them that they can trust, or at least believe they can trust, their therapist.

That goes back to belief again. Then Carl talks about the family unconscious. I don't like the word "unconscious"; I usually use the word "implicit." Since we have so many implicit ideas, implicit feelings, and implicit behaviors, we in RET (rational-emotive therapy) are easily conscious of most of them if we look for them as we teach. They are not deeply hidden in any unconscious. They can be brought up fairly easily. They are part of the implicit ways of thinking and behaving and feeling which the family has. They bring to the situation, just as they brought to their original family situation, ways of being, especially ways of philosophizing. Some people call it "inferring," and we had better be in touch with how clients infer and how they can change their self-defeating, and sometimes unconscious, inferences.

Carl also said that clients are human. I would agree that clients are human and not werewolves, or anything like that. Even families are human. Sometimes they seem a little off, to say the least. But I would say the individual, too, in the family is what we forget about; all individuals in families are humans and live as fallible mortals. They are individuals and they are all different, but in terms of their humanity they have some surprising likenesses. If we didn't realize that and have some glimmering of what those likenesses were, we would waste time for years in any therapeutic situation and get nowhere.

We therapists have theories and ideas and sometimes a few facts about the human condition that are brought to any family and any therapeutic situation. By having those ideas, we are able to zero in much more effectively and efficiently than if we just considered every person in individual therapy or every family in family therapy as different. They are different but they are also the same.

I very much like Carl's term *bio-psycho-social-family*. I like it particularly since so many therapists, especially family therapists but others too, ignore the biological elements. We are all reared in many different ways, but basically we are human and have a lot of similarities and a lot of *tendencies*—not innate ideas, nor behaviors, nor even feelings, but strong biological *tendencies*—which we *bring* to any family because we are biosocial animals. A great deal of what we do to upset ourselves is prejudiced by biological conditions. Don't forget that biologically we are humans, all of us, and we are biological in regard to our bodily processes—in the way we think, in our neurotransmitters, and in everything about us. Unless we get to some of those biological aspects and at least consider how they affect us and our therapies, we are not going to really understand what is going on and we are going to assume, which is the old psychoanalytic hypothesis, that practically everything is the result of environment and forget the pronounced biophysical and psychological and social, or biosocial, tendencies that we bring to situations.

Carl said that family members do psychotherapy with each other all the time. I think it a very important concept that psychotherapy doesn't just consist of a therapist and his or her clients. That is formal psychotherapy. Psychotherapy is done by people all the time in their own social groups, in their families, with each other, and within their own heads. Consequently, we had better face the fact that family members are continually indoctrinating each other, influencing each other, helping each other, and, yes, hindering each other—often doing poor psychotherapy, we might say. We had better see that this is going on. In RET family treatment especially, as well as in RET individual treatment, we try to show individuals how to be more effective therapists to each other—not just to themselves but to each other—to learn about some of the fundamental disturbances that all of us tend to have, and also to learn how to deal with these disturbances. We try to help clients see precisely what they are doing at any one moment to upset themselves—and not to merely assume that *others* upset them. We try to teach them in the therapy sessions to remind each other of RET principles when they are participating in their own family life and help them to use these principles of therapy to become more efficient therapists to themselves and, preferably, also to those with whom they intimately live.

Carl said, rightly I thought, that we should not get too invested in the process of therapy as a therapist. He described some of his own unique techniques. I am not sure I would use that much myself but I would say, yes, keep from getting too invested by facing the fact that you are a person in this family therapeutic situation and you do have your own biases and prejudices, your own belief system. Consequently, you had better stop at least every once in awhile to ask yourself why you are doing this, why you are trying to get over this concept or teach them this skill or this behavior. The answer frequently is, "Because of my own hang-ups I bring to the situation, I had better watch that and be invested, but not overinvested." I think a good therapist can be involved but not overinvested. Not overinvolved.

Carl also said that you as a therapist had better draw a line between being a therapist and the client's family and social living. Again, I would say yes, you are working with the family in order to help them in their lives, not in your life, and you had better watch your own ego processes and bigotries which you may bring to the therapeutic sessions.

Carl said that anything that is worth knowing can be taught. That goes with another corollary—that anything you believe can be disbelieved if you work at it. If you really want to know something and will work at it as a therapist and as a client, normally you can teach it to yourself or can understand it and use it. Therefore, as a therapist you had better be interested in self-teaching as well as teaching others. My prejudiced view is that therapy is still largely not only relating and being yourself, which have their great advantages, but knowing a little more about family dynamics and family and individual treatment than the clients know.

Now, as might be expected, I have a few disagreements with Carl, so let me just briefly go through those.

One, he said that single parents are insane, if I heard him correctly, which sounds like a fairly nutty statement. Two, Carl is a pioneer, along with John Warkenton, in multiple therapy, which has its great advantages. However, it is expensive and takes time and very few clients are really able to support it, except maybe in a research setting. Three, Carl also said that the language of the therapist is the language of inference. That is partly true, but the language of the client is also very largely the language of inference. The therapist had better make the client's, as well as his or her own, inferences clear and show clients how they very frequently are making inferences which don't follow from the data and are upsetting themselves by these inferences.

Four, Carl said that he had never treated an Italian family without an Italian cotherapist. You could run this into the ground because it follows that he would never see a Jewish family without a Jewish cotherapist, and he would never see any kind of a family without cotherapists

who were raised in that family's ethnic setting. Of course, there is a great advantage to knowing the standards of the family. These are very frequently ethnic or regional and community differences, and unless you know something about the ethnicity and the region, you are not going to understand those standards too well. Yet the standards are often not that important. We would teach in rational-emotive therapy that people get upset not because of the nutty standards they have or because they get taught by their families and communities, but because they take any standard and have, I would hypothesize, an innate tendency to escalate it into a demand.

The illustration I usually give is that of American boys who are taught to be interested in football and baseball and British boys who are taught to be interested in cricket. In both places, as well as all over the world, they take as their standard, "Let us do well at this sport in our country at this time." This is a good idea because they will play the game better and thereby obtain advantages. Then they say, "Because it is preferable to play cricket well or baseball well, therefore I *have* to, therefore I *must*." And the musts and the shoulds and the oughts—the tyranny of the shoulds, as Karen Horney said years ago—are not learned. They are innate. Humans are frequently out of their heads and will bring absolutistic musts, shoulds and oughts to any standard that they are taught.

Therefore, I can see Italians very nicely without a cotherapist and I can see Eskimos or whomever without a cotherapist because whatever their original standard, this is not my standard, I was not raised with it. It would be nicer if I understood theirs more fully. But I can practically guarantee their often escalating it into a demand, an autocratic and dogmatic *must*. And if I zero in on their musts about the standard, then I can accept their standards, whatever they are. I can show them not how to change the standards, but how to keep their standards, values, goals, and interests while giving up their whining and screaming that these standards *must* definitely be fulfilled. That is their craziness.

Five, Carl said we should be clear about the process and not get confused about the results. That's a very nice understanding of process, but you had better understand the results and check on them and do research as to which process leads to which results. This will certainly help you as a therapist and particularly help the client, we hope. The only criteria of successful psychotherapy, he says, is if you enjoy the hour. Well, that is a quaint view! It may be true, but as a hopeful scientist I would say "Let's test that hypothesis." We can study 100 therapists who have a great time during the therapy hour and 100 therapists who sweat and strain and do not have a great time. Then we can see if the first group gets better results than the second. I am entirely skeptical!

So these are some of the main agreements and disagreements, but I particularly like the fact that Carl was truly comprehensive. He covered all the major aspects of the biological, as well as of the psychological and the social, which interact with the biological. They all interact with each other, and his viewpoint is truly a comprehensive one. He gives us a lot to think about.

QUESTIONS AND ANSWERS

Question: Could you discuss the violent family and whether the danger of injury alters your concept in any way?

Whitaker: That is a great question. One of the problems of being a psychotherapist is this character structure which makes us play the fool. Let me give you an example. Some years ago they started a marital court in Madison (Wisconsin) and every new divorce case had to be interviewed by a therapist. About six or eight weeks later I began to get these social workers in for psychotherapy because they were

being destroyed. Thay sat there six or seven hours a day with two people hating each other and they tried to help. Yet the solution was so simple. If you are working for the judge and you are doing an examination, don't try to be the therapist. You say to the couple, "Look, I am hired by the judge. Don't say anything to me that you don't want reported to him. I have an hour to see you to find out whether you really want to get a divorce or whether you are trying to play games with each other in order to get to a therapist. I am not your therapist. I will only be seeing you for one hour. If you want a therapist, I will be glad to give you some names. We have an official list." And then you go ahead with the interview. In separating the function of being a therapeutically trained detective from the function of being a therapist, a helper, their symptoms disappeared. They didn't lie awake at night worrying about what they should have done and never would do again.

I think the same is true here. If you are dealing with a violent family, you ought to find out and decide before you start if you are going to be an enforcement agent for the police or a loving mother who is trying to help. It is very difficult to be both. If you are in the middle of the interview and violence takes place, the solution is very simple: Just walk out. Say, "Call me when you guys are through with the war. I am not your Supermama. I am just a professional therapist and if you want to have a bedroom fight, I will be glad to leave so you can have it, or you can go home and have it there." If you are in danger, don't try to be a therapist at all. My karate teacher told me that if you are accosted by a patient with a gun, there is no karate answer. Run like hell. I think we need to be very careful that our delusion system doesn't make us assume we are Superman. We aren't. We are like anybody else.

Question: Dr. Whitaker, you said that to be a single parent is insane. What would you recommend for those people who are?

Whitaker: That you find somebody to team with. Another single parent with her kids, your mother, your mother-in-law. Your boyfriend to whom you are trying to make clear that there are two systems—that you belong to an older generation system and the children belong to their generation. I think this is the inference that Ellis was talking about—the inference of a mother and child living together is that neither one is where she belongs. The mother is a 24-hour babysitter and the daughter is a 24-hour partner. Neither one knows if she is adult or child and it becomes like an A.A. Milne story about the "halfway up the stair. It isn't in the nursery and isn't in the town, but sometimes my head goes round and round and I don't know what I am."

The mysterious thing to me is that single parents don't find someone to team with. Divorce that stops the marital problem is not the same thing as stopping the parental problem. Parents are forever. What I do as a therapist to protect myself is to fight like hell to keep from being "the new man" in somebody else's life.

Question: Dr. Ellis, we live in a world that is not always rational, particularly in discussing the family but also in individual counseling. If a family is invested in irrational beliefs, how do you intervene with rational ones?

Ellis: That would take the whole history of rational-emotive therapy to answer, but I will answer it briefly. The family is normally invested with two kinds of irrational beliefs. One might be irrational standards that they have. For example, they believe that because the people in their culture should never get a divorce, they are not allowed to do so. Therefore, they adopt the standard of the culture. This might be OK for most people most of the time, but they may rigidly stick to that standard. Therefore, a therapist might question whether that standard is right for them or whether they hold it too rigidly.

Another standard in our culture is that you only marry when you are romantically in love, instead of first hopefully being in love but also assessing the values and the companionship and the other aspects of marriage that frequently go with a good marriage. As I frequently tell my clients, you had better not marry anybody you don't love, but you had also better not marry everybody you do love! Consequently, that standard of romantic love is one that I take a skeptical view of. That old Hollywood standard that you marry the one you are madly in love with and live happily ever after is decreasing today. So you can dispute, question, challenge, inquire into those standards and ask if they are good for this individual at this particular time in this family or in this nonfamily about to be a family.

Another standard that I hypothesize that practically all humans have in every kind of family and all over the world—both individually about themselves and about what should happen when they are married and in a family—is that they *have to* achieve their goals no matter what these are. They feel that they *must* do well or that others know and *must* treat them nobly and kindly, especially when they are married to them. They believe that conditions, including family and apartment and monetary conditions, *must* be easy, and it is horrible when they are not. Almost all humans, especially those in families, have some of those *shoulds* and *oughts* and *musts* and in RET we would very frequently say to them, "Let's assume that it is desirable that you do well and be approved by other members of your family, that it is highly desirable that your family members and others treat you kindly and considerately and that conditions be easier than they are in terms of health factors and money and environmental conditions. Why do they *have* to be? Why *must* you get what you want?" And we show them cognitively by using the scientific method which says, "Prove it. Where is the evidence? Tell me." And we get them to work emotively on their negative views, especially the feelings of hate, rage, and vindictiveness which ruin innumerable family relationships, and show them how to work behaviorally on their dysfunctional behaviors, their goofings, avoidances, procrastinations, or compulsions, such as addiction to alcohol. We get them to work on these and to dispute their negative ideas in all these basic ways. We don't always succeed but at least we try.

Whitaker: Let me give you an example of the language of inference. The speaker asked what to do *if* you see an irrational family. I have never in my life seen a family that wasn't irrational.

Question: I would like to follow up on the first question. In California we have a compulsory reporting law for child abuse. I often find myself in the position where I am counseling with the mother and father and there is abuse of a young infant. I am required by law to report any instances of child abuse. As soon as I do that, I destroy my counseling relationship with that family. Do you have any advice in that area?

Whitaker: There are two obvious tricks. One is to find out before you start and tell them to go report to the police first, after which you will be glad to see them. The other one is, if you find abuse, to say you are now through being their therapist and tell them, "You will have to go find another therapist because I have to report you. I am going to double-cross you here and now because of the law."

Question: I would like to ask all of the panel members if they would comment on how you use self-disclosure in your therapy. How and when do you make that decision to use self-disclosure?

Ellis: You use it very cautiously. You don't indulge in it and tell them everything about your life that you would enjoy telling them, even when they ask you direct questions.

When I was a psychoanalyst many years ago, patients would ask: "Are you married?", "How many women do you go to bed with a week?" or something like that. And I would use the old psychoanalytic ploy of replying, "Why are you asking that question?" That gets me off the hook. However, now I normally answer. I don't fill in all the gory details and go on at length. I know, since I am presumably a therapist, that certain people under certain conditions would traumatize themselves by certain of my answers. I do reveal much more than most therapists because I don't care what my clients think of me. I am presumably rational, so I watch my disclosures and don't reveal everything all of the time.

Satir: When we were children, we hardly were ever able to ask the questions we needed to ask. Therefore, when developing a treatment context, people will ask questions. Sometimes this is in the interest of getting an experience they didn't have when they were children. On another level, I may, myself, present some experience of my own which indicates some different way of coping with something or a way of understanding some things. Often I use my personal examples in a funny way when I want to reduce some kind of anxiety but at the same time I have clients take a fresh look at something that seems so weighty. That is a good way to do it for me.

Whitaker: I am very excited about my participating in the therapeutic process and I frequently tell clients, "You know, I am not doing this because I am trying to help you. I am really trying to grow myself, so you should be suspicious of everything I say." But I think that what Ellis said is very critical. Don't cut your own throat. Patients are not bound by confidentiality. Whatever you say in that interview is public information and you had better stay aware of that. Within the limits of that kind of clinical judgment, I think you ought to respect your free associations, your impulses, your fantasies, but be very suspicious of them. If you don't protect yourself, you can expose fragments of yourself.

I think the reason Freud was so concerned about this is that he didn't have a very good therapist. If you have a good therapist, I don't think you are going to get into the problem he was concerned with—that if you expose yourself, you become the patient. I think that is the problem. You can share yourself without becoming the patient, but if you parentify the patient as some mothers and fathers parentify the child, you ought to get some help from a therapist or work with a cotherapist.

Let me go back to the business of a cotherapist because Ellis raised this subject and the question of money. I think it was very important and fortunate for me that I was in a setting where I could have full-time cotherapists. However, you need not have them full time. In fact, you don't even have to have a real one, although a real one for ten minutes at the beginning of the second interview is critically important. You can do like the couple I know up in the wilds of Minnesota. If things get tough, he buzzes the secretary and asks will you get Minuchin on the phone for me (he never calls Whitaker). She buzzes back and he says, "Sal, this is Joe. Let me tell you about this. Do you have a minute?" No answer, of course, because there is nobody on. "Now let me tell you about this family. I have seen them five times and the father is a typical cold fish and the mother is a typical real sucker for her kids and, I guess, for her husband. I don't know what to do. I don't think I am getting any place. What did you say? I shouldn't see them? For three months? Hey, look, Sal, these are nice guys. It is a very nice family. You really mean it? You didn't have a fight with your wife,

Pat? You are really talking about this case? What do I do after three months, Sal? I can see them twice more and then I should call you again? You know you get awful mean sometimes. You think it is the way I should treat the family. Well, thanks, I guess, OK, OK."

So he has had this consultant for years and he says to the family, "Well, Sal says I should not see you for three months and then I can see you twice more and then call him. I think probably that is the best thing to do. I hope we can make it." You can always pull that, you know, if you have a secretary. You don't have to have a cotherapist full time. You just need to make it clear to the people you are seeing that you are not a single parent, you don't belong to them, you belong to another generation and have a world that they aren't a part of, that they can look at but not be captured by it.

E. Polster: Just one more word about self-disclosure. I agree with what has been said about being careful about what one says. I usually answer questions because I can't think well enough to decide whether to do it, so I just answer questions, but I won't answer things I don't want to answer. But another aspect of disclosure is what you would contribute yourself in terms of some experience that would show the person the recognition of your own realization that what they are doing is also a part of your life. I think it makes for a common bond. Another thing that used to happen is that people would say, "This is not a fair relationship. I do all the talking about myself and you don't say anything about yourself." On the few occasions when I took them seriously and started talking about myself, I discovered very quickly that that is not what they were interested in.

"If You Desire to See, Learn How to Act"

Paul Watzlawick, Ph.D.

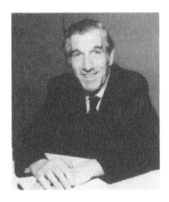

Paul Watzlawick, Ph.D.
Paul Watzlawick received his Ph.D. from the University of Venice in 1949. He has an Analyst's Diploma from the C.G. Jung Institute for Analytic Psychology in Zurich.

Watzlawick has practiced psychotherapy for more than 30 years. Currently, he is research associate and principal investigator at the Mental Research Institute. He is Clinical Professor at the Department of Psychiatry and Behavioral Sciences, Stanford University Medical Center.

Watzlawick is a noted family therapist; he is recipient of the Distinguished Achievement Award from the American Family Therapy Association. Also, he is the author, co-author or editor of eight books on the topics of interactional psychotherapy, human communication and constructivist philosophy.

Ever erudite, charming and incisive, Watzlawick argues against simplistic "linear causality." Circular causality can be applied to human systems to promote effective change.

This title is borrowed from an essay by the famous cybernetician, Heinz von Foerster. He calls it his *Aesthetic Imperative*. Although postulated in a different context (von Foerster, 1973), it nevertheless expresses what I consider an important aspect of the evolution of therapy. (The omission of the prefix *psycho-* before the word *therapy* is no slip, which I hope to be able to explain in the course of my presentation.)

I do not know how exactly the inverse of von Foerster's Imperative—the idea that in order to *act* differently, one must first learn to *see* the world differently—arose and acquired dogmatic dominance in our field. For as different and even as contradictory as the classic schools and philosophies of psychotherapy are among themselves, one of the assumptions they firmly share is that the understanding of the origin and the evolution of a problem in the past is the precondition for its solution in the present. Undoubtedly, *one* compelling reason for this perspective is that it is embedded in the model of *linear* scientific thought and inquiry, a model that must be credited with the vertiginous progress of science during the last 300 years.

Until the middle of our century, relatively few people questioned the supposedly final validity of a scientific worldview based on strictly deterministic, linear

91

causality. Freud, for instance, saw no reason to doubt it. "At least in the older and more mature sciences, there is even today a solid ground work which is only modified and improved, but no longer demolished" (Freud, 1964). This statement is of more than historic interest. Seen from the vantage point of the year 1985, it makes us aware of the evanescence of scientific paradigms—whether we have read Kuhn (1970) or not.

One would naïvely believe that the history of the twentieth century alone should leave no doubt about the horrifying consequences produced by the illusion of having found the ultimate truth and, therefore, the final solution. But the evolution of our field—since it usually is 30 years in arrears—has not quite arrived at this realization. Endless hours of "scientific" debates and tens of thousands of pages in books and scientific journals are still wasted in order to show that since my way of seeing reality is the right and true one, anybody who sees it differently is necessarily wrong. A good example of this fallacy is Edward Glover's book, *Freud or Jung?* (1956), in which this eminent author employs approximately 200 pages to say what could be said in one sentence, namely, that Jung was wrong because he did not agree with Freud. This, incidentally, is what Glover finally does himself on page 190 when he states, "As we have seen, the most consistent trend of Jungian psychology is its negation of every important aspect of Freudian theory." Clearly, to write such a book would have to be considered a waste of time, unless the author and his readers are convinced that their view is right and any other view *therefore* is wrong.

There is something else that our professional evolution no longer lets us disregard. The dogmatic assumption that the discovery of the real causes of the present problem is a *conditio sine qua non* for change creates what the philosopher Karl Popper has called a self-sealing proposition; that is, a hypothesis is validated both by its success and its failure and thus becomes unfalsifiable. In practical terms, if a patient improves as a result of what in classical theory is called *insight*, this obviously proves the correctness of the hypothesis about the need to lift forgotten, repressed causes into consciousness. If the patient does not improve, this *proves* that the search for these causes has not yet proceeded deep enough into the past. The hypothesis wins either way.

A related consequence of the belief in possessing the ultimate truth is the ease with which the believer can dismiss any evidence to the contrary. The mechanism involved here is well known to philosophers of science, but usually not to clinicians. A good example is the review of a book dealing with the behavior therapy of phobias. It culminates in the reviewer's statement that the author defines phobias "in a way that is acceptable only to conditioning theorists and does not fulfill the criteria of the psychiatric definition of this disorder. Therefore, his statements should not apply to phobias, but to some other condition" (Salzman, 1968, p. 476). The conclusion is inescapable: A phobia that improves as result of behavior therapy is *for this reason* no phobia. One gets the impression that it sometimes seems more important to save the theory rather than the patient, and one is reminded of Hegel's dictum: If the facts don't comply with the theory, so much the worse for the facts. (Hegel was probably far too great a mind to have meant this in any other than a facetious sense. But I may be wrong. Hegelian Marxism certainly means it dead seriously—and, again, the word *dead* is not to be taken as a mere slip of the tongue.)

Finally, we can no longer afford to remain blind toward yet another *epistemological error*, as Gregory Bateson might have called it. Only too often we find that the limitations inherent in a given *hypothesis* are attributed to the *phenomena* which that hypothesis is supposed to elucidate. For instance, within the framework of psychodynamic theory, symptom removal must necessarily lead to symptom substitution and exacerbation—not be-cause this complication is in some sense inherent in the nature of the human *mind,* but because it imposes itself logically and necessarily from the premises of that *theory.*

In the midst of such complicated thoughts, don't we all occasionally have a disconcerting fantasy: If that little green man from Mars arrived and asked us to explain our techniques for affecting human change, and if we then told him, would he not scratch his head (or its equivalent) in disbelief and ask us why we have arrived at such complicated, ab-struse and far-fetched theories, rather than first of all investigating how human change comes about naturally, spontaneously, and on an everyday basis? I, for one, would try to point out to him that there have been at least some historic forerunners of that eminently reasonable and practical idea which Heinz von Foerster so well summarized in his Aesthetic Imperative.

One of them is Franz Alexander to whom we owe the important concept of the *corrective emotional experience.* He explains (Alexander & French, 1946, p. 22):

It is not necessary—nor is it possible—during the course of treatment to recall *every* feeling that has been repressed. Therapeutic results can be achieved without the patient's recalling all important details of his past history; indeed, good therapeutic results have come in cases in which not a single forgotten memory has been brought to the surface. Ferenczi and Rank were among the first to recognize this principle and apply it to therapy. However, the early belief that the patient "suffers from memories" has so deeply penetrated the minds of the analysts that even today it is difficult for many to rec-ognize that the patient is suffering not so much from his memories as from his incapacity to deal with his actual problems of the moment. The past events have of course prepared the way for his present difficulties, but then every person's reactions are dependent upon behavior patterns formed in the past.

And a little further on he states that

"this new corrective experience may be supplied by the transference relationship, by new experiences in life, or by both" (Alexander & French, 1946, p. 22). While Alexander attributes a far greater impor-tance to a patient's experiences in the transference situation (because these are not chance events but are provided by the analyst's refusal to let himself be forced into a parental role), he is quite aware also to what extent the outside world may provide just such random events that will affect profound and lasting change. In fact, in his *Psychoanalysis and Psychotherapy* (Alexander, 1956, p. 92), he mentions spe-cifically that "such intensive revelatory emotional experiences give us the clue for those puzzling therapeutic results which are obtained in a considerably shorter time than is usual in psychoanalysis."

In this connection, Alexander (Alex-ander & French, 1946, pp. 68-70) refers to Victor Hugo's famous story of Jean Valjean in *Les Misérables.* Valjean is a violent criminal who, upon his release from a long jail sentence which brutalized him even more, is caught stealing the bish-opric's silver. He is brought before the bishop; but instead of calling him a thief, the bishop asks him very kindly why he left behind the two silver chandeliers that were part of the bishop's gift to him. This kindness totally upsets Valjean's world-view. In the mental imbalance produced by the bishop's reframing of the situation, Valjean meets a little boy, Gervais, who is playing with his coins and drops a 40-*sous* piece. Valjean puts his foot on the coin and refuses to let Gervais have it back. The boy cries, desperately pleads for his money, and eventually runs away. Only then does it dawn on Valjean how hideously cruel his behavior—which only an hour earlier would have been a matter of course for him—now appears in the light of the bishop's kindness towards him. He runs after Petit-Gervais but cannot find him.

Victor Hugo explains,

He felt indistinctly that the priest's forgiveness

was the most formidable assault by which he had yet been shaken; that his hardening would be permanent if he resisted this clemency; that if he yielded he must renounce that hatred with which the actions of other men had filled his soul during so many years, and which pleased him: that this time he must either conquer or be vanquished; and that the struggle, a colossal and final struggle, had begun between his wickedness and that man's goodness. One thing which he did not suspect is certain, however, that he was no longer the same man; all was changed in him, and it was no longer in his power to get rid of the fact that the bishop had spoken to him and taken his hand.

We must bear in mind that *Les Misérables* was written in 1862, half a century before the advent of psychoanalytic theory, and that it would be a bit preposterous to assume that the bishop was simply an early-day analyst. Rather, what Hugo shows is the timeless human experience of profound change arising out of an unexpected and unexpectable action by somebody.

I do not know whether another eminent psychiatrist and author, Michael Balint, has explicitly incorporated Franz Alexander's concept of the corrective emotional experience into his own work. However, in his book, *The Basic Fault* (1968, pp. 128–129), he mentions the classic somersault incident which provides an excellent illustration of such an experience. He was working with a patient, "an attractive, vivacious, rather flirtatious girl in her late 20s, whose main complaint was an inability to achieve anything." This was due, in part, to her "crippling fear of uncertainty whenever she had to take any risk, that is, take a decision." Balint describes how after two years of psychoanalytic treatment

... she was given the interpretation that apparently the most important thing for her was to keep her head safely up, with both feet firmly planted on the ground. In response, she mentioned that ever since her earliest childhood she could never do a somersault; although

at various periods she tried desperately to do one. I then said: 'What about it now?'—whereupon she got up from the couch and, to her great amazement, did a perfect somersault without any difficulty.

This proved to be a real breakthrough. Many changes followed, in her emotional, social, and professional life, all towards greater freedom and elasticity. Moreover, she managed to get permission to sit for, and passed, a most difficult postgraduate professional examination, became engaged, and was married.

Balint then proceeds to use almost two pages to prove that this remarkable, immediate change was, after all, not in contradiction to object-relations theory. "I wish to emphasize" he concludes, "that *the satisfaction did not replace interpretation, it was in addition to it*" (p. 134).

The first comprehensive shift in the evolution of our understanding of human change occurred in 1937, when Jean Piaget published his seminal work *La construction du réel chez l'enfant,* which became available in English in 1954 under the title *The Construction of Reality in the Child.* Here, Piaget proves on the basis of painstaking observations that the child literally *constructs* his reality by exploratory *actions*, rather than first forming an image of the world through his perceptions and *then* beginning to act accordingly. Only a few passages from his enormously detailed study can be quoted here to support this contention. In what Piaget calls the third stage of the development of object concepts, between three and six months of age, "the child begins to grasp what he sees, to bring before his eyes the objects he touches, in short to coordinate his visual universe with the tactile universe" (Piaget, 1954, p. 13). Later, in the same chapter, Piaget states that these actions lead to a greater degree of assumed object permanence (p. 41).

A greater degree of permanence is attributed to vanished images, since the child expects to find them again not only in the very place where they were left but also in places within the extension of their trajectory (reaction to falling, interrupted prehension, etc.). But in comparing this stage to the following ones we prove that this permanence remains exclusively connected with the action in progress and does not yet imply the idea of a substantial permanence independent of the organism's sphere of activity. All that the child assumes is that in continuing to turn his head or to lower it he will see a certain image which has just disappeared, that in lowering his hand he will again find the tactile impression experienced shortly before, etc.

And again, a little further on (pp. 42–43),

In effect, at this stage the child does not know the mechanism of his own actions, and hence does not dissociate them from the things themselves; he knows only their total and undifferentiated schema (which we have called the schema of assimilation) comprising in a single act the data of external perception as well as the internal impressions that are affective and kinesthetic, etc., in nature.

... The child's universe is still only a totality of pictures emerging from nothingness at the moment of the action, to return to nothingness at the moment when the action is finished. There is added to it only the circumstance that the images subsist longer than before, because the child tries to make these actions last longer than in the past; in extending them either he rediscovers the vanished images or else he supposes them to be at disposal in the very situation in which the act in progress began.

The importance of Piaget's findings for our work can hardly be overrated. In the gradual unfolding of his research results, Piaget shows how not only the idea of a world "out there," independent of oneself, is the outcome of exploratory *actions,* but also the development of such basic concepts as causality, time, and eventually, as he calls it, *the elaboration of the universe.* If this be so, then, obviously, different actions may lead to the construction of different "realities." However, before

arriving at this subject, some further milestones along the evolutionary path of therapy must be mentioned.

It may seem far-fetched, indeed, that in order to arrive at the next milestone I go back in time to Blaise Pascal who, in his *Pensée 223,* developed an argument that has become known as *Pascal's wager.* It is of interest to us therapists because, although theological in form, it deals with a problem very close to home. Pascal examines the age-old question of how a nonbeliever can arrive, by and through himself, at a state of faith. His suggestion is intriguing: *Behave as if you already believed*—for instance by praying, using Holy Water, partaking in the sacraments, and so forth. Out of these actions, faith will follow. And since there is at least a probability that God exists, to say nothing of the potential benefits (peace of mind and final salvation), your stakes in this game are small. "*Qu'avez-vous à perdre* (what do you have to lose)?" he asks rhetorically.

Pascal's *wager* gave rise to innumerable arguments, speculations, and treatises. Let me mention just one of them. In his fascinating book, *Ulysses and the Sirens,* Norwegian philosopher Jon Elster (1979, pp. 47-54) takes up Pascal's thought and goes on to show that one cannot decide to believe something without the necessity to *forget* the decision: "The implication of this argument is that the decision to believe can only be carried out successfully if accompanied by a decision to forget, viz. a decision to forget the decision to believe. This, however, is just as paradoxical as the decision to believe. ... The most efficient procedure would be to start up a single causal process with the double effect of inducing belief *and* making you forget that it was ever started up. Asking to be hypnotized is one such mechanism ..." (p. 50).

This seems crucial to my subject. To forget on purpose is one thing, and it is impossible. But to do something because the reason, impulse, or suggestion for this action comes from the outside, either as the result of a chance event or of a deliberate action or suggestion by someone else—in other words, in communicative interaction with another person—is quite another thing.

At this point I have to take up the evolution of modern family therapy, which no longer asks, "*Why* is the identified patient behaving in this bizarre, irrational fashion?," but rather, "In what sort of human system does this behavior make sense and is perhaps the only possible behavior?" and "What sort of solutions has this system so far attempted?" But these considerations would make my address mastodontic. Let me merely point out that at this juncture therapy has little, if anything, to do with concepts beginning with the prefix *psycho-*, such as psychology, psychopathology, psychotherapy. For it is no longer just the individual, monadic *psyche* that concerns us here, but the superindividual structures arising out of the interactions between individuals. Regrettably, it has to do with something that I already mentioned here in Phoenix two years ago (Watzlawick, 1985), and repetitions are admittedly boring.

What I mean is the fact that in their vast majority, the problems we want to change are not problems related to the properties of objects or of situations—to the *reality of the first order* as I have proposed to call it (Watzlawick, 1976, pp. 140–142)—but are related to the meaning, the sense, and the value that we have come to attribute to these objects or situations (their *second-order reality*). "It is not the things themselves that worry us, but the opinions that we have about those things," said Epictetus some 1900 years ago. And most of us know the answer to the question about the difference between an optimist and a pessimist: The optimist says of a bottle of wine that it is half full; the pessimist says that it is half empty. The same reality of the first order—a bottle with some wine in it—but two very different second-order realities, resulting in fact, in two different worlds. Seen in this way, one may say that all

therapy is concerned with bringing about changes in the way people have constructed their second-order realities (which they are totally convinced are the *real* reality).

In traditional psychotherapy one attempts to achieve this through the use of *indicative* language, that is, the language of description, explanation, confrontation, interpretation, and so forth. This is the language of classical science and of linear causality. However it does not lend itself very well to the description of nonlinear, systemic phenomena (e.g., human relationships); and it lends itself even less to the communication of new experiences and realizations for which the past provides no understanding and which lie outside a given person's reality construction.

But what other language is there? The answer is given, for instance, by George Spencer Brown (1973) in his book *Laws of Form*, where, almost as an aside, he defines the concept of *injunctive* language. Taking mathematical communication as his point of departure, he writes (p. 77):

It may be helpful at this stage to realize that the primary form of mathematical communication is not description, but injunction. In this respect it is comparable with practical art forms like cookery, in which the taste of a cake, although literally indescribable, can be conveyed to a reader in the form of a set of injunctions called a recipe. Music is a similar art form, the composer does not even attempt to describe the set of sounds he has in mind, much less the set of feelings occasioned through them, but writes down a set of commands which, if they are obeyed by the reader, can result in a reproduction, to the reader, of the composer's original experience.

And a little later (p. 78), he comments on the role of injunctive language in the training of scientists,

Even natural science appears to be more dependent upon injunction than we are usually prepared to admit. The professional initiation of the man of science consists not so much in reading the proper textbooks, as in obeying injunctions such as "look down that microscope." But it is not out of order for men of science, having looked down the microscope, now to describe to each other, and to discuss amongst themselves, what they have seen, and to write papers and textbooks describing it.

In other words, if we manage to get somebody to undertake an action which in and by itself was always possible, but which he did not perform because in his second-order reality there was no sense or reason to carry it out, then through the very performance of this action he will experience something that no amount of explaining and interpreting may ever have led him to see and to experience. And with this we have arrived at Heinz von Foerster's imperative: If you desire to see, learn how to act.

Needless to say, people may strenuously resist the request to perform such an action. The classical example is Galileo Galilei's contemporaries who disdained to look through his telescope because they *knew* without looking that what he claimed to see *could* not be the case (within the limits of their second-order reality, i.e., geocentricity). Remember—if the facts don't comply with the theory, so much the worse for the facts.

To anybody acquainted with Milton Erickson's work, the concept of injunctive language, if not the designation, is nothing new. In the second half of his professional life, Erickson increasingly utilized direct behavior prescriptions outside trance states in order to achieve therapeutic change. Being a master in dealing with resistance, he gave us the important rule: Learn and use the patient's language. This, too, is a radical departure from classical psychotherapy, where a great deal of time is spent in the beginning stages of treatment in the attempt to teach the patient a new "language," that is, the conceptualizations of the particular school of therapy that the therapist subscribes to. Only when the patient has begun to think in terms of this epistemology, to see himself, his problems, his life in this perspective, is therapeutic change then attempted within this framework. Needless to say, this process may take a long time. In hypnotherapy the opposite takes place; it is the therapist who learns the patient's language, his reality construction (as we would call it nowadays), and then gives his suggestions in this language, thereby minimizing resistance (and time).

Outside its therapeutic applications, the study of injunctive language had its origins in the work of the Austrian philosopher Ernst Mally. In his book *Grundgesetze des Sollens* (1926), Mally developed a theory of wishes and commands that he called *deontic* logic.

Another important contribution to this subject can be found in the work of the British philosopher of language, John L. Austin (1962). In his famous Harvard Lectures (in 1955), he identified a particular form of communication which he called *performative speech acts* or *performative sentences*. "The term *performative* will be used in a variety of cognate ways and constructions, much as the term *imperative* is. The name is derived, of course, from *perform*, the usual verb with the noun *action*: it indicates that the issuing of the utterance is the performing of an action—it is not normally thought of as just saying something" (p. 6).

For instance, if I say, "He promises to return the book tomorrow," I describe (in indicative language) an action, a speech act, by that person. But if I say, "I promise to return the book tomorrow," saying "I promise" *is itself* the promise, the action. In Austin's terminology, the first example (the description) is called a *constative*, while the second is a *performative* speech act. In Lecture IV, Austin points to the difference between the statements "I am running" and "I apologize." The former is a mere report of an action; the latter is *itself* the action, *is* the apology. Other examples from everyday life are: "I take this woman to be my lawful wedded wife," "I name this ship *Queen Elizabeth*," "I give and bequeath my watch to my brother." In all of these and in countless analogous speech acts, a concrete result is achieved, while my saying "Winter is coming" does not make the winter come. Of course, a number of preconditions have to be met for a performative speech act to obtain or be effective. For instance, past disappointment or lies may make me doubt the promise; the apology must not be offered in a sneering, sarcastic tone of voice; the ceremony of naming a ship has to be an established procedure in a given culture. But if and when these preconditions are met, a reality is literally created by the performative utterance, and whoever subsequently referred to that ship as the *Joseph Stalin* would be considered somewhat deranged.

With these remarks I have barely scratched the surface of Austin's work in this specialized area of linguistics, that is, his ideas on "how to do things with words." But I hope that even these brief references will reveal some of the richness and the relevance of it for our work.

Of a particular mind-boggling effect are the so-called self-fulfilling prophecies, known to unorthodox therapists and stock brokers alike—but not to weather forecasters: Imagined effect produces concrete cause; the future (not the past) determines the present; the prophecy of the event leads to the event of the prophecy (Watzlawick, 1984).

I am convinced that injunctive language will acquire a central place within the frame of modern therapeutic techniques. Of course, it has always occupied this place in hypnotherapy. For what is a hypnotic suggestion if not an injunction to behave *as if* something were the case— something which does become the case (i.e., becomes "real") as a result of having been carried out. But this is tantamount to saying that injunctions can literally *construct* realities, just as chance events can have this effect not only in human lives, but are known to have it in cosmic as well as biological evolution. In this connection, it would be tempting to go off on a tangent, into questions of self-organi-

zation, or what Prigogine (1980) called *dissipative structures*—a subject that would exceed the limits of my competence and my time.

But, why is there a crucial difference between something originating within myself and an impulse that comes from the outside? Several answers offer themselves, but none seems convincing. *That* it is so, is no secret. In our own lives we have little difficulty creating the same disasters as our so-called patients do in their lives, and to tickle oneself is never as ticklish as being tickled by somebody else.

However, to go back to Pascal. There are two little words in his behavior prescription that merit attention: Behave *as if* you already believed. They clearly point to the initially quite fictional nature of this class of interventions. And it is this fictionality that creates doubts. The common objection is that even if they are successful, their effect cannot last. After all, they are only make-believe, an as-if fiction. Sooner or later, probably sooner, they must run up against the hard facts of reality and be defeated. Here is the counter-argument:

The idea of introducing an as-if assumption into a situation and thereby arriving at concrete results is by no means a recent one. It goes back at least to the year 1911 when the German philosopher Hans Vaihinger published his *Philosophie des Als Ob*, whose English title is *The Philosophy of "As If"* (1924). If it were not for the fact that Alfred Adler (and to a lesser degree also Freud) had already recognized the importance of these ideas, their application to our field could very well be called the Therapy of As If, or the therapy of "planned chance events."

Again, I do not see how I can avoid repeating here something that I already mentioned two years ago: What Vaihinger presents in a mere 800 pages is an astounding richness of examples, drawn from all branches of science as well as from everyday life, showing that we *always* work with unproven and unprovable assumptions which, nevertheless, lead to concrete, practical results. There is not and there never will be any proof that man is *really* endowed with free will and therefore responsible for his actions. However, I know of no society, culture, or civilization, past or present, in which people did not behave *as if* this were the case, because without this fictitious assumption practical, concrete social order would be impossible. The idea of the square root of minus one is totally fictional. It is not only intellectually unimaginable, but also it violates the basic rules of arithmetic; yet, mathematicians, physicists, engineers, computer programmers, and others have nonchalantly included this fiction into their equations and have arrived at very concrete results, such as modern electronics.

The rules and patterns of interaction that a family or systems therapist believes to observe are quite obviously *read* by him into the observed phenomena—they are not *really* there—and yet, to conduct therapy *as if* these patterns existed can lead to practical and quick results. Thus, the question is no longer, "Which school of therapy is *right*?" but it is, "Which as-if assumptions produce better concrete results?" Maybe the decline of dogma is approaching.

Maybe not. However, what can be said—by way of an outlook on the evolution of our field—is that this way of conceptualizing and of trying to resolve human problems is gaining increasing attention as the traditional techniques of problem resolution seem to be reaching the limits of their usefulness. We are beginning to apply these methods to what may be called the specific pathologies of large systems. It does not seem totally utopian to imagine their application even to some of the most pressing and threatening problems of our planet, such as the maintenance of peace or the preservation of our biosphere. However, these attempts are too often beset by the same basic mistake that plays havoc in clinical work, namely, the assumption that since the problems are of enormous proportion, only some equally enormous,

transcending solution has any chance of succeeding.

The opposite appears to be the case. If we look at the history of the last few centuries, beginning with the French Revolution or even with the Inquisition, we see that invariably and without exception the worst atrocities were the direct result of grandiose and utopian attempts at improving the world. What the philosopher Karl Popper calls a policy of small steps is unacceptable to idealists and ideologists. Remember the aphorism that Gregory Bateson often mentioned: "He who would do good must do so in minute particulars. The general good is the plea of patriots, politicians and knaves."

To convince ourselves, we only have to look at nature. Great changes are always catastrophic and cataclysmic. Negentropy—or *anotropy*, as my friend George Vassiliou in Athens prefers to call it in order to avoid the double negative—works patiently, silently, in small steps; yet it is the force behind evolution, self-organization and higher and higher complexity in the universe. I think that if we, as therapists, begin to see ourselves as the servants of negentropy, we will fulfill our function better than we do as supposed world-improvers and gurus. Heinz von Foerster (1973) defined this function in his Ethical Imperative: Act always so as to increase the number of choices.

Many centuries ago this same outlook was already expressed in a charming story: After his death, the Sufi Abu Bakr Shibli appeared to one of his friends in a dream. "How has God treated you?," the friend asked. And the Sufi answered, "As I stood before His throne, He asked me, 'Do you know why I am forgiving you?' And I said, 'Because of my good deeds?' And God said, 'No, not because of those.' I asked, 'Because I was sincere in my adoration?' And God said, 'No.' I then said, 'Because of my pilgrimages and my journeys to acquire knowledge and to enlighten others?' And God again replied, 'No, not because of all this.' So I asked Him, 'O Lord, why then have you forgiven me?' And He answered,

'Do you remember how on a bitterly cold winter day you were walking through the streets of Baghdad and you saw a hungry kitten desperately trying to find shelter from the icy wind, and you had pity on it and picked it up and put it inside your fur and took it into your home?' I said, 'Yes, my Lord, I remember.' And God said, 'Because you were kind to that cat, Abu Bakr, because of that I have forgiven you' " (Schimmel, 1983, p. 16).

REFERENCES

Alexander, F. and French, T. (1946). *Psychoanalytic therapy*. New York: Ronald Press Co.

Alexander, F. (1956). *Psychoanalysis and psychotherapy*. New York: W.W. Norton.

Austin, J.L. (1962). *How to do things with words*. Cambridge: Harvard University Press.

Balint, M. (1968). *The basic fault*. London: Tavistock.

Brown, G. S. (1973). *Laws of form*. New York: Bantam Books.

Elster, J. (1979). *Ulysses and the sirens*. Cambridge: Cambridge University Press.

Foerster, H. von. (1973). *On constructing a reality*. In E. Preiser (Ed.), *Environmental design*. Stroudberg: Dowden, Hutchinson & Ross. (Reprinted in P. Watzlawick (Ed.) (1984), *The invented reality* (pp. 41–61). New York: W.W. Norton.)

Freud, S. (1964). *New introductory lectures on psycho-analysis*. London: Hogarth Press (Standard Edition, vol. 22).

Glover, E. (1956). *Freud or Jung?* New York: Meridian Books.

Kuhn, T. (1970). *The structure of scientific revolutions*. Chicago: University of Chicago Press.

Mally, E. (1926). *Grundgesetze des Sollens*. Graz: Leuscher & Lubensky.

Piaget, J. (1954). *The construction of reality in the child*. New York: Basic Books. (Original work published 1937)

Prigogine, I. (1980). *From being to becoming*. San Francisco: Freeman & Co.

Salzman, L. (1968). Reply to critics. *International Journal of Psychiatry*, 6, 473–476.

Schimmel, A. (Ed.). (1983). *Die orientalische Katze*. Cologne: Diederichs. (Adapted from the German translation)

Vaihinger, H. (1924). The philosophy of '*as if*'. A system of the theoretical, practical and religious fictions of mankind. Transl. C.K. Ogden. New York: Harcourt Brace.

Watzlawick, P. (1976). *How real is real?* New York: Random House.

Watzlawick, P. (1984). Self-fulfilling prophecies. In P. Watzlawick (Ed.), *The invented reality* (pp. 95–116). New York: W.W. Norton.

Watzlawick, P. (1985). Hypnotherapy without trance. In J. Zeig (Ed.), *Ericksonian psychotherapy: Vol. I, Structure* (pp. 5–14). New York: Brunner/Mazel.

Discussion by Ernest L. Rossi, Ph.D.

◆

It is a profound pleasure to be able to discuss Paul Watzlawick's presentation. Each time I hear him or read a paper or book he has written, I learn something genuinely new. There is no question in my mind but that he is one of our most creative thinkers in the entire field of therapy. I am thankful for this all too rare opportunity to learn from him today.

Let me say that his presentation is so rich and complex that I will not be able to do justice to all of it here. Since I do not want to deal in vague generalities, however, I will discuss what was most meaningful to me.

Paul's introduction of the relevance of John Austin's concept of *performance speech* is what was most new, creative, and stimulating. It solves a very serious misgiving I have had all these years about the work of Milton H. Erickson. Erickson was quite content to be "manipulative." He liked to say that manipulating people for their own good was just as satisfactory an approach as the way we manipulated food by cleaning it, cooking it, putting salt on it, eating it, and, hopefully, digesting it.

I could never accept this reasoning. In our work together, I agreed that I would quote him accurately, but in my own thinking and writing I would make a few humanistic substitutions: Instead of *manipulate*, I would *facilitate;* instead of *control*, I would *evoke;* and instead of using hypnotic *techniques*, I would use hypnotic *approaches*. I hoped thereby to create a *humanistic hypnotherapy* more in tune with the realities of twentieth-century consciousness.

If I had heard this talk by Dr. Watzlawick 15 years ago, I could have saved myself a lot of effort and perhaps understood Erickson's genius with more insight and less stress. It used to horrify me when I saw Erickson request absolute *obedience* from certain patients before he would proceed with their therapy; he literally would not continue unless they immediately promised to obey him no matter what.

Such authoritarian requests for obedience often embarrassed me. I would apologize for Erickson to anyone who would listen by saying that he was, after all, a transition figure in the history of hypnosis. Although Erickson had invented the "permissive modern approach" to hypnosis, he was himself only human and would occasionally regress back to the authoritarian methods of the past.

Now, profoundly, Dr. Watzlawick has shown that Erickson's request for obedience was not necessarily a regression nor an error. Requesting obedience was actually a way of requiring the patient to engage in a bit of *performance speech*. By having the patient say, "I will obey you no matter what" as a precondition for therapy, Erickson was doing a number of things that Watzlawick talks about: He was initiating the beginning of a self-ful-

filling prophecy; he was making use of von Foerster's aesthetic imperative, "If you desire to see, learn how to act"; he was laying the foundation that enabled patients to follow his "behavioral prescriptions," which in turn enabled them to break out of their "learned limitations" and create a more adequate and healing "second-order reality."

Of course, Erickson would not ask just anyone for this performance speech of obedience. He asked it only of those he knew would abide by it. When I asked him about it, he said that there were people who, because of their religious background or previous character training, would actually obey if they promised to obey. From Erickson's point of view, he was simply *utilizing* the patient's character structure or belief system to facilitate the process of change. So, even though Erickson probably never heard of *performance speech*, he was playing by the rules for its effective use. The concept of *performance speech* as a way of *creating our psychological reality* opens up possibilities for a new step in the evolution of *psycho*therapy.

The only quibble I have with Dr. Watzlawick is that I do not want to throw out the "psych" in *psycho*therapy. It really seems to me that that would be throwing out the baby with the bath water. After all, it is the psyche that constructs these new realities; Piaget's research was on the child's construction of *psycho*logical reality. I believe that what Dr. Watzlawick is really against is (1) the unwarranted assumptions of the psychodynamically oriented therapies, and (2) the "psychobabble" that clings to them. In this regard I could not agree more. I, too, want to give these things up.

Rather than wasting time on that single caveat, however, I would prefer to ask Dr. Watzlawick if he can tell us something more about how we can learn to use *performance speech* effectively in therapy. Since I am interested in this approach, what must I now do to train myself in its use? How are you, Dr. Watzlawick, learning to use this approach? Do you have any exercises or practical suggestions for us who want to use it?

A second and equally important area concerns the application of the concept of *performance speech* to our current global social conflicts. Dr. Watzlawick, how would you train international leaders such as Reagan and Gorbachev? What behavioral prescriptions would you give them?

RESPONSE BY DR. WATZLAWICK

How can one use performative techniques? I must, unfortunately, tell you I have just begun to think of it more seriously and I will let you know in about five years, if I can.

Coming to the question of the superpowers, there are two difficulties. First of all, there is nobody who can play the role of the therapist. Admittedly, if you look at their behavior, it is a classical illustration of family and couples dynamics. The moment the identified patients, Nazi Germany and Japan, didn't exist anymore, the tenuous alliance between the two parents broke down and the Cold War started. This is something we see in family therapy over and over again. As we now look at these two parents whose children have gone out and started lives of their own, we are absolutely flabbergasted by the similarities of the behavior of these two superpowers.

There is one suggestion I could make, if they would only listen to me, and it isn't even mine; it was postulate and I have said this many times so forgive me for repeating it. It was postulated by Anatole Rappaport in his book *Fights, Games and Debates* that came out, I think, in the early 1960s, in which he bases himself on a suggestion made to him, I believe, by Carl Rogers. Rappaport says, a rule of procedure should be introduced in all international or similar conferences, and the rule of procedure would be that before anything substantive may be discussed, the two delegations must represent, must define, must explain, the viewpoint of the other delegation to the full satisfaction of the other delegation. In other words, for instance, the American delegation would have to present the Soviet viewpoint in all detail so that the Soviets would say, "Yes, you have presented our viewpoint correctly and fully." It would then be the turn of the Soviets to present the U.S. viewpoint until the U.S. delegation says, "Yes, you have presented our viewpoint fully and correctly."

Rappaport says, and I have no doubt that he is right, that if this were possible, 50 percent of the so-called problems would already have disappeared before they even started talking about them.

The second suggestion in the Geneva meeting that I would have made would be to request President Reagan to ask Gorbachev if he, the Soviet leader, were willing to accept an SDI mechanism that was foolproof and was communicated to the Soviets in all detail; there would be no secrets. I think it would have been a very clever move because Gorbachev could hardly have afforded to say no to that one.

QUESTIONS AND ANSWERS

Question: Dr. Watzlawick, in the history of the development of the importance of action as a measure to correct someone's perception, there was in the 50s an American experimental psychologist by the name of Adelbert Ames who had constructed a distorted room at Princeton University. When you looked at that room from just one point of view with your chin in the chin piece, you could not detect that this was a distorted room and you would make all kinds of false assumptions about the sizes of people and how they changed when they walked across the room. Without actually acting within the situation, he would give people a long stick and ask them to touch the far corner of that room and to walk in the room. Then they would understand that it was distorted. If they didn't do any of that, they could not determine that the room was distorted. I think that that's a tremendous example that has not been sufficiently used in this development.

Watzlawick: I stand corrected, yes. Gregory Bateson has mentioned again and again the Ames experiments and he even speculated that if a so-called schizophrenic could be made to undergo this experience it might help more than anything else. I should have mentioned Vygorski and his experiments on the psychology of preferences or experiments on noncontingent reward. Things like that are absolutely pertinent here.

Question: Dr. Watzlawick, I'm having trouble putting together some of the points you've made and seeing them as consistent. You were critical of the linear deterministic model of traditional science. Yet, I heard you appealing to the indubitability of data, to the givenness of data which I would see as part of that traditional, linear deterministic world view. Can you say how those statements fit together?

Watzlawick: I'm not certain that I used the word data at all. Facts, yes. I'm fully aware that facts come from *factare* in Latin that means *to make, to do*. Facts are for me the things that people communicate. If someone says I see the situation a certain way, that to me is a communication. I don't think there are any facts beyond communicated information.

Question: I was wondering what you do with the past. You referred to the past as a way of elucidating some of your points and you referred to history, to what happened when people followed a linear deterministic model and the trouble that got us into. That reference was supposed to make us remember something, to pull us toward a certain construction of reality. When I listen to you speak and to many others here, I feel as if I'm starting now, from now to then, and I wonder how to integrate where I was before and how you integrate what has happened before. This is not to say that I am quarreling with the notion of looking into the future or of constructing a reality geared toward the future, but I feel that there is a mythology about the past also that needs to be constructed for people to feel satisfied. How do you deal with that?

Watzlawick: I'm not sure if there is this need. Some people may insist that there is, perhaps because they've spent $25,000 on retrospective, introspective, intrapsychic therapy. If I ask someone, "Suppose that your problem changed as a result of a few sessions here, suppose that your problem improved and you never found out why, would that be acceptable?" I've yet to find somebody who says no. I would have to understand it in terms of my past. If I mention the past here, in this context, it is not because I believe that I could not have given my lecture without the references to the past. My address would then have been subject to the very criticisms that I hope I have somewhat mitigated by saying I'm aware of what people have said in the past. But what I want to show you is what can be done in the here and now.

Question: If I imagine myself going to see a therapist, I see myself, because of my acculturation, speaking in indicative language about the problem which I'm presenting. Since the patient expresses himself in indicative language in explaining his problem or describing his condition or symptoms, I wonder how the translation into injunctive language takes place in the therapist's mind. How do we know that the therapist is, in fact, bilingual and that he can make an accurate translation into injunctive language?

Watzlawick: If you read Erickson, especially, or if you had the chance to watch Don Jackson do therapy, you would wonder how on earth the man got this idea to ask the patient to do such and such or to say such and such at that moment. It seems to me miraculous; it seems to imply some kind of particular gift. Sometimes people say, well even though you no longer work as a Jungian, you are a Jungian, you are therefore intuitive, you just don't know it. I say, "No." If you are aware of the solutions attempted previously, of what people have so far done to cope with their problem, then you know that this is where our intervention is applied. We try to block what people have done so far because this perpetuates the problem and it goes on and on in a circular fashion.

Question: I very much like the reflection of a leaf rising from a pool to meet its falling counterpart. Could Dr. Watzlawick talk more about this, about the interaction of the therapist/client, the teacher/student, about the performer/audience relationship in terms of creating a performative act, a speech act as it were? I think giving a prescription encourages the false self. How do you address the actual practice of giving a prescription and assessing for this rising/falling meeting of therapist/client language act?

Watzlawick: That's the point where the therapist is supposed to learn the client's language. It is not a meeting halfway. If a therapist gives a behavior prescription and if the idea behind it fits the context as he, the therapist, sees it, then in carrying out the behavior prescription the client may have something that might be called the equivalent of classical insight. That's really all I can answer you.

Question: Two brief points. One is from Gestalt therapy where it seems to me that there is a very specific emphasis on turning indicative language into performative language. When the patient says, "I can't do something," which is for the patient a description in indicative language, "This is a fact about me." The therapist asks this person to say, "I won't," which makes the patient aware that he or she is indeed using performative language. I think that using this is what you were talking about. My other point is that your emphasis is basically on using what works, what is useful. Therefore, I wonder why you would throw out the use of a psychic change if this is what works. I can understand adding to techniques, but I can't understand saying that this whole theory, some of which works for some people at times, why that should also not be used when it works?

Watzlawick: The fact that I haven't mentioned, for instance, the parallelism to Gestalt therapy or Behavior therapy is merely due to limitations of time and space. I would agree with you on the other question. I don't know whether your question points in that direction, but I am definitely not a guru. Being a therapist does not mean that I have a better idea of what existence is about, where we come from, where we go to. I have mentioned this very often, let me repeat it, I don't want to be a guru. I want to be a mechanic.

SECTION II

♦

Cognitive/Behavioral Approaches

The Evolution of Rational-Emotive Therapy (RET) and Cognitive Behavior Therapy (CBT)

◆

Albert Ellis, Ph.D.

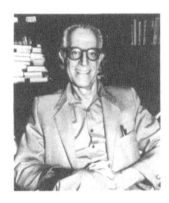

Albert Ellis, Ph.D.
Albert Ellis is the Executive Director of the Institute for Rational-Emotive Therapy in New York. He has practiced psychotherapy, marriage and family counseling and sex therapy for more than 40 years. Ellis received the Humanist of the Year Award from the American Humanist Association; the Distinguished Professional Contribution to Knowledge Award from the American Psychological Association; and an award from the Academy of Psychologists in Marital and Family Therapy. Ellis has authored or edited approximately 50 books and monographs and more than 500 papers and chapters in psychological, psychiatric and sociological publications. His Ph.D. in clinical psychology was granted from Columbia University in 1947.

Ellis presents the fundamentals of the school of psychotherapy that he developed, Rational-Emotive Therapy. Emphasized is the importance of realizing and correcting negative internal dialogue—the "shoulds" that disrupt effective living.

The organizers of this conference on the Evolution of Psychotherapy have given a list of questions to all the invited speakers. Since these questions appear to me unusually relevant, I shall now attempt to answer them.

QUESTION 1: *HOW DO YOU DEFINE PSYCHOTHERAPY? WHAT ARE ITS GOALS? HOW DO YOU DEFINE MENTAL HEALTH?*

Psychotherapy, as viewed by rational-emotive therapy (RET), has two main as-

pects. First is helping clients (and, as far as I am concerned, virtually the whole human race) to minimize their irrational thinking, inappropriate feelings, and dysfunctional behaviors. In RET, we assume that these three major aspects of what is commonly called "emotional disturbance" are integrally interrelated, and that one virtually never exists entirely in its own right but also includes aspects of the other two. Thus, when people have severe "emotional" problems (such as anxiety and depression), RET assumes that they have irrational ideas and self-defeating behaviors that accompany and to some significant degree create these problems. But it also assumes that self-sabotaging irrational beliefs follow from inappropriate affects and behaviors and that self-destructive behaviors stem from dysfunctional cognitions and emotions (Ellis, 1958, 1962, 1984a, 1984b).

According to RET, the first important part of psychotherapy, is to zero in on clients' needless injurious thoughts, feelings, and behaviors—with which they sabotage their own happiness and effectiveness as well as the well-being of other members of the social group in which they choose to live—and to help them clearly see what they have done and are still doing to foolishly upset themselves. The therapist then endeavors to show clients how to significantly change their own dysfunctional activities.

The second part of psychotherapy—which begins in RET from the first session and continues onward—consists of helping clients to actualize themselves more fully and to achieve a greater degree of happiness, pleasure, joy, and self-fulfillment than they would otherwise tend to achieve. This is an important part of therapy, because even people who do not specifically sabotage themselves and others frequently, by reason of their human tendency to habituate themselves to comfort rather than to adventure and creativity, tend to lead quiet, uninspired lives. They get by all right—at home, at work, and socially. But they do little more than just "get by." The finer things they could do and could create for themselves—and I mean the things that they, personally, would more thoroughly enjoy—they fail to think about, to plot and scheme to generate, and to actively launch.

Effective and efficient psychotherapy, therefore, at least in the view of RET, not only helps and teaches people how to minimize (and, hopefully, extirpate) their gratuitous emotional and behavioral problems, but also assesses their potential for having a more vibrant existence, and tries to show them how they can enjoy themselves more fully (Ellis, 1971a, 1971c, 1976a, 1979a; Ellis & Dryden, in press).

Mental health can be, and often has been defined in many different ways. Rational-emotive therapy adopts and adapts several of these definitions and then adds a few of its own (Ellis, 1962, 1973, 1983). Let me briefly summarize some of RET's views on the goals of mental health that seem to be desirable for most—though not, of course, all—people.

SELF-INTEREST

Emotionally healthy people are primarily true to themselves and do not masochistically subjugate themselves to or unduly sacrifice themselves for others. They tend to put themselves at least a little before others, realizing that if they do not primarily take care of themselves, who else will? But they also put a few selected others a close second and the rest of the world not too far behind.

SOCIAL INTEREST

Mentally healthy people are usually somewhat gregarious and choose to try to live happily in a social group. Because they desire to live successfully with others, and usually to relate intimately to a few of these selected others, they work at feeling and displaying a considerable degree of what Adler (1927, 1964) called social interest and what Sullivan (1953) termed interpersonal competence. They take the "I'm OK; you're OK" position of Berne (1964, 1972) and Goulding and Goulding (1979). While primarily interested in their personal survival and enjoyment, they also strive to be considerate and fair to others; to avoid needlessly harming these others; to engage in collaborative and cooperative endeavors; at times to be somewhat altruistic; and to distinctly enjoy interpersonal and group relationships.

SELF-DIRECTION

Emotionally healthy people largely assume responsibility for their own lives, enjoy the independence of working out their own problems, and while often wanting others' approval, do not think that they absolutely *must* have such support for their effectiveness and well-being.

TOLERANCE

Healthy people give others the right to be wrong—as Dr. Robert A. Harper and I urged in the original edition of *A New Guide to Rational Living* (Ellis & Harper, 1961a). While disliking or abhorring others' *behaviors*, they refuse to condemn *them*, as total *persons*, for behaving poorly or badly. They accept the fact that all of us humans are remarkably fallible and they refrain from unrealistically demanding and commanding that any of us be perfect and they resist damning people globally for their obnoxious acts.

ACCEPTANCE OF AMBIGUITY AND UNCERTAINTY

Emotionally mature individuals accept the fact that, as far as has yet been discovered, we live in a world of probability and chance and that this world does not, nor probably ever will, contain absolute necessities or complete certainties. They have a philosophy that enables them to live in this probabilistic world quite tolerably and to see it in terms of adventure, learning, and exciting striving.

FLEXIBILITY

Emotionally sound people are intellectually flexible, tend to be open to change, and are prone to take an undogmatic and unbigoted view of the infinitely varied people, ideas, and things in the world around them. They can be firm and passionate in their thoughts and feelings, but they can also look comfortably at new evidence and often revise their notions of "reality" to conform with this evidence.

SCIENTIFIC THINKING

According to RET, emotionally sensitive and stable people are reasonably objective, rational, and scientific. They construct hypotheses about how they would like to see themselves and others behave and they check the validity of these hypotheses by applying the rules of logic and of the scientific method to their own lives and to their interpersonal relationships. Science is thoroughly antidogmatic and open to change; so are emotionally undisturbed people (Ellis, 1973, 1985a; Ellis & Bernard, 1985; Mahoney, 1985; Popper, 1972; Russell, 1950).

COMMITMENT

As I have noted in several of my writings on RET, emotionally healthy and happy people are usually absorbed in something outside of themselves, whether this be people, things, or ideas. They usually lead better lives when they have at least one major creative interest, as well as some profound human involvements, which they make very important (but not sacred!) to themselves and around which they structure a good part of their lives (Ellis, 1957a; Ellis & Becker, 1982; Ellis & Harper, 1975).

RISK-TAKING

People who have good emotional health are able to take risks, to ask themselves what they would really like to do in life, and then to try to do this, even though they have to risk defeat and failure. They are reasonably adventurous (though not foolhardy); are willing to try almost anything once, if only to see how they like it; and look forward to some different or unusual breaks in their everyday routines.

SELF-ACCEPTANCE

Emotionally healthy individuals are glad to be alive and to accept themselves as "deserving" of continued life and happiness just because they exist and because they have some present or future potential to enjoy themselves. In accordance with one of the main principles of RET, they *fully* or *unconditionally* accept themselves—or give themselves what Rogers (1961) calls unconditional positive regard and what Tillich (1953) calls "the courage to be." They try to perform adequately or competently in their affairs and to win the approval of others; but they do so for enjoyment and not for ego gratification or self-deification. They consequently try to rate their acts, deeds and traits only in the light of their chosen goals and values; and they rigorously try to avoid rating their *self*, their *being*, their *essence*, or their *totality* (Ellis, 1972, 1973, 1976b).

LONG-RANGE HEDONISM

Well adjusted people tend to seek both the pleasures of the moment and those of the future, and do not often court future pain for present gain. They are hedonistic—that is, happiness-seeking and pain-avoidant—but they assume that they will probably live for quite a few years and that they had therefore better think of both today and tomorrow, and not be obsessed with immediate gratification (Ellis, 1979a, 1980a).

NONPERFECTIONISM AND NONUTOPIANISM

Healthy people accept the fact that they (and other humans) will most probably never act perfectly and that even when perfectionism (as in art or science) is worth striving for, it never *has to be* achieved. They also accept the reality that utopias are probably unattainable and that no humans are likely to get everything they want and to avoid all pain. They may try to get close to, but never really expect to achieve, total joy, happiness, or perfection, and they do not expect complete lack

of anxiety, depression, self-downing, and hostility.

SELF-RESPONSIBILITY FOR OWN EMOTIONAL DISTURBANCE

Healthy individuals tend to accept a great deal of responsibility for their own disturbance, rather than defensively blaming others or social conditions for their own self-defeating thoughts, feelings, and behaviors.

Healthy people, in other words, unconditionally accept themselves because they *choose* to do so, regardless of how well or badly they perform and regardless of how much approval they receive from others. They distinctly *prefer* to act competently and to win others' favor; and they accordingly assess and criticize their own *behaviors* when they fail in these respects. But they don't believe that they absolutely *must* do well or be approved; and they therefore don't conclude that they, in toto, are *good people* when they succeed and are *rotten individuals* when they fail (Ellis, 1962, 1972, 1976b, 1985b; Ellis & Grieger, 1977; Ellis & Whiteley, 1979).

QUESTION 2: *HOW DO PEOPLE CHANGE IN THERAPY? WHAT ARE THE BASIC PREMISES AND UNDERLYING ASSUMPTIONS IN THE RET APPROACH TO FACILITATE CHANGE?*

RET holds that people change in therapy by doing or experiencing many kinds of things, ranging from being empathically loved to being objectively directed by a therapist, and ranging from being passively heard to being actively taught and pushed. Many kinds of strokes work with many kinds of folks. For more lasting and effective change, however, RET claims that most clients had better do three major things: (1) Acknowledge that they mainly are responsible for their own disturbed thoughts, feelings, and actions, and stop copping out by blaming their parents, their culture, or their environment. (2) Clearly see how they are thinking, feeling, and behaving when they needlessly upset themselves. (3) Work hard, forcefully, and persistently to change their neurotic cognitions, emotions, and performances.

From the start, RET has favored insight as the most important mode by which people can bring about personality change. But the insight that it favors is hardly Freudian or psychoanalytic, which hypothesizes that if you fully understand the origins or history of your emotional problems you will surely help yourself to resolve them. On the contrary, the more time you spend in gaining such understanding, the more you may sidetrack yourself from doing anything effective to change your dysfunctional ways.

The three insights, instead, that RET has always promoted are: (1) No matter what happened to you in your childhood or your early family life, you brought your own individual reactivity to these early experiences, and therefore you largely—though not completely—overreacted or underreacted to the stimuli of your childhood, and thereby mainly upset yourself. (2) No matter when and how you originally disturbed yourself, and no matter how you reacted to your parents, your teachers, and the conditions under which you first lived, you are maladjusted today not because of these early reactions but because you *still* largely react in a similar fashion *today*. Your past doesn't *cause* your present malfunctioning, though it may have originally *contributed* to it. (3) Because you *naturally* and *easily* think crookedly and behave defeatingly, because you have a strong biological as well as sociological tendency to disturb yourself, and because you are the kind of human animal who *habituates* yourself to self-sabotaging conduct and who therefore usually has a difficult time rehabituating yourself to more fulfilling ways of living, there is normally no way but hard work and practice—yes, *work and practice*—to change yourself and to keep yourself

less miserable and more functional (Ellis, 1962).

What are the basic premises and underlying assumptions in the RET approach to facilitate change? These include the following:

THE ABCs OF IRRATIONAL THINKING AND DISTURBANCE

Humans, as Adler particularly noted (1927, 1964), have goals, purposes, and ideals; and RET assumes that they do practically anything they do (including avoidances) because they want to survive and to be reasonably happy while surviving. More particularly, they usually have the basic goals of being happy (1) when they are alone; (2) when they live and socialize with other people; (3) when they are intimately involved with a few selected individuals; (4) when they have some vocation or profession and are able to take care of themselves economically; and (5) when they engage in various kinds of recreational pursuits, such as art, music, literature, sports, crafts, and games.

Starting, then, with their basic goals *(G)*, people frequently encounter blocks or frustrations that tend to prevent them from reaching these goals. In RET, we call these blocks or hassles negative Activating Events (*A*s). Once these negative Activating Events (*A*s) occur, people have the choice of feeling appropriately or inappropriately, of behaving self-helpingly, self-defeatingly at point *C* (their emotional and behavioral Consequences). In order to survive and be reasonably happy, they tend to react appropriately most of the time to the negative *A*s in their lives. Thus, when they fail and get rejected at some important task—for example, getting a good job or establishing a love relationship—they generally feel appropriately frustrated, disappointed, and sorry; and these feelings, though negative and unpleasant, are good in the sense that they spur people who fail and get rejected to return to their Goals *(G)* and to the Activating Events (As) that block these goals and to try to change the latter so that they can later succeed and get accepted and thereby achieve their goals.

The main reason, RET holds, that humans feel and act appropriately when they are confronted with frustrating Activating Events is because they have, at point B, rational or realistic Beliefs (rBs), such as: "I don't like failing at this task, and I hope that I am able to succeed at it next time. And I distinctly prefer getting accepted rather than rejected by significant others; but if I do get rejected, that's only unfortunate, and hardly the end of the world, and I can try again and do my best to get accepted next time."

RET theorizes, in other words, that whenever people feel badly and therefore act appropriately to change the frustrating Activating Events of their lives, it is not these events, in their own right, that drive them to feel and behave in this self-helping manner. Rather, it is mainly their rational, sensible Beliefs (Bs) about such events (As).

More importantly, if we look at human disturbance, RET holds that self-defeating feelings and behaviors largely (not completely) stem from people's irrational Beliefs (iBs) at point B. Thus, when they fail and get rejected, at point A (Activating Event), they consciously or unconsciously tell themselves something like, "I absolutely should not have failed and ought not have got rejected. Because I did fail and get rejected, as I must not, it is awful, I can't stand it, I am an inadequate person, who deserves to fall on my face; and I am so inadequate that I'll doubtless always fail in the future and never get accepted by significant others!"

Virtually all the other cognitive-behavioral therapies basically agree with The ABCs of RET but with some significant differences:

1. Although almost all cognitive and cognitive-behavior therapies follow my lead—just as I followed that of Epictetus (1890), Marcus Aurelius (1890), and other early philosophers—and hold that irrational Beliefs (iBs) lead to human disturbance, they often imply that any and all irrationalities produce emotional upsets (Beck, 1976; Burns, 1980). This is hardly true, for as John Dewey (1915) pointed out early in this century, people can believe the craziest things and often not make themselves needlessly suffer. Indeed, as Richard Lazarus (Lazarus & Folkman, 1984) has correctly indicated, people's irrational and unrealistic thinking—such as their ideas that they have a non-fatal illness when they really have a fatal one—may at times even help them to be less disturbed than they might otherwise be.

Noting this, RET hypothesizes that people mainly—perhaps only—upset themselves with evaluative irrational Beliefs rather than with nonevaluative ones. Thus, if you devoutly believe that your fairy godmother looks out for you and is always ready to help you, you may live happily and undisturbedly with this highly questionable and unrealistic Belief. But if you evaluate your fairy godmother's help as extremely desirable and go even further to insist that because it is desirable, you absolutely must at all times have her help, you will almost certainly make yourself anxious (whenever you realize that her magical help that you must have may actually be absent) and you will tend to make yourself extremely depressed (when you see that in your hour of need this help actually does not materialize).

RET, then, does not concern itself with any or all irrationalities but only with those that are evaluative and that are tied up with your strong desires and commands. Unlike a teacher of logic who might try to help you give up all your unrealistic and illogical thinking, a rational-emotive therapist only deals with your iBs about what you think you want and what you believe you therefore need. It explains and disputes only those irrationalities that interfere with your goals, desires, purposes and ideas; and it thereby aims for relatively brief and efficient therapy (Bard,

1980; Dryden, 1984; Ellis, 1984e, 1985a; Ellis & Abrahms, 1978; Ellis & Harper, 1975; Walen, DiGiuseppe, & Wessler, 1980; Wessler & Wessler, 1980).

2. RET makes a special attempt to operationally define rational Beliefs (rBs) and to distinguish them clearly from irrational Beliefs (iBs). By the same token, it is practically the only popular school of therapy that precisely distinguishes inappropriate from appropriate feelings and self-helping from self-defeating behaviors. Following Dewey's (1915) pragmatism, RET mainly defines rational Beliefs as those that tend to help people better achieve their personally chosen goals and values and therefore abet their self-interest, as well as preserve the social group in which they choose to live. Irrational Beliefs (iBs) are evaluations that tend to sabotage people's goals and values and lead them to experience needless pain, suffering, lack of pleasure, and sometimes premature annihilation.

Usually, rBs that help people are logical and realistic while iBs that harm people are illogical and unrealistic. But not necessarily! For, as noted above, illogical Beliefs—such as, "Because the person whom I love rejected me, there must be something wrong with me"—may be followed by highly rational Beliefs—such as, "Even if there is something wrong with me, I can most probably find some other suitable person to love me." And unrealistic or antiempirical Beliefs—such as, "Now that I have been rejected by the person I love, everyone I love will surely reject me"—can also be followed by a rational Belief—such as, "Even if everyone I ever love rejects me, I can still live without love and lead a pretty happy life."

Only certain kinds of iBs—especially godlike demands and commands on yourself, on other people and on the universe—almost always will cause you severe feelings of anxiety, depression, rage, and self-downing. For example: "Because no person whom I love must reject me, and this particular one did, I am a rotten, worthless individual who can never be loved by any suitable partner! Therefore, I never can be happy at all!" This Belief is both illogical (an overgeneralization and a nonsequitur) and unrealistic (opposed to reality). But what makes it really irrational is that it will almost always lead its believer to be depressed and self-hating and, instead of trying for a new love relationship, encourage him or her to withdraw from future involvements.

In RET, then, we are not looking merely for iBs but for those that lead to inappropriate feelings of anxiety, depression, rage, and self-hatred that often lead to self-defeating behaviors and that therefore bring people needless pain and minimal happiness.

3. Where the cognitive behavioral therapies of Beck (1976), Maultsby (1984), Meichenbaum (1977), and other cognitivists emphasize quite a number of unrealistic and illogical inferences and assumptions that are normally false, and that can fairly easily be disputed by therapists, RET assumes that these are indeed irrational Beliefs (iBs) and that they truly tend to cause disturbances, but that they would rarely exist without being derived from unconditional and absolutistic musts. Therefore, therapists who try to uproot these iBs without getting to and extirpating their musturbatory core may indeed help their clients, but will probably do so in a somewhat superficial and inelegant way.

Thus, if you refuse to date me or marry me, when I strongly want you to do so, I can unrealistically and illogically infer, (a) "There is something radically wrong with me," (b) "I am a totally rotten person," and (c) "I'll never be able to date or to marry anyone whose love I truly want to win." The first of these inferences is probably wrong, because you may reject me for a good many reasons other than there being something radically wrong with me. The second inference is clearly an illogical overgeneralization, because even if there is something wrong with me and I am not very good at winning people's love, that hardly makes me a totally rotten individual. The third inference is also false—or at least unprovable—because even if you and many other potential partners reject me, that doesn't prove that I'll *never* be able to date or to marry anyone whose love I truly desire to win.

All my inferences, therefore, are unrealistic and/or illogical; and you, as my therapist, could fairly easily rip them up and convince me that I am foolishly upsetting myself by invalidly making them. In doing so, however, you would be helping me in a highly inelegant way. For you would not be getting at my basic irrational demands on myself—my unconditional and absolutistic musts.

For the underlying, and highly important, reason why I am falsely concluding that, "There is something radically wrong with me" when you reject my overtures for dating or for marriage, is because I bring to your rejection (at point *A*, my Activating Event), the conscious or unconscious premise that you (and every other person in whom I am truly interested) absolutely *must*, at all times and under all conditions, approve of me. And when I don't get your approval, as I unconditionally *must*, I *then* infer that there must be something radically wrong with me—as, of course, I think that there *must* not be.

Again, the basic reason why I probably conclude, "I am a totally rotten person," when you reject me is because, when I ask for your (or anyone else's) acceptance, I fundamentally believe that I completely *must* be able to win it. And since I am not doing what I thoroughly *must* do, I *therefore* falsely conclude that I am *totally* rotten—instead of more sanely concluding that I am a *person who* badly failed this time, but that that never makes me a wholly *rotten person.*

Still again, the main reason why, when you reject me for dating or for marriage, I mistakenly conclude, "I'll never be able to date or to marry anyone whose love I truly want to win" is because this overgeneralized idea is largely a *derivative* of my *must.* What *must*? Well, pretty ob-

viously, my view that I absolutely *must* win every significant person whose love I crave; and that *therefore* if I fail to do this, fail to do what I *have to do*, I am "obviously" a person who will *never* be able to date or to marry anyone whom I truly find desirable.

So RET contends that just about all the main irrationalities that I have described in my writings and papers since 1956 and that are also included in those of other leading cognitive-behavior therapists seem to be derivatives of underlying, conscious or unconscious, absolutistic and dogmatic *shoulds* and *musts.* As Karen Horney (1945) correctly stated, we all tend to upset ourselves by the "tyranny of the shoulds." RET, going even further than Horney, holds that this is the main and the most important, way in which we basically create our own disturbances. Unless we acknowledge this, we can indeed discover and uproot our self-defeating irrationalities; but not as elegantly or permanently as when we do fully see our unconditional *musts* and forcefully and actively undermine them.

4. Because of its emphasis on the importance of *must*urbatory thinking in the creation of emotional disturbances, RET employs all the methods of Disputing irrational Beliefs that the other cognitive-behavioral therapies employ. But it also tried to get to and to help clients surrender the main derivative *iB*s that they commonly (though not always) derive from their *musts.* These *iB*s include: "Because I *must* succeed at important tasks and *have to* get accepted by significant people, (1) It's *awful* and *terrible* when I fail and get rejected, (2) I *can't stand* failure and rejection, (3) I'm an *inadequate* and *unlovable* person for failing and being disapproved, (4) I'll *always* fail and *never* get accepted, (5) I am so bad that I really don't *deserve* to have a good life and only *merit* continued pain and suffering.

As RET practitioners help clients to clearly perceive and actively Dispute (at point D) their *must*urbatory Beliefs, they also show them that they derive these main illogical and unrealistic inferences from their *musts*—and they teach clients how to surrender these, too. But in so doing, they practically never neglect—as other cognitive-behavior therapists often do—clients' absolutistic shoulds, oughts, and musts.

ACTIVE-DIRECTIVE DISPUTING OF IRRATIONAL BELIEFS

Because I derived the cognitive aspects of RET largely from philosophy rather than from psychology and because philosophers, from the time of Socrates and Plato, have actively disputed their students' mistaken ideas, I incorporated active disputation of irrational Beliefs in RET when I first began to use it in 1955. Behavior therapy, of course, also uses active teaching and demonstration methods, so I had a good active-directive model from that source. Finally, my previous experience of six years with the passive and nondirective methods of psychoanalysis convinced me that sitting and waiting for clients to fully understand themselves and thereby supposedly change their ways got them (and me!) practically nowhere. So I certainly was not going to fool around with that kind of passivity any longer!

Even more importantly, experimentation and research with my first attempts at RET showed me that clients with whom I had been doing psychoanalysis for several years and with whom I had made minimal progress often improved quickly and dramatically when I started to use RET (Ellis, 1957b). So while other cognitive-behavioral therapies take pride in slow and cautious (or I would say, namby-pamby) disputing, RET maintains that many (though hardly all) clients can quickly learn how to see, explore and Dispute their irrational Beliefs. So I, as well as many other, RETers Dispute clients' *iBs* in a highly active-directive manner from their first session onward. If this kind of fast-paced RET seems too rapid for some clients, we then slow down appreciably.

But not before we test out the more active-directive modes of Disputing, to see if they soon begin to work (Ellis, 1962, 1971a, 1973, 1985a).

THE USE OF THE SCIENTIFIC METHOD IN RET

As noted above, RET sees human disturbance—or at least neurosis—as being almost synonymous with absolutistic, dogmatic, rigid thinking. It also sees modern science as being flexible, probabilistic, and ever willing to change its theories for more accurate and better versions—or even to surrender them completely. RET, therefore, not only uses the scientific method to evaluate its own theories and practices, but is virtually the only major therapy that specializes in teaching clients, whenever they are capable of learning and using it, how to apply the scientific method to their own thinking and behaving. Not that science is sacred or infallible, for it isn't. But RET hypothesizes that using it rigorously provides the best current method of understanding our disturbance-creating dogmas and of efficiently uprooting them.

COGNITIVE, EMOTIVE AND BEHAVIORAL EMPHASIS

Some cognitive therapists—such as Paul Dubois (1907) and Alfred Adler (1927)—almost exclusively used intellectual techniques like persuasion and teaching. Other cognitivists, such as George Kelly (1955), mainly stress emotive techniques like fixed role playing. Still other cognitive-behavioral therapists, such as Emmelkamp (Emmelkamp, Kuipers, & Eggeraat, 1978), mainly use behavioral methods like *in vivo* desensitization. From the start, RET has always emphasized all three of these modalities, thus becoming the first major school of therapy to be truly multimodal. But it is not multimodal for the reason noted by Arnold Lazarus (1981), namely, that technical eclecticism is pragmatic and often works. Instead, the theory of RET states (as noted above) that cognitions, emotions and feelings are inexorably intertwined and that, as I stated in my first paper on RET (Ellis, 1958) and restated in *Reason and Emotion in Psychotherapy* (Ellis, 1962, pp. 38–39, 52):

> The theoretical foundations of RET are based on the assumption that human thinking and emotion are *not* two disparate or different processes, but that they significantly overlap and are in some respect, for all practical purposes, essentially the same thing. Like the other two basic life processes, sensing and moving, they are integrally interrelated and never can be seen wholly apart from each other.

> In other words: none of the four fundamental life operations—sensing, moving, emoting, and thinking—is experienced in isolation. If an individual senses or perceives something (e.g., sees a stick), he also tends, at the very same time, to do something about it (pick it up, kick it, or throw it away), to have some feelings about it (like it or dislike it), and to think about it (remember seeing it previously or imagine what he can do with it). Similarly, if he acts, emotes, or thinks he *also* consciously or unconsciously involves himself in the other behavior processes.

> Instead, then, of saying that "Smith thinks about this problem," we had better more accurately say that "Smith senses-moves-feels-THINKS about this problem."

> The rational therapist believes that sustained negative emotions—such as intense depression, anxiety, anger, and guilt—are almost always unnecessary to human living, and that they can be minimized if people learn consistently to think straight and to follow up their straight thinking with effective action. It is his or her job to show clients how to think straight and act effectively.

QUESTION 3: *WHAT ARE SEEN AS THE BENEFITS AND LIMITATIONS OF RATIONAL-EMOTIVE THERAPY?*

As I think I clearly noted in the final chapter of *Reason and Emotion in Psy-*

chotherapy (Ellis, 1962), all modes of psychotherapy, including RET, have their serious limitations. People *easily* and *naturally* disturb themselves, and often have difficulty making significant—let alone radical—personal changes. Virtually none of them, even with the effective use of RET, ever get completely cured, although they often appreciably improve. For, at least in part, disturbance or self-defeating behavior is the human condition and never is completely and intrinsically erased (Ellis, 1976c, 1985a).

RET holds, for example, that its own (and other therapies'!) benefits are limited by several basic, innately predisposed irrationalities: (1) Because people's disturbed feelings are often profoundly experienced, they falsely think they are inevitable and unchangeable and they only weakly (and meekly!) work to change them. (2) Because they feel badly almost immediately after Activating Events occur, they are sure that these *A*s indubitably cause their emotional Consequences (*C*s) and that they can only change their Cs by changing their *A*s. (3) Because harmful feelings, such as severe anxiety, guilt and anger, lead to *some* good results, people think that they are good or useful and should be cherished rather than minimized. (4) Because some feelings, such as legitimate concern and caution, overlap with some inappropriate negative feelings, such as severe anxiety and panic, people (and therapists!) confuse the two and have great trouble keeping the former while surrendering the latter. (5) Some RET techniques—such as taking responsibility for one's poor performances but refusing to damn oneself for indulging in them—require subtle and discriminative thinking by clients, and a number of such clients are not too capable of that kind of thinking. (6) RET requires a certain age level and intellectual capacity (such as a chronological age of eight *and* average intelligence) before clients can adequately understand and use it—and especially before they can use it in any elegant manner.

But many individuals, of course, do not have these capacities.

In addition to these common interferences with RET—and with other kinds of therapy—most people seem to have many biological predispositions that encourage them to *easily* disturb themselves and to encounter *great difficulty* in making themselves less disturbed. As noted in *Reason and Emotion in Psychotherapy* (Ellis, 1962) and in *Overcoming Resistance* (Ellis, 1985a), some of the main resistances to change include: (1) A tendency to habituate themselves to dysfunctional thoughts, feelings and behaviors and to have trouble dehabituating and unlearning these self-defeating practices. (2) A tendency to surrender to physical, emotional and intellectual inertia. (3) A propensity to be short-sighted and to be short-range rather than long-range hedonists. (4) An inclination to strongly desire and be greatly excited by many acts and substances (such as gambling and boozing) in spite of their obviously harmful aspects. (5) An exceptionally powerful tendency to be highly suggestible, gullible, and over-conforming. (6) A penchant for overvigilance and panic instead of normal caution and concern. (7) A predilection for grandiosity. (8) An affinity for extremism and all-or-none thinking. (9) A predisposition for arrant wishful-thinking. (10) An incredibly powerful appetite for procrastination and avoidance. (11) A frequent refusal to persist at desirable personality and other changes. (12) An erroneous tendency to overgeneralize and to fall prey to many other logical fallacies. (13) A pronounced proclivity for unthinkingness and rashness. (14) An immense susceptibility for disturbing themselves and downing themselves for their disturbances. (15) A ubiquitous talent for dogmatic, absolutistic, rigid, antiscientific thinking.

These are only a few of the major cognitive, emotive and behavioral propensities that virtually all humans have for easily disturbing themselves and for stubbornly resisting self-helping change (Ainslie, 1974; Ellis, 1962, 1976b, 1985a, 1985d; Frankel, 1973; Frazer, 1959; Hoffer, 1951; Kahneman & Tversky, 1973; Korzybski, 1933; Levi-Strauss, 1970; Pitkin, 1932; Rachleff, 1973; Tversky & Kahneman, 1981, 1983).

This is not to say that the prospect of humans drastically changing themselves is hopeless. On the contrary! For as Maslow (1962), Rogers (1961), Berne (1972), and others have shown, and as I have repeatedly emphasized in RET (Ellis, 1962, 1971a, 1973; Ellis & Harper, 1975), virtually all people have strong self-actualizing as well as self-defeating tendencies. They are born and reared to think, to think about their thinking, and to think about thinking about their thinking. Therefore, in spite of their cognitive-emotive-behavioral limitations they can also, if they work hard enough at it, make profound philosophic changes. Otherwise, psychotherapy, including RET, would be useless.

So I take an optimistic instead of pessimistic view of the possibilities of psychotherapy. But I think we had better also realistically admit its distinct limitations and imperfections. Including those of RET!

In spite of its limitations, RET has some unique benefits, including these:

1. It is an intrinsically brief therapy, since it almost always tries to zero in, as quickly as possible, on clients' *basic* irrational Beliefs, and to show them how to dispute and act against them. It therefore often helps people in a few sessions and, if clients will work at using it, rarely fails to help them make significant gains within three to six months.

2. It aims not only for effectiveness but efficiency—and for using mainly those techniques that work but also those that potently and economically work with the majority of clients—such as active disputing of *iB*s, rational-emotive imagery, shame-attacking exercises, and *in vivo* desensitization. If these techniques do not prove to be effective with some clients, RET then has at its disposal scores of other cognitive, emotive, and behavioral

methods that may be uniquely effective for special or difficult clients (Ellis, 1985a).

3. Although it is most effective with intelligent, educated and well-motivated clients, RET can be toned down, put in very simple language and taught to young children, to dull and uneducated clients, and to resistant individuals (Bernard & Joyce, 1984; Ellis, 1985a; Ellis & Bernard, 1983, 1985). It may well be more applicable to a wider range of individuals than any of the other popular schools of therapy.

4. While first designed for regular psychotherapy clients, RET has now been incorporated into many teaching, business, communication, recreational, and other psychoeducational applications and has been incorporated into many self-help materials. It consequently has been helpful to literally millions of individuals who have had little or no psychotherapy (Bingham, 1982; Ellis, 1957a, 1973, 1976a, 1977a; Ellis & Becker, 1982; Ellis & Bernard, 1985; Ellis & Knaus, 1977; Hauck, 1973, 1974; Knaus, 1974; Powell, 1976).

5. While many popular schools of therapy—such as psychoanalysis, Gestalt therapy, client-centered therapy, and experiential therapy—have very few outcome studies that show they are effective when used in controlled research studies, RET and CBT now are backed by over 200 controlled experiments, the vast majority of which show that they have greater effectiveness than other forms of therapy and other waiting list control groups (DiGiuseppe, Miller & Trexler, 1979; Ellis, 1979c; McGovern & Silverman, 1984; Meichenbaum, 1977; Meichenbaum & Jaremko, 1983; Miller & Betman, 1983).

6. Although I first created RET as a method of individual therapy, on a one-to-one basis, it has now been successfully adapted to a number of other therapeutic modes, including group therapy, rational encounter marathons, large-scale workshops, rational training intensives, public demonstrations, computer-assisted therapy, crisis intervention, and other forms of therapy (Ellis, 1969, 1973; Ellis &

Abrahms, 1980; Institute for Rational-Emotive Therapy, 1985–1986).

QUESTION 4: *HOW DOES RET TRAIN STUDENTS? WHAT ARE THE QUALITIES THAT ARE IMPORTANT IN A PSYCHOTHERAPY TRAINEE?*

The Institute for Rational-Emotive Therapy has been training students in RET since its founding in 1959, at first with one, two- and three-day workshops and, since 1968, on a three-level certificate-granting basis. At present, primary certificates in RET have been granted to more than a thousand professionals, all of whom have at least a master's degree in psychology, counseling, social work, or an allied field and who then take an intensive five-day practicum (or its equivalent) in the theory and practice of rational-emotive therapy and who pass a test showing that they have some degree of competence in RET.

Holders of primary certificates, however, are not considered to be well-trained RETers. Trainees are qualified for referrals only after they have become Associate Fellows or full Fellows of the Institute. These two groups qualify only after they have had two more years of intensive RET training, including supervision of at least 25 sessions of individual and/or group therapy and also a considerable number of theoretical seminars and knowledge of the main RET writings and recordings. To date, several hundred therapists have received Associate Fellowship certificates and are on the Institute's referral list.

On the highest level of training, full Fellows of the Institute are required to come to the Institute's main branch in New York for two years and be intensively supervised in individual, group, workshop, and other modes of RET. Associate Fellows and Fellows are then eligible for the special supervisory training which may qualify them to become qualified supervisors of RET trainees.

As I have noted in *Overcoming Resis-*

tance: Rational-Emotive Therapy with Difficult Clients (Ellis, 1985a), virtually all therapy trainees had better have several important characteristics. Thus, they must be vitally interested in helping their clients; unconditionally accept their clients as people; have a wide knowledge of therapeutic theories and practices and be flexible and undogmatic in using various techniques; be effective at communication; be patient and persistent in their therapeutic endeavors; be ethical and responsible and use therapy for the benefit of clients rather than for personal indulgence; freely refer to other therapists clients they think they can't help; and try to be neither underinvolved nor overinvolved with clients they retain.

In addition to these and other general therapeutic qualities, RET practitioners had better have the following characteristics: (1) Enjoy being active and directive. (2) Be devoted to philosophy, science, logic, and empiricism. (3) Be skilled teachers and communicators. (4) Have high frustration tolerance and unconditional self-acceptance. (5) Enjoy problem-solving. (6) Be experimental and risk-taking. (7) Have a good sense of humor. (8) Be energetic and forceful. (9) Be well informed about the theory and practice of RET and be willing to apply it in a consistent but unrigid manner (Ellis, 1984a, 1984b, 1985a; Wessler & Ellis, 1980, 1983). Naturally, all rational-emotive therapists will not ideally have all these characteristics. But it would be nice if they did!

QUESTION 5: *HOW IS THE EFFECTIVENESS OF RET EVALUATED? WHAT IS THE PLACE OF THERAPY RESEARCH?*

Effectiveness of RET (and of CBT) is mainly evaluated by controlled experimental studies, especially those that include legitimate control groups. It is *not* evaluated by case tests or anecdotal material. At the Institute for Rational-Emotive Therapy in New York (and at several of our affiliated institutes in U.S. and abroad), we keep evaluating RET in a number of ways, including these:

1. We regularly question our clients and ex-clients to see how they are improving—and not improving—and what they find helpful and unhelpful in working with our therapists.

2. We have been engaged for the last year in a comprehensive research study that evaluates, with several standard tests and special rationality questionnaires, how our clients at the Institute think, feel, and behave when they enter therapy and how they progress—or retrogress—every month they continue in therapy.

3. We evaluate our workshops and intensives to see how they are received by the participants and how helpful they are to them. We use these evaluations to modify our future presentations.

4. We retain the Biographical Information Forms that all our clients fill out before they enter therapy at the Institute and feed data from them into our computer, to keep researching several important psychological and sociological variables that the data on these forms include.

5. We have a research requirement for all our Fellows of the Institute and a number of them have published RET studies based on the work they have done to fulfill their requirement.

QUESTION 6: *HOW HAS RET EVOLVED, AND WHERE DO YOU SEE IT EVOLVING? WHERE DO YOU SEE PSYCHOTHERAPY EVOLVING?*

RET has evolved in many important ways since I first created and started to use it early in 1955. These ways include:

1. Beginning purely as individual one-to-one therapy, it soon grew into group RET as well, and now group RET is very popular with RETers and is one of its most important aspects. We now have eight therapy groups at the Institute and many

other RET groups exist in various parts of the world.

2. A few years after beginning to do RET, I also began to give public workshops in which I presented it to large public groups—ranging from 30 to 2,000 people. I have now given over 1500 of these public workshops, and many other RETers have given thousands.

3. Beginning in 1955, I presented several public talks on RET; since that time I and other RET professionals have given hundreds of such talks every year. In addition, scores of RETers keep making radio and TV presentations on its theory and practice, and the Institute for Rational-Emotive Therapy distributes many of these presentations on audio and video tapes.

4. Since 1955, I have published close to 50 books and over 500 articles on RET, many of which are specially designed for self-help purposes. Other authors have presented RET in hundreds of books and thousands of articles. Many millions of readers have been reached through this medium.

5. RET has been taught for the last 30 years in many high schools, colleges and graduate classes and is often one of the most popular courses on college campuses.

6. Since 1983 RET has been available as computer software. The Institute in New York now has plans to present it on educational laser disks for mass presentation to businesses, schools, clinics, and individuals who have access to computers.

7. While RET was first developed for therapists and their clients it has such broad general applications that it has now been applied to many other fields, including politics, the law, communication, leadership, corporate services, criminology, philosophy, education, anthropology, sex and marriage relations, parenting, and other areas (Ellis & Bernard, 1985).

8. When I started to use RET in 1955, I formulated ten major irrational Beliefs (iBs) that lead to human disturbance and these have been cited in hundreds of books and thousands of articles. More than 20 standardized tests of irrationality have been derived from these beliefs and about 250 research studies have been done so far, almost all of which show that people with more serious disturbances acknowledge holding more irrational Beliefs than those who are less seriously disturbed. These tests have also been found useful in a great number of psychotherapy outcome research studies (DiGiuseppe, Miller, & Trexler, 1979; Ellis, 1979c).

9. As I worked over the years with RET, I discovered that all the basic irrational Beliefs that people hold can be condensed into three major unconditional musts and that musturbatory thinking underlies virtually all the 20 or more unrealistic and illogical ideas that tend to create human disturbance (Ellis, 1976c, 1977a, 1979a, 1984d, 1985a, 1985b; Ellis & Becker, 1982; Ellis & Grieger, 1977; Ellis & Harper, 1975). As noted previously in this paper, the new developments in RET shoulds and musts have helped make RET a briefer but at the same time more philosophic and more profound form of therapy.

10. Although RET was confrontative, evocative, and emotive from the start, it has become even more emotive and forceful over the years and now employs a number of experiential and encounter methods that did not exist in 1955 but that fit beautifully into RET theory and practice. In the 1960s I invented a number of experiential exercises—such as my rather famous shame-attacking exercise—and incorporated them into RET group therapy and encounter therapy (Ellis, 1969). I also began emphasizing forceful self-dialogues and other vigorous and vivid methods of RET (Dryden, 1984; Ellis, 1971a, 1985a; Ellis & Abrahms, 1978; Ellis & Becker, 1982; Maultsby & Ellis, 1974). Although originally accused of being too "rational" and too "unemotive," RET is now actually the most emotive of the major cognitive therapies and in many ways stresses vigorous and dramatic techniques more than many of the experiential therapies.

11. As mentioned above, RET has al-

ways used homework assignments—cognitive, emotive and behavioral. The first systematic cognitive homework forms were devised by Jon Geis, myself, and Charles Stark in the 1960s. Maxie Maultsby (1971) particularly pushed cognitive homework when he began to do RET in the late 1960s and early 1970s. The Institute for Rational-Emotive Therapy began to use self-help report forms with most of its clients when it began its psychological clinic in New York in 1968 (Ellis, 1971b) and it has revised and simplified its regular form over the years and encourages all its clients to use the latest version of the Rational Self Help Form (Sichel & Ellis, 1984).

12. RET has always specialized in humorously ripping up people's irrational Beliefs, because its theory holds that people had better take themselves and their lives seriously and be committed to vital and absorbing interests (Ellis & Harper, 1961a, 1961b, 1975). But it also contends that emotional disturbance arises when people take things *too* seriously and give themselves and others *highly exaggerated* or *sacrosanct* importance. Beginning in 1976, at the annual meeting of the American Psychological Association (Ellis, 1977a, 1977b) in Washington, I sang some of the rational humorous songs that I had been using with clients for a few years before that. These songs became such an instant hit that I and many other RETers have used them with many clients and at talks and workshops since that time, and we have found them to be quite helpful to many depressed, anxious, and hostile individuals (Ellis, 1981, in press - b).

13. As noted above, RET disagrees with some of the claims of family systems therapists that changing the system in which people reside will profoundly change the personality of those in the system. But it has developed its own comprehensive form of systems therapy which it employs, first, to help change the irrational Beliefs, inappropriate feelings and dysfunctional behaviors of all the people in a family (or other) system and then *also* to change some of the important dysfunctional aspects of the system itself. In this respect, RET has now become perhaps the most systematic of all the various schools of systems therapy (Ellis, 1985a).

14. RET included the teaching of unconditional acceptance to clients when I first did it in 1955, after I had derived this idea from some of the existential philosophers, particularly from Paul Tillich (1953). So I taught people to unconditionally accept themselves just because they are human, just because they exist (Ellis, 1957a, 1962; Ellis & Harper, 1961a, 1961b). I later realized, however, that this is a good practical solution to the problem of human worth because anyone who adapts it cannot possibly hate himself or herself, but that it is philosophically unsound because there is no way of proving or falsifying the proposition, "I am good because I exist," nor is there any way of proving or falsifying the contrary proposition, "I am bad because I exist." Rating one's *self*, *existence*, *being* or *totality*, moreover, is always inaccurate, as Korzybski (1933) has shown, since it is an overgeneralized abstraction. You *are* so many things, traits, deeds, and performances that you have no way of giving a single, global rating to your *you-ness* or *yourself.* Modern RET, therefore, is probably the only system of therapy that tries to help people *only* rate their thoughts, feelings and behaviors (in regard to how effectively they fulfill people's chosen goals and purposes) and not to rate their *selves* or *being* at all (Ellis, 1972, 1973, 1976b).

Where do I see RET evolving? First of all, I think and, of course, fondly hope that some of its most important aspects—especially showing people that they mainly upset themselves by rigidly holding dogmatic *shoulds* and *musts* and teaching them how to surrender their antiscientific thinking—will be incorporated into virtually all schools of therapy. This is already happening, so that even psychoanalysis, Gestalt therapy, and systems therapy are being much more rational-emotive and cognitive-behavioral than they previously have been

(Bieber, 1981; Goldfried, 1980; Kraft, 1969; Wachtel, 1978).

Second, I see RET specifically and psychotherapy in general evolving away from their present emphasis on individual and small group therapy and mightily expanding into the field of educational and mass media therapy. RET is already largely a form of active-directive teaching: because its practitioners, from the first session onward, show clients the ABCs of human disturbance; teach them how to use the scientific method to dispute their irrational Beliefs; guide them into accepting and devising for themselves cognitive, emotive and behavioral homework assignments; give them thinking and experiential exercises to do during and in between therapy sessions; use a great deal of bibliotherapy and audiovisual therapy; and employ a number of other psychoeducational methods. Consequently, RET is uniquely suited to mass media applications. And it is my prediction—and, again, fond hope—that in the future it will be widely used for individual and group therapy and even more widely taught in homes, schools, colleges, campuses, social institutions, political organizations, community centers, hospitals and other centers where both healthy and disturbed individuals can learn how to stubbornly refuse to seriously upset themselves about virtually anything—yes, anything!—and thereby live happier and more self-actualizing and socially involved lives (Ellis & Dryden, in press).

REFERENCES

Adler, A. (1927). *Understanding human nature*. New York: Greenberg.

Adler, A. (1964). *Social interest*. New York: Capricorn.

Ainslie, G. (1974). Specious reward: A Behavioral theory of impulse and impulse control. *Psychological Bulletin, 82,* 463–496.

Bard, J. A. (1980). *Rational therapy in practice*. Champaign, IL: Research Press.

Beck, A. T. (1976). *Cognitive therapy and the emotional disorders*. New York: International Universities Press.

Bernard, M. E., & Joyce, M. (1984). *Rational-emotive therapy with children and adolescents*. New York: Wiley.

Berne, E. (1964). *Games people play*. New York: Grove.

Berne, E. (1972). *What do you say after you say hello?* New York: Grove.

Bieber, I. (1981). *Cognitive psychoanalysis*. New York: Aronson.

Bingham, T. R. (1982). *Program for affective learning*. Blanding, UT: Metra.

Burns, D. (1980). *Feeling good*. New York: Morrow.

Dewey, J. (1915). Quoted in M. Davidson, Pragmatism, cognitive theory, and American clinical casework. Unpublished paper, 1985.

DiGiuseppe, R. A., Miller, N. J., & Trexler, L. D. (1979). A review of rational-emotive therapy outcome studies. In A. Ellis & J. M. Whiteley (Eds.), *Theoretical and empirical foundations of rational-emotive therapy* (pp. 218–235). Monterey, CA: Brooks/Cole.

Dryden, W. (1984). *Rational-emotive therapy: Fundamentals and innovations*. London: Croom Helm.

Dubois, P. (1907). *The psychic treatment of nervous disorders*. New York: Funk & Wagnalls.

Ellis, A. (1957a). *How to live with a neurotic*. New York: Crown. Rev. ed., North Hollywood, CA: Wilshire, 1975.

Ellis, A. (1957b). Outcome of employing three techniques of psychotherapy. *Journal of Clinical Psychology, 13,* 334–350.

Ellis, A. (1958). Rational psychotherapy. *Journal of General Psychology, 59,* 35–49.

Ellis, A. (1962). *Reason and emotion in psychotherapy*. Secaucus, NJ: Citadel.

Ellis, A. (1969). A weekend of rational encounter. In A. Burton (Ed.), *Encounter* (pp. 112–127). San Francisco: Jossey-Bass.

Ellis, A. (1971a). *Growth through reason*. North Hollywood, CA: Wilshire.

Ellis, A. (1971b). *Homework report*. New York: Institute for Rational-Emotive Therapy.

Ellis, A. (1971c). Problems of daily living workshop. In R. J. Menges & F. Pennington (Eds.), *A survey of 19 innovative educational programs for adolescents and adults* (pp. 49–51). Minneapolis: Youth Research Center.

Ellis, A. (1971d). Sexual adventuring and personality growth. In H. Otto (Ed.), *The new sexuality* (pp. 94–109). Palo Alto: Science and Behavior Books. Reprinted: New York: Institute for Rational-Emotive Therapy.

Ellis, A. (1972). *Psychotherapy and the value of a human being*. New York: Institute for Rational-Emotive Therapy.

Ellis, A. (1973). *Humanistic psychotherapy: The*

rational-emotive approach. New York: McGraw-Hill.

Ellis, A. (1976a). *Sex and the liberated man.* Secaucus, NJ: Lyle Stuart.

Ellis, A. (1976b). *RET abolishes most of the human ego. Psychotherapy, 13*(4), 343–348. Reprinted: New York: Institute for Rational-Emotive Therapy.

Ellis, A. (1976c). The biological basis of human irrationality. *Journal of Individual Psychology, 32,* 145–168. Reprinted: New York: Institute for Rational-Emotive Therapy.

Ellis, A. (1977a). *Anger—how to live with and without it.* Secaucus, NJ: Citadel.

Ellis, A. (1977b). Fun as psychotherapy. *Rational Living, 12*(1), 2–6. Also: Cassette recording. New York: Institute for Rational-Emotive Therapy.

Ellis, A. (1977c). *A garland of rational songs.* (Songbook and cassette recording.) New York: Institute for Rational-Emotive Therapy.

Ellis, A. (1979a). *The intelligent woman's guide to dating and mating.* Secaucus, NJ: Lyle Stuart.

Ellis, A. (1979b). Discomfort anxiety: A new cognitive-behavioral construct. Part 1. *Rational Living,* 14(2), 3–8.

Ellis, A. (1979c). Rational-emotive therapy: Research data that support the clinical and personality hypotheses of RET and other modes of behavior therapy. In A. Ellis & J. M. Whiteley (Eds.), *Theoretical and empirical foundations of rational-emotive therapy* (pp. 101–173). Monterey, CA: Brooks/Cole.

Ellis, A. (1980a). Discomfort anxiety: A new cognitive-behavioral construct. Part 2. *Rational Living,* 15(1), 25–30.

Ellis, A. (1981). The use of rational humorous songs in psychotherapy. *Voices, 16*(4), 29–36.

Ellis, A. (1983). *The case against religiosity.* New York: Institute for Rational-Emotive Therapy.

Ellis, A. (1984a). Rational-emotive therapy. In R. J. Corsini (Ed.), *Current psychotherapies* (pp. 197–238). Itasca, IL: Peacock.

Ellis, A. (1984b). Foreword to W. Dryden, *Rational-emotive therapy: Fundamentals and innovations* (pp. vii–xxvi). London: Croom Helm.

Ellis, A. (1984c). Is the unified-interaction approach to cognitive-behavior modification a reinvention of the wheel? *Clinical Psychology Review,* 4, 215–218.

Ellis, A. (1984d). Maintenance and generalization in rational-emotive therapy (RET). *Cognitive Behaviorist,* 6(1), 2–4. Rev. ed.: *How to use RET to maintain and enhance*

your therapeutic gains. New York: Institute for Rational-Emotive Therapy.

Ellis, A. (1984e). Use of personal computers in rational-emotive therapy. In R. A. Wakefield (Ed.), *The home computer, families, and the mental health professions* (pp. 18–20). Washington, DC: American Family, Inc.

Ellis, A. (1985a). *Overcoming resistance: Rational-Emotive Therapy with difficult clients.* New York: Springer.

Ellis, A. (1985b). Intellectual fascism. *Journal of the Institute for the New Man, 1*(1), 39–54. Reprinted: New York: Institute for Rational-Emotive Therapy.

Ellis, A. (1985c). A rational-emotive approach to acceptance and its relationship to EAP's. In S. H. Klarreich, J. L. Franeck, & C. E. Moore (Eds.), *The human resources management handbook* (pp. 325–330). New York: Praeger.

Ellis, A. (1985d). Two forms of humanistic psychology: Rational-emotive therapy vs. transpersonal psychology. *Free Inquiry, 15*(4), 14–21.

Ellis, A. (1985e). Expanding the ABC's of RET. In M. J. Mahoney & A. Freeman (Eds.), *Cognition and psychotherapy* (pp. 313–323). New York: Plenum.

Ellis, A. (in press-a). Fanaticism that may lead to a nuclear holocaust: The contributions of scientific counseling and psychotherapy. *Journal of Counseling and Development.*

Ellis, A. (in press-b). The use of rational humorous songs in psychotherapy. In W. A. Salemeh & W. F. Fry (Eds.), *Handbook of humor and psychotherapy.* San Diego: Professional Resource Exchange.

Ellis, A., & Abrahms, E. (1978). *Brief psychotherapy in medical and health practice.* New York: Springer.

Ellis, A., & Abrahms, E. (Speakers). (1980). *RET and crisis intervention* (Cassette Recording). New York: Institute for Rational-Emotive Therapy.

Ellis, A., & Becker, A. (1982). *A guide to personal happiness.* North Hollywood, CA: Wilshire.

Ellis, A., & Bernard, M. E. (Eds.). (1983). *Rational-emotive approaches to the problems of childhood.* New York: Plenum.

Ellis, A., & Bernard, M. E. (Eds.). (1985). *Clinical applications of rational-emotive therapy.* New York: Plenum.

Ellis, A., & Dryden, W. (in press). *The practice of rational-emotive therapy (RET).* New York: Springer.

Ellis, A., & Grieger, R. (Eds.). (1977). *Handbook of rational-emotive therapy.* Vol. 1. New York: Springer.

Ellis, A., & Harper, R. A. (1961a). *A guide to*

rational living. Englewood Cliffs, NJ: Prentice-Hall.

Ellis, A., & Harper, R. A. (1961b). *A guide to successful marriage.* North Hollywood, CA: Wilshire.

Ellis, A., & Harper, R. A. (1975). *A new guide to rational living.* North Hollywood, CA: Wilshire.

Ellis, A., & Knaus, W. (1977). *Overcoming procrastination.* New York: New American Library.

Ellis, A., & Whiteley, J. M. (Eds.). (1979). *Theoretical and empirical foundations of rational-emotive therapy.* Monterey, CA: Brooks/Cole.

Emmelkamp, P.M.G., Kuipers, A.C.M. & Eggeraat, J.B. (1978). Cognitive modification versus prolonged exposure in vivo: A comparison with agoraphobics as subjects. *Behaviour Research and Therapy, 16,* 33–41.

Epictetus. (1890). *The works of Epictetus.* Boston: Little, Brown.

Frankel, C. (1973). The nature and sources of irrationalism. *Science, 180,* 927–931.

Frazer, G. (1959). *The new golden bough.* New York: Braziller.

Goldfried, M. R. (1980). Toward the delineation of therapeutic change principles. *American Psychologist, 35,* 991–999.

Goulding, M. M., & Goulding, R. L. (1979). *Changing lives through redecision therapy.* New York: Brunner/Mazel.

Hauck, P. A. (1973). *Overcoming depression.* Philadelphia: Westminster.

Hauck, P. A. (1974). *Overcoming frustration and anger.* Philadelphia: Westminster.

Hoffer, E. (1951). *The true believer.* New York: Harper.

Horney, K. (1945). *Our inner conflicts.* New York: Norton.

Institute for Rational-Emotive Therapy (1985). *September 1985–March 1986 catalogue.* New York: Institute for Rational-Emotive Therapy.

Kahneman, D. & Tversky, A. (1973). On the psychology of prediction. *Psychological Bulletin, 80,* 237–250.

Kelly, G. (1955). *Psychology of personal constructs.* 2 vols. New York: Norton.

Kendall, P., & Hollon, J. (Eds.). (1979). *Cognitive-behavior interventions.* New York: Academic Press.

Knaus, W. (1974). *Rational-emotive education.* New York: Institute for Rational-Emotive Therapy.

Korzybski, A. (1933). *Science and sanity.* San Francisco: Institute for General Semantics.

Kraft, T. (1969). Psychoanalysis and behaviorism: A false antithesis. *American Journal of Psychotherapy, 23,* 482–487.

Lazarus, A. A. (1981). *The practice of multimodal therapy.* New York: McGraw-Hill.

Lazarus, R. S., & Folkman, S. (1984). *Stress, appraisal, and coping.* New York: Springer.

Levi-Strauss, C. (1970). *Savage mind.* Chicago: University of Chicago Press.

Mahoney, M. J. (1985). Psychotherapy and human change processes. In M. J. Mahoney & A. Freeman (Eds.), *Cognition and psychotherapy* (pp. 3–48). New York: Plenum.

Marcus Aurelius. (1890). *Meditations.* Boston: Little, Brown.

Maslow, A. H. (1962). *Toward a psychology of being.* New York: Van Nostrand Reinhold.

Maultsby, M. C., Jr. (1984). *Rational behavior therapy.* Englewood Cliffs, NJ: Prentice-Hall.

Maultsby, M. C., Jr. (1971a). *Handbook of rational self counseling.* Lexington, KY: Rational Self Help Books.

Maultsby, M. C., Jr. (1971b). Systematic written homework in psychotherapy. *Psychotherapy, 8,* 195–198.

Maultsby, M. C., Jr., & Ellis, A. (1974). *Technique of using rational-emotive imagery.* New York: Institute for Rational-Emotive Therapy.

McGovern, T. E., & Silverman, M. S. (1984). A review of outcome studies of rational-emotive therapy from 1977 to 1982. *Journal of Rational-Emotive Therapy, 2*(1), 7–18.

Meichenbaum, D. (1977). *Cognitive-behavior modification.* New York: Plenum.

Meichenbaum, D., & Jaremko, J. B. (Eds.). (1983). *Stress reduction and prevention.* New York: Plenum.

Miller, R.C., & Berman, J.S. (1983). The efficacy of cognitive behavior therapies: A quantitative review of the research evidence. *Psychological Bulletin, 94,* 39–53.

Pitkin, W. B. (1932). *A short introduction to the history of human stupidity.* New York: Simon and Schuster.

Popper, K. (1972). *Objective knowledge.* London: Oxford University Press.

Powell, J. (1976). *Fully human, fully alive.* Niles, IL: Argus.

Rachleff, O. (1973). *The occult conceit.* New York: Bell.

Rogers, C. R. (1961). *On becoming a person.* Boston: Houghton Mifflin.

Russell, B. (1950). *The conquest of happiness.* New York: Pocket Books.

Sichel, J., & Ellis, A. (1984). *RET self-help form.* New York: Institute for Rational-Emotive Therapy.

Sullivan, H. S. (1953). *The interpersonal theory of psychiatry.* New York: Norton.

Tillich, P. (1953). *The courage to be*. New York: Oxford.

Tversky, A., & Kahneman, D. (1981). The framing of decisions and the psychology of choice. *Science, 211*, 453–458.

Tversky, A., & Kahneman, D. (1983). Extensional versus intuitive reasons: The conjunction fallacy in probability judgment. *Psychological Review, 90*, 293–315.

Wachtel, P. (1978). *Psychoanalysis and behavior therapy*. New York: Basic Books.

Walen, S. R., DiGiuseppe, R., & Wessler, R. L.

(1980). *A practitioner's guide to rational-emotive therapy*. New York: Oxford.

Wessler, R. L., & Ellis, A. (1980). Supervision in rational-emotive therapy. In A. K. Hess (Ed.), *Psychotherapy supervision* (pp. 181–191). New York: Wiley.

Wessler, R. L., & Ellis, A. (1983). Supervision in counseling: Rational-emotive therapy. *Counseling Psychologist, 11*(1), 43–49.

Wessler, R. A., & Wessler, R. L. (1980). *The principles and practice of rational-emotive therapy*. San Francisco: Jossey-Bass.

Discussion by Mary McClure Goulding, M.S.W.

◆

It's a delight to be here on the platform with Dr. Ellis. I hope that all of you will take back with you the word "musterbation." I think that when clients and all of us come into therapy, there are three things we want: We want to grow, to change to live more fulfilled lives; that's one of them. The second is that, although we don't admit it, we sort of want to be told we're absolutely perfect just the way we are. Third, if we're not absolutely perfect just the way we are, it ought to be the fault of the people we're living with, or the people who raised us. It's a breath of fresh air to hear Ellis hew to the line all of these 25 years that I've heard of you that *we* are the ones who distress ourselves, *we* are the ones in charge of ourselves, and *we* are in charge of our own thinking, feeling and behavior. I think that's the bottom line for any change for anyone.

I'm delighted to hear that you're using all kinds of techniques. I've read your paper carefully, I like the broad range, and I'm still struck by the important part—the fact that we're in charge. I think that yours was a voice in the wilderness 25 years ago and I think that more and more

people accept this as the bottom line for therapy: that therapy isn't just empathy and caring and all that hot air, because that's stroking people for their pathology, that's taking their money without giving them good service. I've said that the first profession, "rent a lover," is much more honorable than the second, "rent an ever loving mommy or daddy." I like the briefness of your therapy and I don't have more to say. I'd like to hear from the audience. I'm just thrilled that more and more therapies are using your basic beliefs.

QUESTIONS AND ANSWERS

Question: Coming into this session, in a way I feel like I'm coming home, in that I have been most familiar with Dr. Ellis' work before this conference and so I feel a strong desire, "Yeh, that's the way I want to go, I want to give myself to that style of work." But then, in the past couple of days, I've been deeply moved and intrigued by other works: Masterson, on the one hand goes into much more of a diagnostic approach to understanding borderline and narcissistic patients and has a compelling rationale for how to do therapy. I feel like, "OK, I've got to read all of Masterson's books and maybe divert from the cognitive stuff." Then, I hear Whitaker, or the Ericksonians. How would you decide, if you were a student today, what kind of therapist you were going to be? How would you decide? How would you decide not to use the other approaches?

Ellis: Let me give my answer to that. The answer is, you would decide the best way, probably, and the most scientific way by experimenting. That's the way you normally decide anything, whether you're conscious of it or not. So you would take what you personally consider are the best of each or all of these approaches and you'd use it with your clients. You would, therefore, get more familiar and adept at it and then you would finally decide with controlled studies and with clinical observations of what works best with you for your clients. And you would either end up by abandoning all those techniques and using an original one of your own, or by abandoning most of them and focusing on one of them; or you could even end up by having a theory that is basically close to one of them. But, you would experimentally and experientially use a variety of techniques that you test in your own practice. There is no absolute answer to the question of what to use and what works for you and your client. So again, I say, "Experiment, experiment, experiment."

Question: You mentioned, Dr. Ellis, that 20 years ago or so you had a very long list of irrational behaviors and thoughts, and so forth. Now you have mentioned that you sort of worked it down to three. I would be interested in what those three are.

Ellis: I have them in the rest of my paper, but I thought that I might not have time to read the whole paper, so I omitted them. Let me say what they are. At first I pre-

sented 12 in my first paper on RET in 1956, at the American Psychological Association. Then I added another and got up to 13 and people added others. But I felt that practically all those that were added beyond the original 12 were just variations on the 12. Then, as I worked more and more in RET, I found to my surprise, that there were only really three. The others are subheadings under the three. Here are the three:

One, I *must* do well and be approved by *significant* others, and if I don't do as well as I *should* or *must*, there's something really rotten about me. It's terrible that I am this way and I am a pretty worthless, rotten person. That irrational belief leads to feelings of depression, anxiety, despair and self-doubting. It's an ego *must*. *I* have to do well or *I'm* no good.

The second irrational belief is, "You, other humans with whom I relate, my original family, my later family that I may have, my friends, my relatives, and people with whom I work, *must, ought,* and *should* treat me considerately and fairly and even *specially,* considering what a doll I am! Isn't it *horrible* that they don't and they had better roast in hell for eternity!" That's anger, that's rage, that's homicide, that's genocide.

Then the third irrational belief, "Conditions under which I live—my environment, social conditions, economic conditions, political conditions—*must* be arranged so that I easily and immediately, with no real effort, have a free lunch, get what I command. Isn't it horrible when those conditions are harsh and when they frustrate me? I can't stand it! I can't be happy *at all* under those awful conditions and I can only be miserable or kill myself!" That's low frustration tolerance.

Under these three major musts, which are all commands and demands, not merely strong preferences when people are disturbed, we have 10 to 20 subheadings. I deal with many neurotic persons (many of them to this day, since I have right now about 300 individual clients whom I fairly regularly see and five therapy groups. I also demonstrate with volunteers at my Friday night workshop and at presentations all over the world. So I may see more clients than any other therapist in the world). I find that every single time my clients talk about their depression, obsession, or compulsion, I can quickly, when using RET, within a few minutes, zero in on one, or two, or three of their major musts: "I *must* do well; you *must* treat me beautifully; the world *must* be easy." I then show these clients that they have these *musts* and teach them to surrender them. Now, they have many subheadings and variations on their musts but they all seem to be variations on a major theme, which I call "musterbation, absolutistic thinking or dogma," which, I hypothesize, is at the core of human disturbance.

Canter (moderator): Might I add, for myself I use the rubric, "Quit the musterbation, start the experimentation." Would that be fair, Al?

Ellis: That would be very good, Aaron. I said many years ago, that masterbation is good and delicious, but musterbation is evil and pernicious.

Question: You mentioned the educational applications with RET. I was wondering if you could comment how some of those applications are either being used now in some public school settings, for instance, maybe high school, or how you might envision the application of this in a general way in a high school situation?

Ellis: Well, we had a school for elementary school children for five years to test RET taught by teachers, not by therapists. The therapists supervised the teachers in their own little school and we found out, to my surprise, that Piaget was right and I was wrong. Below the age of eight, the children could learn the RET, they learned that activating events didn't upset them, that they upset themselves. They could tell you the difference between rational and irra-

tional ideas. But they didn't use it. They have low frustration tolerance and, as Piaget would have said, "They haven't reached good judgment yet."

But, above the age of eight, we found that the children were not only able to understand it, but to use it and do fairly well with it. So we experimented and we (the Institute for Rational-Emotive Therapy) published a book, in fact several, on Rational-Emotive Education, by William Knaus (1974).* Currently Thomas Bingham (1982), in California, has a syllabus for using RET for teaching in the classroom from about fourth grade upward.

Bingham is doing a good deal of research that he hasn't published yet, showing that when teachers teach RET in accordance with his syllabus in the classroom, the children feel better and act better and their parents like it as well. There have been about ten controlled studies teaching RET to children in the classroom, some in high schools, some in elementary schools, a few in the colleges. When tested with a control group, these studies, as I recall, show that children or students who learn the RET from teachers and by reading material, not from therapists, do significantly improve. So there's a good deal of research showing that RET works educationally. But we hope to perfect especially the educational mass media materials on it, which would consist of VCRs, audio cassettes, and laser discs, and bring RET more and more to the public in a systematic and researched way.

Question: Could you give us an example of shame-attacking exercise and the irrational song?

Ellis: The shame-attacking exercise gets to one of the main essences of human disturbance—embarrassment, shame, self-downing, or shithood. Most people feel like a worm when they do something wrong

---

* This and other references cited in this discussion can be found in the Reference List at the end of Dr. Ellis' paper.

or foolish in public. You say, "I feel ashamed," but you really mean, "I feel badly about myself." So we get people to go out in public and do some shame-attacking exercises. You can do anything that you feel is shameful as long as, first, you do not harm anybody, like slapping someone in the face; or, second, you don't get into trouble, such as getting arrested. Thus, you could walk naked in the streets of Phoenix, but the police would take a dim view of that, so I wouldn't advise that. So you do a shame-attacking exercise many times while working on your feelings so that you do not feel ashamed.

For example, one of the things you can do is go out on a bright, Sunday afternoon, like today, and walk a banana and feed it with another banana. Or you can go out on a sunny day with a raincoat and a black umbrella over your head. Or try the simpler one that a lot of people select, because it's fast and easy: You go into this convention center, or into the Hyatt or Hilton hotels, or on the streets of Phoenix, and you stop a stranger and say, "I just got out of the looney bin, what month is it?" Again, let me repeat the one I mentioned the other day, one of our famous ones. You go into a drugstore at a crowded hour and you say in a loud voice, preferably to a female clerk, "I'd like a gross of condoms, and since I use so many of them, I should get a special discount." Or you can walk down the street singing at the top of your lungs one of our rational-emotive songs or any song you feel like singing.

So there are many shame-attacking exercises you can figure out, but you had better use something that you personally would feel ashamed about. Don't do something that you enjoy and that you're not ashamed of.

You could also do a practical one. I'll give you an example. A woman in one of my therapy groups was ashamed to wear pants to work in her very distinguished law office. In her own garden on Long Island, she always wore pants; with her friends, that was OK. Her shame-attacking exercise was that on Monday morning she would go back to work wearing pants. And she did. She felt very ashamed at the beginning, but then she got over her shame after she did it a few times. And then she often wore pants to work, which she had always wanted to do. So it can be something practical that you're ashamed of doing that you'd like to do but hold yourself back from doing it.

You said you wanted an example of one of my rational humor songs. Well, let's see. I don't think you have songsheets. We have some extra ones that I have. So I'll sing you right now one of my rational humor songs. These songs are designed to show people how ridiculous their irrational ideas are. I hear somebody asking for the whining song. OK, I'll do the famous whining one, which is one of the favorites. It was the Yale Whiffinpoof song, whose tune happened to be written by a Harvard man in 1896. Yale took the tune and made it into "Ba Ba Ba." So our rational humorous version is:

> I cannot have all of my wishes filled.
> Whine, whine, whine.
> I cannot have every frustration stilled.
> Whine, whine, whine.
> Life really owes me the things that I miss!
> Fate has to grant me eternal bliss!
> Since I must settle for less than this,
> Whine, Whine, Whine.

Anyone who wants a songsheet and doesn't have one, can send to the Institute for Rational-Emotive Therapy, 45 East 65th Street, N.Y. N.Y., and we'll be glad to send you a songsheet, as well as our latest catalogue that has all kinds of RET material in it.

M. Goulding: May I make a comment? The songs are just wonderful. This is when I first fell in love with you, Dr. Ellis. When I was in the second grade, the teacher told me to only move my lips, because I couldn't sing and I threw everyone off. I didn't know that before and was horrified. I started singing again when my son was a little boy and he came home from nursery school and said, "Mother, you know all the songs but you don't sing them right. Let me show you." Then I heard you in a cast of thousands and you're not operatic material, naturally. Just singing and not being ashamed. And I thought, wow, this is really some guy.

Question: Dr. Ellis, in my understanding of mental disturbances, low self-esteem plays a very significant part in most disorders. Could you comment again about your concept of self-esteem?

Ellis: Yes, our concept is different from Nathaniel Branden's and that of most other people, who wrongly say, according to us, that if you esteem yourself, you have high self-regard and you're a healthy individual. And if you hate yourself, you're obviously unhealthy. Now the second is true, but we think that self-esteem is not good, either. We go along with Carl Rogers, who says it differently, but he goes for what is called "Unconditional Positive Regard."

Now, in RET we don't even like the term "regard," because regard is a rating and humans really can't rate themselves. You can rate any trait, any behavior, anything that you do, once you set a goal or purpose. If you want to walk across the street safely, you'd better look to the right and the left and watch the cars. Now, if you want to kill yourself while walking across the street, it would be good behavior not to look. Whatever your goal is, when you get to it and achieve it and abet it, that's good behavior; and whenever you defeat yourself, act against your own interests and goals and, as Alfred Adler said, against the interests of the social group in which you live, which you wouldn't want to harm because you will suffer indirectly, if not directly, that's poor behavior. But you cannot say, because I act well, I am a good person. That's what Nathaniel Branden is really saying: "I'm competent, and I act well, I know what I'm doing, therefore, I am OK." Because

if you say that, then when you're incompetent, as you will be, because you're a fallible human; and when you act poorly and do unethical things, back to shithood you will go. Even when you're competent, you worry about being incompetent *later.* I use with my clients the illustration of Thomas Eagen who wrote *Mr. Roberts* at the age of 28. This was a novel that sold very well. It was a play and became a movie with Henry Fonda. The author made millions and he killed himself. He committed suicide, as did Ross Rockridge, another novelist, and as did Malcom Lowry, who drank himself to death, because they were all afraid they couldn't repeat their first successful performance.

So even when you do well, and say, "Therefore, I'm OK," you have to keep being OK all the time. As Eric Berne pointed out, if you do anything like that and you say I'm OK, then you're implying that others are not OK. You aren't truly self-accepting unless you get to the I'm OK, You're OK position, which is a different position. In RET we say, "All human beings are OK, simply because they're alive, because they're human." But you'd have a hard time, philosophically, proving that because it's just an assumption, a statement. It'll work OK, it'll work practically. But the better philosophic solution, we think, is that no one is OK or Non-OK. As long as people are alive, they can choose to rate their acts, deeds, and performances to *enjoy* themselves—not to *prove* themselves, but to *enjoy* themselves. They had better not rate themselves, their being, their essence at all. Only rate their acts, deeds and performances, and that we call self-acceptance.

This is pretty much the same as Eric Berne's I'm OK, You're OK and as Carl Rogers' unconditional positive regard. But we assume that unconditional self-acceptance had better be taught, because it's so difficult for humans not to rate themselves. I contend that they have a strong innate tendency to jump from "I did well" to "I'm a good person" and "I did poorly, so I'm a rotten person." So they had better be taught, over and over, not to do this and preferably to have no self-rating at all, just to rate again their acts and deeds. They can legitimately rate their aliveness, and say, "My aliveness is good because I am able to live and enjoy; and if I cannot be happy at all, which would be very, very rare, being alive would not be good. But I am *not* just my traits, I am I, a holistic human who has many traits, deeds, acts and performances, all of which change. So I'd better only rate my *acts* and not my *self*. Self-acceptance means I'm alive, I'm determined to stay alive, and to enjoy aliveness. Now let's see how I can do that." In RET there's no rating at all of the *self* or the *person*—only of his or her behavior.

Question: I'd like to address this to Mary Goulding. I have used both RET and TA in my own practice and found them very compatible. I wonder if you'd comment briefly on the differences you see, or the way you use them differently.

M. Goulding: I find the basic assumptions compatible. I haven't studied with Ellis, so I don't know all of the techniques. It sounds to me as if you use a wider and wider range of methods, but I think that you do not go into the past to have people redecide that they can give up their irrational beliefs. We use fantasy trips to the past to do that.

Ellis: I'll just say that as far as I can see, and I've read the book by Mary and Bob Goulding, that they do TA and a combination of other things pretty much in an RET manner. Now, that's not TA because TA does it in a different manner and TA will spend a lot of time talking about your being a parent, and an adult and a child, and imply, though not say, that you received the tapes, your childish tapes, from your parents. On the other hand, we would say that you received standards from your parents, but your disturbed tapes, the musts, the shoulds and oughts, you largely made up yourself. You are responsible for

them. You not only tell yourself, from childhood onward, what you'd better do in this world to please your parents and other people, but foolishly tell yourself that you *have* to do what's better. So RET holds, probably more than Eric Berne believed, that humans have innate tendencies to think childishly and construct their own self-defeating tapes. But what the Gouldings do is very similar to RET.

M. Goulding: We broke with Eric on that whole business of his saying that parents planted electrodes and if your parents said you could go to a shrink when you're 22, you'll go to a shrink. We say, people make their own decisions based on what's going on around them when they're kids.

Question: On the concept of self-acceptance, would you, Dr. Ellis, consider that the theological concept is very close to what you're talking about? That is, the concept of reverence, that each person is made in the image of God and is, therefore, to be revered, to evoke within us a sense of solidarity with one another.

Ellis: Yes, I'm glad you brought up the term reverence. I don't usually use that term, but I do talk about grace and several other people have done so too—especially John Powell, who has written the book, *Fully Human, Fully Alive* (1976). He is a Jesuit priest. His book is pure RET. He accepts it and we have other ministers and rabbis, some who practice therapy and others who don't, who accept it.

Father Powell says, and I've said for years, that the concept of self-acceptance is equivalent to the concept of grace. In the Christian religion, and several other religions, you get grace no matter what you've done. Don't forget that the Bible says, "You accept the sinner, but not the sin," which is what we are saying as well. Grace means that if you accept the Christian teachings, if you accept Jesus fully, then you get what you have described as reverence and that you can always accept yourself, even when you've acted poorly.

Now we say, in RET, that you can do that without the Christian religion. You can do it just because you do it. When you do it through the Christian religion, you choose to get grace by believing in Jesus and God, and thereby you choose reverence, or you choose grace. We say you can choose it under any condition, whether you are a Christian or non-Christian. But it is the same basic concept. You decide that "Because I'm alive, because I choose to accept myself, self-choosing, therefore, I am acceptable," which would be our concept and the overlapping concept of several other groups.

Question: In observing RET being taught in the hospital setting, and also in group settings, I've noticed some people will buy into it right away and accept the responsibility, where other people will have a real hard time seeing that, initially. I'm wondering if any studies have been done to correlate locus of control, internal or external, with people's ability to adapt or use that theory.

Ellis: Yes, there are a good many studies of locus control, hundreds of them, and they tend to validate RET. Some people in the locus of control movement, which was originated by Julian Rotter, do what might be called locus of control therapy, which overlaps with RET. It has been found in studies of depression and anxiety that once you accept the responsibility for creating your own disturbance and you put the locus of control in you, rather than in the external world, then you have a much higher probability of changing. Because if you put it in the world, you're going to have to change the world. If you put it in you, you can always change yourself to some degree, as I keep telling people much of the time. Anything that you believe, you can choose to disbelieve, just because you are the believer and because you acknowledge that your beliefs create your feelings.

What we are really doing in RET and what Aaron Beck is doing in his form of cognitive therapy, and what all cognitive behavior therapy is saying is that you have much more locus of control than you think you have and you learn helplessness by assuming, again, that when conditions are difficult, you have no control over them, when actually you do have considerable control. Frequently, you can't control the conditions, but you can always change your reaction to them. So, when people are successful with RET, they really have changed their locus of control. When they change their locus of control, they're on their way to RET.

Question: Dr. Ellis, I'd like you to expand on your reference to Piaget's developmental ideas in psychology. Kendall and Hollon (1979), as well as Meichenbaum (1977), in the last 10 or 15 years have been doing research on teaching children and adolescents to think before they act. It seems to me, RET assumes intact judgment. How would RET teach acting-out, impulsive, antisocial children and adolescents past eight years of age to think before they act?

Ellis: Well, first let me say that we have three books on the subject, two edited by me and Michael Bernard (1983, 1985) and one written by Michael Bernard and Marie Joyce (1984). They show how RET is applied. My book with Michael Bernard (1985) has many chapters showing how RET is applied to children by different RET therapists. Bernard and Joyce (1984) also apply RET to children and adolescents. These techniques of RET overlap with the ones used by Meichenbaum and Kendall and Hollon. They take the RET concepts and put them in very simple language and dramatize them. They show how RET may be incorporated into stories and plays. And we teach the children, as Tom Bingham does in his lesson plans, what would often be called rational, coping statements. Each of his lessons emphasizes one rational coping statement and the first one is, "It's OK to make a mistake, but just try to correct it."

Now, we would change that around a little bit because it's really not OK to make a mistake. We would put it, "It's too bad but not horrible to make a mistake. Just try to correct it." So, rather than teach children to use the scientific method at the age of eight or nine, we mainly use what Meichenbaum calls "self-instructional training," what Richard Lazarus calls "coping statements," what we call "rational beliefs or rational self-statements." We teach them, over and over, the main rational statements. We also use behavioral exercises and emotive exercises and we try to get children to adopt a rational philosophy of life applied to things that are meaningful to them as children.

Question: Beck makes a distinction between automatic thoughts and cognitive schema which are supposed to underlie the automatic thoughts. Adler makes a distinction between private logic and life-style, which sounds like what you're talking about when you discuss the basic philosophical musts. My question is, do you find and regard them as primarily unconscious or nonconscious, as the Adlerians would say, and how do you attack them directly and immediately?

Ellis: That's a very good question and, again, I made that clear in my longer paper. We assume that people have an implicit philosophy which is most of the time largely unconscious. Very bright people explore it, and they know what their philosophy is; they'll come right out and say, "Of course, it's terrible to be rejected. You *must* not reject me, I must *always* be accepted." But most people would just conclude that it's terrible and they can't stand it, because implicitly and unconsciously in what Freud calls their pre-conscious (not their deep repressed unconscious) they have this philosophy.

So we think that most of the time people are unaware of their basic automatic thoughts or unconscious processes which lead to disturbance. However, they're just below the surface of consciousness; and within a few minutes we can get them to see their underlying musts, shoulds, oughts, commands, awfulizing, I can't stand ititis, and self-downing that stem from the *musts.* When we show them their unconscious or implicit *shoulds* and *musts,* they almost always agree, right away, that they hold them. So we usually reveal them rapidly and directly, and then we quickly show them how to dispute their *musts.* Most of the basic philosophies that lead to emotional disturbances are semiconscious, but not deeply repressed, very rarely deeply hidden. RET specializes in quickly revealing, examining, and disputing them—as well as disputing the misperceptions and unrealistic inferences which largely seem to be derived from explicit and implicit dogmatic *musts.*

The Promotion of Scientific Psychotherapy: A Long Voyage

◆

Joseph Wolpe, M.D.

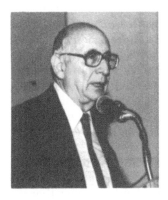

Joseph Wolpe, M.D.
Joseph Wolpe received his M.D. in 1948 from the University of Whitwatersrand in Johannesburg, South Africa. He is Emeritus Professor of Psychiatry and former Director of the Behavior Therapy Unit at Temple University Medical School. He is Professor of Psychiatry at the Medical College of Pennsylvania. One of the leading practitioners of behavior therapy, he has authored three books and co-edited two, and has more than 200 professional publications. He cofounded the Journal of Behavior Therapy and Experimental Psychiatry. *He is recipient of the Distinguished Scientific Award for the Applications of Psychology from the American Psychological Association.*

Wolpe persuasively argues for the widespread use of behavioral techniques. He addresses myths and misconceptions that have plagued this school, and presents case studies and cites research that support his arguments.

At this remarkable conference, nothing is more remarkable than the wide spectrum of its offerings. There are on stage a score of authority figures, each advancing a different viewpoint, and each proclaiming that his or her psychotherapeutic light is the true light. An outside observer would be surprised to learn that this is what the evolution of psychotherapy has come to—a babel of conflicting voices. Evolution implies modification and growth—whether of an organism or of a system or a technology. Chemistry, for example, has in this sense evolved in the past century, developing and elaborating its original concepts. What has made this evolution possible is the systematic accumulation of empirical data that have tested its concepts and enabled their elaboration. We have seen the growth of a single science of chemistry, and not two or three competing systems jostling for recognition. The result has been increasing strength of this single field and applicability to human use. The same is true of physics or botany, and of the healing professions generally.

Within the domain of the healing

Portions of this address have been taken from an article entitled, "Misrepresentations and Underemployment of Behavior Therapy," published in *Comprehensive Psychiatry, 1986, 27*, 192–200.

professions, psychotherapy is the stark exception. Instead of the growth of a single ramifying system of tested propositions, psychotherapy presents the pre-scientific spectacle of viewpoints that differ on fundamentals, schisms within viewpoints, and the frequent blossoming of new viewpoints, with a crop every year from California!

Why is psychotherapy different? It is common to hear the self-comforting answer that it is because the human mind is so complex. However, the human body is also complex, and so is the whole of nature. The truth is that lack of conceptual discipline is always counterproductive. The real reason why psychotherapy is different lies in the fact that therapists are deceived by their own success. As has been known for many years, every therapist can obtain recovery or marked improvement in 40-50 percent of his cases (Landis, 1937; Wilder, 1945; Eysenck, 1952). It is natural to be confident, and even militant, about one's approach if a large proportion of one's patients do well. It is natural to attribute the success to one's methods. But there is no escaping the fact that the baseline level of benefit is quite uniform and any success is, therefore, not attributable to the specific methods, but rather to some process that is common to all therapies. This common process is related, apparently, to the emotional impact of therapist on patient. The psychoanalysts have called it transference. In any case, nobody can claim potency for his specific interventions unless they yield either a percentage of recoveries that is substantially above the common level or greater rapidity of recovery.

So far only for behavior therapy is there substantiating evidence. Skilled behavior therapists obtain in an average of about 25 sessions recoveries or marked improvements in over 80 percent of patients, without relapse or symptom substitution (Wolpe, 1958; Paul, 1969). In 1973, a task force of the American Psychiatric Association concluded from the evidence that, "Behavior therapy has much to offer in the service of modern clinical and social psychiatry."

However, behavior therapy's therapeutic success has not received due recognition (Andrews, 1984; Brady, 1973; Brady & Wienckowski, 1978; Latimer, 1980). This is largely due to the existence of misconceptions about it. It is widely believed that behavior therapy is simplistic and unconcerned with human feelings or dignity, and of value only for phobias and simple sexual difficulties. These misconceptions are maintained by a stream of misinformation from many sources.

This presentation will: (1) review some sources of misinformation about behavior therapy of the neuroses; (2) outline the basic assessment and treatment practices; (3) provide a summary of recent outcome data; (4) indicate the uses of behavior therapy in complex neuroses, and finally, (5) discuss the implications of making full use of behavior therapy's potentialities.

SOURCES OF MISINFORMATION

Misinformation about behavior therapy has a long history. The earliest reports elicited a great deal of scorn from the psychiatric establishment. A seven-page review in 1959 by Edward Glover (1959) of my *Psychotherapy by Reciprocal Inhibition* (1958) decried almost everything in the book—from its parallels between human and animal neuroses to its nonacceptance of what Glover called "painfully acquired psychological insights." In his critique he made many factual errors, such as including "laying on of hands" as a behavior therapy method.

Misreporting, often with pejorative overtones, has been the rule ever since (e.g., Rotter, 1959; Patterson, 1966; Locke, 1971). To this day, practically all nonbehavioristic writers, including many who are regarded as impartial judges of the psychotherapies, such as Frank (1973), Bergin (1971), Strupp (1978), and Garfield (1981), have played down behavior therapy and have consistently ignored positive data such as presented below. Marmor, in a pivotal chapter in the book he edited to reconcile behavior therapy and psychoanalysis (Marmor & Woods, 1980), made several substantive errors, including the statement that behavior therapists "assume that what goes on subjectively within the patient is irrelevant and that all that matters is how he behaves" (p. 44).

In recent years serious misinformation has come from people who have had various kinds of association with behavior therapy, "insiders," so to speak. The earliest of these was Arnold Lazarus (1971), who became a militant detractor of behavior therapy about 15 years ago. He based his antipathy largely on a 36 percent relapse rate he had found in 112 patients he had treated by what he called behavior therapy. Lazarus' results must be contrasted with Paul's (1969, p. 159) review of nearly 1,000 different clients treated by 90 different therapists. Paul states, "Relapse and symptom substitution were notably lacking, although the majority of authors were attuned to these problems." So Lazarus was condemning behavior therapy in general for a high relapse rate that was unique to his own mode of practice (Wolpe, 1984c). Much more important damage, especially among psychiatrists, was done by the British psychiatrist, Isaac Marks (1976), who at a keynote address to the American Psychiatric Association in 1975 made the statement that behavior therapy "can help perhaps 10 percent of all adult outpatients when used as the chief agent of change." Although totally unable to support this claim, either privately or in print, he continued to state it for years. More recently the "cognitivists" (Beck, 1976; Ellis, 1974; Mahoney, 1977) have revived in a new way the idea of behavior therapy being simple and mechanistic. They have promoted certain idiosyncratic cognitive techniques that they claim have improved the results of behavior therapy. (However, a survey by Latimer & Sweet (1984) has found no support for their claim.) At the same time, cognitivists assert that stan-

dard behavior therapy overlooks thoughts and feelings. Beck (1976), for example, has stated that behavior therapists "selectively exclude information regarding patients' attitudes, beliefs and thoughts." This echoes the passage I quoted from Marmor, but Beck's identification with behavior therapy greatly increases the impact of this mistaken belief.

A BIRD'S EYE VIEW OF BEHAVIOR THERAPY OF THE NEUROSES

We start from a point of basic agreement with Freud (1933)—that anxiety* is the centerpoint of the neuroses. We define a neurosis as a persistent unadaptive learned habit of which anxiety is the central constituent (Wolpe, 1958, p. 32). While anxiety is the most common presenting feature of neuroses, it often has secondary effects which, for the patient, may take precedence, such as sexual inadequacy, stuttering, blushing, migraine, obsessional behavior, neurotic depression or "existential" problems. Eliminating the underlying anxiety response habits removes the secondary manifestation (Wolpe, 1958, 1982).

There are two types of neurotic fear: (1) classically conditioned and (2) cognitively based (Wolpe, 1981; Wolpe, Lande, McNally, & Schotte, 1985).

CLASSICALLY CONDITIONED NEUROTIC FEAR

Classically conditioned fear in humans may result from a single event or be progressively built up in the course of a series of events. A familiar example of fear conditioning is the war neurosis, but civilian examples are much more common: A 34-year-old man's four-year fear of being in automobiles started when his car was struck from behind while he was waiting for a red light to change. At that moment

---

* "Fear" and "anxiety" are used synonymously in this paper because they are psychophysiologically indistinguishable.

he felt an overwhelming fear of impending death; subsequently he was afraid to sit inside even a stationary car. That the fear was purely a matter of classical autonomic conditioning (automatic response to the ambience of a car's interior) was evidenced by the fact that he had no expectation of danger when he sat in a car.

In experimentally induced neurotic fears in animals, treatment often consists of arranging for weak anxiety responses to be inhibited by the competition of feeding (Wolpe, 1958), a measure also successfully used against children's fears (Jones, 1924). The most widely used inhibitor of fear in human adults is the calmness produced by deep muscle relaxation, usually in the context of systematic desensitization. However, sexual responses, anger and a considerable number of other responses have also been successfully used to overcome anxiety response habits (Wolpe, 1982). There are, in addition, some methods, such as flooding, that are based on other paradigms (Wolpe, 1982).

COGNITIVELY BASED NEUROTIC FEAR

The second category of neurotic fears stems from erroneous beliefs. As a matter of background, a great many *nonneurotic fears*, i.e., those that have a foundation in reality, are based on beliefs; they have been acquired by information and not by classical conditioning. We fear lightning or a reckless driver not because we have had frightening experiences with them, but because we know them to be dangerous. Fears elicited by *erroneous* beliefs are just as distressful. A man may fear masturbation because he was led to believe that it would injure his health, and a woman may be afraid of sexual arousal because of horror stories her mother told her about it. People may fear worms, flying insects, doctors or hospitals because they have observed a parent consistently show fear of these things. Some wrong beliefs are based on erroneous inferences and not on wrong messages. For example, a person

who has a bizarre and unusual sensation may fearfully infer that his personality is disintegrating.

Cognitively based fears call for correction either verbally or by demonstration. A fear of attacks of dizziness in the belief that it bodes insanity, for example, may be overcome by demonstrating that the dizziness is caused by hyperventilation (Wolpe, 1982). The correction of misconceptions is, in general, easier than the elimination of classically conditioned fear.

BEHAVIORAL ASSESSMENT OF NEUROTIC PATIENTS

The general atmosphere of the behavioristic interview is shaped by the therapist's conception that the neurotic patient's problems consist of maladaptive habits whose core is a response of anxiety that was established during stressful experiences; it is an atmosphere of total permissiveness and absence of blame. The patient is given to understand that the therapeutic enterprise will be a collaboration of therapist and patient directed towards the reversal of the patient's maladaptive habits. The assessment focuses upon identifying and analyzing the triggers to the untoward responses. The therapist takes a history of each complaint from its beginning through its changes over time. He responds to the patient's disclosures with suitable follow-up comments and questions. He empathizes with the patient's problems and makes this empathy evident. The history of complaints is followed by the gathering of background history encompassing family relations, education and love life, and so forth (Wolpe, 1982). The combined information gives the therapist a wide conspectus of the patient's life and problems, on the basis of which therapeutic interventions are planned. The popular image of a detached behavior therapist interested in behavioral mechanics but not in the human being and his problems is simply a fabrication!

RECENT OUTCOME STUDIES

As I mentioned earlier, across the spectrum of the neuroses well-trained behavior therapists achieve lasting recovery or marked improvement in more than 80 percent of neurotic cases in an average of about 25 sessions, with relapse and symptom substitution rarely occurring.

The special efficacy of behavior therapy was disputed by Luborsky et al. (1975) and by the meta-analysis of Smith & Glass (1977), which purported to show equal outcomes for all psychotherapies. Recent reviews have overturned the conclusions of both sets of critics. A reexamination of Luborsky et al.'s work by Giles (1983) led him to conclude that the data were, in fact, substantially in favor of behavior therapy. Andrews & Harvey (1981), in a reanalysis of Smith & Glass' original data, found that in *neurotic patients* the outcome of behavior therapy was superior to that of psychodynamic treatment at the level of .001.

Recent documentation of the effectiveness of behavior therapy has focused mainly on individual syndromes. The following is a partial listing of diagnoses in which striking success has been achieved: agoraphobia (McPherson et al., 1980; Mathews et al., 1981; Emmelkamp & Kuipers, 1979); simple phobia (Paul, 1966; Gillan & Rachman, 1974); sexual dysfunction (Wolpe, 1982; Mathews et al., 1976); obsessive-compulsive disorders (Foa et al., 1983; Milby & Meredith, 1980; Rachman & Hodgson, 1980); marital discord (Jacobson, 1978; Stuart, 1969); stuttering (Brady, 1971; Azrin et al., 1979); migraine headache (Friar & Beatty, 1976; Mitchell & Mitchell, 1971; Mitchell & White, 1977); tension headache (Budzynski et al., 1973; Kondo & Canter, 1977; Philips, 1978); and primary insomnia (Ascher & Turner, 1979; Steinmark & Borkovec, 1974). To these may be added type A behavior (Friedman et al., 1982; Suinn, 1982), although its basis is an excessive proclivity to anger and not anxiety.

Details of three of the listed studies will exemplify the results obtained. Of 56 agoraphobic patients treated by McPherson et al. (1980), 47 were either symptom-free or markedly improved after treatment and at follow-ups between 3.0 and 6.3 years later, with correlated improvement in other symptoms, such as depression. Foa et al. (1983) found that of 50 patients with handwashing compulsions, 58 percent were much improved after 3 to 4 weeks of more or less daily treatment, and also at follow-ups ranging from 3 months to 3 years. In a study of migraine, Mitchell & Mitchell (1971) found a 66.8 percent overall reduction of attacks in subjects treated with desensitization and assertiveness therapy, but no change in no-treatment controls. The benefit was maintained at a 4-month follow-up.

THE BREADTH OF BEHAVIOR THERAPY'S RELEVANCE IN THE NEUROSES

Impressive as the numbers presented above may be, they will not change the evaluation of behavior therapy by individuals who regard its scope as circumscribed. On the contrary, the listing of successes in the treatment of particular syndromes may, to some, actually *consolidate* the impression of behavior therapy as being symptom-oriented and irrelevant to the "neurotic core." This impression is actually accurate only in relation to certain practices, such as conventional biofeedback treatments or *ad hoc* uses of relaxation (Wolpe, 1984a, b), neither of which qualifies as behavior therapy because the target is symptom control and not habit change. Certainly, until now evidences of success have not altered the psychiatric image of behavior therapy nor increased its participation in psychiatric residency training programs.

As a step towards dislodging these widely held misconceptions, it is necessary to provide a picture of what standard behavior therapy practice really does include. To begin with, it may be noted that only a minority of the neurotic anxieties treated by behavior therapists are classical phobias: They made up only 14 of 68 hierarchies treated by systematic desensitization (Wolpe, 1982), most of the others being social fears, such as devaluation, rejection or guilt.

The really important question is *whether there are certain neurotic problems for which behavior therapy misses the mark or is inadequate, and for which psychodynamic approaches provide the answer.* Related to this is the question whether in neurotic cases generally a breadth of recovery is obtained by psychodynamics that is beyond the scope of behavior therapy.

Most psychiatrists would probably give an affirmative answer to both questions, to which the natural corollary is, why tinker with superficial remedies when you should be working toward fundamental solutions? This would be a persuasive argument if it were supported by facts. Unfortunately, the available facts are not very supportive.

In an early study of 402 psychoanalyzed cases, Knight (1941) reported that 40.5 percent were either apparently recovered or much improved (62 percent of cases having terminated after less than six months of psychoanalysis are excluded from the tally). Similarly, out of the 595 patients reported by Brody (1962) from the study of the Fact-Gathering Committee of the American Psychoanalytic Association, 210 were followed up after completing their analyses, and 126 of them (60 percent) were stated to have been cured or much improved. This success rate is within the bounds of what might be obtained by any therapist through "non-specific effects" (Wolpe, 1958). Kernberg et al. (1972), reporting on the Menninger Foundation Psychotherapy Research Project, found that out of 42 patients given psychoanalytic psychotherapy or psychoanalysis, only ten were much improved and 11 were worse either at termination or at a two-year follow-up, a picture even less favorable than the earlier studies.

Despite these unflattering results, there is wide confidence in the basic correctness of psychodynamic theories, and firm reliance on the methods. Sometimes the consequence is years of therapy without real benefit, which probably happens nowadays as often with psychoanalytically oriented therapy as with formal psychoanalysis. Schmideberg (1970), a leading psychoanalyst, writes of patients who "have been made to feel that analysis is the only worthwhile therapy, and that there must be something quite specially wrong with them if it cannot help them as it has helped others." She gives the example of a woman of 28 whom she saw after 12 years of ineffective psychoanalysis. The patient had embarked on the treatment without definite symptoms but in the hope of leading a fuller life and making a happy marriage. Having developed a progressively worsening agoraphobia during her first analysis, she later continued with two other analysts, steadily deteriorating, becoming more and more obese and losing all hope of marriage.

When psychoanalytic treatment goes on for long periods without substantial benefit, it is a reason for turning to behavior therapy as a practical alternative. The literature contains numerous examples of behavior therapy succeeding, usually in a modest length of time, after prolonged psychodynamic therapy failed. I personally reported many instances of this (Wolpe, 1958, 1982). Two that have been described in considerable detail are a 56-year-old woman with a complex "character neurosis" who had had 25 years of psychoanalysis; and a 36-year-old woman with lifelong anxiety and depression and nine years of psychoanalysis (Wolpe, 1964).

The potentialities for a switch into behavior therapy are often perceptible in published accounts of psychoanalytic treatments of neurotic patients. This is apparent, for example, in each of three extremely well-presented cases that Gustafson (1984) uses to illustrate brief "dynamic psychotherapy." In the third case, a young man with an eight-year history of severe migraine headaches, it became clear that these were related to emotional tension "whenever others made demands for performance." The distress was easily aroused by small confrontations that would make the patient "full of the worst inclinations for revenge." The therapist states, "If he were not to have headaches, he would have to live with his own ferocity. ... Given his new capability for recognizing his flood of anger at stupid assignments, it is unlikely that he can be the model student that he was." He continues:

Before long, this will certainly bring on various confrontations with his teachers, which will be very emotional, since he wants them to accept him as he actually is. Whether these counterattacks can be negotiated by him, rendering something unto Caesar, keeping something for himself, remains to be seen, but it is certain that these powerful tests of his new bridging capability, these tests of "dynamic change" will come.

Everything here is left to insight and its consequences, and one can only agree with Gustafson that under these circumstances an uphill road lies ahead. The prospect could undoubtedly be lightened if at this point the interpersonal sources of stress were subjected to a behavioral analysis and appropriate treatment prescribed. From the information given in the transcripts, the patient would almost certainly profit from assertiveness training; and oversensitivity to devaluation and disapproval are likely targets for systematic desensitization. Noticeable beneficial change should occur within a few weeks.

Such favorable expectations come from day-to-day experience with neurotic patients, both those whose neurotic anxieties are apparent from the start and those in whom they have to be ferreted out, as in Gustafson's case. The role of anxiety was similarly "covert" in a personal case of hysterical blindness in a 50-year-old artist, precipitated by his mother-in-law having begun legal action against him "for mishandling her husband's will." He was profoundly upset by this action, in keeping with extreme lifelong general fear of "doing the wrong thing." Central to his therapeutic program was desensitization to an extreme sensitivity to social disapproval. An early hierarchy item displays the degree of sensitivity: It was refusing a hostess' offer of a second bowl of soup that he had not enjoyed. In correlation with the overcoming of this and related neurotic sensitivities, his vision began to return after about five months, at first in spurts and finally totally. He went through the court hearing (which absolved him), defending himself against his mother-in-law with minimal anxiety. Recovery has now lasted two years.

THE IMPLICATIONS OF REEVALUATING BEHAVIOR THERAPY

Skill in behavioral assessment and in the use of behavior therapy techniques is a demonstrable asset in the treatment of neuroses. A great many patients who today spend months or years in inconclusive psychotherapy could, through behavior therapy, look forward to relatively rapid and lasting improvement.

For this reason, adequate instruction in behavior therapy should be a standard part of residency training. But even without it, psychiatrists should know when referral for behavior therapy would be advantageous. Lack of this knowledge could, under certain circumstances, lead to litigation. For example, a Los Angeles psychiatrist, who had for two years blocked the attempts of a patient with premature ejaculation to switch to behavior therapy, was successfully sued by the patient when eventual behavior therapy overcame the problem. Psychiatrists, no less than other physicians, need to be up to date with "the state of the art."

Obviously, the provision of adequate training in behavior therapy poses practical problems. In departments of psychiatry both in the United States (Brady,

1973) or Canada (Brady & Wienckowski, 1978), it is usually provided in token form. Efforts to introduce programs of high quality will certainly prove highly rewarding, as has been the experience at the Departments of Psychiatry at Temple Medical School and the University of Southern California, where such programs have been in place for many years. There is a roster of trained professionals to which one can refer (Behavior Therapy and Research Society, 1983).

It would also be well to provide postgraduate courses in behavior therapy. Many informal programs are offered and advertised, but many of them, unfortunately, are conducted by inadequately trained teachers. The psychiatrist who "coopts" behavior therapy need not abandon his own ideology or orientation. He can make use of behavioral methods as a technical resource—just as I would use a nonbehavioral method for which there is empirical support without changing my standpoint, for example, paradoxical intention.

My hope is that this presentation will be an effective step toward dispelling the falsehoods that have for so long deflected psychiatrists from learning behavioral skills, and that some psychiatric and psychological training programs will be influenced by it. Such a development would provide one more instance of the truth of Freud's (1938, p. 945) observation that often in the history of science "the very assertion which, at first, called forth only opposition received recognition a little later."

REFERENCES

American Psychiatric Association. (1973). Task Force Report: *Behavior Therapy in Psychiatry*: 5.

Andrews, G. (1984). On the promotion of non-drug treatments. *Br Med J, 289,* 994–995.

Andrews, G., & Harvey, R. (1981). Does psychotherapy benefit neurotic patients? *Arch Gen Psychiatry, 38,* 1203–1208.

Ascher, L.M., & Turner, R.M. (1979). Paradox-ical intension and insomnia: An experimental investigation. *Behav Res Ther, 17,* 408–411.

Azrin, N., Nunn, R., & Frantz, S. (1979). Comparison of related breathing versus abbreviated desensitization on reported stuttering episodes. *J Speech Hear Disorders, 44,* 331–339.

Beck, A.T. (1976). *Cognitive therapy and the emotional disorders.* New York: International Universities Press.

Behavior Therapy and Research Society Roster of Clinical Fellows. (1983). *J Behav Ther Exp Psychiatry, 14,* i–x.

Bergin, A.E. (1971). The evaluation of therapeutic outcomes. In A.E. Bergin & S.L. Garfield (Eds.), *Handbook of psychotherapy and behavior change: An empirical analysis.* New York: Wiley and Sons.

Brady, J.P. (1971). Metronome-conditioned speech retraining for stuttering. *Behav Ther, 2,* 129.

Brady, J.P. (1973). The place of behavior therapy in medical student and psychiatric resident training: Two surveys and some recommendations. *J Nerv Ment Dis, 157,* 21–26.

Brady, J.P., & Wienckowski, L.A. (1978). Update on the teaching of behavior therapy in medical student and psychiatric resident training. *J Behav Ther Exp Psychiatry, 9,* 125–127.

Brody, M.W. (1962). Prognosis and results of psychoanalysis. In J.H. Nodine & J.H. Moyer (Eds.), *Psychosomatic medicine.* Philadelphia: Lea and Febiger.

Budzynski, T., Stoyva, J., Adler, C., et al. (1973). EMG biofeedback and tension headaches: A controlled outcome study. *Psychosom Med, 35,* 484–490.

Ellis, A. (1974). *Humanistic psychotherapy: The rational-emotive approach.* New York: Julian Press.

Emmelkamp, P.M.G., & Kuipers, A.C.M. (1979). Agoraphobia: A followup study four years after treatment. *Br J Psychiatry, 134,* 352–355.

Eysenck, H.J. (1952). The effects of psychotherapy: An evaluation. *J. Consult. Psychol., 16,* 319.

Foa, E.B., Grayson, J.B., Steketee, G.S., et al. (1983). Success and failure in the behavioral treatment of obsessive-compulsives. *J Consult Clin Psychol, 51,* 287–297.

Frank, J.D. (1973). *Persuasion and healing* (rev. ed.). Baltimore: The Johns Hopkins University Press.

Freud, S. (1933). *New introductory lectures on psychoanalysis.* New York: W.W. Norton.

Freud, S. (1938). The history of the psychoanalytic movement, Part I. In A.A. Brill (Ed.), *The basic writings of Sigmund Freud.* New York: Modern Library.

Friar, L., & Beatty, J. (1976). Migraine: Management by trained control of vasoconstriction. *J Consult Clin Psychol, 44,* 46–50.

Friedman, M., Thoreson, C., Gill, J., et al. (1982). Feasibility of altering type A behavior pattern after myocardial infarction. *Circulation, 66,* 83–92.

Garfield, S.L. (1981). Psychotherapy: A 40-year appraisal. *Am Psychol, 36,* 174–183.

Giles, T.R. (1983). Probable superiority of behavioral interventions-II: Empirical status of the equivalence of therapies hypothesis. *J Behav Exp Psychiatry, 14,* 189–196.

Gillan, P., & Rachman, S. (1974). An experimental investigation of behavior therapy in phobic patients. *Br J Psychiatry, 124,* 392–401.

Glover, E. (1959). Critical notice. *Br J Med Psychol, 32,* 68–74.

Gustafson, J.P. (1984). An integration of brief dynamic psychotherapy. *Am J Psychiatry, 141,* 935–944.

Jacobson, J. (1978). Specific and non-specific factors in the effectiveness of a behavioral approach to the treatment of marital discord. *J. Consult Clin Psychol, 46,* 442–452.

Jones, M.C. (1924). Elimination of children's fears. *J. Exper. Psychol., 7,* 382.

Kernberg, O., Burstein, E., Coyle, L., et al. (1972). Psychotherapy and psychoanalysis. Final report of the Menninger Foundation's Psychotherapy Research Project. *Bull Menninger Clin, 36,* Nos. 1/2.

Klein, M.H., Dittmann, A.T., Parloff, M.B., & Gill, M.M. (1969). Behavior therapy: observations and reflections. *J. Consult. Clin. Psychol., 33,* 259–266.

Knight, R.P. (1941). Evaluation of the results of psychoanalytic therapy. *Amer. J. Psychiat., 98,* 434.

Kondo, C., & Canter, A. (1977). True and false electromyographic feedback: Effect on tension headache. *J Abn Psychol, 86,* 93–100.

Landis, C. (1937). A statistical evaluation of psychotherapeutic methods. In L. Hinsie (Ed.), *Concepts and Problems of Psychotherapy.* New York: Columbia University Press.

Latimer, P. (1980). Training in behavior therapy. *Can J Psychiatry, 25,* 26–27.

Latimer, P.R., & Sweet, A.A. (1984). Cognitive versus behavioral procedures in cognitive-behavior therapy. *J Behav Ther Exp Psychiatry, 15,* 9–22.

Lazarus, A.A. (1971). *Behavior therapy and beyond.* New York: McGraw-Hill.

Locke, E.A. (1971). Is behavior therapy behavioristic? *Psychol Bull, 76,* 318.

Luborsky, L., Singer, B., & Luborsky, L. (1975). Comparative studies of psychotherapy: Is it true that "Everyone has won and all must have prizes"?. *Arch Gen Psychiatry, 32,* 995.

Mahoney, M.J. (1977). Reflections on the cognitive-learning trend in psychotherapy. *Am Psychol, 32,* 5–13.

Marks, I.M. (1976). Current status of behavioral psychotherapy: Theory and practice. *Am J Psychiatry, 133,* 253–261.

Marmor, J., & Woods, S.M. (1980). *The interface between the psychodynamic and behavioral therapies.* New York: Plenum Press.

Mathews, A., Whitehead, A., Hackmann, A., et al. (1976). The behavioral treatment of sexual inadequacy: A comparative study. *Behav Res Ther, 14,* 427–430.

Mathews, A., Gelder, M., & Johnston, D. (1981). *Agoraphobia: Nature and treatment.* New York: Guilford.

McPherson, F.M., Brougham, L., & McLaren, L. (1980). Maintenance of improvements in agoraphobic patients treated by behavioral methods in a four-year followup. *Behav Res Ther, 18,* 150–152.

Milby, J., & Meredith, R. (1980). Obsessive-compulsive disorders. In R. Daitzman (Ed.), *Clinical behavior therapy and behavior modification.* New York: Garland.

Mitchell, K., & Mitchell, D. (1971). Migraine: An exploratory treatment application of programmed behavior therapy techniques. *J Psychosom Res, 15,* 137–143.

Mitchell, K., & White, R. (1977). Behavioral self-management: An application to the problem of migraine headaches. *Behav Ther, 8,* 213–220.

Patterson, C.H. (1966). Theories of counselling and psychotherapy. New York: Harper & Row.

Paul, G.L. (1966). *Insight versus desensitization in psychotherapy.* Stanford: Stanford University Press.

Paul, G.L. (1969). Outcome of systematic desensitization. In C.M. Franks (Ed.), *Behavior therapy: Appraisal and status.* New York: McGraw-Hill.

Philips, C. (1978). Tension headache: Theoretical problems. *Behav Res Ther, 16,* 249–261.

Rachman, S., & Hodgson, R. (1980). *Obsessions and compulsions.* Englewood Cliffs, NJ: Prentice Hall.

Rotter, J.B. (1959). Substituting good behavior for bad. *Contemp Psychol, 4,* 176–178.

Schmideberg, M. (1970). Psychotherapy with failures of psychoanalysis. *Br J Psychiat, 116,* 195–200.

Smith, M., & Glass, G. (1977). Meta-analysis of psychotherapy outcome studies. *Am Psychol, 132,* 752–760.

Steinmark, S., & Borkovec, T. (1974). Active and placebo treatment effects of moderate insomnia under counterdemand and positive demand instructions. *J Abn Psychol,* *83,* 157–163.

Strupp, H. (1978). Psychotherapy research and practice: An overview. In S.L. Garfield & M. Lambert (Eds.), *Handbook of psychotherapy and behavior change.* New York: Wiley and Sons.

Stuart, R.B. (1969). Operant-interpersonal treatment for marital discord. *J Consult Clin Psychol, 33,* 675.

Suinn, R.M. (1982). Intervention with type A behaviors. *J Consult Clin Psychol, 50,* 933–949.

Wilder, J. (1945). Facts and figures on psychotherapy. *J. Clin. Psychopath., 7,* 311.

Wolpe, J. (1958). *Psychotherapy by reciprocal inhibition.* Stanford: Stanford University Press.

Wolpe, J. (1964). Behavior therapy in complex neurotic states. *Br J Psychiatry, 110,* 28–34.

Wolpe, J. (1981). The dichotomy between classical conditioned and cognitively learned anxiety. *J Behav Ther Exp Psychiatry, 12,* 35–42.

Wolpe, J. (1982). *The practice of behavior therapy* (3rd ed.). New York: Pergamon Press.

Wolpe, J. (1984a). Tension control for coping and for habit change. In F.J. McGuigan, W.E. Sime, & J.M. Wallace (Eds.), *Stress and tension control 2.* New York: Plenum Press.

Wolpe, J. (1984b). Deconditioning and ad hoc uses of relaxation. An overview. *J Behav Ther Exp Psychiatry, 15,* 299–304.

Wolpe, J. (1984c). Behavior therapy according to Lazarus. *Amer. Psychol., 39,* 1326–1327.

Wolpe, J., Lande, S.D., McNally, R.J., & Schotte, D. (1985). Differentiation between classically conditioned and cognitively based neurotic fears: Two pilot studies. *J. Behav. Ther. & Exp. Psychiat., 16,* 287–293.

Discussion by Judd Marmor, M.D.

◆

Let me begin by paying tribute to Dr. Wolpe as the founder of behavior therapy. His place in the history of psychotherapy is a secure one and I want to acknowledge my own personal respect for his contribution. I underline this because if in the course of the remarks that I am about to make, I take issue with many of the things he has said, I want to assure you that it is not out of any rancor, but rather out of a genuine wish to clarify some of the issues and some of the misconceptions which I think you have heard here.

As I try to hear and understand what is going on in Dr. Wolpe's mind, I have a feeling that he has been traumatized by the extreme antagonism that his work originally aroused in the 50s from the psychoanalytic establishment and that he is stuck in a time warp. He is still fighting that battle and is refusing to recognize that events have changed, that there has been a great deal of overlap now between the dynamic and behavioral therapies and a great deal of coming together, and that the enemy he is fighting is still the orthodox psychoanalytic form of treatment, which itself is undergoing constant modification. Indeed, the prevailing trend in contemporary psychiatry and psychotherapy is an eclectic one in which individuals are borrowing the best things that are available in each field and not a polarization which Dr. Wolpe's remarks seem to indicate.

Basic to his remarks is the assumption that there can and should be a single science of psychotherapy and that that science rests with the behavioral approach which he espouses. Both implicitly and explicitly, he indicates that dynamic psychotherapy is outside of that scientific paradigm.

Let me examine some of his premises.

To begin with, one of his first misstatements is that "in the realm of the healing professions, psychotherapy is the only exception to the rule of a single ramifying system of tested proposition." Nothing could be farther from the truth. In the field of internal medicine, there are profound disagreements about how hypertension should be treated, how diabetes should be treated, how arthritis should be treated, whether surgery or drugs should be used in any particular form, whether radiotherapy should be used or surgery should be used, whether lumpectomies should be done or total mastectomies, to say nothing of the competing schools of naturopathy, osteopathy, chiropractic and laying on of hands. There are all kinds of different approaches in the healing arts, and psychotherapy is not unique in this regard.

The problem with psychotherapy is not, as Wolpe said, simply that the human mind and body are so complex. Psychotherapy is not just a question of how the human body and mind work, but rather the question of how two or more people can relate to one another in such a way as to bring about certain desired modifications of thought and behavior in one or more of the other people. In this respect, psychotherapy is more like teaching, and teaching involves not just a particular teaching method but also particular teachers and particular pupils and particular subject matter. And just as no teacher or teaching method is optimal for all students, so no psychotherapeutic method is necessarily optimal for all patients and all disorders that patients present.

Wolpe tends to dispute this in his remarks. He honestly believes that the behavioral approach is the optimal one, the best one for a wide range of psychiatric disorders, not only for symptom neurosis but even, he implies, for complex characterological disorders.

Now what is the evidence that he presents in this regard? Early in his paper he states, correctly, I believe, that one of the major problems in our field is that therapists are deceived by their own suc-

cess. It is natural to be confident and even militant about one's approach if a large portion of one's patients do well. But isn't that exactly what he has done this morning, isn't that exactly what he is doing? No, he would argue that that is not so. He believes that the success of others does not exceed the baseline of benefits that is attributable to nonspecific practices in psychotherapy, while his own higher percentage proves that it is the specific superiority of the behavioral approach that accomplishes this. He asserts that *skilled* (and mind you, I underline *skilled*) behavior therapists get 80 percent improvement in an average of 25 sessions. This is an astounding statement. I will point out later why I think there are a lot of holes in that assertion. Many groups, however, make similar assertions about their high success rate and when there are lower success rates they also attribute the lower rate to unskilled therapists, as he does for lower success rates among behavior therapists.

Secondly, the question of improvement can never be decided by the evaluation of the therapists themselves. In all of the figures he gives, there are no indications whether outside evaluators checked these results or what criteria were used. Sometimes it is like comparing apples and oranges; when psychoanalysts compare improvement, they are talking of a whole different nature of behavioral and psychological changes than behavior therapists are talking about. This kind of superficial and broad statement really fails to advance the art and science of psychotherapy.

I think that an interesting fact that Wolpe doesn't mention is that his 80 percent rate is dated 1958. My goodness, I would expect a later date than that, but the fact is that there was a very careful study (Klein, Dittman, Parloff & Gill, 1969)* which made a detailed, day-by-day study

---

* This and all other references cited in this discussion can be found in the Reference List following Dr. Wolpe's presentation.

of the work of Wolpe and his group. They reported that, as a result of the success Wolpe was having with the more or less simpler phobias and anxiety states he was then treating, he and his group were beginning to see more complicated disorders that were being referred to them. As a result of that, these careful and objective investigators reported, behavior therapy was becoming longer and more complicated, and its success rate was diminishing and beginning to approach that of many other therapies in these complicated character disorders.

We have seen the same thing happen in the treatment of sexual disorders. When Masters and Johnson first came out with their behavioral approach to the treatment of sexual dysfunctions, the success rates were extremely high because they were dealing with performance anxiety cases. But more and more, as time goes on and as the easy cases are being treated by people who first encounter these problems as gatekeepers, the more complex sexual dysfunctions, based on more serious psychological disorders, psychoneurotic disorders, are beginning to emerge. Those problems take longer to treat and the success rate is not as high as achieved by the simple behavior treatment of performance anxiety.

When respected behavior therapists, like Arnold Lazarus and Sir Isaac Marks take cognizance of these limitations of a purely behavioral approach, what Wolpe does is to arbitrarily dismiss them or accuse them of being poor behavioral therapists and he reads them out of the behavior therapy book. I was president of a meeting some 20 years ago at Temple University when Arnold Lazarus first indicated that the results were not all as perfect as Wolpe implied. Wolpe at that point, in a way that was very reminiscent of the way that Freud read Jung and Adler out of the psychoanalytic movement, promptly read Lazarus out of the behavior therapy movement.

Another of Wolpe's major points is that there has been no careful or comparable

scientific research in the area of psychodynamic therapy as compared to behavioral therapy. I think in making this statement he ignores the careful work done by people like Lester Luborsky (1975), Hans Strupp (1978), and Smith and Glass (1977). Especially surprising, I think, is his omission of a careful study done by Bruce Sloane, who was originally one of his devoted followers at Temple University and is still an ardent proponent of behavior therapy and whose residents, now that he is chief of psychiatry at the University of Southern California, are being taught behavioral therapy. Dr. Wolpe mentioned it in his remarks. Dr. Sloane and his group published a study they did at Temple University in 1975 in which they took some 94 clients who came to the clinic and randomly assigned them to three groups: one treated by behavior therapy, one treated by dynamic therapy, and the third in a control group. The control group had a careful initial interview and then at intervals through the next four months they would be called by a clinic assistant who simply assured them they were still on the waiting list, that they hadn't been forgotten, and, indeed, if they had any real emergency, they could come in. However, they got no formal therapy. In other words, it was kind of a nonspecific approach. There were 30 in that group, and 30 in each of the other two groups. The other two groups were treated, each of them, by three experienced therapists. What were the results?

At the end of four months of therapy in which they were seen once a week for an average of 14 or 15 visits, both treated groups improved consistently better than the untreated group. In other words, there was evidence that both behavioral therapy and dynamic therapy worked, and both worked better than nonspecific therapy. At the end of a year, those results continued to show a distinct advantage over the untreated group. Moreover, there was no significant difference between the behaviorally treated group and the dynamically treated group. These patients were all carefully assessed, not by their own therapists but by objective tests and by three experienced observers from the outside.

But there was something else that was very significant and relevant to what we are talking about today. There was a remarkable overlap in the techniques of both groups; indeed, I will show you that there is an overlap in what Dr. Wolpe himself does. Both groups, the behavior therapists and the dynamic therapists, took complete case histories, they formulated the patient's problems, they reconstructed possible causes for the problem, they looked for continuing causes in the present, they corrected misconceptions, they made use of every action and of suggestion. Interestingly enough, the behavioral therapists made just as many interpretive statements as did the dynamic psychotherapists. So what people do and what they say they do are often quite contradictory.

How did the patients in both groups explain their improvement? In both groups, when the patients were asked, "What made you feel better?", they mentioned: (1) the nonpossessive warmth and the awareness that their therapists showed them; (2) their feeling that the therapist had helped them understand themselves and their problems better; (3) the ability to confide and talk to an understanding person; and (4) being encouraged to practice facing things that they had been avoiding.

Now, when you compare this with Wolpe's own description of what he does, it is exactly the same. He is warm, he is caring, he is genuine. He is a good psychotherapist and he takes a complete history; he tries to understand what is going on. He even makes use of analytic interpretations. Just yesterday, in giving us a demonstration on how he works with a patient, he said to the patient, "Do you know what you are doing?" He was talking about the patient's feeling that other people didn't like him. Dr. Wolpe said, "You know what you are doing? You don't like yourself and you are attributing the fact that you don't like yourself to somebody

else, and you are, therefore, thinking they don't like you." What he was describing there was a phenomenon of projection, a clearly psychoanalytic defense mechanism. He uses that and I am sure he uses others too. He works in a combined behavioral and psychodynamic way; indeed, psychodynamic therapists of the contemporary type are doing the same thing.

Interestingly enough, Dr. Wolpe described a psychoanalyst who failed to make use of sex therapy when it was indicated in a certain case. I think he is absolutely right and I think the analyst was mistaken in failing to make use of the latest forms of the art. But I was a little amused to hear Dr. Wolpe describe a case of hysterical blindness that he treated for over five months; at the end of five months, the blindness gradually began to improve. To describe that kind of approach at a meeting sponsored by the Milton H. Erickson Foundation is somewhat surprising because the fact is that most cases of hysterical blindness can be relieved rather rapidly by hypnotic therapy. I remember one case of hysterical aphonia who walked into my office, whom I put on the couch immediately and hypnotized. I got rid of the aphonia in the first visit and was then able to proceed with dynamic psychotherapy. So, perhaps Dr. Wolpe himself failed to make use of the most advanced techniques available because he is so wedded to what he conceives of as a single approach.

I think we must all get away from the Procrustean bed of feeling that we must fit all patients to our own particular technique. We must be ready to adapt our own techniques flexibly to the particular needs of the patient. I would venture to say that nine times out of 10 that is exactly what Wolpe himself does.

Please understand, therefore, that in this critique I am not detracting from Dr. Wolpe's superb clinical ability and his own results. I believe he has honestly reported that. I am concerned with his polarization of behavior therapy versus dynamic or analytically oriented therapy and his failing to take note of the fact that, indeed, there has been a tremendous bridging and coming together of the two techniques. The war is over, the time now is to try to find ways of peaceful coexistence and collaboration so that we can really develop the kind of scientific therapy that does not promote one therapy over all others, but rather tries to find out which therapeutic approach is best for which patient under which circumstances. My plea at this point is for an end to the kind of adversarial antagonism and attacks of one school on the other. This is a time for peaceful coexistence and collaboration. We expect this of our political leaders in the field of international relations; surely, we in the mental health field can do no less.

RESPONSE BY DR. WOLPE

While I appreciate Dr. Marmor's kind remarks and thank him for them, it is sad that I have so much to disagree with. At several points he seems not to have been listening to my paper. For example, from his references to Luborsky et al. (1975) and Smith & Glass (1977), he was obviously oblivious of the critiques of their studies that I featured in the paper, in particular Andrews & Harvey's (1981) demonstration that in neurotic cases the Smith & Glass data show behavior therapy as superior to psychodynamic therapy at the level of .001. Similarly, he could not have heard me say that Lazarus had become a militant antibehaviorist after obtaining a 36 percent relapse rate in practicing his particular mode of behavior therapy, in contrast to the 1000 cases surveyed by Gordon Paul two years earlier in which relapse had hardly ever occurred. So inferentially the problem was not with behavior therapy, but with how Lazarus had been doing it (see Wolpe, 1984). Dr. Marmor also said that I had arbitrarily repudiated Isaac Marks, though the explicit objection in my paper was that Marks had been making damaging statements, such as that only 10 percent of adult outpatients benefit from behavior therapy—

a statement he has never vindicated either in print or in personal communication. Dr. Marmor may adulate Marks and Lazarus, but the harm they have done to the image of behavior therapy is considerable.

What Dr. Marmor says about behavior therapy and psychoanalysis performing equally in the Sloane study is another instance of the misreporting which I complained about. Giles (1983) pointed out that actually in eight of nine measures made in the Sloane study, the behavioral group did better than the psychodynamic group, including in duration of change. I can only ask you to look at the original study and not just accept second-hand accounts. It is quite true that there is a certain overlap between what all of us do, but that does not make the differences inconsequential.

In the case of hysterical blindness I described, the behavioral analysis showed that the blindness had been precipitated by an intense emotional experience in a very hypersensitive person, and that the most basic task was to remove the oversensitivity. The belief that symptoms can be removed by direct suggestion is very largely a myth, and I am surprised to hear it endorsed by Dr. Marmor. But even if that could have happened, it would have still been necessary to overcome the underlying social sensitivity. For this, in the event, systematic desensitization was markedly successful, with recovery from the blindness as a logical by-product.

With regard to my demonstration patient here, there was actually no evidence of what Dr. Marmor calls the psychoanalytic defense mechanism of projection. The patient felt uncomfortable in situations where he didn't have a specific role. He volunteered that in such circumstances he felt as if the audience were rejecting him, as if they were making negative judgments about him. He was not projecting onto them his feelings of hostility. There is no evidence that he had such feelings. It was also not a case of the unconscious becoming conscious. He told me of it without any interpretative help.

I reject Dr. Marmor's assertion that behavior therapy obtained better results early on because only simple cases were treated early on. The whole range of neuroses was treated from the start, as is clearly reflected in my *Psychotherapy by Reciprocal Inhibition* (Wolpe, 1958). Dr. Marmor rests his assertion on the report of Klein, Dittman, Parloff & Gill (1969) on the basis of five days they spent in the Behavior Therapy Unit. These authors acknowledged that they had no concrete data and presented their impressions with proper reserve.

If behavior therapy is admitted to be a valuable part of psychotherapy, it certainly ought to be incorporated in training programs. Yet the great majority of departments of psychiatry and many departments of psychology simply do not include it. The departments of psychiatry with which Dr. Marmor has been associated are exceptions.

I am very glad that openminded psychoanalysts like Dr. Marmor have been increasingly adding nonanalytical techniques to their practices, and that some, like Dr. Marmor, include behavioral techniques. His flexibility is very much to his credit. But it does not answer the challenge that I have for many years been posing to my psychoanalytic colleagues. The most basic truth in psychotherapy is that virtually every therapist can get recovery or marked improvement in 40 or 50 percent of his patients. I am talking about recovery from the suffering and impaired quality of life that have brought the patient to treatment in the first place. The basis of such recovery must be some factor common to all therapies, probably related to what psychoanalysts call "transference" (see Wolpe, 1958, p. 193).

The case for adding behavior therapy techniques to psychotherapeutic repertoires is the existence of evidence that their use significantly increases the baseline recovery rate—to over 80 percent— and in much less time. My challenge to the psychoanalysts is whether they, too, can show percentages of recovery from neuroses significantly in excess of the 50 percent baseline. When they can show this,

I will have to agree that they have something that adds to "transference" effects. I have yet to see them providing evidence of this kind. If such evidence were to appear, I would be very happy to resort to psychoanalytic methods as a positive addition to my repertoire. I emphasize this to contest Dr. Marmor's allegation that I am "fighting" psychoanalysis. I will welcome with open arms any procedure for whose effectiveness evidence is produced. My acceptance of certain of Victor Frankl's paradoxical methods illustrates this (Wolpe, 1982, p. 247).

COMMENTS BY DR. MARMOR

I don't want to unnecessarily prolong the controversy. We can throw statistics around. Unless the nature of those statistics are known and the case material discussed and the kinds of cases we are talking about and who the evaluators were and how the evaluations were made, such ex cathedra statements about reports of success are really essentially meaningless.

I want to talk about training. You know, Dr. Wolpe decries the fact that there is not more training in behavior therapy and implies that the dominant form of training today is still psychodynamics. I think that is another indication of the time warp that he is caught in because the fact is that psychoanalytic training and psychodynamic training are at a low ebb now in the departments of psychiatry throughout the country, and the main emphasis today in most of the medical schools is on biological approaches to therapy. This is simply an indication of the fact that he hasn't kept up with what is happening in the field.

I believe very strongly that there should be behavioral methods taught. And when I was chief of the Department of Psychiatry at the Cedar Sinai Medical Center in Los Angeles, I saw that my residents were exposed to behavioral therapy techniques, at least so that they knew what those techniques could do and where they were most effective, and had the ability to use them or to refer people for them when they couldn't treat them themselves. I think that is the benefit of eclectic training. That is why we should not get hooked on just one method and then feel that that is the only way to treat people; that means fitting patients to a Procrustean bed.

Finally, with regard to what is going on in the psychodynamic field, let me just say this. There are comparable results being reported and being very carefully studied. For example, in the area of short-term dynamic psychotherapy, people like Sifneos and Davenloo are doing very care-

ful studies in short-term approaches using a psychoanalytic framework and reporting results which are quite comparable to those of the behavioral school. We are in a profession which is evolving and growing and I think that if we can get away from the assumption that our own particular method is superior to any other and if we can maintain the willingness to listen, learn and read about what is going on in our field, and try to learn from one another and integrate our knowledge, I think we will all be better off.

Cognitive Therapy

Aaron T. Beck, M.D.

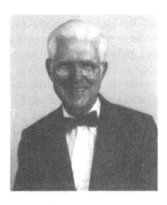

Aaron T. Beck, M.D.
Aaron T. Beck is a pioneer in the areas of cognitive therapy and depression. Having received his M.D. from Yale University in 1946, currently, he is both a University Professor of Psychiatry and a Professor at the Graduate School of Education at the University of Pennsylvania. He is also an adjunct professor of Psychiatry at Temple University.

Beck has written a number of important books on cognitive therapy and its use in emotional disorders such as depression, anxiety, and phobias and in suicide prevention. He has authored more than 150 articles in professional and scientific journals and is the recipient of Awards from the American Psychiatric Association, American Psychopathological Association and American Association of Suicidology.

Beck comprehensively presents fundamentals of the theory and practice of cognitive therapy. Special attention is placed on the dynamics of depression and anxiety. Also addressed are the role of the therapist and the mechanisms by which all psychotherapy is effective.

DEFINITION OF COGNITIVE THERAPY

Cognitive therapy is a short-term, focused form of psychotherapy developed from the finding that psychological disturbances frequently involve habitual errors in thinking, or cognition. The theoretical structure is related to cognitive psychology, information processing theory, social psychology, evolutionary biology and psychoanalysis. The underlying theoretical rationale stipulates that the way an individual feels and behaves is determined by the way he structures his experiences. When, for example, an individual interprets a situation as dangerous, he will feel anxious and want to escape.

The cognitions, or verbal or pictorial events in one's stream of consciousness, are related to underlying beliefs, attitudes and assumptions. Patients may judge themselves too harshly due to a belief that they are inadequate; they may fail to generate plans or strategies to deal with problems because of a belief that they are helpless; or they may reason on the basis of self-defeating assumptions.

The therapy, which is active, structured and time-limited, has been used successfully in the treatment of depression, anxiety, phobias, psychosomatic disorders, eating disorders, and chronic pain problems. A combination of verbal procedures and behavioral modification techniques are used within the framework of a cognitive model of psychopathology. The techniques are designed to help the patient identify and correct the distorted assumptions and dysfunctional beliefs that underlie the cognitions. Patients experience an improvement in symptoms by thinking and acting more realistically and adaptively with regard to their present psychological and situational problems.

MODEL OF ABNORMAL BEHAVIOR

The model of psychopathology is based on the premise that excessive dysfunctional reactions are exaggerations of normal adaptive responses. The four basic emotions are evoked by specific conceptualizations of events. Sadness is evoked when there is a perception of loss, defeat, or deprivation. Frequently the loss takes the form of disillusionment or disappointment due to unfulfilled positive expectations. The response to loss is withdrawal of emotional investment from the source of disappointment and cessation of activity toward the goal. In contrast, elation is evoked by a perceived gain and reinforces activity toward the goal.

Anxiety and anger are elicited by perceived threats to the individual. The person experiencing anxiety is compelled to withdraw for fear of being hurt or killed. In anger, the individual focuses on the offensive qualities of the threat rather than on his own vulnerability. The angry individual seeks to destroy the threat by attack.

The psychopathological syndromes represent exaggerated and persistent forms of normal emotional responses. In depression, the sense of defeat or deprivation, the sadness, and the withdrawal of investment in previous goals become all pervasive and unremitting. In mania, on the other hand, investment in expansion and goal-seeking behavior are increased. In

anxiety disorders, we find a generalized and intensified sense of vulnerability and a resulting inclination toward self-defense and escape. In paranoid disorders, by contrast, what is generalized is the perception of being mistreated, and the consequent inclination is to counterattack.

All emotional responses are understood to be mediated by primal cognitive processes analogous to Freud's concept of the primary process. A person's initial conceptualization of a situation tends to be global and somewhat crude. In the "normal" individual, a higher level of cognitive processing, comparable to Freud's secondary process, provides reality testing and corrects the initial global conceptualization of the event. In psychopathology, however, the corrective function of the higher level of cognitive processing appears to be impaired. As a result, the normal "floor" under sadness and "ceiling" over elation, anger, and anxiety no longer exist for the individual. The primal responses escalate into the psychopathological syndromes when the secondary process is not functioning properly.

The question of causality is not addressed by this analysis of the cognitive mechanisms; proximal and ultimate *causes* are not to be found in cognitive structures or processes. The causes of the psychological syndromes are best understood to lie in the interaction of innate, biological, developmental, and environmental factors.

BASIC PRINCIPLES OF THE COGNITIVE MODEL

The cognitive model is based on eight specific principles. The first of these is that the way an individual structures a situation determines how he behaves and feels. For example, when a person interprets a situation as dangerous, he will feel anxious and take measures to protect himself or escape. The cognitive structuring triggers a particular affect which either mobilizes the individual to action or demobilizes him. The affects triggered are anxiety, anger, sadness, or affection; their behavioral correlates are flight, attack, withdrawal, and approach.

The second principle is that interpretation is an active, ongoing process comprised of appraisals of the external situation, coping capacities, and the potential benefits, risks, and costs of different strategies. When an individual makes the judgment that his vital interests are at stake, he is inclined to make egocentric, global and somewhat crude assessments relative to danger, loss, and self-enhancement.

The third principle of the cognitive model is that each individual has idiosyncratic sensitivities and vulnerabilities which result in psychological distress. Those events which result in great stress for one person may not create stress for another. The particular sensitivities of an individual generally are triggered by a class of specific stressors.

Fourth, some of the wide variations in individual sensitivities are attributable to basic differences in personality organization. *Autonomous* personalities respond to one class of stressors, while *sociotropic* personalities respond to another. Therefore, psychiatric disorders are, to a great extent, contingent on vulnerabilities related to the individual's personality structure.

Fifth, the normal activity of the cognitive organization is adversely affected by stress. The primitive, egocentric cognitive system is activated when one determines that his vital interests are threatened. The individual is then primed to make extreme, one-sided, absolutist, and global judgments. In addition, the individual becomes less able to ignore intense, idiosyncratic thinking due to the loss of voluntary control over his thinking processes. With this loss of voluntary control, there occurs a significant reduction in the person's ability to reason, remember, and concentrate.

The sixth principle of the cognitive model is that psychological syndromes, such as depression and anxiety disorders,

consist of hyperactive schemas with idiosyncratic content that characterizes the particular syndrome. A specific cognitive constellation controls each syndrome and results in characteristic affects and behavioral tendencies. The cognitive content of psychological syndromes is on a continuum with the content that triggers similar affects and behavior in normal experience.

Seventh, stressful interactions with other people create a mutually reinforcing cycle of maladaptive cognitions. Mechanisms such as framing, polarization, and the egocentric cognitive mode result in increased activation of the mechanisms associated with the psychological syndromes.

A final principle is that the individual will exhibit the same *somatic* response to threat whether the threat itself is physical of symbolic. The same cognitive-motoric systems are involved in mobilization to *Fight-Flight-Freeze* whether the meaning of the challenge or threat is "physical attack" or "social criticism."

THE COGNITIVE MODEL OF DEPRESSION

THE COGNITIVE TRIAD

Three major cognitive patterns are triggered in depression. As a consequence of the activity of this *cognitive triad*, the patient sees himself, his experiences, and his future in a negative way.

The first component of the triad consists of the individual's negative view of himself. The person considers himself defective, inadequate, deprived, or deficient and tends to attribute his unpleasant experiences to presumed mental, physical, and moral defects. The patient rejects himself because of these defects and concludes that he is worthless and undesirable. Further, he decides that he lacks the qualities he considers essential to attain happiness and contentment. This component is present in most depressed individuals.

The second component of the triad consists of the patient's tendency to interpret experience in a negative manner. He sees the world as making exorbitant demands on him, as presenting unsurmountable obstacles to his ability to achieve his life goals, and as lacking in pleasure and sources of gratification. The patient construes his experiences in a negative way and interprets interpersonal interactions in terms of defeat and deprivation. It often seems as if the depressed person tailors the facts to fit his own preformed negative conclusions.

The third component of the cognitive triad consists of regarding the future in a negative way. This symptom is present in almost all depressed patients. When the depressed person looks into the future, he expects that his current difficulties and suffering will continue indefinitely. The individual envisions a life of unremitting hardship, frustration, and deprivation. When he considers undertaking a particular task in the immediate future, he anticipates failure.

RELATION TO SYMPTOMS

The motivational and behavioral symptoms of depression stem from the negative cognitive patterns. The *increased dependency* is a consequence of the patient seeing himself as inept and undesirable. He overestimates the difficulty of ordinary tasks in life and expects that things will not turn out well for him. He looks for help from people whom he considers more competent than himself. The *indecisiveness* seen in depression comes from the patient's conviction that he is not capable of making the right decision.

Paralysis of the will develops from the depressed patient's pessimism and hopelessness. Because he expects his efforts to result in failure, he is unwilling to commit himself to a goal and his level of activity drops. He seeks to avoid new situations

since he is convinced he does not have the capacity to cope with them or to control their outcome. The desire to escape from what seem to be uncontrollable and unbearable problems reaches its extreme in the *suicidal wishes* experienced by depressed patients. Because the patient sees himself as a worthless burden, he can come to believe that everyone would be better off if he were dead.

Some of the physical symptoms of depression may also be related to the cognitive patterns. Apathy, low energy, easy fatigability, and inertia appear to be derived from the negative expectations. When a patient in therapy is encouraged to initiate an activity, his retardation and sense of fatigue are often reduced.

COGNITIVE SCHEMAS

The cognitive model of depression uses the concept of the *schema* to explain the vulnerability of some individuals to depression. The thinking that predisposes an individual to depression is developed early in life. It is shaped by the individual's personal experiences, identifications with significant others, and perceptions of the attitudes of other people toward him. Inherited factors have also been implicated. A particular concept formed by the individual may then influence the formation of subsequent concepts. If the concept persists over time, it will become an enduring cognitive structure or schema.

An underlying schema which is normally latent will be activated by particular circumstances. A situation analogous to the original experience responsible for embedding the negative concept will trigger a depression in the individual. For example, if someone lost a parent during childhood, the disruption of a close interpersonal relationship in adulthood is likely to activate the schema of irreversible loss that was embedded by the early experience of loss. The kinds of events that can precipitate depressions include not performing up to one's expectations on an examination, being demoted at work, contracting a disease, or encountering severe difficulties or frustrations in attaining life goals. There is not always a specific stressful situation to which a depression may be attributed; sometimes depression is the reaction to a series of nonspecific traumatic experiences.

While the precipitating events mentioned would be painful to any person, the average person would be able to maintain interest in many aspects of his life, despite the trauma in one area. If the person is especially sensitive to the situation because of a predisposition, he will experience a negative shift in his view of every aspect of his life and become depressed. As the depression deepens, the person's thinking becomes permeated with depressive themes regardless of the immediate situation. The depressed individual gradually loses the ability to view his negative thoughts objectively as the activated schemas interfere with the operation of the cognitive structures involved in reasoning and reality testing. The systematic errors which result in the distortion of experience (arbitrary interpretation, selective abstraction, etc.) are attributable to the activity of the hypervalent schemas.

In addition to the concept of the schema, a feedback model helps explain the phenomena encountered in depression. Unpleasant life circumstances trigger cognitions related to defeat or deprivation, negative expectations, and self-blame. The cognitions produce the corresponding affects of sadness, apathy, and loneliness, as well as reduced activity. Both the affect and the inertia are then interpreted as further indications of loss or failure, and the negative feelings are reinforced.

THE COGNITIVE MODEL OF ANXIETY DISORDERS

The basic mechanisms of the anxiety disorders may be viewed as derived from certain evolutionary strategies. These strategies were adaptive at an earlier period in the history of our species, but they are not well-suited to our current environment. They may be analyzed in terms of their cognitive, affective, physiological, and behavioral components.

The cognitive appraisal of danger triggers (a) the affective component—fear; (b) the motor component designed for coping with threats—fight, flight, freeze, or faint; and (c) the physiological component—the autonomic nervous system—which facilitates the action of the motor component. The symptoms of anxiety disorders are the subjective experience of the specific systems involved: nervousness (affective), muscular tension (motor), wish to flee (motivational), inhibition of speech and movement (behavioral), and multiple fears, inhibition of memory, and selective focus (cognitive).

Subjective anxiety provokes the organism to take protective action in response to danger. An immediate response to danger, such as freezing, occurs almost instantly; the anxiety has the function of impelling the individual to select an appropriate strategy after he has appraised the dangerous situation. Anxiety stimulates the individual to mobilize active coping mechanisms to reduce the actual danger. The anxiety itself has an important protective function for the organism: It increases as one approaches a dangerous situation and decreases as one withdraws from the danger. The motivation to reduce the danger by withdrawing from the situation is reinforced by the reduction of the anxiety.

The individual with an anxiety disorder experiences anxiety even when there is no objective threat; his assessment of the dangerousness of a problematic situation is erroneous or exaggerated. There is no possibility for the individual to develop and to apply coping skills because there is no objective danger for which the coping could be effective.

The autonomic nervous system and the somatic nervous system reflect the kind of action that has been selected by the organism (run, freeze, crouch, etc.) rather than the goal of the action (attack or escape). The type of autonomic innervation depends on the particular behavioral (motor) pattern mobilized and not on the affect (anxiety, anger, love) or the ultimate purpose of the activity. The autonomic activity serves to facilitate the motor activity by regulating blood supply, metabolism, and body temperature. The cognitive set is reflected in the activity of the autonomic nervous system. For example, a hypervigilant set (preparation for fight, flight, or defense) will be reflected in a rigid, crouching posture ("freeze") and an increase in heart rate and blood pressure; while a "helpless" set will be evidenced in a slump or fall, accompanied by a decrease in heart rate and blood pressure. The sympathetic nervous system is dominant in the active coping set; whereas the passive set created by an unanticipated and overwhelming threat is associated with the dominance of the parasympathetic system.

Physical and psychosocial threats trigger the same type of response. Negative evaluation by one's superior at work, for example, can trigger a response similar to what one would experience if physically attacked. In response to either type of threat, the same autonomic-motor pattern, such as defensive stiffening accompanied by sweating and pulse and blood pressure alteration, would take place. The inhibition of action is reflected in the tonic immobility associated with sympathetic dominance; whereas demobilization is reflected in the atonic immobility associated with parasympathetic dominance. The impulse for self-protection and self-regulation is expressed by muscular and vocal inhibition.

Anxiety disorders, like depression, are best understood as expressions of the excessive function or malfunction of normal mechanisms. The basic mechanism for coping with a threat is identical for the normal person and the anxious patient. The difference is that the anxious patient's perception of danger is inaccurate or excessive, while the normal person's response to threat is based on a reasonably accurate assessment of the possibility of harm. When the normal individual incorrectly identifies a situation as dangerous and becomes unnecessarily mobilized, the misperception is readily amenable to reality testing and subsequent alteration. The response returns to the base level when the perception of danger is modified. On the other hand, the anxious patient perceives danger when there is no objective threat and is insensitive to cues which are indicative of safety. Once he has perceived danger, his reality testing is impaired.

The thoughts of the individual with an anxiety disorder are dominated by the notion of danger and how to deal with danger. When the patient contemplates an ambiguous or problematic situation, he considers only the most negative possible consequences. Because the anxious patient is fixated on extreme outcomes, he is constantly over-mobilized to deal with physical or psychosocial threats. For example, an individual with public speaking anxiety will become fixated on the disaster of being rejected by his audience. The thoughts of failure and rejection will permeate the individual's thinking, despite their lack of relevance to the performance task at hand. Thoughts that are central to the perceived danger are enhanced; while concentration, planning, and recall relevant to the task are blocked because they are extraneous to the danger. Thus, selective focus and memory retrieval are actively blocked by the individual. In panic there appears to be an analogous selective inhibition of reflective activity and reality testing.

COGNITIVE TECHNIQUES

Cognitive therapy approaches the treatment of psychiatric disorders by seeking to reduce the activity of the dominating dysfunctional schemas and by supporting the patient's adaptive behavior. Structural change may be achieved through the analysis of *rules* and imperatives which have governed the person's responses. The therapy seeks not only to alter the cognitive patterns associated with the specific syndrome but also to change the organization of assumptions, formulas, and rules that result in the misperception of events. Some of the particular cognitive techniques utilized are identifying automatic thoughts, recognizing cognitive errors and distortions, and reality testing through collaborative empiricism.

IDENTIFYING AUTOMATIC THOUGHTS

Most people are barely aware of the automatic thoughts which precede unpleasant feelings or automatic inhibitions. The automatic thoughts, or cognitions, do not always appear in verbal form; they may also be visual images or pictures. With some training, people can increase their awareness of automatic thoughts and learn to focus on them and evaluate them, just as one can identify and reflect on physical sensations.

The patient receiving cognitive therapy learns to identify his automatic thoughts by learning to observe the sequence of external events and his reactions to them. There is a gap which occurs between a stimulus and an emotional response. Ellis (1961) refers to the sequence as the ABC. A is the activating stimulus, and C is the excessive or inappropriate response. B is the blank in the patient's mind which he fills in. An excessive or inappropriate emotional response becomes more comprehensible when the individual becomes able to recollect the thought that occurred during the gap.

Consider the following illustration: A patient saw an old friend cross the street and then experienced considerable anxiety. The anxiety seemed incomprehensible until the patient played back his thoughts: "If I greet Bob he may not remember me. He may snub me—it's been so long, he won't know who I am. Maybe I'll just walk by and ignore him."

Automatic thoughts have several char-

acteristics distinguishing them from the flow of thoughts in ordinary reflective thinking or free association. The automatic thoughts occur rapidly and are generally at the fringe of consciousness. The individual takes it for granted that the thoughts are accurate because they seem completely plausible. For the person experiencing a pathological syndrome such as depression or an anxiety disorder, the automatic thoughts have an imperative quality which makes them persist and recur despite the individual's efforts to block them out. Most of the patient's automatic thoughts will reflect the thematic content characteristic of the specific syndrome. The thoughts will precede such affects as anger, sadness, or anxiety, and their content will be consistent with the affect.

RECOGNIZING COGNITIVE ERRORS

Depressed and anxious patients interpret situations in negative ways even though more plausible interpretations are available to them. The patient may realize that his interpretation was biased or rested on an incorrect inference when he is asked to reflect on alternative explanations. He will then be able to recognize that he adjusted the facts to conform with preformed negative conclusions. There are a number of typical conceptual or inferential errors found in psychopathology.

Selective abstraction consists of focusing on a set of details taken out of context. In this process the person may ignore salient features of the situation and conceptualize the entire experience on the basis of a single set of data. Thus, the depressed patient may single out the negative and exclude the positive aspects of a situation, the anxious person may focus exclusively on symbols of danger, and the paranoid person may selectively extract instances of abuse.

Arbitrary inference is the process of drawing a conclusion without evidence to support it, or in the face of evidence which is contrary to it. *Overgeneralization* is the process of using a single incident to draw general conclusions considered operative across all situations. *Magnification and minimization* refer to the polarized assessment of events, skills, etc. For example, a patient may magnify the difficulty of a task and minimize his ability to accomplish it. *Personalization* is the tendency to relate external events to oneself when there is no basis for making such connections. *Dichotomous thinking* refers to the patient's tendency to interpret on an either-or, black-or-white basis. The depressed person sees himself exclusively as competent or incompetent, as a success or a failure.

REALITY TESTING THROUGH COLLABORATIVE EMPIRICISM

Through a process of *collaborative empiricism*, the cognitive therapist and the patient work together to frame the patient's conclusions in the form of a testable hypothesis. The patient's thinking becomes more realistic through this process because objectivity and perspective are increased. For example, a patient thought he would evoke a noxious response from a cashier if he took time to count his change carefully. He and the therapist framed the following hypothesis: "When I count my change, the cashier will glare at me in a peculiar way." When the patient tested the hypothesis, he found that was correct only 5 percent of the time; 95 percent of the time his negative expectation was wrong. Another patient believed everyone would notice him and disapprove of him if he dressed in an unconventional manner. This patient's belief that he was the center of attention is typical of most depressed and anxious individuals. When the patient followed the therapeutic plan of not shaving for a day, not dressing in his usual neat manner, and walking down the street with a gangling and uneven gait, he discovered that, in fact, few people seemed to pay any attention to him.

BEHAVIORAL TECHNIQUES

ACTIVITY SCHEDULING

Because a substantial amount of the success of cognitive therapy is a result of the patient's application of the principles outside of the therapy session itself, it is important that the therapist help the patient structure his day and week in a way that will maximize the effect of the therapy. Behavioral techniques are especially important in the early stages of therapy with profoundly depressed patients who are not yet capable of the introspection required to work with automatic thoughts and assumptions. At first, the therapist obtains necessary baseline information by asking the patient to complete a *Daily Schedule of Activities*. Using this report as a basis, the therapist and patient begin to schedule homework assignments. The assignments vary depending on the particular phase of therapy and the needs of the patient.

GRADED TASK ASSIGNMENTS

At first, the therapist and patient agree on scheduling activities that will help mobilize the patient and counteract the inertia so often present, especially in depressed patients. Because most patients need to proceed by small steps, graded task assignments are developed to enable patients to experience progressively greater amounts of success without overextending themselves. The patient completes *mastery and pleasure* ratings for each activity. This allows him to grade each experience according to the amount of self-mastery demonstrated and satisfaction obtained. This reinforces successful activity.

When patients are apprehensive about undertaking assignments, preparatory work is carried out during the therapy session in the form of *behavioral rehearsal*. The rehearsal activities enable the patient to practice techniques, giving him the opportunity to evaluate the negative automatic thoughts activated by the activities. Behavioral techniques also are used in devising experiments to test hypotheses formed from the patient's negative automatic thoughts.

The behavioral technique used in *exposure* therapy for agoraphobics is used in the therapy of patients with clinical anxiety. Most anxious patients are accustomed to thinking of their anxiety as being constantly at a high level. However, anxiety usually occurs in waves. If the individual recognizes that the anxiety has a beginning, a peak, and then a tapering off, he is able to handle the anxiety more effectively. He learns that if he is in a social situation, for example, he merely has to "wait it out" until the wave of anxiety passes.

Patients are given assignments that allow them to experience anxiety for increasing amounts of time without having to use "props," such as taking a pill, finding a helper, making a phone call, or escaping from the situation. Patients discover through these assignments that they can stay in anxiety-producing situations for successively longer periods of time without experiencing continuing escalation of their distress.

THE THERAPEUTIC RELATIONSHIP

The cognitive therapist functions as a guide in helping the patient acquire the understanding that will enable him to cope more effectively with his problems. The therapist also functions as a catalyst enabling the patient to have experiences outside of the therapy session that will enhance his adaptive skills. Like the Rogerian or client-centered therapist, the cognitive therapist manifests genuine warmth and nonjudgmental acceptance toward the patient. However, the cognitive therapist takes a more active role than Rogerian and psychoanalytic therapists do. He collaborates actively with the patient in pinpointing problems, focusing on important

areas, and proposing and rehearsing the specific cognitive and behavioral techniques.

While the therapist attempts to maintain an optimal level of warmth and rapport during the therapy, this does not preclude uncovering the patient's negative reactions and "resistances." Negative reactions are often a valuable part of the therapy and are dealt with in terms of the underlying assumptions and dysfunctional beliefs.

Transference reactions also are valuable and can be used to demonstrate the distortions embedded in the patient's cognitive reactions to the therapist.

Most of the therapist's verbal statements are in the form of questions. This reflects the empirical orientation of cognitive therapy and the immediate goal of changing the patient's closed belief system into a more open one. Questioning also provides the patient with a model for introspection which he can use on his own when the therapist is not present and after the termination of formal treatment. Through questions, the therapist helps the patient uncover and modify cognitive distortions and dysfunctional assumptions.

FORMULATION AND TREATMENT PLAN

The first step in preparing a treatment plan is conceptualization of the case. The therapist seeks out the common denominators among the patient's dysfunctional reactions. By working on these, he hopes to solve many problems simultaneously.

For example, a woman in treatment for anxiety was handicapped by a multitude of fears. She was afraid of elevators, tunnels, hills, closed spaces, riding in open cars, taking airplanes, swimming, walking fast, running, strong winds, and hot, muggy days. After analyzing each of these problems with the patient, the therapist determined that the common denominator was a fear of suffocation. The woman was afraid she would suffocate in elevators, tunnels, closed cars, and closed spaces generally. Her fantasy of being in an airplane was that there would be a leak or sudden drop of oxygen. She was afraid that while riding in an open car "the wind would be swept out of my mouth." Lying on the beach on a hot, muggy day made her think she would suffocate. During treatment, the patient learned to pay attention to her respiratory cues, and she began to realize that she would get the sense of suffocation simply by thinking about being in one of these situations.

The initial formulation of the case forms a fabric into which are woven the threads of the individual's habitual patterns of reaction, his particular vulnerabilities, and the specific stresses that impinge on these vulnerabilities and therefore activate the apparent pattern of symptoms. The formulation also includes an abstract of early developmental factors in the patient's background and some notion of the influence of these factors, the patient's relationships, and his adjustments on his present personality structure. Ideally, the formulation would also include an explanation of how the individual is handling current problems and stresses in light of his past history.

RESULTS OF COGNITIVE THERAPY

The theory of cognitive therapy was first operationalized and tested in the treatment of unipolar outpatient depression at the University of Pennsylvania. The first systematic outcome study indicated that the treatment produced major improvement in depression over a 12-week period in 80 percent of the patients and was superior to the results of treatment with imipramine. These results still held at a one year follow-up.

Additional studies conducted at the University of Pittsburgh, the University of British Columbia, the University of Manitoba, and the University of Edinburgh revealed cognitive-behavioral or behavioral cognitive therapy to be superior

to, or equal to, treatment with antidepressant medication. Studies undertaken at the University of Minnesota and Washington University showed that cognitive therapy was equivalent to treatment with antidepressant drugs; while a study at the University of Edinburgh revealed that the combination of cognitive therapy and medication was superior to either form of treatment alone. Additional controlled clinical treatment trials have supported the superiority of cognitive therapy when compared to standard treatments (Johns Hopkins University and Oxford University).

Four follow-up studies (University of Pennsylvania, University of Edinburgh, Washington University, and University of Minnesota) showed that cognitive therapy has a lower relapse rate one to two years after termination of treatment.

APPLICATIONS AND LIMITATIONS

Cognitive therapy programs have been adapted to a variety of clinical disorders. Systematic controlled studies have demonstrated the effectiveness of cognitive therapy in the treatment of anxiety disorders, social anxiety, anorexia nervosa, migraine headaches, public speaking anxiety, test anxiety, anger control, and chronic pain. Cognitive therapy also has been shown to be an effective addition to the standard treatment of heroin addiction. In addition, cognitive therapy has been substantially effective in obtaining compliance with a lithium regimen from manic patients.

Some preliminary studies suggest that the combination of cognitive therapy and pharmacotherapy may have a special application in treating the delusions of schizophrenic patients and helping these patients regulate their bizarre thinking and behavior. Additional studies have indicated a role for cognitive therapy in the treatment of drug abuse and anorexia nervosa.

Some types of depression, such as psychotic depression and melancholia, have been shown to be relatively unamenable to cognitive therapy alone. A recent report indicates, however, that depressions resistant to antidepressant medication or cognitive therapy alone may be more responsive to a combination of the two methods of treatment.

HOW PSYCHOTHERAPY WORKS

The previously outlined principles of cognitive therapy may be extended into the more general questions of how psychotherapy works and what mechanisms produce change.

The specific ingredients for a durable change are, first, *a comprehensive framework*. The framework may be the implicit rationale in systematic desensitization; namely, that the successive approximations to a most threatening scene, when accompanied by muscular relaxation, result in a neutralization of the inappropriate or *conditioned* fear (reciprocal inhibition). The *rationale* in cognitive therapy is that recognition of automatic thoughts, followed by a test of their logic or relevance to available data, modifies the dysfunctional belief and thus results in affective change. One of the many rationales in psychoanalysis is that the uncovering of early memories or unconscious material allows them to be assimilated, as it were, by the conscious ego.

The second facet is the patient's *engagement* in the actual problematic situation (either real, fantasied, or recalled). For engagement to be effective, the individual must experience the situation as if there was a definite threat. The indicator of engagement would be the patient's experience of affect.

The final ingredient appears to be the individual's either implicit or explicit *reality-testing* of the induced memory, image, or actual exposure experience. In this way he is able to forcibly discriminate a true danger from a pseudo-danger.

Various therapies can be compared according to the above three components:

Psychoanalysis. Two aspects of psychoanalytic treatment consist of lifting the veil of the childhood amnesia and developing the transference neurosis. According to the previous formulation, the reliving of a childhood experience provides the ego with an opportunity to observe in a more mature way a trauma that could not be readily absorbed and also to discriminate a past reality from a current reality. Similarly, the transference neurosis enables the patient to relive early experiences in relationship to the context of his or her reactions to the therapist and thus to make distinctions and discriminations between reality and fantasy.

Cognitive Therapy. Cognitive therapy utilizes procedures from both behavior therapy and psychoanalysis. There is more emphasis on actual *behavior* (that is, behavioral assignments) than in psychoanalysis and much more emphasis on introspection than in behavior therapy. The theory of cognitive therapy encompasses ingredients of both. The arousal of affect associated with problematic situations is achieved through a variety of techniques such as role-playing, exposure, and use of imagery.

Other therapies seem to encompass features similar to those already expressed. Perhaps a common feature of relationship therapies is the *corrective emotional experience*. Although this is not explicitly stated, it is probably a factor in abreactive or experiential therapies such as rational-emotive therapy, psychodrama, or Sifneos' short-term psychodynamic therapy, as well as nondirective Rogerian treatment. The experience of arousal or catharsis is also central in the popular approaches such as EST or primal scream.

HOW CHANGES OCCUR IN SPECIFIC DISORDERS

How people change has been a subject of speculation and debate by philosophers since ancient times. Despite the plethora of schools of psychotherapy and the conflicting theories regarding how these therapies produce change—when they work—there seem to be some common denominators that cut across the effective treatments for the various conditions. I should emphasize that, as psychotherapists, all we can possibly know is how we behave towards the patient (the input) and how the patient behaves (the output). What happens outside the "black box" may be totally different from what the patient reports and from what we speculate takes place.

My basic theory of change is that certain cognitive constellations that produce symptoms or dysfunctional behavior may be modified only if they can be made accessible.

Depression

Take, for example, the cognitive therapy of depression. The depressed patient comes to the interview saturated with negative thoughts about himself, his past, and his future, and with considerable unpleasant affect. Thus, his dysfunctional beliefs are available at the time of the interview not only for inspection but for modification. It is thus possible to have him examine the data to see if he is leaving out some important pieces; to examine the logical processes leading up to conclusions; and to examine the conclusions themselves. The therapist can empirically test the conclusions by conducting an experiment right in the office.

For example, a depressed woman was convinced that she had lost the ability to function at all on her job and that she was incapable of even writing some important letters to be sent out the next day. When I asked her to dictate the letter to me, we found that she was able to do so with a great deal of fluency and she articulated precisely what she wanted to say. This experiment, conducted at the peak of her despair, was able to penetrate the constellation of negativity and changed

her belief from "I can't do it" to "I can do it." This particular disconfirmation then spread to a general notion that she was capable of doing anything.

Various other disorders can be analyzed in terms of the relevance of arousal with affect during therapy.

Traumatic Neurosis

At least since the time of Freud it has been recognized that reliving a traumatic experience under a specified structured condition can lead to an attenuation of the painful memories as well as the associated symptoms. In Freud's report of the case of Anna O., reliving the experiences and nursing her father produced a *catharsis* and her symptoms dissipated. We have observed similar successes in treating traumatic neuroses associated with both combat and civilian accidents.

Anxiety Disorders

Unlike the depressive, the patient with generalized anxiety disorder may feel comfortable when he enters the office. The anxiety, as he experiences it in this situation, may or may not be relevant to his major anxiety problem. When he experiences anxiety in reference to the therapist's presumed reactions to him, his constellation may be penetrated on the spot. When this is not the case, the anxiety may be evoked by focusing on some forthcoming event that is problematic. Furthermore, anxiety can be evoked by role-playing a particular type of encounter that is threatening to the patient. For instance, if the patient has a forthcoming interview, the therapist can role-play the interviewer.

The point of this maneuver is not to produce anxiety per se but to evoke the specific cognitive constellation or fears that lead to the anxiety. In the language of cognitive therapy we try to produce *hot cognitions*. Ultimately, of course, the patient has to expose himself to the situations which he fears and which he is likely to avoid. It is only after repeated exposure and application of what he has learned in therapy that he is able to work through the dysfunctional beliefs.

Phobia

As in the activation of the specific constellations in generalized anxiety disorder (GAD), the approach to phobia consists of inducing an experience relevant to the individual's fear. Sometimes this can be implemented in the office by exposing the patient to the specific phobic stimulus (for example, a small animal). Similarly, the individual can be exposed to a picture of the threatening stimulus. In cases of social phobias, the patient can be induced to make a phone call in the office or to carry on a simulated telephone conversation with the therapist. The classical behavioral approach is the induction of scenes in a hierarchical sequence (systematic desensitization). The common denominator of all of these procedures is the confrontation with the frightening stimulus.

Another quite effective way to start exposure therapy is to have the patient imagine the frightening scenes. This can be done in a graded way, as in systematic desensitization, or the patient can simply be asked spontaneously to imagine the situation and possibly to carry it to its ultimate "disaster." Alternatively, a *flooding* technique can be used. This involves presenting an extremely frightening scenario relevant to the patient's fear. Imagery can be very effective in the treatment of phobias. Ultimately, of course, the patient has to confront the real life situation.

Panic Attacks

Panic disorders often can be treated in the office after preparing the patient with information on the nature of panic. Sometimes the actual attack can be activated through a variety of techniques, such as overbreathing, rapid exercise, infusion of sodium lactate, or breathing a combination of carbon dioxide and oxygen. During and after the induced panic attack the individual can "work through" the psychological constellation, which consists of a fear of some internal catastrophe such as a heart attack, stroke, loss of control, or precipitation into insanity.

Conjoint Therapy

In order to enable each partner in a couple to modify his or her own "internal workings," it is often important to provide a stimulus for them to get into one of their characteristic, interpersonal conflicts while seeing the therapist in the office. When the conflict is at its peak the therapist can then work with the *hot cognitions* of one partner, while the other partner temporarily withdraws from the action. He can then turn his attention to the *hot cognitions* of the second partner. In this way the anger-producing beliefs are made accessible and can be identified and evaluated.

From the foregoing, it is obvious that some type of intellectual framework is important if the cathartic, flooding, or emotional experience is to have a therapeutic effect. It is apparent that people go through catharses or abreactions, such as those described above, continuously throughout their lives—without any benefit. What seems to be offered within a therapeutic milieu is the patient's ability to experience simultaneously the *hot cognitions* and to step back, as it were, and observe this experience objectively. The framework, whether it is couched in the terminology of learning theory, cognitive therapy or psychodynamic therapy, is a crucial factor in providing the patient with the necessary objectivity.

The framework is important because it provides both engagement in the problematic situation and distancing. As pointed out previously, we don't know how things are finally sorted out. The mind has its own system for integrating corrective feedback. For most circumstances in our lives we do not need a therapeutic framework for modifying our erroneous or dysfunctional beliefs. In the area of our particular chronic psychological problems, however, the usual corrective feedback provided by ordinary experience does not seem to be effective. Thus, the type of psychotherapeutic interventions described above are necessary. When therapy is effective, the essential components are the production of *hot cognitions* and affect within a therapeutic structure and the opportunity to reality-test these cognitions—whether the therapist is employing psychoanalysis, behavior therapy, cognitive therapy, or one of the experiential therapies.

COMMON DENOMINATORS OF CHANGE

I don't believe that simply arousing the affect is a sufficient cause for change. When the affect is aroused, there is an activation of the underlying cognitive constellation. For example, take a person who becomes anxious when he enters social situations. What is activated, what is producing his anxiety is his fear of disapproval—looking like a "jerk," being rejected by people, or being treated like a nonentity. Once these thoughts of being socially undesirable are powerful enough to arouse the affect, then it is possible for the patient to start reality-testing his interpretation of the situation and to reappraise the exaggerated cognitive response that was not accessible before.

In cognitive therapy and rational-emotive therapy, the reality-testing is highly organized. The patient begins to recognize at an experiential level that he has misconstrued the situation. Thus, one of the mechanisms of change, with many of the patients who do respond to therapy, centers around making accessible those constellations which produce the nonadaptive behavior or the excessive symptomatology. In a way, this mechanism is perhaps analogous to what the psychoanalysts call *making the unconscious conscious.*

In order to fully understand processes of change, we should look at how the organism uses available data to provide a reasonable fit to the environment. All organisms depend on information processing to provide for their delicate adjustment to external situations and also to facilitate internal homeostasis. If we did not appropriately extract and synthesize information from the environment, we would not live very long. We would go about like individuals who are deaf, dumb, blind, and lacking other sensory receptors.

Thus, we are by and large, tuned into our environment and we make the appropriate inferences that enable us to act appropriately. In cases of psychopathology, however, information processing is skewed. The aggravating factors may be simply from within, based on some internal upset in our biochemical homeostasis; or the precipitating factors may be due to the impact of specific environmental effects. The end result, in terms of disturbing the information processing, may be the same, irrespective of whether the instigating factor is biochemical or psychosocial.

For example, we can see individuals with profound depressions developed after the ingestion of antihypertensive drugs. We find that their information processing system shifted towards the negative; they have as many negative misconstructions as the individual who becomes depressed after, say, a severe loss. It is interesting that it is not necessary to utilize another drug in order to reverse the negative thinking in a drug-induced depression. The disorder may be immediately alleviated through the same type of "psychological antidepressants" that are used in "psychologically-induced depressions."

It seems likely that although different methods work through different channels, they all ultimately produce a positive result through the effect on the information processing system. For example, some studies comparing cognitive therapy with the use of antidepressant drugs in the treatment of depression have shown that for those patients who improve under cognitive therapy there is a marked shift in the way they perceive themselves, their future, and their personal world. This may not be surprising, but what may be more surprising is that under drug therapy the improved patients react the same way; that is, they show the same cognitive improvement.

Why should two procedures that are so far apart—the ingestion of a particular molecule versus hearing some statement from a therapist—produce similar end results? It seems likely that completely different systems are involved initially in the various types of therapies. However, all these systems are related to one another by a kind of internal circuitry or internal feedback loops. Thus, it is impossible to make a clean *surgical* intervention in one system without its spreading to another system. All systems work together in much the same way as do the heart and lungs. Thus, you can effect the cognitive systems through cognitive therapy, but you will also get a spread to the affective motor and physiological systems. Similarly, physiological systems may be directly affected through procedures such as relaxation, but this may lead to a reverberation throughout all the other systems.

REFERENCE

Ellis, A. (1961). *Reason and emotion in psychotherapy*. New York: Lyle Stuart.

The Need for Technical Eclecticism: Science, Breadth, Depth, and Specificity

◆

Arnold A. Lazarus, Ph.D.

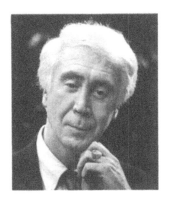

Arnold A. Lazarus, Ph.D.

Arnold Lazarus is Distinguished Professor at the Graduate School of Applied and Professional Psychology at Rutgers University. Lazarus serves on the editorial boards of ten professional journals. He was president of the Association for Advancement of Behavior Therapy and received the Distinguished Service to The Profession of Psychology Award from the American Board of Professional Psychology. His Ph.D. was granted in 1960 from the University of the Witwatersrand, Johannesburg, South Africa. He has authored four books; co-authored, edited or co-edited seven; and authored or co-authored more than 150 professional papers and chapters.

In a thoughtful and witty manner, Lazarus calls for a broad-based systematic technical eclecticism. Procedures and tenets of his Multimodal approach are described, including the diagnostic, treatment-oriented BASIC ID methodology.

PREAMBLE

Before journeying to Phoenix, I had discussed the magnitude and significance of this conference with some of my students. I pointed out that this unparalleled assemblage of so many pre-eminent psychotherapists placed the entire field in tremendous jeopardy. "Can you just imagine," said I, "what would happen if an anti-mental health terrorist organization bombed the building?" While I was musing how this catastrophic event could under-

mine virtually every facet of our profession, one of the students interrupted me. "Not necessarily," she said. "Perhaps by clearing away the debris, a new and freer wind would blow, and from the ashes would come forth . . . " I cut her off at this point and made a mental note to deal with her in some cruel and inhuman manner as soon as I could conceive of a punishment or torture befitting such heresy!

In a similar discussion with one of my postdoctoral fellows, I adopted a different position. I discussed the history of Franz Gall's studies on organology, physiognomy, and craniology, which his erstwhile student, assistant, and disciple, Spurz-

Acknowledgement: My grateful thanks to Allen Fay, M.D., for his constructive criticism of the initial draft of this Invited Address.

heim, popularized as *Phrenology*, a term coined by Thomas Foster in 1815. The medically educated Dr. Gall had specialized in neurology, after receiving the best training that his generation afforded. Indeed, his system was based upon the most advanced physiology and psychology of his day. His lectures proved to be very popular; students flocked to him. His *science of personality* was acclaimed not only by the laity, but by many scientists, scholars, and professionals in France, Germany, Switzerland, Scotland, England, Ireland, and America.

In 1823, *The British Phrenological Journal* was launched, and in 1838, the New York Institute of Phrenology founded *The American Phrenological Journal* which endured for over 70 years, finally ceasing publication in 1911 after its 124th volume. Nevertheless, the American Institute of Phrenology was still in existence in 1925. Phrenology, once endorsed by eminent scholars and scientists, enjoyed its greatest popularity in the 1850s. Today it is but a roost for charlatans.

After some further reflections on the rise and fall of Phrenology, I asked my postdoctoral trainee whether he agreed with me that within 50 to 100 years from now, psychotherapists are likely to display the same respect for each of our current theories and methods that we now show for Dr. Franz Gall's quaint, misguided, and naive belief in Faculty Psychology. I stressed the high probability that most of our ideas about the mechanisms of human learning and the resolution of affective misery, will be as significant and as accurate as Gall's and Spurzheim's ascriptions of the relevance of various bumps and indentations in the skull. My trainee's prediction surprised me. He stated that in the years to come, even greater chaos will prevail as new claims and counterclaims proliferate and compete with one another, as charismatic leaders spawn dozens of additional psychotherapeutic systems, schools, and eclectic jumbles. "By the year 2085," said he, "I fear that the most eminent psycho-

therapists will look back to this era and say that we really knew a thing or two at this stage in history!"

The remainder of my chapter will endeavor to remedy my student's blasphemy and my trainee's pessimism. By underscoring the virtues of technical eclecticism and the dangers of theoretical eclecticism, I hope to pave the way for a sincere appreciation of the scientific method, the significance of breadth versus depth approaches, and the overriding need for specificity.

Prior to 1950, psychotherapy and psychoanalysis were virtually synonymous. By the 1940s, many splinter groups had formed, and deviations in psychoanalysis were numerous (e.g., the writings of Adler, Stekel, Jung, Rank, Ferenczi, Reich, Horney, and Sullivan). Nevertheless, the predominant theme remained essentially *psychodynamic*. Trenchant criticisms of the psychoanalytic position (Wohlgemuth, 1923; Salter, 1949) went almost completely unheeded. Gradually, during the 1950s, we witnessed the emergence of several approaches or systems that seriously challenged the technical and theoretical underpinnings of the psychoanalytic movement. Carl Rogers developed his "Client-Centered Therapy," Fritz Perls cultivated "Gestalt Therapy," Albert Ellis presented what he then called "Rational Psychotherapy," and Joseph Wolpe wrote about "Psychotherapy by Reciprocal Inhibition." During the 1960s and 1970s, the proliferation of psychotherapeutic methods, systems, and schools was such that Herink (1980) published a handbook describing more than 250 different therapies. It is difficult to determine whether this represents an evolution or a devolution!

ECLECTICISM

Surveys (Garfield and Kurtz, 1974; Smith, 1982) have indicated that the majority of clinicians are eclectic. The limitations of orthodoxy have become apparent. Nevertheless, the dangers of unsystematic, synthetic, or theoretical eclecticism must be emphasized. Eclectic therapists who select theories and techniques largely on the basis of subjective appeal tend to foster chaos and confusion. The theories and assumptions that underlie the numerous psychotherapeutic systems often reflect fundamental differences in ideology and epistemology. These differences are not merely terminological or semantic. A close examination usually reveals basic paradigmatic incompatibilities.

For example, there appears to be considerable overlap between some of the central conceptions of Berne's (1961) "Transactional Analysis" and Adler's (1924) "individual psychology." Among their apparent commonalities is their emphasis on the importance of *scripts* and *life-plans*. The theoretical eclectic who borrows freely from both Berne and Adler and who uses their respective concepts interchangeably, or blends them into a seemingly harmonious entity, would be making an egregious error. The Adlerian concept of a life-plan or a lifestyle is not the same as the transactional view of a script. Adler (1963) wrote: "The life-plan remains in the unconscious, so that the patient may believe that an implacable fate and not a long-prepared and long-mediated plan for which he alone is responsible is at work." Berne (1972, p. 59) stressed "(1) that the life-plan is usually not unconscious; (2) that the person is by no means solely responsible for it." Indeed, according to Adlerian precepts and transactional ideologies, the entire manner in which the life-plan is attained and expressed is construed quite differently and irreconcilably. The attempt to integrate divergent theories usually results in syncretistic muddles.

I have long held (Lazarus, 1967) that a therapist who wishes to be effective with a wide range of problems and different personalities has to be flexible, versatile, and *technically* eclectic. An ethical therapist will administer seemingly helpful techniques, regardless of their provenance. But in so doing, he or she is urged to exercise extreme caution before subscribing to the theories that spawned the particular procedure. Indeed, methods or techniques may be effective for reasons other than those that initially gave rise to them. Useful techniques may be garnered from any source and, if necessary, totally divorced from their origins. Thus, a technically eclectic practitioner draws on a wide range of interventions while adhering to a consistent theoretical structure that is open to verification or disproof. Eventually, a super-organizing theory may emerge, a superstructure under whose umbrella present-day differences can be subsumed and reconciled. Meanwhile, it is well to remember that we presently function in a preparadigmatic phase that demands astuteness and caution in the face of any of our existing theories.

Psychotherapy is in dire need of broader integrative theoretical bases. In my opinion, all of our current theoretical underpinnings have significant lacunae. We need a clinical thesaurus that would cross-reference an objective body of actual operations of patient-therapist interactions across many conditions. We need to operationalize and concretize therapist decision-making processes. All of this requires a systematic prescriptive eclecticism (Norcross, 1986), which is different from an eclectic orientation that remains open to every new development so that its practitioners fall prey to every fad. The hodge-podge eclectic is no better than those who remain dogmatically, narrowly, and rigidly fixated to a particular orthodoxy. Random or unsystematic eclecticism cannot give birth to the much-needed tests and measurements that predict responses to specific treatments, nor can it yield instruments with predictive validity and high reliability for clinical decision-making. This calls for *science*, which is the next topic of discussion.

SCIENCE

As I have endeavored to emphasize, a therapist who wishes to achieve constructive results with a wide range of problems has to be technically eclectic. However, rigorous scientists in laboratory settings cannot afford to be eclectic—technically or otherwise. In laboratories, it is essential to test one or two variables at a time in order to separate the inert and incidental ingredients from those that are active and specific. Scientific research often requires withholding potentially helpful methods in order to determine what actually works and to discover *why* it works. In clinical practice, withholding potentially helpful methods often would be unprofessional and inhumane.

Nevertheless, it is impossible to overstate the need for all psychotherapists to place great value on meticulous observation, careful testing of hypotheses, and continual self-correction on the basis of empirically derived data. Too many clinicians fail to display due regard for scientific objectivity. In many circles, there appears to be too much emphasis on clinical experience, intuition, and similar subjective factors. This is not to discredit the important realm of clinical judgment. There is an artistic dimension to the therapeutic enterprise that may always exist beyond the delimited frontiers of science. Nonetheless, we must all remain extremely cautious in the face of conjecture and speculation; we must guard against persuasion and hearsay. The boundaries of knowledge pertaining to effective treatment call for a rigorous process of deduction from testable theories.

Some theorists and therapists forget that it is possible to be *scientific* without being *scientistic*—that is, totally committed to the proposition that the methods of the natural sciences should be used in all areas of investigation. What is needed, of course, is reciprocity between laboratory and clinic (Woolfolk & Lazarus, 1979). Many would agree that a chasm exists between laboratory research and clinical practice, and that it is important for the future of the field to find increasingly more instances wherein experimental knowledge coincides with clinical wisdom. The creative clinician can generate many testable hypotheses that the laboratory researcher can subject to controlled investigations. Without productive dialogues between practitioners and experimenters, the field is likely to stagnate.

All effective therapists must straddle the fence between science and art. In a patient with bipolar affective disorder in a florid manic phase, psychopharmacologists have demonstrated that lithium carbonate, alone or combined with neuroleptics, is strongly indicated. The *art* consists of persuading the patient to comply with the medical prescription, as well as addressing intrapersonal factors or interpersonal networks that might require attention.

As another example, consider a patient with encrusted obsessive-compulsive symptoms. Clinical research indicates that if this individual is treated by a practitioner well-versed only in family systems therapy, or by a therapist whose expertise lies in unraveling complex intrapsychic dynamics, or if hypnosis, systematic desensitization, self-monitoring, or any combination thereof is administered, the obsessive-compulsive rituals most probably will not abate. In the successful treatment of obsessive-compulsive disorders, *response prevention and flooding techniques are often a sine qua non* (Steketee, Foa, & Grayson, 1982). But it is erroneous to assume that *response prevention and flooding* are standardized, unitary, simple, or uniform in their implementation. It requires clinical skill to motivate patients (i.e., gain their compliance and diminish resistance) and to teach them to cope with the heightened anxiety that typically occurs during flooding and response prevention.

Psychotherapy looks to a variety of sciences for help with its problems, drawing on social sciences (psychology, sociology, and communication theory) as well as biological sciences (biochemistry, physiology, and pharmacology). The artistic component usually depends on apprenticeships—the trainee will do best by modeling experts who are able to articulate the hidden rules of clinical algorithms and heuristics.

BREADTH

We are beings who move, feel, sense, imagine, think, and relate to one another. At base, we are biochemical, neurophysiological entities. Consequently, comprehensive treatment calls for the correction of maladaptive and deviant behaviors, unpleasant feelings, negative sensations, intrusive fantasies, dysfunctional beliefs, stressful relationships, and biochemical imbalances. To the extent that problem identification (diagnosis) systematically explores each of these modalities, whereupon therapeutic intervention remedies the major deficits and maladaptive patterns that emerge, treatment outcomes are likely to be positive and long-lasting (Lazarus, 1981). The acronym BASIC I.D. is a convenient mnemonic for recalling the seven discrete but interactive pillars of human temperament and personality: B=Behavior, A=Affect, S=Sensation, I=Imagery, C=Cognition, I.=Interpersonal relationships, D.=Drugs/Biology.

Every patient-therapist interaction involves *behavior* (be it lying down on a couch and free associating, or actively role-playing a significant encounter), *affect* (be it the silent joy of nonjudgmental acceptance, or the sobbing release of pent-up anger), *sensation* (be it the spontaneous awareness of bodily discomfort, or the deliberate cultivation of specific sensual delights), *imagery* (be it the fleeting glimpse of a childhood memory, or the contrived perception of a calm-producing scene), and *cognition* (the insights, philosophies, ideas, and judgments that constitute our fundamental attitudes, values, and beliefs). Each of the foregoing takes place within the context of an *interpersonal* relationship, or several interpersonal relationships. An added dimension with many clients is their need for *drug* therapy (e.g., neuroleptics, antidepressants, and anxiolytic agents).

To know the principal ingredients of a person's BASIC I.D. is to know a great deal about that person and his or her social network. Moreover, appreciation of the interactions of the various modalities—how certain behaviors influence and are influenced by affects, sensations, images, cognitions, and significant relationships—achieves a level of prediction and control that leaves as little as possible to chance. Self-knowledge implies an awareness of the content of one's own BASIC I.D. as well as insight into the interactive effects therein.

In my opinion, to ignore any aspect of the BASIC I.D. is to practice a therapy that is incomplete. Of course, not every case requires attention to each modality, but this conclusion can be reached only after each area has been carefully investigated. The thorough, systematic, and deliberate assessment of the BASIC I.D. has been termed *multimodal therapy* (Lazarus, 1973, 1981, 1985). Many clinicians embrace multidimensional and multifaceted assessment and treatment procedures which they often term "multimodal therapy." Yet while all multimodal therapists are eclectic, few eclectic therapists are "multimodal" in the sense of thoroughly and systematically traversing the entire BASIC I.D. It is an exemplar of what is implied by *breadth*. A major premise of this broad-spectrum orientation is that the more coping responses a person learns in therapy, the less likely will he or she relapse.

An allied assumption is that patients are usually troubled by a multitude of specific problems that should be dealt with by a similar range of specific treatments. What a multimodal clinician might term "a broad-based, intricate, interactive problem," more traditional therapists might call *deep*. To my way of thinking, "depth conceptualizations" have inherently negative effects. Let us examine the "depth phenomena."

DEPTH

Too many therapy theories appear to compound simple elements into complex entities. Some clinicians even manage to pathologize straightforward problems, pulling intricate dynamics or putative collusions out of thin air the way a magician pulls rabbits from hats. Instead of complicating matters, efficient theories should reduce complex and seemingly involved factors to their simplest elements. The use of metaphysical expressions, such as *primitive masochistic needs* or *identity crises*, obfuscates matters and tends to increase mystification and confusion. When problems are labelled "serious" or "deep-seated," an aura of hopelessness often ensues, and this is inclined to elicit a negative self-fulfilling prophecy. When a patient refers to his or her problem as being "very deep," Fay (1978) is apt to respond paradoxically, "You mean like in the spleen or pancreas?" He answers a question such as "Don't we have to go deep into the past?" with "You mean back to the dinosaur era?"

The term *deep* as applied to psychological factors usually implies that subtle events in early childhood are responsible for the genesis of a given habit or current difficulty, and that attention only to recent antecedents and maintaining factors will not properly address the situation. This is the temporal meaning of *deep*. The deeper it goes, the more involved and perhaps hopeless it feels. Consider the following example:

Mr. N.C., a single, white, 32-year-old accountant had been labelled "masochistic, self-destructive, passive-aggressive, and borderline" as a consequence of "deep-seated problems" stemming from an over-punitive father and an overprotective mother. Despite his more than adequate academic credentials, he was functioning at a level far below his qualifications, trapped in a work situation by exploitative employers who supposedly took full advantage of his alleged "fear of success." At age 26, he had sought help from several counselors, a psychiatrist (who used a combination of antidepressant medication and psychodynamic psychotherapy), and later, from a family therapist of the Bowenian persuasion—all to little, if any, avail. He was referred to me for "multimodal therapy" by a maternal aunt whose daughter had been in therapy with me.

The *broad-based* multimodal assessment revealed several excesses and deficits in most areas of his BASIC I.D., but the *imagery* modality yielded especially fertile information. He reported specific images of parental mishandling, images of ridicule and abuse from peers, and a host of self-defeating images in many areas of his past and present functioning. Equally important was the absence of significant coping images—when trying to picture himself succeeding at virtually any task, pictures of defeat and failure invariably took over. Accordingly, an immediate therapeutic focus was aimed at modifying his self-defeating imagery. This called for two basic procedures:

1) Using a "time machine," I had him traveling back to specific incidents that troubled him. For example, he had dwelled on a particular incident when he was nine years old and his father, in a fit of temper, had allegedly flung N.C.'s brand new bicycle against a wall, damaging it beyond repair. The reparative image had him at age 32 going back to upbraid his father and comfort his nine-year-old alter ego. Several "time trips" back to critical events were enacted, the rationale being that by modifying the image, one "desensitizes" the individual to their negative sequelae.

2) Success images were cultivated by having Mr. N.C., in piecemeal fashion, picture himself coping in stages with various tasks and activities. Confidence develops when seemingly overwhelming situations are sequentially dissected into their component parts, with each specific step along the way being successfully completed.

The breadth-formation of the multimodal spectrum provides a holistic "blueprint" that enables the therapist to address excesses and deficits in each mode of interaction. Thus, in addition to the imagery modality which revealed self-defeating representations, the interpersonal modality indicated a dire need for assertiveness and social skills training; the cognitive modality was replete with dysfunctional beliefs (e.g., perfectionism, dichotomous reasoning), calling for considerable restructuring, disputation, and factual information. When therapy ended after 14 months of weekly sessions, each relevant facet of the client's BASIC I.D. had been carefully scrutinized. The behaviors that had led previous therapists to label him "self-destructive, masochistic, and borderline" were conspicuously absent. He had expanded his personal and professional dealings, had stopped smoking, was more "health conscious," had changed jobs and was no longer functioning as a "bookkeeper" but was employed as a Certified Public Accountant.

Individual cases prove nothing, of course, but my reason for presenting Mr. N.C. is to point out the essential differences between depth and breadth approaches. The wide range of problems across a client's BASIC I.D. can seem so formidable at times that one may be puzzled about where to start intervening. Clinicians should adopt the same piecemeal strategy that Mr. N.C. was taught to employ, thereby systematically whittling away, problem by problem. This approach does not seem to have the same ominous implications that the sallow-faced gloom permeating diagnoses of deep masochism or borderline personality tend to generate.

Apart from the term *deep* connoting that which goes way back in time, other implications are that the issues are profound, intense, or highly personal. Whatever the implication, the message usually conveys complexity, or inaccessibility. In my view, this militates against the confident, hopeful outlook that successful psychotherapy usually requires of both client and therapist alike. Notice that the next time you encounter a therapist proclaiming a problem to "go very deep," the speaker invariably adopts a somber expression and shakes his or her head negatively from side to side!

SPECIFICITY

The points of emphasis throughout the preceding sections all coalesce into what

might be termed an overriding emphasis on *specificity*—namely, a concerted effort to determine "*what* treatment, by *whom*, is most effective for *this* individual with *that* specific problem, and under *which* set of circumstances" (Paul, 1967). In theory, most clinicians agree that every client is unique and treatment has to be tailored to his or her specific problems; yet in practice, the consumer is all too often fitted to preconceived treatment modes, whether or not this is what he or she requires.

It is an age-old dictum that appropriate treatments for particular patients are apt to be successful, whereas procrustean maneuvers that force one and all into the same mold are apt to yield inferior results. A clinician, fully cognizant of specificity, will ask the following questions:

Am I well-suited to meeting the needs of this client?
Would it be in the client's best interests to be referred elsewhere?
Do we appear to have established rapport?
Do I feel confident that my ministrations will prove effective?
Have I deduced what treatment style, form, speed, and cadence to adopt?
Have we agreed upon the initial frequency and duration of treatment sessions?

The foregoing are some crucial issues that need to be addressed if the therapy can legitimately be regarded as "custom-made." But there is more.

Let us assume that therapy has been progressing satisfactorily, and the therapist, at this juncture, deduces that the client will derive benefit from relaxation training. In keeping with the specificity notion, a new set of questions arises:

Which of the many types of relaxation training programs is this particular client likely to respond to most favorably?
How frequently, and for what length of time, should the client practice the selected sequence?
Will compliance be augmented or atten-

uated by the supplementary use of cassettes for home use?

Note the level of treatment specificity that is being addressed here. The foregoing questions are generally not pondered by Freudians, Adlerians, Jungians, Sullivanians, Rogerians, or by most practitioners of psychotherapeutic disciplines. In place of vague constructs, omnibus theories, overgeneralizations, and inferred dynamics, I am saying that our survival as a scientific discipline calls for specific answers to highly specific questions. Indeed, at all levels of diagnostic or therapeutic discourse, it is only by asking the right questions that clinicians are likely to arrive at rational and effective solutions.

Let me offer a final example of the degree of precision that is made possible by the breadth of the BASIC I.D. Two patients present with seemingly identical problems: they both suffer from "anxiety attacks" which they claim "come out of the blue." Using a procedure called *tracking* (Lazarus, 1981) the client is encouraged to examine how these anxiety attacks actually arise.

The first patient discovered, upon introspection and careful self-scrutiny of his behavior, a fairly consistent and predictable *modality firing order*.

"First I seem to have some funny body sensations, something unpleasant—it could be anywhere in my body. Perhaps my head feels tight, or I notice a pain, a tremor, or my knees feel weak. I seem to pay attention to this negative sensation, which only makes it grow worse, and pretty soon I am aware of other unpleasant feelings in my body. At this point I start *thinking* about all the terrible things that might be wrong with me. I have an overactive mind! I also have a vivid imagination, and pretty soon I am *picturing* all sorts of horrible things, like having a heart attack or a stroke or some sort of seizure. At that point my anxiety starts to peak!"

Here, an S-C-I firing order, Sensation—Cognition—Imagery, is reported to cul-

minate in a dysfunctional affective reaction—anxiety.

The second patient reported a different *firing order:*

"Things will be going along just fine, when I start *thinking* about all the different things that may go wrong. As I tune into each horror, I can just *visualize* these things occurring. By that time, I notice that my heart is pounding away, my jaws are *tense*, and pretty soon I have a full-blown anxiety attack."

Here, a C-I-S pattern, Cognition—Imagery—Sensation, precedes the anxiety reaction.

The simple tracking procedure revealed that two individuals who initially presented with seemingly identical problems actually had distinctive differences. Of course, the way a person tunes into or punctuates his or her sequence is highly subjective and arbitrary, and some clients alternate or vacillate among their identified patterns of response. Others report predictable firing orders when anxious, but they notice a different combination when depressed.

Clinically, the relevance of this tracking procedure is that it enhances the accuracy of technique selection. Let us assume that Case Number Two (the person with the C–I–S sequence) is first treated with biofeedback and relaxation. These are *sensory* procedures applied to someone for whom this modality is perceived as being third in line. Theoretically, if the client's catastrophic cognitions and terrifying images go unchecked, by the time the sensory system holds sway, the mitigating powers of biofeedback and relaxation are unlikely to offset the problem. In Case Number One, where Sensation appeared first on the firing order, the use of biofeedback and other sensory techniques as the initial intervention may be expected to "nip it in the bud." While these notions await experimental verification, we have amassed a fair amount of clinical evidence to support them.

It is recommended that technique selection be tailored to the client's self-reported firing order. When treating someone with a Cognition–Imagery–Sensation pattern (C-I-S), the first strategy would be the cognitive component of Meichenbaum's (1977) self-instructional training. Thus, upon becoming aware of the onset of negative thoughts, the client would be trained to say or think: "Stop! I will only dwell on pleasant thoughts. I must think about the positive probabilities. I am doing just fine. I will continue to focus my mind on good, healthy, and calming thoughts." To augment the process, the client would then address the next element of the firing order—Imagery. Here, deliberate pictures of coping, combined with calm-producing scenes, and pleasant memories would become the primary focus (Lazarus, 1984). Next, the Sensory modality would be addressed via biofeedback, relaxation, etc. The client with the S-C-I pattern would commence with sensory techniques, immediately followed by positive self-talk, ending with imagery procedures.

I would like to end with a passage from Seymour Halleck (1978, p. 501) that I have often quoted:

We are too restricted by the parochial teachings of our own past to have learned to use effectively all dimensions of treatment. It is my hope that professionals dedicated to bringing about helpful changes in their patients' behavior will seek and welcome similar changes in their own behavior. We will achieve the goal of multidimensional treatment more quickly to the extent that we approach our patients with open minds and a relentless commitment to study and confront the complexities of human behavior.

REFERENCES

Adler, A. (1924). *The practice and theory of individual psychology*. New York: Harcourt, Brace & Jovanovich.

Adler, A. (1963). Individual psychology. In G.B. Levitas (Ed.), *The world of psychology*. New York: Braziller.

Berne, E. (1961). *Transactional analysis in psychotherapy*. New York: Grove Press.

Berne, E. (1972). *What do you say after you say hello?* New York: Grove Press.

Fay, A. (1978). *Making things better by making them worse*. New York: Hawthorn.

Garfield, S.L., & Kurtz, R. (1974). A survey of clinical psychologists: Characteristics, activities, and orientations. *The Clinical Psychologist, 28*, 7–10.

Halleck, S.L. (1978). *The treatment of emotional disorders*. New York: Jason Aronson.

Herink, R. (Ed.) (1980). *The psychotherapy handbook*. New York: New American Library.

Lazarus, A.A. (1967). In support of technical eclecticism. *Psychological Reports, 21,* 415–416.

Lazarus, A.A. (1973). Multimodal behavior therapy: Treating the BASIC ID. *Journal of Nervous and Mental Disease, 156*, 404–411.

Lazarus, A.A. (1981). *The practice of multimodal therapy*. New York: McGraw-Hill.

Lazarus, A.A. (1984). *In the mind's eye*. New York: Guilford Press.

Lazarus, A.A. (Ed.) (1985). *Casebook of multimodal therapy*. New York: Guilford Press.

Meichenbaum, D. (1977). *Cognitive-behavior modification: An integrative approach*. New York: Plenum Press.

Norcross, J.C. (Ed.) (1986). *Handbook of eclectic psychotherapy*. New York: Brunner/Mazel.

Paul, G.L. (1967). Strategy of outcome research in psychotherapy. *Journal of Consulting Psychology, 31*, 109–118.

Salter, A. (1949). *Conditioned reflex therapy*. New York: Farrar, Straus.

Smith, D. (1982). Trends in counseling and psychotherapy. *American Psychologist, 37*, 802–809.

Steketee, G., Foa, E.B., & Grayson, J.B. (1982). Recent advances in the behavioral treatment of obsessive-compulsives. *Archives of General Psychiatry, 39*, 1365–1371.

Wohlgemuth, A. (1923). *A critical examination of psychoanalysis*. London: George Allen & Unwin.

Woolfolk, R.L., & Lazarus, A.A. (1979). Between laboratory and clinic: Paving the two-way street. *Cognitive Therapy and Research, 3*, 239–244.

Discussion by Cloé Madanes

◆

I would like to emphasize certain aspects of Dr. Lazarus' presentation that I believe constitute a framework which the different schools of therapy can agree upon.

(1) There is a difference between attempting to integrate divergent theories and attempting to utilize helpful techniques regardless of where they come from. We can all agree that certain theories are irreconcilable. For example, the idea that psychopathology stems from the repression of early childhood fantasies is incompatible with the idea that psychopathology originates in a person's current social situation.

However, even though the *interpretation* was a therapeutic technique that developed from the theory of repression, it may be occasionally useful within an interpersonal approach. Within a psychoanalytic approach, the interpretation to a rejecting husband might be that he refuses his wife because she represents his mother whom he idealized and worshiped. Within an interpersonal approach, the interpretation might be that the man is caught in a conflict of loyalties between his wife and his mother and alternates between betraying one or the other.

(2) Methods or techniques may be effective for reasons other than those that gave rise to them. Within the theory of repression, an interpretation is effective because in explaining the truth it lifts repression. Within interpersonal theory, an interpretation is effective because it can motivate a client to follow a therapist's suggestion or directive. In the example of the rejecting husband, a psychoanalytic interpretation would attempt to convey the truth about what the wife represents to the man. Within interper-

sonal theory, the interpretation would be made to motivate the husband to choose between his wife and his mother. Similarly, within a behavior modification approach, when a usually misbehaving and insolent child is polite to his mother, the father might be asked to reinforce the good behavior by rewarding the boy with tokens or money. Within a strategic approach, it might be assumed that the boy is covertly encouraged by the father to be hostile to the mother. The intervention might be that each time that the boy is insolent to the mother, the father should thank him and pay him one dollar. The two interventions are similar, but in one good behavior is rewarded within a theory of positive reinforcement; in the other negative behavior is rewarded within a theory that a child expresses a covert conflict between the parents and that making the conflict overt removes the child from the triangle.

(3) The art of therapy consists of persuading the patient to comply, and that is true no matter what the treatment modality. Compliance is the most difficult problem for all kinds of therapy. Within most schools, experienced therapists can solve a presenting problem if the client comes to the therapy and complies with the instructions, but the reluctance to comply and to change is an essential aspect of the problems presented by our patients. Here is where the different schools of therapy divide. Some insist on treating only those clients who comply with certain rigid rules of therapy, such as who should be present, frequency of sessions, rules about cancellations, and so forth, and refuse therapy to those who cannot or will not comply. Other schools believe in accommodating and bending so as not to refuse treatment and will work

with whoever is available and will even attempt to change someone who does not come to the sessions by working with the relatives.

(4) Training relies heavily on apprenticeships with experts who are able to articulate the hidden rules of therapy and to develop the unique potentials of each trainee. Training institutes such as the one led by Jay Haley and myself in Washington, D.C., are developing throughout the country as students realize that the complexity of therapy requires individual instruction with the use of one-way mirrors and videotapes for live supervision. With these devices, therapy is no longer private and secret, and the work of the therapist becomes accountable.

(5) Dr. Lazarus presented the acronym BASIC I.D. for the seven pillars of human temperament and personality. His idea inspired me to propose my own acronym— HELP, for what I consider the four most important dimensions of therapy: H = Humor; E = Enlightenment; L = Love; P = Play. These are the dimensions that a therapist needs to promote and bring out in himself or herself and in the client for therapy to be successful, comprehensive and long-lasting in its effects.

Humor and spiritual enlightenment provide a respite that makes tolerable the loneliness of the human condition. Humor, or what Koestler calls the *ha ha* experience, has an affective and a physiological component such as the release of tension in laughter. Also there is a cognitive component of self-discovery and self-understanding, but the experience transcends the affective, the biological and the cognitive. It is also different from what Koestler calls the *aha!* experience of sudden insight or illumination. However, the realization that we are all part of what Virginia Satir calls the cosmic joke is probably a combination of the *ha ha* and the *aha!* experience.

Spiritual enlightenment is what Koestler refers to as the *ah* domain and what Maslow calls the *peak experience*. This is the experience of transcending the boun-

daries of the self, of union with others, and of ecstasy. Together with humor, the search for shared spiritual enlightenment helps us to transcend the loneliness of our situation.

Humor is what makes it possible to tolerate the paradox of living. The search for enlightenment is the essential hope that there is meaning to life even though that question will never be answered. Love and forgiveness are part of the experience of spiritual enlightenment. To give and receive love is what gives us strength. Unity with others on relatively rare occasions is also experienced through sexual ecstasy, play, and shared grief. Play is the basis of creativity and discovery. The greater a person's ability to experience humor, to strive for enlightenment, to give and receive love and to enjoy play, the greater the chances of tolerating life's difficulties and of finding fulfillment.

(6) I was interested in Dr. Lazarus' use of the "time machine" in the example where the man travelled back to specific incidents that troubled him and repaired negative images of the past by asserting himself and comforting his old alter ego. This case reminds me of my favorite therapy by Milton Erickson that is a therapy of humor, enlightenment, love and play. I would like to summarize it for you from Haley's book *Uncommon Therapy* (New York: Norton, 1973:

A young wife approached Erickson and said that she was an only child of rich parents who had neglected her so that she was raised by servants and lived a lonely and loveless childhood. Her problem was that she was afraid of having children for fear of being a bad mother due to not knowing anything good about childhood. Erickson describes how he hypnotized the young woman and regressed her to the age of "somewhere around four or five years." To quote Erickson (Haley, 1973):

She was given the instruction that upon regression to that age she would come "downstairs to the parlor," where she would "see a strange man" who would talk to her.

She regressed in a satisfactory fashion and looked at me with the open-eyed wonder of a child and asked, "Who are you?" I answered, "I am the February Man. I am a friend of your father's. I am waiting here for him to come home. Would you be willing to talk to me?" She accepted the invitation and told me that her birthday was in February. She talked quite freely at the level of a four- or five-year-old girl who was rather lonesome, and she manifested a definite liking for the "February Man." After about a half-hour visit, I said that her father was arriving and that I would see him first while she went upstairs. She asked if the February Man would return, and I assured her that he would. The February Man appeared in April, in June, and a little before Thanksgiving and Christmas.

This therapy continued over a period of several months, sometimes twice a week. She had spontaneous amnesia for the trance events, but in the regressive hypnotic states she was allowed to remember previous visits with the February Man. As therapy continued with her, she was regressed from year to year and there were longer and longer intervals between the February Man's visits, so that when she reached the age of 14 it was possible to meet by "accident" in actual places where she had been at various times in her life. This was frequently done by having the February Man appear just a few days before some real memory in her life. As she approached her late teens, she continued her visits with the February Man, evincing definite pleasure in seeing him again and again and talking about teen-age interests. With this method, it was possible to interject into her memories a feeling of being accepted and a feeling of sharing with a real person many things in her life. When she requested presents, things were offered that were very transient in character. Thus she was given the feeling that she had just eaten some candy or that she had just been walking with the February Man past a flower garden. By having her doing all these various things, I felt that I was successfully extrapolating into her memories of the past the feelings of an emotionally satisfying childhood.

As this therapy continued, the patient in the ordinary waking state began showing less and less concern about her possible inadequacy as a mother. She repeatedly asked what I was doing with her in the trance state to give her a feeling of confidence that she would know how to share things properly with children of any age. She was always told, in the waking state and also in the trance state, not to remember consciously anything that had occurred in the trance state so far as its verbal meaning was concerned. But she was to keep the emotional values, to enjoy them, and, eventually, to share them with any possible children she might have. Many years later I learned that she had three children and was enjoying their growth and development.*

In the therapy of Milton Erickson, boundaries are illusions. The reality of no-boundary was to him a matter of everyday living. By introducing himself as the memory of a new loving person in the patient's past, Erickson eliminated the boundary between past and present, client and therapist, fantasy and reality. Where many therapists would have chosen to encourage the woman to face the reality of her past, Erickson chose to introduce a fantasy into her memory and so to create a new reality for her.

To conclude, I agree with Dr. Lazarus' emphasis on the principle of simplicity and on his call for specific answers to specific questions. Yet, is it possible to teach how to innovate in therapy as Erickson did in the case of the February Man? Oscar Wilde said, "Nothing that is worth knowing can be taught." And Albert Einstein once commented, "Imagination is more important than knowledge." It is *that* imaginativeness that is so worth knowing and so difficult to teach that makes it possible for therapists to create new realities.

---

* Reprinted from *Uncommon Therapy: The Psychiatric Techniques of Milton H. Erickson, M.D.*, by permission of W.W. Norton & Company, Inc. Copyright © 1973 by Jay Haley.

SECTION III

◆

Humanistic/Existential Therapies

Rogers, Kohut, and Erickson: A Personal Perspective on Some Similarities and Differences

◆

Carl R. Rogers, Ph.D.

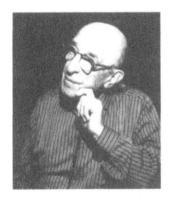

Carl R. Rogers, Ph.D.
Carl Rogers received his Ph.D. in 1931 from Teachers College, Columbia University. He is the founder of the client-centered approach to psychotherapy. Currently he is resident fellow at the Center for Studies of the Person in La Jolla, California. Rogers has served as president of the American Psychological Association, the American Association for Applied Psychology, and the American Academy of Psychotherapists. He is the recipient of eight honorary doctorates and the Humanist of the Year Award from the American Humanist Association. The American Psychological Association afforded him two awards: the Distinguished Scientific Contribution Award for research in the field of psychotherapy and the first Distinguished Professional Contribution Award. Rogers also received the Award of Professional Achievements from the American Board of Professional Psychology. He is the author or co-author of 12 books and numerous articles in psychological, psychiatric and educational journals dating from 1930.

Carl Rogers is probably the world's most eminent and influential clinical psychologist. The reverence and respect afforded him were quite evident at the Conference. He received a five-minute standing ovation . . . before he began to speak. In this chapter, Rogers compares and contrasts his therapeutic method and principles with those of Heinz Kohut and Milton Erickson. Similarities are more apparent with Erickson, but differences still exist between those two practitioners. Rogers also discusses the role and function of theoretical formulations.

INTRODUCTION

I have several purposes in these remarks. I wish to present some of the major elements in my work, especially elements which I feel have been often misunderstood. I wish to acknowledge the fact that the work that I and my colleagues have done is being increasingly compared with the work of Heinz Kohut, a major innovator in psychoanalysis, and Milton Erickson, an innovator who went far beyond hypnotherapy (Stolorow, 1976; Graf, 1984; Gunnison, 1985; Kahn, 1985). Finally, from

179

my limited knowledge of the work of these two men, I should like to give my view (undoubtedly biased) of some similarities and differences between my contributions and theirs. I hope I can do this in a way that will provoke fresh thought about some of the basic issues of psychotherapy.

FUNDAMENTAL HUMAN NATURE

The importance of the perception of fundamental human nature has been underestimated. Thirty years ago I wrote:

My views of man's most basic characteristics have been formed by my experience in psychotherapy. . . . I have discovered man to have characteristics inherent in his species, and the terms which have at different times seemed to me descriptive, are such terms as positive, forward moving, constructive, realistic, trustworthy. (Rogers, 1957, p. 199)

My belief in that statement has been confirmed by continued experiences in individual therapy, in small groups, in large groups, and in groups consisting of antagonistic factions. It is borne out by experience with severely troubled and psychotic individuals and individuals with deep defenses. If one is able to get to the core of the person, one finds a trustworthy, positive center.

I am pleased to find that on this point Kohut and Erickson agree with what I have stated. Kohut specifically rejects the idea that the most basic element of human nature is a "wild beast." He maintains, "We are born as an assertive whole, as an affectionate whole, not as a bundle of isolated biological drives—pure aggression or pure sexual lust—that have to be gradually tamed" (Graf, 1984, p. 74).

Erickson used the term "unconscious" to represent the core of the person. For him, the therapeutic task was to arrange the conditions that would encourage and facilitate the emergence of the unconscious as a positive force. He said, "Unconscious processes can operate in an intelligent, autonomous and creative fashion. . . . People have stored in their unconscious all the resources necessary to transform their experience" (Gilligan, 1982, pp. 87–103).

This similarity of views—seeing the human organism as essentially positive in nature—is profoundly radical. It flies in the face of traditional psychoanalysis, runs counter to the Christian tradition, and is opposed to the philosophy of most institutions, including our educational institutions. In psychoanalytic theory our core is seen as untamed, wild, destructive. In Christian theology we are "conceived in sin" and evil by nature. In our institutions the individual is seen as untrustworthy. Persons must be guided, corrected, disciplined, punished, so that they will not follow the pathway set by their inherent natures.

THE ACTUALIZING TENDENCY

It is my experience that in the nurturing climate I endeavor to create the actualizing tendency becomes evident. * In client-centered therapy, the person is free to choose *any* direction but actually selects positive and constructive pathways. I can only explain this in terms of a directional tendency inherent in the human organism—a tendency to grow, to develop, to realize full potential:

It is confirming to find that this is not simply a tendency in living systems but is part of a strong formative tendency in our universe, which is evident at all levels.
Thus when we provide a psychological climate that permits persons to *be*—whether they are clients, students, workers, or persons in a group—we are not involved in a chance event. We are tapping into a tendency which permeates all of organic life—a tendency to become all the complexity of which the organism is capable. And, on an even larger scale, I

* Note that the *self*-actualizing tendency may be opposed to the more basic actualizing tendency (see Rogers, 1959, pp. 196–197).

believe we are tuning in to a potent, creative tendency which has formed our universe, from the smallest snowflake to the largest galaxy, from the lowly amoeba to the most sensitive and gifted of persons. And perhaps we are touching the cutting edge of our ability to transcend ourselves, to create new and more spiritual directions in human evolution. . . . This kind of formulation is, for me, a philosophical base for a person-centered approach. It justifies me in engaging in a life-affirming way of being. (Rogers, 1980, p. 134)

One aspect of this basic tendency is the capacity of the individual in a growth-promoting environment to move toward self-understanding and self-direction.

When I look at Erickson's work, I find that he also seems to trust this directional aspect in the person. This is indicated in the aforementioned quotation. Both of us have found that we can rely, in a very primary way, on the wisdom of the organism.

I believe Kohut's trust was of a more limited nature. He made it clear that it is the *analyst* who is responsible for movement in therapy, not the patient. In a talk given a short time before his death (Kohut, 1981), he stated that the analyst *cures* by *giving explanations*. He was wedded to the medical model of therapy. His trust in the actualizing tendency was sharply limited.

THE SIGNIFICANCE OF EMPATHY

I wish now to turn to what I consider one of the most important elements in therapy.

The way of being with another person which is termed empathic has several facets. It means entering the private perceptual world of the other and becoming thoroughly at home in it. It involves being sensitive, moment to moment, to the changing felt meanings which flow in this other person, to the fear or rage or tenderness or confusion or whatever, that he/she is experiencing. It means temporarily living in

his/her life, moving about in it delicately without making judgments, sensing meanings of which he/she is scarcely aware, but not trying to uncover feelings of which the person is totally unaware, since this would be too threatening. (Rogers, 1980, p. 142)

To my mind, empathy is in itself a healing agent. It is one of the most potent aspects of therapy because it releases, it confirms, it brings even the most frightened client into the human race. If a person can be *understood*, he or she *belongs*.

Kohut, too, was greatly interested in this aspect. Consider this beautiful statement: "Empathy, the accepting, confirming, and understanding human echo evoked by the self, is a psychological nutrient without which human life as we know and cherish it, could not be sustained" (Kohut, 1978, p. 705). I read this carefully and felt very much in tune with him. Then I came across a most contradictory statement, published later.

Empathy is employed only for data gathering; there is no way in which it could serve us in our theory building. In the clinical situation, the analyst employs empathy to collect information about specific current events in the patient's inner life. After he has collected these data with the aid of empathy, he orders them and gives the patient a dynamic or genetic interpretation. (Goldberg, 1980, pp. 483–484)

Here is where we part company. This cold, impersonal use of the capacity for understanding is abhorrent to me.

We differ in another way. It is my practice to test my empathic understanding by checking with the client. Sometimes I tie together or integrate some of these understandings into a more general picture. I am especially careful to check these, to see if this is actually the way the client sees it.

Kohut, too, makes tentative tests of the interpretation he wishes to give. He says, "The analyst may use empathic testing maneuvers [once he has] tentatively formulated his dynamic and, especially, his genetic interpretations, before he decides to communicate them to the analysand" (Goldberg, 1980, p. 484).

I believe that a transcript of one of my integrative responses would seem similar in form to one of Kohut's preliminary tests of an interpretation. But the *intent* would be quite different. I would be testing to see if I was deeply in tune with my client because this *in-tune-ness* is in itself healing, confirming, growth-promoting. Kohut's intent would be to see if his patient was ready to accept his explanation, the explanation which cures.

Erickson, though he worked in ways very different from my own, gave great importance to sensitive understanding. He believed that "An attitude of empathy and respect on the part of the therapist is *crucial* to insure successful change" (Erickson & Zeig, 1980, p. 335).

Gunnison (1985) describes the manner in which Erickson was empathic:

Erickson expressed his understanding of the inner world of his patients in a way different from Rogers. It was "through the use of the client's own vocabulary and frames of reference, pacing, and matching, a powerful kind of empathy developed that forms the interpersonal connection." He recognized that this was similar to the approach Rogers took to therapy (p. 562).

INTUITION

In recent years, I have given more importance to another aspect of my functioning.

As a therapist, I find that when I am closest to my inner, intuitive self, when I am somehow in touch with the unknown in me, when perhaps I am in a slightly altered state of consciousness in the relationship, then whatever I do seems to be full of healing. Then simply my *presence* is releasing and helpful. There is nothing I can do to force this experience, but when I can relax and be close to my transcendental core, then I may behave in strange and

impulsive ways in the relationship, ways which I cannot justify rationally, which have nothing to do with my thought processes. But these strange behaviors turn out to be *right* in some odd way. At those moments it seems that my inner spirit has reached out and touched the inner spirit of the other. Our relationship transcends itself and has become a part of something larger. Profound growth and healing and energy are present. (Rogers, 1986b, pp. 188–189)

One has only to read some of Erickson's cases to realize the masterful quality of his intuitive reactions and responses to his patients. He seems to be unmatched in his ability to sense their deepest feelings and to react to these in ingenious, spontaneous, creative ways. *

Due to his own early suffering and pain, Erickson discovered for himself much about altered states of consciousness. This undoubtedly helped him to be intuitively sensitive to his patients. "He was so *in touch* with his own inner experience and so trusted the 'wisdom of *his* unconscious,' that he was capable of incredible understandings of his patients' worlds" (Gunnison, 1985, p. 562).

THE PERSONAL QUALITIES OF THE THERAPEUTIC RELATIONSHIP

Therapy is a person-to-person experience. Of the various conditions I have described as essential to effective psychotherapy, the outstanding element is congruence—a genuineness or realness in which the therapist is being him/herself. This not only means striving to understand the client when that is the purpose being experienced; but it also means a willingness to communicate other feelings—even negative ones—when they are being persistently experienced. Thus, boredom, anger, compassion, or other feelings may be expressed when they are a

---

* In analyzing Erickson's every move, in studying "pacing," "matching," "seeding," and other detailed aspects of his work, his followers may run a risk of losing the *spontaneity* of his intuition.

significant and continuing part of the therapist's experience.

So, for me, therapy proceeds most effectively when the relationship contains the therapist's experiencing of sensitive, even intuitive, empathy; of prizing or caring for the client; and, above all, of congruence, in which the therapist is willing and able to be his/her true feelings.

It is strikingly clear that for Erickson, too, therapy was a highly personal affair, different for each person, a deeply involving experience. He thought about his patients, he reacted to them in personal ways—challenging, abrupt, patient, soft, hard—always being himself in the interest of his client. He sometimes took individuals into his home, or used pets, or told of his own life—doing whatever would keep him in close personal touch.

It appears equally clear that for Kohut the therapeutic relationship was cooler, less personal. The analyst was observing, gathering data through his empathy, preparing for the all-important explanations. His attitudes are perhaps most transparently shown in an incident where he departed from his usual style and was more personal. He described this in one of his last talks, where he discussed his work with a woman who was strongly suicidal.

In one session she was so badly off that I thought, "How would you feel if I let you hold my fingers for a little while?" I am not recommending it, but I was desperate, so I gave her two fingers to hold. I immediately made a genetic interpretation to myself. It was of the toothless gums of a very young child, clamping down on an empty nipple. . . . I reacted to it even then as an analyst to myself. . . . I wouldn't say that it turned the tide, but it overcame a very difficult impasse at a dangerous moment. (The analysis went on for years and was reasonably successful.) (Kohut, 1981)

In this interaction Kohut experienced desperation, caring, and compassion. He found a beautifully symbolic gesture that enabled him to express something of what he was feeling. Yet, in his statement, he was apologetic about this act, about giving her his fingers to hold. Even more astonishing—and sad—is his interpretation to himself that he was giving her a dry nipple. He seemed unaware that by having given something of himself—his own deep and persistent feelings—he gave her the nourishing human caring and compassion which she so desperately needed. Having been open with his feelings with her was most therapeutic. Yet, he appeared to be unaware that this act was the most healing thing he could have done.

I differ deeply from Kohut in the value I give to being one's own whole person in the therapeutic relationship.

THE REORGANIZATION OF THE SELF IN THERAPY

One of the satisfactions of my professional career has been to advance a theory that is later confirmed by research. This pattern was evident in my thinking about the reorganizing of the concept of self as a central aspect of therapeutic change.

In 1946 I was elected president of the American Psychological Association. During the ensuing year, I prepared my presidential address, which centered on the changes in perception of self and reality that took place in therapy. It was with real trepidation that I wrote this paper, for it seemed totally unlike the presidential presentations which preceded it. With some inner uncertainty, I led up to the statement that in the therapeutic relationship it is the absence of threat and "the assistance in focusing upon the perception of self, which seem to permit a more differentiated view of self, and finally the reorganization of self" (Rogers, 1947, p. 368). The paper was received with polite acceptance.*

* The acceptance was *very* minimal. When the chairman of the meeting, John Anderson, and I went to the men's room after the address, we could hear the loud buzz of comment and conversation as we opened the door. As I entered, the sound dropped to absolute silence. There was not a word of greeting or comment. As we left, I could hear the loud buzzing recommence. Never have I experienced so vividly being a "loner" in my profession.

I had no hard evidence for my statement in 1947. I could only support my theory with illustrations from recorded interviews. It was therefore immensely satisfying to be able to publish research findings on the subject in 1954 (Rogers & Dymond, 1954). Using Stephenson's new *Q-technique* in an original adaptation, we were able to objectify this very subjective entity (the concept of self) and to measure in great detail the changes that took place during therapy.

We found, much as I had hypothesized earlier, that clients showed certain characteristic change in self-perception during therapy. They became less anxious, guilty, driven, hostile, dependent. They became more secure, self-confident, more aware of experiences and conflicts previously denied to awareness, more able to give and receive love. This reorganization of the self was clearly in a direction perceived as healthy (Rogers & Dymond, 1954, especially Chapters 4 and 15).

Erickson used different words, but it is clear that these changes in perception were also important to him. He spoke of the process of therapy as a loosening of the cognitive maps of the patient's experience, "helping them break through the limitations of their conscious attitudes to free their unconscious potential for problem-solving" (Erickson, Rossi & Rossi, 1976, p. 18). This is very similar to my view that in a sound therapeutic relationship "all the ways in which the self has been experienced can be viewed openly, and organized into a complex unity" (Rogers, 1947, p. 366).

Kohut is in general agreement. The restructuring of the self is central to his whole concept of therapy, and we share many common ideas.

THE PLACE AND NATURE OF THEORY

There is another element of my work which I feel is not completely understood. It is the kind of importance I give to theoretical hypotheses and the way I see the place of theory. I spelled out some of my views quite explicitly in the major presentation of my theoretical views (Rogers, 1959).

I see the formulation of a theory as "the persistent, disciplined effort to make sense and order out of the phenomena of subjective experience" (Rogers, 1959, p. 188). To be of value, such formulations should be tentative. This makes them more stimulating to further creative thought. They should also be testable, since a theory has minimal truth value until it is subjected to some sort of rigorous test, through empirical or phenomenological research (see Rogers, 1985b).

It was and is important to me in my exposition of the theory of client-centered therapy that all of the major statements are testable through empirical means. It is gratifying that a considerable number have been so tested, with generally confirmatory results. (For a review of the studies of the therapeutic conditions, see Paterson, 1984.) To me there seems little value in a theory which cannot be tested; such theory must remain static. There is no possibility of growth or correction. I emphasized this in my 1959 article: "There is only one statement which can accurately apply to all theories—and that is that at the time of its formulation, every theory contains an unknown (and perhaps at that point unknowable) amount of error and mistaken inference" (Rogers, 1959, p. 190).

I see science itself, where our theories and research find their place, as a directional flow. "If the movement is toward more exact measurement, toward more clear-cut and rigorous theory and hypotheses, toward findings which have greater validity and generality, then this is a healthy and growing science. If not, it is a sterile pseudoscience. . . . Science is a *developing* mode of inquiry, or it is of no particular importance" (Rogers, 1959, p. 189).

One aspect of my purpose in formulating theory is often overlooked. Throughout my professional life I have been interested in the *process of change* in personality and behavior, and this is the major focus of both my theory and practice. I have been much less interested in the way in which personality develops or in its structure. These two are, however, the major foci of Freudian theory, so comparison is often difficult.

Neither Erickson nor Kohut had such a commitment to science as I feel. Erickson did place great value on flexibility of thought and action, and he warned against too much loyalty to a method, a school of thought, a mentor, or a technique. He said, "Remember that whatever way you choose to work must be your own way, because you cannot really imitate someone else" (Haley, 1967, p. 535). This is similar to a statement I have often made to students and those in training: "There is one *best* school of therapy. It is the school of therapy you develop for yourself based on a continuing critical examination of the effects of your way of being in the relationship."

Kohut was much interested in the formulation of a theory of the development of personality. His concepts are intriguing and complex. What troubles me is his lack of interest in testing his theories.

Let me give an example. Kohut sees the self as developing along two lines, beginning in infancy: the *grandiose self* and the *idealized parent image*. He postulates "that in early self-development the infant's narcissistic exhibitionism and idealization become established as independent constituents of a 'nuclear' self: the grandiose and the reinternalized ideal parent image" (Graf, 1984, p. 82).

Without quibbling about definitions, this is an interesting basic theory. It can never be disproved. By the same token, however, it can never be proven nor validated. There is no known way by which we can enter the infant's conceptual world to discover if in fact there are these two lines of development. So this theoretical formulation, like most psychoanalytic theories, exists only in a speculative space. It thus becomes a matter of belief or disbelief, rather than a matter of confirmation or disconfirmation.

I have been puzzled by the lack of interest in testability of theories exhibited by Kohut and others. I see it as perhaps due to two factors.

The first is a European tradition which sees theory as an entity in itself, rather than as a step toward more solid knowledge. (Einstein's theory of relativity was only that—a theory—until it was confirmed by observational findings.)

The second factor is Kohut's belief that a *genetic* explanation of his patient's behavior is essential to cure. This means that the analyst must know and understand the patient's past. Hence there must be theories concerned with the way in which behavior develops. The analyst must *know* the past history—the inner and outer history—of the patient's infancy and childhood in order to make a useful and valid genetic interpretation.

But this overlooks a most important fact. We can never *know* the past. All that exists is someone's current *perception* of the past. Even the most elaborate case history, or the most complete free association about the past, reveals only memories present *now*, "facts" as perceived *now*. We can never *know* the individual's past. I pointed out earlier that "the effective reality which influences behavior is at all times the perceived reality. We can operate theoretically from this base without having to resolve the difficult question of what *really* constitutes reality" (Rogers, 1959, p. 223).

I believe Kohut is mistaken in thinking that data gathering—through empathy or otherwise—is a key to an accurate and helpful causal explanation of present behavior.

I do not minimize the importance of dealing with the past as it is remembered in the present. But my client is the one best able to see the significant patterns in this remembered past. I cannot, no matter how much I desire it, give my client an account of his/her *real* past.

Because of this assumed importance of *genetic* interpretations, Kohut must know the patient's past and the course of his/her development. This leads to theories about personality development which are of necessity speculative and untestable.

Thus, Kohut and I differ sharply over the nature of theory and particularly over our ability to know and interpret a *real* past history of any client/patient.

THE APPLICATION OF THERAPEUTIC PRINCIPLES

In one respect, the work that I and my colleagues have done is completely different from that of Erickson, Kohut, and most other psychotherapists. This point of difference is my interest in using the principles I feel I have learned in therapy, in fields quite divergent from those in which they originated.

Why have I been involved in the application of therapeutic learnings? I believe it is partially due to the fact that an important part of me is a scientist. I understand the enthusiastic exaggeration of Archimedes when he discovered that the forces operative in the lever could be described in a mathematical formula. "Then," he said, "If I have a lever long enough, I can move the world!" I, too, have dreamed of that long lever!

I expressed something of this sort a decade ago, when I was in a large workshop in which I felt we were discovering important things.

If we can find even one partial truth about the process by which 136 people can live together without destroying one another, can live together with a caring concern for the full development of each person, can live together in the richness of diversity instead of the sterility of conformity, then we may have found a truth with many, many implications. (Rogers, 1977, p. 175)

Since writing that I have had increasing opportunity to test some facilitative principles in practice. There have been many cross-cultural workshops, a number of interracial groups, and more and more groups containing antagonistic factions (Rogers, 1977, Chapters 6 and 7; 1984).

It was a privilege and a challenge to deal with a group from Belfast, with militant Protestant and Catholic members (Rogers, 1977); a group in Dublin with persons from Northern and Southern Ireland as well as participants from many other countries; a black/white group in South Africa (Sanford, 1984); a group of international leaders from Central and South America and other interested countries, focused on "The Central American Challenge" (Rogers, 1986a). In my wildest dreams I could not have imagined participating in such an exciting series of events.

In each of these groups I learned a great deal. In each one there have been disappointments; in no case have there been miracles. However, in each of these situations there occurred a decrease in bitterness, an improvement in communication, and constructive actions taken by members after the workshop.

I find a deep satisfaction in discovering that some of my basic learnings in psychotherapy apply in other areas of life. This is not a one-way street. I learned about therapy from my experiences in these different fields. I found that the sort of climate which is so important in the therapeutic relationship is also important in education, in administration, in dealing with interracial, intercultural, and even international tensions and conflicts. This was a richly rewarding experience. To have the opportunity to test such principles in three of the world's "hot spots"—Northern Ireland, Central America, and South Africa—has been incredibly special. I am well aware that these opportunities have been small in scale—test-tube experiments, really—but I hope they have helped to set precedents for a more human interaction that may move us in the direction of peace.

REFERENCES

Erickson, M.H., Rossi, E.L., & Rossi, S.I. (1976). *Hypnosis realities: The induction of hypnosis and forms of indirect suggestion.* New York: John Wiley.

Erickson, M. H. & Zeig, J. K. (1980). Symptom prescription for expanding the psychotic's world view. In E. L. Rossi (Ed.), *The collected papers of Milton H. Erickson on hypnosis: Vol. 4* (pp. 335–337). New York: Irvington.

Gilligan, S. G. (1982). Ericksonian approaches to clinical hypnosis. In J. K. Zeig (Ed.), *Ericksonian approaches to hypnosis and psychotherapy* (pp. 87–103). New York: Brunner/Mazel.

Goldberg, A. (Ed.) (1980). *Advances in self-psychology.* With summarizing reflections by Heinz Kohut. New York: International Universities Press.

Graf, C. L. (1984). *Healthy narcissism and new-age individualism: A synthesis of the theories of Carl Rogers and Heinz Kohut.* Unpublished doctoral dissertation, State University of New York, Stony Brook.

Gunnison, H. (1985, May). The uniqueness of similarities: parallels of Milton H. Erickson and Carl Rogers. *Journal of Counseling and Development, 63,* 561–564.

Haley, J. (Ed.) (1967). *Advanced techniques of hypnosis and therapy: Selected papers of Milton H. Erickson, M.D.* New York: W. W. Norton.

Kahn, E. (1985, August). Heinz Kohut and Carl Rogers: a timely comparison. *American Psychologist, 40,* 893–904.

Kohut, H. (1978). The psychoanalyst in the community of scholars. In P. H. Ornstein (Ed.), *The search for self: Selected writings of H. Kohut* (Vols. 1–3). New York: International Universities Press.

Kohut, H. (1981, October 4). *Remarks on empathy* [Film]. Filmed at Conference on Self-Psychology, Los Angeles.

Paterson, C. H. (1984). Empathy, warmth, and genuineness in psychotherapy: A review of reviews. *Psychotherapy: Theory, Research and Practice, 21,* 431–438.

Rogers, C. R. (1947, September). Some observations on the organization of personality. *American Psychologist, 2,* 358–368.

Rogers, C. R. (1957). A note on the nature of man. *Journal of Counseling Psychology, 4,* 199–203.

Rogers, C. R. (1959). A theory of therapy, personality and interpersonal relationships as developed in the client-centered framework. In S. Koch (Ed.), *Psychology: A study of a science, Vol. III. Formulations of the person and the social context* (pp. 184–256). New York: McGraw-Hill.

Rogers, C. R. (1977). *Carl Rogers on personal power.* New York: Delacorte.

Rogers, C. R. (1980). *A way of being.* Boston: Houghton Mifflin.

Rogers, C. R. (1984). One alternative to nuclear planetary suicide. In R. Levant & J. Shlien (Eds.), *Client-centered therapy and the person-centered approach: New directions in theory, research and practice* (pp. 400–422). New York: Praeger Publishers.

Rogers, C. R. (1985a, May). Reactions to Gunnison's article on the similarities between Erickson and Rogers. *Journal of Counseling and Development, 63,* 565–566.

Rogers, C. R. (1985b, Fall). Toward a more human science of the person. *Journal of Humanistic Psychology, 25,* #4, 7–24.

Rogers, C. R. (1986a). The Rust Workshop: A personal overview. *Journal of Humanistic Psychology,* Summer 1986, *26,* in press.

Rogers, C. R. (1986b). Client-centered therapy. In I. L. Kutash & A. Wolf (Eds.), *Psychotherapist's casebook: Theory and technique in practice* (pp. 197–208). San Francisco: Jossey-Bass.

Rogers, C. R., & Dymond, R. F. (Eds.) (1954). *Psychotherapy and personality change.* Chicago: University of Chicago Press.

Sanford, R. (1984). The beginning of a dialogue in South Africa. *Counseling Psychologist, 12,* 3, 3–14.

Stolorow, R. D. (1976). Psychoanalytic reflections on client-centered therapy in the light of modern conceptions of narcissism. *Psychotherapy: Theory, Research and Practice, 13,* 26–29.

An Inquiry into the Evolution of the Client-Centered Approach to Psychotherapy

◆

Ruth C. Sanford, M.A.

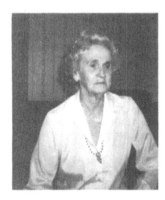

Ruth C. Sanford, M.A.
Ruth C. Sanford (M.A., Teachers College, Columbia University, 1938) was chosen by Carl Rogers as his co-faculty member. She is adjunct professor at three universities: Long Island University, Hofstra, and the Union of Experimenting Colleges and Universities in Cincinnati; she resides in Seaford, New York. As a longtime co-worker of Carl Rogers, Sanford is quite conversant with the central tenets of the person-centered approach. She describes personal and professional perspectives on the evolution of its key concepts and addresses the issue of elitism as it applies to psychotherapy.

In this joint presentation of the client-centered approach to psychotherapy, Carl Rogers has chosen to review some of his current thinking and applications of the client/person-centered approach in a wider field of psychological and social endeavors. With the theme of this conference in mind, he has also chosen to point out and further clarify comparisons and contrasts between his work and that of Milton Erickson and of Heinz Kohut.

It is my intention to look into my own experience and into the literature as I trace the evolution that has occurred *within* the client/person-centered approach to psychotherapy and extended to include other significant relationships during the period from the 1940s to the present.

Because I think of my life as a journey I am, in reality, inviting you to fall into step with me as I retrace a few steps before setting forth on this new part of our journey together.

Not only do many of the paths, the highways, the flights of my experience become fresh again in my "mind's eye," but also companions who have walked with me, some briefly, others for years. As I began writing, two companions came to mind, each with a message that, at this moment, seems relevant to what I am about to do.

The first was a college professor whom

I would not have considered a "significant other" in my life. She was my English composition teacher in my freshman year of college. I was attracted to her but I didn't like her very much, and I have reason to believe that she didn't like me either. At the end of the year I had written my crowning piece of work, a research paper well documented, written in my best style, neatly copied, carefully edited and on time. I was sure the paper deserved an A. I was being considered for selection as a sophomore assistant in the English Department for the following year, so the term paper was especially important.

At the next meeting of the class it came back to me with a "B-" and, written in firm hand, diagonally across the front fold, "Fluent, well-written. A patchwork, a clever compendium of other people's ideas."

How cruel and how right she was!

Only just now has a second experience involving my daughter during her junior year in high school became significantly related to the earlier one and, I now realize, to this presentation.

My daughter, Mei-Mei, wrote a paper on Herman Melville relating his work to the Transcendentalists. It seemed to me a well-written paper, advancing some original thoughts on the subject, and quite remarkable for one so young. Her teacher called her to the office of the department and confronted Mei-Mei sternly with, "What is the authority on which you base this interpretation?" Mei-Mei's answer was "Sixteen years of living. These are my own opinions based on my readings and observations." With the final comment, "That is no authority!" the paper was returned to her with a low grade.

From both of these experiences, one personal and one vicarious, I have learned about myself and about the facilitation of learning. In this presentation I shall refer to the work of persons who are widely recognized for their contributions in their fields and from whom I have learned. I shall also rely heavily on my own experience, the only experience I can truly know. For the most part I shall not use the impersonal third person of academe.

Over a period of 13 years I have found in the client-centered approach to psychotherapy and in the person-centered approach to a wide range of personal, professional relationships a compatibility with my own philosophical approach to living and being with myself and other—I was about to say people. But I am moved to include other living beings and the world about me. Before 1972 I held many of these values and used them in my work as a counselor and administrator, and, with more difficulty, in my intimate family relationships. Acquaintance with the person-centered approach brought more focus, more affirmation, more meaning, more wholeness to my complex, demanding, and often fragmented days.

For many years I had been a caring, conscientious, certified, trained, competent, in some ways effective counselor and teacher with my share of error and success—even some special recognition and awards.

But it was when I *unlearned* the how-to's and formalized theory of much of my professional training that I could sit down facing a client or student, with my head and my eyes clear of clutter, look into the eyes of another *person*, feel their presence and be free to enter into the experience of the other person, undistracted. It was a fresh and energizing experience.

So I have put aside a whole heap of techniques, therapies, expectations, rules, how-to's, methods, strategies, tests, case studies, case histories, theories, et cetera, et cetera, et cetera. They are all in here, somewhere, a part of me; but I do not pull them out for use, one by one, choosing which one is at the moment appropriate, or will *work* on this person or in that situation. I have no way of knowing just what fertile seeds will grow from the compost heap of my making, but they continue to grow.

EVOLUTION WITHIN THE CLIENT-CENTERED APPROACH TO PSYCHOTHERAPY

I. FROM NON-DIRECTIVE TECHNIQUE TO CLIENT-CENTERED PSYCHOTHERAPY TO A PERSON-CENTERED WAY OF BEING

Over a period of 40-years, the growth that began with the non-directive technique evolved first to client-centered therapy, to a person-centered approach to interpersonal relationships.

It is the changing organismic quality, the vitality of the growing edge that appeals to me in this approach. Emphasis on *non-directive technique* in the early 1940s, although still rooted in the diagnostic-prescriptive approach, was one of the early buds on this new plant. Rogers in *A Way of Being* (1980, p. 37) says of these years, the early 1940s:

I began to realize that I was saying something new, perhaps even original, about counseling and psychotherapy, and I wrote the book of that title. My dream of recording therapeutic interviews came true, helping to focus my interest on the effects of different responses in the interview. This led to a heavy emphasis on technique—the so-called non-directive technique.

It was during those years that the word "reflective" was rather widely used in describing the *non-directive* response of the therapist. Both terms were sometimes seen as passive and indicative of a person who put himself away and repeated accurately what the client said and nodded or said "um hum" to let the client know he was listening.

What happened next is for me part of a pattern of growth that has characterized the evolution of the client/person-centered approach. The early emphasis was on recording, observing, and evaluating not only the therapeutic process but also the part of the therapist and the client in the process—similar to the way a scientist works.

It was this unfamiliar method of giving order to experience in the therapeutic relationship that opened up the possibility by the lay and professional public of oversimplification of a very complex, very active way of interacting in a very delicate relationship. Such oversimplification resulted in mechanical responses on the part of some practitioners who adopted the designation "Rogerian." Only last year I heard a university professor refer to this kind of response as "orthodox Rogerian"!

Concluding the earlier quotation, Rogers continues, "I found that I had embarked not on a new *method* of therapy but a sharply different *philosophy* of living and relationships" (pp. 37–38).

Here the two metaphors come into focus, that of the growing plant and that of the journey, the two metaphors best characterizing the client-centered/person-centered approach: the potato sprout growing toward the light even in a dark cellar and the therapist walking beside the client as they set out on a journey into self and toward becoming a fully functioning person, more fully functioning within the self and more fully functioning as a responsible resident of the planet Earth.

Rogers, in *A Theory of the Fully Functioning Person* (1959, pp. 234–235), wrote:

Certain directional tendencies in the individual and certain needs have been explicitly postulated in the theory thus far presented. . . . There is already implicit in what has been given a concept of the ultimate in the actualization of the human organism. This ultimate hypothetical person would be synonymous with "the goal of social evolution," "the end point of optimal psychotherapy," etc. We have chosen to term this individual the fully functioning person. It should be evident that the term "the fully functioning person" is synonymous with optimal psychological adjustment, optimal psychological maturity, complete congruence, complete openness to experience, complete extensionality as these terms have been defined.

Since some of these terms sound somewhat static, as though such a person "had arrived," it should be pointed out that all the charac-teristics of such a person are *process* charac-teristics. . . . The only statement which can be made is that the behaviors would be ade-quately adaptive to each new situation, and that the person would be continually in a pro-cess of further self-actualization.

II. FROM FULLY FUNCTIONING SELF TO FULLY FUNCTIONING SELF WITHIN THE SOCIETY: SELF TO SOCIAL AWARENESS/INVOLVEMENT

Similar to the quiet process of growth in other life forms, we have moved almost unnoticed to another facet of the evolution within this process—the evolution that took place between the 1940s and 1983, from emphasis on the fully functioning person, the inner self of that person, to the inclusion by the self-fulfilling, more fully functioning person, of the *Other* or Others, in relationship. I shall call this the *movement toward socialization.*

Within the context of evolution or or-ganismic growth, I find quite illuminating a statement by Rogers in 1983 on the same subject:

Here, then, is my theoretical model of the per-son who emerges from therapy, *from the best of education*, the individual who has experi-enced optimal psychological growth—the per-son functioning freely in all the fullness of his organismic potentialities; a person who is de-pendable in being realistic, self-enhancing, so-cialized, and appropriate in his behavior; a creative person, whose specific formings of be-havior are not easily predictable; a person who is ever-changing, ever developing, always dis-covering himself and the newness in himself in each succeeding moment of time. . . .
Let me stress, however, that what I have de-scribed is a person who does not exist. He is the theoretical goal, the end-point of personal growth. We, the persons moving in this direc-tion from the best of experience in education and from the best experience in therapy, from the best of family and group relationships . . . . But what we observe is the imperfect

person moving toward this goal. [Italics added for emphasis] (p. 295)

The organismic growth in the concept of the therapeutic experience brought with it not only a wider field of functioning for the client, but a broadening of the concept of the therapist, functioning in the climate of the person-centered approach, and com-patible with the metaphor of companion on a journey—a more experienced and mature companion, but quite different from an expert or a doctor who prescribes a remedy, or a wise person who knows the "solution" and will bring the patient around to it in due time, or at least will reveal in the process the causes of the illness or dilemma.

We are seeing the experienced thera-pist, a fallible human being, psychologi-cally and emotionally mature, secure enough within her/himself to be real and open in the relationship, trustful enough of self to enter into the world of the other and move about comfortably in it without losing him/herself, and holding her/him-self in sufficient respect, not only to accept the client with nonpossessive, nonjudg-mental caring, but to communicate that attitude accurately to the client.

We are seeing the therapist (and read-ing in the literature about the therapist) as a facilitator of change, of growth, of learning, of self-empowerment for the other. We are seeing the facilitator who can work with individuals or groups in an academic institution, an agency, a busi-ness organization, a center of conflict, in less depth and intensity over a shorter period of time but with many of the same results as a therapist working with *a client*, one-to-one in a traditional setting. As the therapist is a companion on the journey of a client, so the teacher is a companion to the student, and the group facilitator is a companion to each member of a group on the journey of self-discovery and growth. Other members of the inten-sive group, in turn, become companions in the search, and in the experience of hundreds of participants, the experience is even more powerful in its own way than psychotherapy alone, and also can lead to long-lasting changes.

In retrospect, an excerpt from Rogers (1970, p. 116) was prophetic:

Doubtless there are other ways in which this loneliness can be allayed. I have simply tried to present one way, the encounter group or the intensive group experience, in which we seem to be creating a means of putting real individuals in touch with other real individuals. It is, I believe, one of our most successful modern inventions for dealing with the feeling of unreality, of impersonality, and of distance and separation that exists in so many people in our culture. What the future of this trend will be I do not know. It may be taken over by fadists and manipulators. It may be superceded by something even more effective. At the present time it is the best instrument I know for healing the loneliness that prevails in so many human beings. It holds forth the hope that isolation need not be the keynote of our individual lives.

III. BEYOND THE ELITISM OF TRADITIONAL PSYCHOTHERAPY

My own personal experience in an intensive week-long seminar at the Universidad Iberoamericana in Mexico City in 1982 speaks clearly and eloquently not only of my own process of growth, but also of the process of evolution within the living, growing organism of the whole approach we are examining. It was at the close of a morning panel in which six or seven panelists representing analysts, behavioral psychotherapists and humanistic psychotherapists (by their own self-descriptions) presented the basic tenets of their approach or system, the structure of their practice, and practical situations illustrating their success and problems. There was some discussion among them before questions from participants, in a group of about 250, were invited. The questions were serious and probing.

A graduate student who came from and worked among the underprivileged of her

city spoke with a strong Spanish accent. She directed a question to me: "We are a part of the so-called *third world*, a developing country. We have millions of people who struggle every day to survive, who feel powerless, many emotionally distraught, isolated, parents trying to do well for their children, living in strife, who desperately need the kind of help and support you on the panel have been describing. But only a very few of our more educated and affluent can afford the fees you charge. And even for those who could, with hardship, pay—there are not enough therapists of all kinds to help them. Some of you have said one of the criteria for selecting patients is 'Can they pay for one, two, three or more sessions a week for a determined period of time!' What has the person-centered approach to offer in our country?"

In a flash I saw what I had learned and experienced over many years about short-term therapy, ability-to-pay fees and, above all, our work and research with intensive groups. It was instantaneous, the turning of a kaleidoscope of happenings like subliminal images projected on a screen, and through it all came the word *elitism*. Her direct, piercing, very human question had penetrated the facade of fine-sounding words and preoccupation with theory and brought us back to people.

In response I spoke of the elitism of all psychotherapies, not only in Mexico and *the third world*, but also in the U.S., and *for the first time* ever I addressed the issue in light of the evolution toward socialization within the client/person-centered approach. It was as if suddenly I saw something as *new*, so clearly that the concept and the words emerged together. It was, for me, one of those rare moments of insight that brings about irreversible personal change. Out of that moment came the term *beyond elitism*. "We must move beyond."

For me, moving beyond elitism means moving beyond the hierarchical selectivity of the one-to-one-only, prescribed, long-term, therapist/analyst dominated treatment pattern for patients. It means first moving away from the medical model, labels and diagnoses, prognoses, plans of treatment, quick dependence on drugs, and a "the doctor knows best" attitude, and moving toward trust in the potential of the human organism for growth and positive change, for self-direction, for assuming responsibility for its own growth and actions. It means laying aside the illusion that a psychotherapist, no matter how well-trained or well-grounded in a system, no matter how well-intentioned, can be the expert on another person's life and experience or destiny. It means stepping down from the dais.

Moving beyond elitism means that I acknowledge the efficacy of even a large group of participants interacting in a climate conducive to emotional and psychological growth—facilitated, not dominated by experienced persons—to bring about growthful change in individuals who take the opportunity to empower themselves. It means that I accept many avenues by which a client or group participant can enter a growth-promoting or therapeutic relationship, and thereafter can find other ways of continuing the growthful change alone, in other groups or in a client-therapist relationship. It means that I trust that the process, once set in motion will continue even if I (the therapist or facilitator) am not there to make it happen or direct its course—or, what may be more wrenching to accept, *because* I am not there to direct or make it happen.

No one can calculate the life-touching effect of the numbers who have been part of intensive groups all over the world, and in turn have touched others in this freeing way.

Our return in January, 1986, to South Africa, by invitation from participants in groups with whom we worked in 1982, for the purpose of facilitating intensive groups for professional people, students, volunteers in helping professions representing all classifications, who want in turn to facilitate groups in their own communities, attests to the potential for pos-

itive change even in groups of 50 to 600. The hope is that as individuals have the experience of listening, caring about one another, and learning to know one another, communication and understanding will grow across lines of conflict, and that individuals will empower themselves and hold both themselves and others in more positive regard.

Add to the process set in motion in intensive groups the same kind of experience in the best of education "taught" by experienced facilitators in elementary, high schools, colleges and universities. Then, without belaboring the parallel, I return to Roger's reference to the end point of psychotherapy.

Is this an answer to the question, "What has the person-centered approach to offer in a 'third-world' country"? It is the best response I have as of today.

IV. FROM ACCEPTANCE TO LOVE TO UNCONDITIONAL POSITIVE REGARD IN THE THERAPEUTIC RELATIONSHIP: RESPONSE TO A HUMAN NEED

Unconditional positive regard, one of the three conditions clearly stated as necessary and sufficient for constructive personality change to take place (Rogers, 1957), has been selected for examination in this presentation because it illustrates the process of evolution of the concept from its use in 1951 to the present. As we trace the evolving meaning of the term, we become involved in the search for an exact word that would best communicate the essence of the concept. This purposeful search for meaning, for testing of hypotheses by research and experience, and a relentless striving for clarity and communication have marked the work of Rogers from the beginning. A second and by far more compelling reason for focusing on this one of the three conditions is stated clearly by Rogers:

As the awareness of the self emerges, the individual develops a *need for positive regard.*

This need is universal in human beings, and in the individual, is pervasive and persistent. Whether it is an inherent or learned need is irrelevant to the theory (1959, p. 223).

The need and the satisfaction of the need are seen as reciprocal in a relationship with a significant other or others. Development of the need for self-regard and development of conditions for worth or of unconditionality are basically important to development of personality. This is a strong statement, and so far as I have learned from the literature, the *need* for positive regard without conditions is the only need so defined in the evolution of the client/person-centered approach.

Our purpose will be well served by going back to the experience in therapy from which the term evolved. In the chapter "The Process of Therapy" (Rogers, 1951, p. 159) we come upon an introduction to the concept in the context of process or experience:

One hypothesis is that the client moves from the experiencing of himself as an unworthy, unacceptable, and unlovable person to the realization that he is accepted, respected, and loved, in this limited relationship with the therapist. "Loved" has here perhaps its deepest and most general meaning—that of being deeply understood and deeply accepted.

The term *nondirective* was being used at the Counseling Center of the University of Chicago at the time that this hypothesis involving acceptance, respect and love was being formulated. Another way of "framing" the same hypothesis is that as the client experiences acceptance on the part of the therapist, he is able to accept and experience the same attitude toward himself and, as he thus begins to accept, respect, like, and love himself, he is capable of experiencing these attitudes toward others.

Oliver H. Bown, a member of the staff, felt strongly that the term love, easily misunderstood though it may be, is the most useful term "to describe a basic ingredient for the therapeutic relationship"

(Rogers, 1951, p. 160). Bown supports his position as follows:

It seems to me that we can love a person only to the extent that we are not threatened by him. . . . Thus, if a person is hostile towards me and I can see nothing in him at the moment except the hostility, I am quite sure that I will react in a defensive way to the hostility. If, on the other hand, I can see this hostility as an understandable component of the person's defense against feeling the need for closeness to people, I can then react with love toward this person, who also wants love, but who at the moment must pretend not to. Similarly, and somewhat more important to me in my experience, I feel that positive feeling expressed by the client toward us can be a very real source of threat, provided again that this positive expression, in whatever form it may take, is not clearly related to these same basic motivations mentioned above (p. 161).

Bown, in his willingness to be open and accepting of his own feelings and to be honest in recognizing those feelings in relationship with the client, found that his clients " . . . moved into more delicate areas which I had been (through fear) shutting off within myself, and the feelings and needs which were involved in these areas could not only be discussed but also experienced freely and without fear" (p. 165). To him, the alternative was a deeply and subtly nonverbally expressed warning, "Do not express your deepest feelings or needs for in this relationship it is dangerous." He adds, "acceptance is an emotional phenomenon, not an intellectual one" (p. 165).

Bown has probed with courage and daring into the relationship of client and therapist as a real human relationship and thereby has challenged me to face my fears, my self-imposed limitations in relationships and to test the depth to which I can trust and accept both myself and the other. Experience of his struggle for realness and acceptance of his deep feeling (his and the other's) becomes more significant when followed by a long detailed statement from the client.

Rogers closes this part of the chapter in this way: "The hypotheses which are implicit in this formulation will be difficult—though not impossible—to put to rigorous test. This is a way of looking at the change which goes on in therapy which cannot be overlooked." So much for the pre-1951 use of "perhaps the purest form of love" as a basic ingredient in the process of positive personality change in therapy! As Bown acknowledged, the term love in our society is so enmeshed in romantic fantasy that misunderstanding easily grew out of oversimplification by both the lay and professional public and could easily have identified this deeply responsible, honest, sensitive, mature and delicate involvement in a relationship by the casual and unknowledgeable or insensitive critic as cheap, unethical and an "anything goes" attitude.

It was in 1954 that Standal first formally introduced the term *positive regard,* which has been in wide use since that time. In 1959 Rogers added the *unconditional,* which in turn caused the casual reader to raise questions that obscured the deeper meaning. An inquiry into the deeper intended meaning of *unconditional positive regard* was reported in a paper, "Unconditional Positive Regard: A Misunderstood Way of Being" (Sanford, 1984), and in Rogers' "Client-Centered Therapy" from *Psychotherapist's Casebook: Theory and Technique in Practice* (1986). The most recent description is ". . . acceptance or caring or prizing—unconditional positive regard."

In my opinion, "acceptance, caring, prizing" without the unconditional positive regard falls short of conveying the essential of unconditionality. There are in our society, in education, in business, in family and intimate relationships, including the relationship between client and therapist, varying levels of acceptance, prizing, caring—but usually with conditions attached. The parent implies, "I love you when you're good."; the teacher, "I accept you when you work hard and get a good grade."; the doctor to the patient in the hospital, "I like you or care more for you when you do as you're told."; the corporation says, "Follow the line and the boss will like you. You'll succeed."

Where and how many times in a lifetime does one know that she or he is unconditionally loved and accepted, valued, held in positive nonjudgmental regard? How many persons from the start have someone or ones significant in their lives who say verbally or nonverbally, "I love you. I respect your personhood even when I disagree or don't like what you do. I know you can't always 'do things right' anymore than I can. Sometimes I'll be angry and sometimes I can't be with you but I'll try to listen to you and understand and I don't stop caring for you or write you off because you do something I don't like." In such an experience, a relationship with another significant human being is great power for healing.

There is nurturance in the response of another to the basic need for positive regard, universal in human beings, and in the individual, pervasive and persistent.

Alice Miller, formerly a teaching psychoanalyst in Switzerland, devotes two chapters of her book *For Your Own Good* (1983) to the effect on Adolf Hitler of the hidden horror of his origin, family, childhood and education. It is evident from her painstakingly researched and documented study (pp. 142–197) that cruel beatings in early childhood by a father who permitted no expression of feeling on the child's part fostered a total denial of the basic, human need for acceptance. She raises the question, "What did this child *feel,* what did he *store up* inside when he was beaten and demeaned by his father every day from an early age?"

She continues, "He knew that nothing he did would have any effect on the daily thrashing he was given. All he could do was to deny the pain, in other words, deny himself and identify with the aggressor. No one could help him, not even his mother for this would spell danger for her too, because she also was battered" (p. 146).

Dr. Miller refers to severe discipline and, again, denial of nurturance in school. "Who knows, perhaps this bright and gifted child might have found a different, more humane way of dealing with his pent-up hatred if his curiosity and vitality had been given nourishment in school. But even an appreciation of intellectual values was made impossible for him" (p. 168).

From a vicarious experience of the life of Adolf Hitler to which I have referred briefly, I am led to raise the question implied by Dr. Miller: If one person, parent, servant, friend or teacher had listened to his pain, anger, frustration and accepted him and his anger before it was turned in upon himself, where it burned out of control, would it have become the fiery cauldron of rage and hate that destroyed millions and himself?

I hear in that question a plea for unconditional positive regard, particularly as it relates to the rearing and nurturing of children. I hear in it a strong statement of the effectiveness, socially and even politically, of meeting the pervasive and persistent need of human beings for unconditional positive regard, somewhere, sometime, from someone, and the terrible consequences of what appears to be a complete lack of response to that need.

Alice Miller has forced me to look with clear eyes at what I have learned about regard for the person by right of being human and to listen to that person deeply before I build a wall of the stuff of my own arrogance against another's reality.

So again the search for the elegance of the finely tuned word, the exact phrase, is evident in the evolution of the client-person centered approach. Perhaps in 1986 a more expressive term or description for this quality will be found.

V. FROM TRADITIONAL LINEAR TO NEW PARADIGM RESEARCH: BRINGING ORDER TO EXPERIENCE

The term that first comes to mind in this aspect of evolution within the client-centered approach is the quest for bringing order to continually growing changing experience. Careful application of scientific procedure to examination of subjective experience during the 1940s at the Counseling Center, University of Chicago, brought to psychotherapy the concept of formulation of hypotheses out of the living stuff of the therapeutic relationship itself—something new in the field of psychotherapy. It moved toward removing the illusion of magic from the therapeutic or analytic phenomenon and studying the relationship between two persons as under a microscope. In the research of this group and the writing of it the conviction of researchers that "a science can never make therapists but it can help therapy" is evident.

Until 1940, objective research studies in any way related to psychotherapy were practically nonexistent—perhaps there were a handful. From 1940 to 1950 workers in client-centered orientations conducted and published more than 40 research studies with half as many again underway at the time. It was a bursting forth of significant research projects, so painstakingly designed, carried out and reported that, in the words of Rogers (1951, pp. 12–13) " . . . each one (is) described in sufficient detail so that any competent worker can verify the findings." It demonstrated that any phase of psychotherapy from heretofore unprobed subtleties of client-centered relationships in therapy to measures of behavioral change and personality development could be researched.

Electrically recorded case material made this painstaking process possible and, by overcoming the taboo of using material in this way, opened up the possibilities of these methods to workers using other approaches to psychotherapy. It was opening a door which had been considered unopenable.

Out of day-to-day experience, then, have grown and are growing theories and hypotheses of the client-centered approach. Thus, in research as well, the use of the term evolution is appropriate. It is impossible here and unnecessary for the informed reader to review the multitude of studies and published results, the Q-Sort, the ratings scales, the employment of trained evaluators uninvolved in the therapy process itself, the willingness of researchers to look honestly at negative as well as positive results, and the work with patients in a mental hospital as well as clients in a counseling center. (For reference to a wider range of early projects, see Rogers, 1951, *Client-Centered Therapy*, Chap. 4. See also Rogers, 1980, *A Way of Being*, Chap. 6; Rogers, 1983, *Freedom to Learn for the 80's*, pp. 197–221; and Rogers & Sanford, 1984, the section on research in the *Comprehensive Textbook of Psychiatry IV*.)

In 1985, in "Toward A More Human Science of the Person," Rogers points to the future and opens another window on research centered in the value of the person and its application in psychotherapy, education, family relationships, and communication between persons and groups in conflict.

My own interest in research centers at present in a year-long project, along with a group of former clients, graduate students and doctoral candidates, in which we are studying, observing the inner process of change in relationship between client and therapist, student and facilitator of learning, family members as well as among ourselves individually and in group from the point of view of the client or learner. This will be, as purely as we can make it so, participatory research (Reason & Rowan, 1981). There is a possibility that we may discover or identify patterns of inner change and growth in the person akin to patterns of growth and change in the more tangible forms that have emerged out of biological research.

We do not know what to expect but we are looking forward to the experience, knowing that in this kind of work the process itself is the research. So, a process that places the value in the person continues, venturing into unknown territory, redefining, testing hypotheses and forming new ones.

REFERENCES

Kirschenbaum, H. (1979). *On becoming Carl Rogers*. New York: Delacorte Press.

Levant, R. F. & Schlien, J. M. (Eds.). (1984). *Client-centered therapy and the person-centered approach: New directions in theory, research, and practice*. New York: Praeger.

Miller, A. (1983). *For your own good*. New York: Farrar, Strauss & Giroux.

Reason, R. & Rowan, J. (Eds.). (1981). *Human inquiry: A sourcebook of new paradigm research*. New York: John Wiley.

Rogers, C. R. (1951). *Client-centered therapy: Its current practice, implications and theory*. Boston: Houghton Mifflin.

Rogers, C. R. (1957). The necessary and sufficient conditions of therapeutic personality change. *Journal of Consulting Psychology, 21*, 95–103.

Rogers, C. R. (1959). A theory of therapy, personality and interpersonal relationships as developed in the client-centered framework. In S. Koch (Ed.), *Psychology: The study of a science: Vol. III, Formulation of the person and the social context* (pp. 184–251). New York: McGraw-Hill.

Rogers, C. R. (1963). A concept of the fully functioning person. *Psychotherapy: Theory, research and practice, 1*(1), 17–26.

Rogers, C. R. (1970). *On encounter groups*. New York: Harper & Row.

Rogers, C. R. (1980). *A way of being*. Boston: Houghton Mifflin.

Rogers, C. R. (1983). *Freedom to learn for the 80's*. Columbus, OH: Charles E. Merrill.

Rogers, C. R. (1985). Toward a more human science of the person. *Journal of Humanistic Psychology, 25*(4), 7–24.

Rogers, C. R. (1986). Client-centered therapy. In I. L. Kutash & A. Wolf (Eds.), *Psychotherapist's casebook: Theory and technique in practice*. San Francisco: Jossey-Bass.

Rogers, C. R. & Sanford, R. C. (1984). Client-centered psychotherapy. In H. J. Kaplan & B. J. Sadock (Eds.), *Comprehensive textbook of psychiatry IV* (pp. 1374–1388). Baltimore: Williams & Wilkins.

Sanford, R. C. (1984). *Unconditional positive regard: A misunderstood way of being*. Unpublished manuscript.

Standal, S. (1954). *The need for positive regard: A contribution to client-centered theory*. Unpublished doctoral dissertation. University of Chicago, Chicago, IL.

Discussion by Miriam Polster, Ph.D.

◆

The common theme I hear in what Dr. Sanford and Dr. Rogers have said centers around this trouble between technique and humanity and the use of the one in order to achieve or support or nourish the other. In a sense, what we are talking about is the struggle each of us undergoes when we come to someone like Dr. Rogers in order to learn for our personal goals. I am talking about the struggle for mastery of our craft. We can see some common aspects of this in all masters, be they in the sciences, in the arts, in the fine arts, wherever they are.

I remember I was in graduate school when research showed that as psychotherapists became more and more experienced they more and more resembled each other. What we are seeing, then, is the paring away of the nonessentials. When we look at some of Picasso's paintings, we see many that are incredibly complicated in construction as they go off in all directions. There is a freedom that surprises us. A Picasso drawing may in three lines—beautifully made and appropriately placed—suggest to us a human figure.

It is that quality of the paring away of the unessentials that makes for something I would hold true of you—what I call an "informed simplicity." Both those words are important. It is not a naivete, not a nonawareness, but rather a very aware, informed, respectful move toward simplicity. What I would like to talk about is what I see as some of the ingredients of simplicity I think we have perceived in Dr. Rogers' work from the beginning. He has shared so much with us of his personal and professional evolution and has linked them for us well. I think we have the right to say we have some sense of what the ingredients of his informed simplicity may be.

The first one for me is that of *precision.* Dr. Rogers has again and again looked at something with insight, separating one element from another and according them their proper place. Thus, in his masterful employment of the Q-sorts, we have a wonderfully precise way to deal with the perception of personal change. It was a brilliant way of investigating that phenomenon, and we also have an insight into what he considers the valid reporting of what has been going on in the process.

We saw another example of his precision when he was discussing what it was like to work with an individual when we investigate the past of the person. He said, and here is an example of the very precision I am talking about, "We do not know the past, we only know our perception of the past."

That sounds like a very simple statement but I think most of you can see what a very clear distinction is being made there and how functional that is in the conduct of therapy.

Another ingredient of informed simplicity is *openness.* Carl was one of the early persons to open the windows and door of the therapy room and examine the process. Therapy at best is a lonely procedure and to be able to bring in light and air and the possibility for openness and disseminating the data is an incredible move out of this small narrow compass. To have devised a way in which we can do it through recordings, Q-sorts and discussion of the conduct of therapy is a move both to respect for technique and to recognition that technique is merely the instrumentality and never deserves the prominence it has sometimes achieved.

This is the public transparency, the public examination of hypothesis and reaction. Carl's speaking often of his own process was an early and inspiring move from technology to humanity.

Another ingredient of informed simplicity is *curiosity*. There is a lively and unprejudiced turn of mind that considers that anything is worth looking at. This is not indiscriminate but rather an engagement with the world outside that finds nothing irrelevant. It can see in what other people might disregard the germ of an important way into the experience of another person or the application of this process to the previously unclaimed field of human endeavor.

Another ingredient of informed simplicity is *clarity*. For me the clarity is revealed over and over in Carl's use of language. His language about therapy is refreshingly untechnical. He uses words that everyday people use in talking about everyday things with everyday companions. This is not special arcane language requiring definition. The interesting thing is that he uses this not so special language in such a way that it is infused by his presence and his wish to understand the person he is talking to. What starts out as not special becomes very special indeed and elevates the ordinary into the sense of extraordinary. This is the kind of exchange that many of us hunger for, that needs to occur more and more often in our world. Carl is a master of this kind of exchange.

This leads to the next point I want to make about the language of informed simplicity—the quiet intensity that Carl often generates. There is an air to the way that Carl listens which amplifies what the individual is experiencing. He listens attentively and quietly and from that listening he produces and offers what it is that he has heard. The person is free to respond to it in a sense of having been adequately heard and understood. In the process there is an amplification of what the person has said that adds to the weight of what might

otherwise have been disregarded. There is a picking up of what might otherwise go unnoticed, and an offering of it back to the person for attention. This process increases the intensity of the exchange and gives it the leverage to move toward change in what seems like a very quiet interaction but one that is tremendously powerful.

Another ingredient in informed simplicity is *courage*. We have heard some examples, as when Dr. Rogers spoke of his address to the American Psychological Association and the resounding silence with which it was received. It takes courage to break a tradition. It is easy to go along using the same techniques and data and data-gathering process. To innovate, to break with tradition, to take a left turn when others are taking a right turn, or, as Ruth said, to have the flowering branch that goes off in its own direction is an extremely courageous act. Courage is not only in the defiance of death; it is frequently in the willingness to take a stand that no one has taken before. Fritz Redl wrote about delinquent behavior. The comparison may amuse you, but Carl performed what Redl called, when he was talking about delinquent adolescents, the magic of the initiatory act. That was something extremely important. Perhaps, Carl, you will become an adult delinquent.

The courage, then, consists of not only the break with tradition, but also the application of his particular perspectives to new populations and new issues. I think you can see in what Carl has been doing the broadening of the applications to territory that has previously been considered out of bounds, moving into it with courage and wisdom and a little sense of maybe, not knowing quite where it is going to go, but going with it anyhow and having faith in the belief, the perspective, the skill, and the humanity of the effort.

Another ingredient in informed simplicity is *the will to union*. This is the wish, somehow, to so fully enter and understand the experience of the other that one is willing to lose one's self. Carl has referred to these as his moments of altered consciousness, but the alteration of consciousness is very often determined by the willingness to lose one's customary sense of self, one's customary connections with what we lovingly call reality, and to let those go in order to meet the person, whoever he or she may be. And Carl's willingness to do that has been demonstrated over and over again—the willingness to give up his own perspective in order to feel the perspective of another.

You can probably add more but the final ingredient of the informed simplicity that I propose is *enthusiasm*. When Carl speaks of the opportunities he has had recently in Ireland, South Africa and Central America, you can see that here is a fresh, lively enthusiasm that looks for a new horizon, finds it and sails towards it. There is the energy and appetite for new experience that is another attribute in informed simplicity.

I would like to end by telling you, Ruth and Carl, of something that I had read. You were talking, Ruth, about changing unconditional love to unconditional positive regard. Someone once said, "Love is not blind, it is generous," and I think that is marvelous. One does not become unperceptive because one loves; as a matter of fact, we could even argue the opposite. You notice details, lovingly. But you are generous and what I want to propose is that Carl is an outstanding example of a generous, large-spirited human being.

QUESTIONS AND ANSWERS

Question: I work in a community with drug addicts, alcoholics and convicts with a current population of 140 people. One of the main tools we use is marathon retreats and I wanted to ask Dr. Rogers about that. During the 60s they were viewed as a very growth-producing experience. Our experience in the last 15 years has been that, when they are not abused, a lot of people can get into the big dimension of tapping their intuitive being. Many people have the opportunity to switch roles between being the therapist and the client, if you will, and it is an excellent tool to bridge gaps between people who think there are large differences. There seems to be an ability to find the similarities between people. In my observations in the last decade, this particular tool of marathon retreats has been used less and less. I wondered if you could comment on that.

Rogers: It sounds to me as though you are asking for confirmation of your own experience and I am very glad to give that. I think that if you have found it useful and effective, you should certainly continue to apply it. I have no special wisdom about marathon groups. I think one reason they have decreased is that often they were misused, but it sounds as though what you are doing is useful and effective and within sensible bounds. I would say, yes, I am glad to add any confirmation to your own experience that I can, simply saying you are trusting your own experience. Fine, go ahead.

Question: I understand, Dr. Rogers, that you are branching out from your work with the self and coming to an awareness of the collective unconscious that we all share within ourselves. I am very interested in Ericksonian work and would like you to speak about the collective unconscious.

Rogers: You are offering me a term that I don't use. There is a term that I do use that might be parallel: I really trust the wisdom of the group. And that was particularly put to test in this recent workshop in Austria with politicians, government officials, ambassadors, and so forth who were not accustomed to the group process. It was only a four-day workshop because you can't get people like that together for very long. It was a concession on their part to be there even for only four days. During the first two days it seemed to me that it was a highly intellectual procedure: People giving little speeches, good speeches, but I thought we were not getting to the heart of it. Yet I felt relatively powerless to change that flow. The only thing I could do was to sit tight in my trust in the wisdom of the group, in my belief that they would come to feel that this was not what they wanted from the meeting. Sure enough, that happened very dramatically at the end of the second day. The next morning we saw a very different workshop. I don't know if that is the collective unconscious, but I felt that the group in its own wisdom realized, "We don't want the same kind of intellectual exchange to which we are accustomed. This is an opportunity for something different. Why don't we make use of it?" And so they most assuredly did. The change from day two to day three was quite electric and I felt justified again in my trust in the group process, in the essential wisdom that exists collectively to move toward goals that individuals inwardly want.

One other minor aspect that might interest you was that many of these people were quite horrified at the fact that there was no set agenda for these meetings. The last day, one man, the vice-president of a Latin American country, said he was very disturbed at first when he learned that there was to be no set agenda, but he had come to realize that that is the most sensible way we could have operated and he now fully approved of it. Well, that is quite a shift, quite an observing of new experience. I feel the whole group went through that, beginning to trust the fact that acting individually in a very diversified fashion somehow made for a collective movement toward greater expressiveness and better communication, everything we are accustomed to in group process. I don't know if that really answers your question, but I think it is relevant.

Question: Could you discuss in a little more detail some of the feedback you re-

ceived from the participants in that workshop? Are you planning to publish any articles on the whole process?

Rogers: Yes, several of us are writing about our experience. I will very soon have completed a fairly brief paper giving an overview of it. One of the fascinating things about it was that I could get cooperation from the most unexpected sources. A major reason we were able to put on that workshop in Austria was that a bank in Vienna paid for all the expenses. At the end of the conference, the president, who had attended the first session and the last and said it was like night and day, offered to publish a book about the workshop in German, English and Spanish. We certainly intend to make use of this offer, so I hope that in the near future there will be more extended descriptions and analyses of the process that went on there.

Question: Dr. Rogers, Freudians pay a lot of attention to something called countertransference. I would be interested in how you have dealt with your unresolved personal problems that might relate to those your client is dealing with.

Rogers: When my unresolved personal problems get big enough, I go for another round of therapy with someone whom I trust. I feel that in regard to transference and countertransference, there is the greatest amount of guff. Yes, the client has feelings which can be preferably defined as transference. I have feelings that don't relate to the situation, that is very true. If I have persistent feelings about the client and about the relationship which are difficult to express, then I had better express them. I think any persistent feelings should be expressed in a relationship, but I simply don't believe in making a whole separate area out of feelings between the client and therapist. I deal with those feelings in the same way I deal with other feelings which arise in the situation. John Schlien has written a very good chapter called "Encounter Theory of Transference" in the recent book by Levant and Schlien, *Client-Centered Therapy and the Person-Centered Approach: New Developments in Theory, Research and Practice* (New York: Praeger, 1984).

It seems to me that this question of transference relates directly to the use in the client-centered approach of a nonmedical model, moving away from the hierarchical which can very easily help to set up that situation in which there is transference and all kinds of complex relationships. The therapist who goes on a journey with the client as a companion and the client who goes with the therapist on that journey can decide together when the time comes that the client wants to go it alone. There is much less expectation, I think, in such a relationship. It seems to me that that is a very important factor in this whole question.

Question: Did you have any critique of your own work that you could offer?

Rogers: I often feel very critical of what I do. However, for a real critique of my work I would rely on others. I value thoughtful criticism by others, but I am not a very good person to offer a critique of my work. Perhaps I will say one thing positive in nature. I quite agree with the statement that one of the most significant things I have done in my professional career is to record interviews. That simple fact really threw open a wide area for study. That is a positive critique. In the negative sense, it is possibly unfortunate that we became so interested in techniques that many people are still understanding my work as it was in 1940, regarded as a technique. I wish they would advance by 10 or 20 years.

Question: A theme throughout all of your work and certainly expressed throughout the presentations by both yourself and Ruth Sanford and Miriam Polster is the warm regard for human beings, seeing them as positive, capable of understand-

ing, forward-looking and trustworthy and seeing the field of traditional psychoanalysis, theology and social institutions, even political ones, as having a different view. I hate to be the ghost at the banquet, but I think that along with that point of view which I warmly respond to is the fact also that there is perversity and evil. If I can use an old term which I think still has, properly understood, some meaning for us, there is original sin. I wish things were like the way you expressed them. As we study history, however, especially in our twentieth century, it seems that it ain't necessarily so. And many of us work with populations where we have to take that into account. Not everyone responds in the way your group in Austria did.

Rogers: I think one of the most frequent and considered criticism of my work is that it takes too positive a view of human nature. I am certainly not blind to all the evil and the terribly irresponsible violence that is going on. There is an enormous amount of evil in the world at the present time. The only word you used that I would really differ with is original sin. There are times that I think I don't give enough emphasis to the shadowy side of our nature, the evil side. Then I start to deal with a client and discover how, when I get to the core, there is a wish for more socialization, more harmony, more positive values. Yes, there are all kinds of evil abounding in the world but I do not believe this is inherent in the human species any more than I believe that animals are evil. I don't think we are. I do feel that as one of the most complex organisms on the planet, we are easily warped, we are easily distorted. We set up social situations, like our slum areas, our ghettos, where we just seem to be in the business of producing alienated individuals who then go in for senseless violence. I am not blind to the things you are talking about. The point I am making is that I do not think it is inherent in the human organism. I think it is what we do to the organism after birth that matters.

The Use of Existential Phenomenology in Psychotherapy

◆

R. D. Laing, M.D.

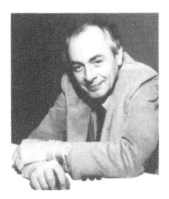

R. D. Laing, M.D.

R. D. Laing received his M.D. from Glasgow University. Laing's name comes to mind when one thinks of practitioners who have been most effective at challenging prevailing medical thinking on schizophrenia. He has practiced psychotherapy for more than 35 years and has authored 11 volumes.

Laing teaches and practices in London. Formerly he served as Chairman of The Philadelphia Association; was associated with the Tavistock Clinic; and was a Fellow of The Foundations Fund for Research in Psychiatry.

Laing's chapter is in two parts. Part one is descriptive: He defines terms and orients us to the idea that praxis and process should not be confused. Part two is experiential: Laing uses vignettes and poetic dialogues to challenge the functional fixedness in which we can entrap ourselves.

I

By "use" I mean efficacy, effective action, skillful means. I might have entitled this paper the pragmatics of existential phenomenology.

At present there is no overall definition or system of phenomenology which is agreed upon by all self-styled phenomenologists. Someone who disclaims phenomenology, such as the French historian Michael Foucault, may nevertheless be regarded as embodying much phenomenology in his theory and method.

By phenomenology I mean the science of description. In order to describe a thing, a process, an event, an action, a set, or a system of things, events or actions, one will avoid confusion if one is correct about what it is one is describing, or, more generally, if one is clear about the domain to which what one purports to be describing belongs. The description of a biochemical process is of a different order than the description of an intention. The description of intentional conduct is of a different order than the description of the unintentional movements of mindless behavior. Descriptions of intentional action, interactions, or transactions, I call *praxis* descriptions, using the word *praxis* to refer to the domain of intentional acts; whereas descriptions of behavior, at any level, of any kind (molecular, biologic, mechanical, or electronic), I call *process* descriptions.

Phenomenology thus takes us into the issue of *what it is* one is describing.

The discipline that addresses itself to *what is* this, that, anything is called ontology.

Phenomenology is a critical discipline for any science. All explanations require descriptions in order to explain.

What we take anything to be profoundly affects how we go about describing it, and how we describe something profoundly affects how we go about explaining, accounting for, or understanding what is what we are, in a sense, defining, by our description.

How do we define, how do we describe, how do we explain and/or understand ourselves? What sort of creatures do we take ourselves to be? What are we? Who are we? Why are we? How do we come to be what or who we are or take ourselves to be? How do we give an account of ourselves? How do we account for ourselves, our actions, interactions, transactions (praxis), our biologic processes? Our specific human existence?

In the light of such accounts as we give of ourselves, in our own complex and often confused ways, we account for our intentions and action, our chemistry and movements, our experience and conduct, our input, central processing and output. The critical reflective monitoring of all this is existential phenomenology; and the use of this discipline, the effective skillful means of this discipline, its pragmatics, its efficacy in the practice of psychotherapy, is what I want to address in the following pages.

The term "psychotherapy" now covers many different divergent, and some apparently antagonistic and mutually exclusive theories, techniques and practices. However, at present, in 1986, all procedures that are subsumed under the term "psychotherapy," maybe, have some elements in common.

People come to psychotherapists because they find themselves, or are found by others to be (1) experiencing themselves, others, or their circumstances or environment in undesired or undesirable ways, or (2) behaving towards themselves, others, or their circumstances or environment in undesired or undesirable ways.

Such patients, or clients, get "into psychotherapy" as the saying goes, with the hope and intention of changing their experience (E), and/or their behavior (B), from an undesired, undesirable starting state to a desired, more desirable end-state.

They wish this change, this transition, this transformation, to occur as quickly, as painlessly, as effectively, as lastingly, and as cheaply as possible. That is, they wish to transit from negative (undesired, undesirable) types or modes of experience (E neg, E minus, −E) to positive (desired, desirable) experience (E positive, E plus, +E); and, similarly, from undesired, undesirable types or modes of conduct or behavior (neg B, B minus, −B) to desired, desirable, types or modes of conduct or behavior (B positive, B plus, +B).

Whether we are naive or sophisticated, as psychotherapists, our procedures to facilitate such transformations and outcomes are necessarily, inevitably, based on the way we construe the problem, on what we take the trouble to be, and on our own willingness, enthusiasm, generosity, in complying with our clients' hopes and intentions, and in our skill in implementing ways and means of fulfilling their hopes and intentions.

We may not be interested in helping someone to be a more ruthless bully, torturer, terrorist, rapist, murderer, hypocrite, liar.

There is room for lengthy discussion here, but I have not the time nor space to go into such issues now. However, I must insist that there has to be *a basic consensus of intention* between therapists and clients. We therapists have to regard the experience and behavior our clients hope for and desire as, basically, desirable. I, personally, am interested in practicing psychotherapy only insofar as I hope that in so doing I am making a contribution to other people, as well as to myself, becoming more fully human, more actual as persons, more real, more true, more loving, less afraid of what it is not necessary to fear, happier, more joyous, more effective, more responsible, more capable of manifesting in everyday ordinary life the desiderata of human existence, courage, faith, hope, loving-kindness in action in the world, and so forth.

In a sense, psychotherapy is applied theology, applied philosophy, applied science. Our psychotherapeutic tactics and strategies are predicated upon, and are permeated by, who and what we take ourselves to be, how and what we wish and do not wish, want and dread, hope and despair, to be, in and through our experience and conduct.

All that is the *theory* and *praxis* of existential phenomenology in psychotherapy.

II

My focus here is to depict and describe what goes on between people's experience (E) as mediated by their behavior (B). I want to convey how I see the interconnections between personal interactions and how different ways of seeing may generate different ways of acting, and vice versa.

To this end, my presentation will presently become less orthodox. I shall mingle theoretical discourse with vignettes and verse, and "straight" talk with irony.

Perhaps you will regard it as "inappropriate" to present a paper in such an idiom. Perhaps it is. It is intended as a friendly provocation. It is evident, I hope, that I am not trying to induce you to adopt a "theoretical model." Rather, I am trying to depict a way of seeing, a way of contemplating what is going on, whether praxis or process, a destructing of destructive constructions, I shall use irony, humor, paradoxical communication, language as a sort of therapeutic *rasayana*,

the yoga of poison as medicine, in serious play rather than in deadly seriousnes: à la Milton Erickson. Here goes!

III

The first act of a teacher is to introduce the idea that the world we think we see is only a view, a description of the world. Every effort of a teacher is geared to prove this point to his apprentice. But accepting it seems to be one of the hardest things one can do; we are complacently caught in our particular view of the world, which compels us to feel and act as if we knew everything about the world. A teacher, from the very first act he performs, aims at stopping that view. Sorcerers call it stopping the internal dialogue and they are convinced that it is the single most important technique that an apprentice can learn. (Castenada, 1974, p. 231)

Don't take it serious.
It's just an experience.

A man had the following problem. He was married. Over a period of 18 months to a year, he became convinced that his wife was having an affair. He did not feel it incumbent on himself to indicate to her that he was aware of this, since she didn't feel it appropriate to mention it. They conducted themselves *as if* she weren't having an affair. Everything was in place just exactly as it always had been.

Then a day came to have one of those "Let's talk about it" conversations.

She: "Let's talk about us."
He: "Let's talk about Ralph as well."
She: "What are you talking about?"
He: "Well, you know."
She: "I don't know. Please tell me what you are getting at, what you are driving at."
He: "Well, you know, come on."
She: "You have to explain to me what you are talking about. I don't know what you are talking about."
He: "This affair you're having with Ralph."

She: "What affair? There is no affair, it's all in your own mind. It's all in your own imagination. You're making it up. There is no affair. Why do you think there is some affair?"

There were no gross indices that he could point to. No "proof." She absolutely insisted that he had it all wrong. He had become absolutely convinced from innumerable microevents that the picture he had constructed (she is having an affair with Ralph) was correct. He couldn't even pin it down to anything in their own intimate sexual relationship. Everything was "in place," *as if* nothing was going on. Indeed, he was at a loss. He wasn't sure. He could have made it all up. He consulted a psychiatrist, a friend. He put this situation to him and asked, "Am I psychotic? If I am making all this up then I must conclude that I am suffering from some sort of a paranoid thing. Maybe I am going paranoid and haven't realized it until now. Am I psychotic?" The psychiatrist replied, "Yes, you are."

This precipitated him into a state of *catastrophic anxiety* at the prospect that he might be paranoid. He came to see me and told me his story. As it happened, I knew that his wife was having an affair. In the social circles where his network and mine overlapped, "everyone" knew his wife was having an affair—except him. So I told him.

This precipitated him into another catastrophic reaction in which he became, not paranoid, but very depressed, for about a year. As he came out of it he said, "What really threw me? I don't think it was jealousy. *I had become terribly attached to my sense of reality.*"

Versions of that situation arise at all levels, international, interracial, between companies, men and women, parents and children. Very often no one knows what the situation is, what is going on, what is the case, and what is not.

Phenomenology is an attempt to release our minds from the blind, uncritical *attachment* to *any* set of miserable meanings—right or wrong, true or false.

The "cure," in this case, was to see the joke. But it is not always funny.

A lady consults me. Her son of 14 was diagnosed as schizophrenic and was referred to a psychiatric unit for treatment. For some time he had not been getting on well with his father. He wouldn't do anything his father asked or ordered and was coming over with "You aren't my father anyway."

The mother's quandary was that, in fact, her husband wasn't the boy's father, but no one knew that except her. Perhaps she would tell her husband and/or her son, "Anything might happen."

Or not. If she did not, she would see her son, diagnosed as schizophrenic, an in-patient, under observation, medicated, and possibly beginning a career as a schizophrenic. She didn't want to see that happen. She eventually did tell her husband, though she was risking everything by doing so. She thought he wouldn't be able to take it. He might beat her, kill her, leave her.

The story had a happy ending, almost too good to be true. She told her husband, she told her son. Her husband was very upset, the son was very relieved. The conduct that had led him to be diagnosed as schizophrenic evaporated; and she and her husband went off for a new honeymoon.

She found the courage to take a chance on truth. Even though all through our lived experience "reality" is constructed (radical constructivism), this striving to construe our reality correctly, which may lead us to radical relative perspectivism and radical constructivism, redeems us from despair and empiricism. Truth should be thought of not as a substance, a thing, but as a *praxis*; grammatically not as a noun for an object, or even for a correspondence between objects or processes, but as a verb for *truthful* speech and action between us.

A description is a definition and a prescription.

A 14-year-old girl is brought before me by her mother because she is

suffering from anorexia. (a *process* description)
She declares
I am not suffering from anorexia.
I am on a hunger strike. (a *praxis* description)
Shall I treat her anorexia?
Shall I try to break her hunger strike?
The plain fact is
She is not eating
She does not eat
One construction is that
She is suffering from anorexia
Another construction is
She is on a hunger strike
She does not sit down
Is she suffering from
no-sitting downness?
Is she on a
not-sitting down strike?

These two ways of describing her not-eating are two ways of defining what is going on—in terms of *process* (suffering from a mental disorder) or in terms of *praxis* (intentional choice-in-action). In such descriptions and definitions, there are, already, by implication, two prescriptions, two strategies of response—in terms of process, treatment of her disorder—in terms of praxis, to treat her as a person. Her treatment is the way we treat her.

An eight-year-old boy
does not read
does not write
Is he suffering from alexia? (process description, definition, prescription, explanation)
Is he on a reading strike? (praxis-description, definition, prescription, understanding)
Is he suffering from agraphia?
Similarly, is he on a writing strike or
anorexia or refusal to eat
alexia or refusal to read
agraphia or refusal to write

These are constructions, in either case explanations of a sort, already not simple descriptions
It is useful to discriminate between

depictions
descriptions, definitions,
constructions,
explanations,
prescription,
but in much clinical terminology all these categories are confounded, all confused. (Read *DSM-III*, alert to these issues)

Epistemologists never tire of telling us that
the map is not the territory,
a menu is not a meal,
the score is not the music,
that that painted pipe is not a pipe, Magritte.
This (1) is not a number.
The radical constructivists do not let us go home, do not let us off so lightly. Whatever I take to be the territory may be a map.
Everyone knows that
A menu is not a meal but many people eat menus.
Waves and particles are not light.
The brain is not the soul.
When my heart stopped it did not attack me.
Death is perfectly safe.
The people we see as patients or clients are seldom in physical pain.
They are in mental misery,
Many are enmeshed in entangled webs of mixed meanings

An incident in couple therapy.
They are arguing.
She gets up and is walking out the door.
He shouts
Why are you walking out the door?
She replies
I am not walking out the door.
He is confused and bewildered.

Do you love me?
If you love me
believe me
Believe me
you don't love me
you don't love anyone
And no-one loves you
except me

Believe me
But
don't believe
because I say so
just look into your heart of hearts
and you will find
that everything I've told you
is true

The therapy here consists in showing the fly the way out of the bottle. It's a simple booby trap. Once you realize, make real to yourself, that it is a trap it ceases to be a trap. Once you see it is a killer, it can't kill you.

You love me
You don't love me
Believe me
Don't believe me

We *learn* what we see and this learning is fraught with complications, contradictions and paradoxes. Sometimes anyone's mind might boggle.

Here are two descriptions of incidents from my own family life. As I did in the book in which they were published (Laing, 1984, pp. 136–138 & p. 144).* I shall withhold the many comments I could make on them. I hope, especially in the context of these present considerations, their relevance will be evident. If you do not see their relevance, then I am sorry to say you do not see what I am trying to point out.

CORFU
AFTERNOON, ON THE BEACH

Adam† sights an unidentified object floating fairly far out to sea. He proposes a "project" with "component operations." Basically, he, Arthur, and I are to swim out to it, identify it, and if "feasible," bring it ashore.

_____
* Reprinted with permission from *Conversations with Adam and Natasha* (1984), Pantheon Books, a Division of Random House, New York.
† Adam is my son, aged eight. Arthur is a friend, about forty. Jutta is my wife, Adam's mother.

The first "component operation" passes uneventfully. Arthur, he, and I stand on an offshore rock. Each throws his goggles and snorkle into the sea, dives in after them, retrieves them, puts them on.

Operation Two is to swim out to unidentified floating object. We set off together. Soon Adam and Arthur were drawing ahead of me, and it was not long before I had swum out further than I had done for at least 25 years. Further was too far. The object, a black shape, looked just as far away as it had done from the shore. Adam and Arthur seemed 30 or 40 feet further out. Then Arthur stopped. Adam was still for going on, but Arthur ordered him back. They swam back together to where I was and the three of us swam back to shore together.

I was grateful to feel the sand under my wobbling knees and very glad to sink back into the safe sand. Arthur looked quite relieved. Adam was livid. I've never seen him so enraged. He was *hopping* mad. He threw himself on the sand and squirmed and twitched around like an eel with vexation.

He blamed it all on Arthur, for turning back.

Arthur: Don't blame me! It was *way* off.
Adam: No it wasn't.
Jutta: *(who had been watching from the shore)* You were only halfway there.
Adam: No we weren't. We were almost there.
Daddy: No we were not almost there. It was still *far* away. Definitely *too* far away.
Adam: It wasn't.
Daddy: It was.
Arthur: Adam! *(he wasn't listening)* Adam!! Your mummy saw it from the shore.
Adam: She did not.
Daddy: It was too far.

Adam looked at us all.

Daddy: I'm telling you. It was too far.
Arthur: It was still far away.
Jutta: You weren't even halfway there.

He was completely surrounded.

Adam: You're all lying.
Arthur: Look. Why should we lie to you Adam. We're all friends.

Adam said nothing.

Arthur: It was too far for me, and it was definitely too far for you.

He still said nothing.

Daddy: Look. You still can't swim further than Arthur, or me, even.
Adam: How do you know?
Daddy: Your mummy saw us from the shore. We were only halfway there.
Jutta: That's right.
Adam: She's lying.
Jutta: No I'm not. You won't listen to anyone, that's your trouble.
Adam: Well I'm not going to listen to you.
Jutta: You'd better watch it. You had better watch it.
Daddy: Do you seriously think that you know better than everyone else?

Adam said nothing.
We all took a short breather. Except Adam, who was still "at it," though he was silent.

Daddy: Anyway. It's not a defeat.
Adam: Yes it is.

And it started up again. After the third full round of the above, with minor variations, Adam's vehemence had in no way abated.

Jutta: It was an optical illusion.
Adam: A what??
Jutta: An optical illusion.
Adam: An optical illusion!? What is an "optical illusion"?
Jutta: Something that looks different from what it is.
Adam: You mean I can't believe my eyes?!
Daddy: Well. Not always. Not just like that. Not without reservations.

Adam: Reservations!?

ITEM 144

March 1977

Jutta is taken aback by coming upon Adam making grandiose magical passes with a stick at our ailing palm tree in the hall.

Jutta: Can I believe my eyes? Can I believe my eyes?
Adam: No.

Later

Jutta: I couldn't believe my ears! I can't believe my eyes!

IV

Everyone knows we are affected by our nearest and dearest. It is devilishly difficult to study the ordinariness of everyday life where most of our clients' happiness and unhappiness arise. Descartean-Galilean natural science does not help us here, for *our* theory must be explicitly designed to *see* the world of personal passions, intentions and actions, that is, *praxis* as well as *process*. Neils Bohr's concept of complementary may help us here.

Any cogent, coherent psychotherapy must both draw on and contribute to the pragmatic knowledge, the knowledge-in-action, of how we affect each other, personally.

There is so much that goes on between us that we can never know. But we do know that the divide between fact and feelings is a product of schizoid constructions, which is not useful in the practice of psychotherapy.

In reality, the reasons of the heart (praxis) and the physiology of the brain (process) coexist and are interdependent.

In this presentation, I tried to depict a way of seeing what is seen or not, what comes into view or not, from whatever point of view. This pragmatic reflexivity, this reflexive pragmatism is necessarily reflected in my style of depiction. It therefore may turn out that the main significance of this presentation lies in the attempt to disclose or reveal a way to look at what we see and do that enables what I describe to be seen and done.

REFERENCES

Castaneda, C. (1974). *Tales of power.* New York: Touchstone Books (Simon & Schuster).
Laing, R.D. (1984). *Conversations with Adam and Natasha.* Pantheon Books, a Division of Random House.

Discussion by Thomas S. Szasz, M.D.

◆

Dr. Laing comes out in this presentation as someone I would characterize, among other things, as a person who fantasizes relativism. He makes a fetish out of relativism. It seems as if everything goes, which is one of the reasons why many critics have recently accused him of changing his position. Well, I don't know if he changes his position, or whether he has so many of them. But I think that this kind of relativism really only applies to the social world and only to some aspects of the social world. In point of fact, in the physical world, our knowledge of physics, chemistry, and mathematics is not nearly as relativistic as modern philosophers make it out, at least not in my opinion. Also, even in the social world it is not nearly as relativistic as it sounds if we take our point of departure somewhere else. In this respect, although some of our views are quite similar, we seem to go at it in different ways. I do not go at it from this very anecdotal, personal point of view, but I look for where the money is, the power. Then things are not so relativistic.

We talk about being teachers and teaching skepticism. But how can you teach skepticism to people until you know something? You can only be skeptical about something you understand. It seems to me,

therefore, that first of all children have to have a certain fund of information. As Archimedes put it, I can move the world if I have a place to stand. When we have a place to stand, then we can begin to be skeptical. I think I know where that place is. That place is having a decent mother and father in childhood, a decent education in adolescence, and courage as a grown-up. Then, we can move things. Then we can be skeptical. Otherwise, we only talk about skepticism. Of course there is also the question that was raised that somehow we want to transcend our frame of reference. We always talk, especially nowadays, in psychotherapy and psychiatry about seeing the world differently. But words are cheap. How many people want to see the world differently? They don't want to do that. I think they want to be left hypnotized.

COMMENT BY DR. WATZLAWICK

Let me try to build a bridge. I remember the day when I read Korzybski and was very taken by this famous quotation, "The map is not the territory." It occurred to me a few years ago that radical constructivism is probably right—the map is the territory. In Korzybski's view, there is a real territory for which the map is an adequate matching. In the perspective of radical constructivism, there are only maps. Of the territory we know nothing. This has important implications for the simple reason that when we talk about reality, it doesn't occur to us that we can only know the real reality, if it exists in terms of what it is not. That is our only reliable knowledge of anything that might be a real reality somewhere because we find out about it only where our reality construction breaks down. Only in the breaking down and the nonfitting of our view of reality do we realize that we are somehow seeing things in a way that is not what they appear to be. That doesn't mean that we therefore know how they are.

As von Glasersfeld says in a book I recently published, *The Invented Reality* (New York: W.W. Norton, 1984), there is a difference between matching and fitting. The transcendental idealist believes that he has a matching view of reality, that somehow his ideas express, contain, and embrace reality as it really is. The radical constructivist, on the other hand, realizes that he has only, at best, a view of reality that fits—just as a key fits the lock. The fitting of the key only tells us that the key fulfills the function for which it was built. It says nothing about the nature of the lock. I think that in therapy we have

to deal with people whose reality constructions have broken down. What therapy can do is to help them to build a new construction or a slightly modified construction.

I would take exception to Dr. Szasz's claim that in the natural sciences we have a more reliable view of reality. I have recently spoken with theoretical physicists who have greatly shaken my view that they are any better off than we are.

As the editor and author of several books on reality, I get angry letters that have to do precisely with what Laing said about nihilism: We, the constructivists, if I may count myself among them, are coming up with a constructive worldview, something in which all values and rules are being made relative. I cannot go into detail, but if you take the idea seriously that we are the architects of our reality, there are three outcomes that seem fairly acceptable. One is that we begin to realize that we are free. If I am the architect of my own reality, it is within my power to construct it one way or the other. The second outcome is that this view makes us responsible, in the deepest ethical sense, because we no longer have the easy way out into the behavior of others or the way things are outside of our control. And the third thing I think a radical constructivist would arrive at is the idea of tolerance.

Therapy in Our Day

◆

Rollo R. May, Ph.D.

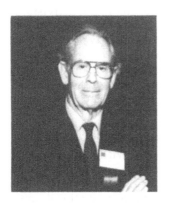

Rollo R. May, Ph.D.
In 1949, Rollo May received the first Ph.D. in Clinical Psychology from Columbia University. In 1938, he was awarded a Master's of Divinity from Union Theological Seminary. Currently, he is in private practice in Tiburon, California. The author or co-author of 14 books, he is the recipient of many awards and honors for distinguished contributions and humanitarian work. He is one of the main proponents of humanistic approaches to psychotherapy and is the principal American interpreter of European existential thinking as it can be applied to psychotherapy.

Rollo May enjoins therapists to attend to meaning rather than emphasizing technique. Adjustment is not a goal if it precludes self-realization based in imperfect values such as integrity, courage and love. Drawing from the humanities, therapy should speak to higher aspirations of the human race—to the values that make life worth living. When individuals in societies are grounded in higher values, therapy may well be obsolete.

When Karl Menninger was visiting our house recently, I asked him how he—as a man who was identified with the mental health movement in this country for 50 years—would define therapy. He answered, "People have been talking to each other for thousands of years. The question is, how did it become worth 60 dollars an hour?!"

You and I are part of a strange phenomenon. The founders of this conference, so Dr. Zeig informed me a year ago, hoped that 3000 people would attend, and he was fearful that that number was a bit ambitious. But before the spring was out, 6000 had already enrolled. The enroll-ments had to be cut off, even though it was known there might well be several thousand more.

A crucial question is, is this great gathering to be part of a three-ring circus? Or is it an important stage in the developing consciousness of a significant new profession?

PART I

We live in an age of therapy. There is a kind of therapy to meet every kind of problem—over 300 kinds at the last count. There is not only psychological therapy;

there are marriage therapists, sex therapists, voice therapists, and even therapists for your pets at home.

If you read history you will discover that therapy, and therapy-like experiences, arise at particular times in the development of each society. This is the time of the disintegration and radical transition that a society goes through. In classical Greece, for example—when Socrates and Plato were in search of goodness, beauty, and truth, when Sophocles and Aeschylus were writing their great dramas, when the Parthenon was being built—it is practically impossible even to find the word "anxiety" among the Greek writers apart from the dramatists of this classical period, which by definition dealt with the Greek myths.

Therapy was thus a part of the normal unarticulated functions of drama, religion, philosophy, dance, and the other forms of communication of the day. In this classical period the society furnished myths and symbols which allayed abnormal anxiety and guilt feelings. People's problems were taken care of by education rather than by reeducation. We see the normal development of the individual toward integration rather than desperate endeavors toward reintegration.

But in the subsequent decline of the Greek period into Hellenism, we see a radical change. And when we go further into the decline of Greek culture in the second and first centuries B.C., we see anxiety and guilt on all sides. The symbols and myths that allayed anxiety earlier are now defunct. We find anxiety and guilt in neurotic degrees. Stoics, Epicureans, Cynics, Hedonists, along with the traditional Platonists and Aristotelians—all of the philosophers—turned to techniques very much like modern psychotherapy. Instead of truth, beauty, and goodness, they talked about how to get over sweating at night; or overcoming nervousness in playing the lyre in front of large audiences. The Epicurean doctrine of *Ataraxia*, seeking tranquility of mind by rationally balancing one's pleasures, was one of their ways

of approaching it. Another was the Stoic doctrine of *Apatheia*, a passionless calm to be attained by being above the conflicts of emotion.

Therapy in this Hellenistic, rather than the classical, period took the form of psychological and ethical systems designed to help the individual find some source of strength and integrity, to enable him to stand securely, to gain some happiness in a radically changing society which no longer lent him that security. Gilbert Murray calls this "failure of nerve" during the second and first centuries B.C.—a term that could be used in any society in need of therapists.

Plutarch (Lucretius, 1951) wrote a book on "the anxious man."

Epicurus. . . . saw . . . men in full enjoyment of riches and reputation, . . . and happy in the fair fame of their children. Yet, for all that, he found aching hearts in every home, racked incessantly by pangs the mind was powerless to assuage and forced to vent themselves in recalcitrant repining. (p. 7)

Written two thousand years ago, this is still a good description of neurosis in the twentieth century.

Philosophers had now largely changed to being therapists. Their lecture halls no longer rang with the pursuit of truth, goodness, and beauty; instead they looked like outpatient clinics.

If you read the history of the disintegration of the Middle Ages, you will find very similar data. Barbara Tuchman's book, *A Distant Mirror* (1978), is a description of the terrible fourteenth century, a mirror of our own times. People called therapists in those days sorcerers, witches, soothsayers, and other fearful names. But they performed functions very similar to what in our days is performed by psychotherapy.

An ideal society ought to furnish symbols and myths to help its members deal with excessive guilt, anxiety, and despair. But when no symbols have transcendent meaning, as in our own day, the citizen of the time no longer has specific aids to transcend the normal crises of life, such as chronic illness, loss of employment, war, death of loved persons, one's own impending death, and the concomitant anxiety and guilt. In such periods, individuals have an infinitely harder time dealing with their impulses, instinctual needs, and drives, and they have a much harder time finding their own identities. Thus, they are prey to neurotic guilt and anxiety.

We do not need to be told in our century that, "The candles in the churches are out. The lights have gone out in the sky." But when Archibald MacLeish (1958) writes this and then adds, "We must blow on the coals of the heart," this also lacks efficacy. The symbols of love have been largely swallowed up by the needs for security and the pseudoexcitement of sex. The myth of success was absorbed by the myth of "the organization man," and that in turn was absorbed by the yuppie who makes a million dollars before he is 35 years old. And even these honored Western symbols are losing their power.

A valedictorian graduating from Stanford University recently wrote about the state of mind and will of his graduating class. He described his class as "not knowing how it relates to the past or the future, as having no life-sustaining beliefs, secular or religious; consequently having no goal and no path of effective action." This condition erodes our purposes and takes away our sense of identity, our sense of self. We feel like the poet Yeats (1950, p. 185):

Things fall apart; the center cannot hold;
Mere anarchy is loosed upon the world . . .
And what rough beast, Its hour come round at last,
Slouches towards Bethlehem to be born?

It is no wonder that in our age, when, with our stockpile of nuclear bombs, no one can be sure of living out even the next ten years.

PART II

I turn now to discuss the importance of loneliness and *presence* in psychotherapy. In our day, we hear much more often, in therapy in general, of the presence of the therapist and the consequent encounter as the hub of the therapeutic hour. The general approval of and relief at the role of the psychiatrist in the film *Ordinary People* is a demonstration of this shift toward a concern with the therapeutic encounter and presence.

In contemporary therapeutic thought, there is a good deal of emphasis on what is called the "narcissistic personality," impelled by the writings of Heinz Kohut and Otto Kernberg. This is the personality described as uncertain of the reality of his own existence, competitive, concerned with the fear of death; a client not having symptoms but being generally purposeless, alienated, and complaining of boredom and compulsiveness in his behavior (Lasch, 1979, p. xv).

This personality type has been called the "existential neurosis" since the 1950s and has been dealt with in existential psychotherapy for the past four decades.

Yeats was not far from the mark when he predicted in his poem that the mechanization of persons was the threat that would destroy us. Techniques and pronouncements of *how to* are an expression of this tendency. You have been hearing a lot about techniques in this conference. However, you will not hear techniques employed in this talk because the existential movement has been against the epiphany of mechanics and techniques. Whereas most therapists ask *how to*, existential therapy asks *what*—in other words, it emphasizes *meaning* rather than mechanics. The *how to* vogue hit its low point on a cover of *Psychology Today* which advised, "Wallow an hour each day in your worries—it helps."

An age of therapy, when the helping professions burgeon so greatly, is not a healthy age. William Whyte (1972) wrote in *The Organization Man*, "Modern man's enemy may turn out to be a mild-talking therapist who was doing what he did to help you."

The great emphasis in this country on making money, on commercialism, on the quick fix by winning millions of dollars in the lottery—these are ideas that existential therapy would regard not as the answer but as the problem.

When we consider the rising suicide rate—suicide has increased 300 percent in the age levels of 15 to 26 during the last two decades—we know that we have to have a life that is worth the effort. The "hot line" is proposed to cut down suicides. This is a typically American technique: Call those who seem suicidal and talk to them. But the long term question is, what do we do that makes life worth living? This should be the effect of the humanities—the study of music, literature, poetry, history, and philosophy. These studies have no goal greater than to enrich life, to give every moment a value and a glow. The humanities can give meaning to each moment in life. "Not life," said Aristotle, "but the *good* life is worth living."

I proposed 30 years ago that students hoping to become therapists should not major in psychology in their undergraduate work; rather they should major in the humanities. For it is the humanities which give them the myths and symbols with which each age sees and interprets itself. The would-be therapist has plenty of time to learn techniques in graduate school. But if the therapist learns the techniques without the meanings, he can lose the greatest help of all in understanding people.

My advice not to major in psychology did not do much good, I am sorry to say. A report of the *National Endowment for the Humanities* (*San Francisco Chronicle*, Nov. 28, 1984) showed that students can graduate without "even the most rudimentary knowledge about history, literature, philosophy or nothing about the roots and growth of our civilization." These students have no knowledge of other civilizations or of the language of other peoples. Philosophy, once the center of the humanities, is now mostly dead. Philosophy was once the main-mast college work, but now it is taught as having nothing to do with values or the problems of everyday life; most college philosophy courses have become linguistic analysis. The humanities have been dropped right and left out of the curricula in American colleges and replaced by technical subjects having to do with computers, accounting, and other topics that purportedly will enable the young person to make money when he gets out of college.

At the University of California in Los Angeles the graduate school takes a poll each year concerning why the student came to college. In 1967, 80 percent of the students gave as their chief reason "to gain a meaningful life philosophy"; only 44 percent said, to become very well-off financially. In 1984, 73 percent stated their chief purpose was to become well-off financially, and only 34 percent said "to gain a meaningful life philosophy."

It is a fortunate thing that Freud was educated in the classics; as a boy he kept his journal in school in the Greek language. Jung, Rank, and other European leaders in new thought in psychotherapy had all read the great works of human history. This had a great deal to do with their great advances in therapy. Bruno Bettelheim's book on fairy tales, *The Uses of Enchantment* (1977), shows his vast acquaintance with the humanities. And Bettelheim's essays (1983) point out that Freud's books were clearly humanistic and had been made excessively technical by successive English translations.

Existential psychotherapy could well be called existential-humanistic, for it stands against the worship of techniques and stands *for* the rebirth of the humanities. Existential therapy does not ask *how to*, rather it looks for the underlying meaning in the statements and the myths and symbols in the client's psychology and being.

PART III

Let us consider how the meaning of the Oedipus myth is sought in existential psychotherapy. It is exceedingly interesting to note that Sophocles, after writing *Oedipus Rex*, wrote another play about Oedipus, *Oedipus in Colonus*. I have never seen a reference to this second play in orthodox psychoanalytic literature. Perhaps this is because in the first play, when the deeds are done, Oedipus finds out the truth—that he has killed his father and married his mother. And when he has been punished by the gods and has gouged out his own eyes in self-horror, this seems to be considered the whole meaning—namely, Oedipus has done his deeds and has been punished for them.

But no. Viewing the myth, in the second play, as the presentation of man's struggle in self-knowledge, to know the reality about his own being, we must indeed go on, as Sophocles does, to see how the man comes to terms with the meaning of these acts. This subsequent drama is Oedipus' struggle for reconciliation with himself and with his fellow men, in the persons of Theseus and the Athenians, and a reconciliation with the ultimate meaning in his life. "For the gods who threw you down sustain you now," as his daughter Ismene phrases it. * In some ways, this drama is more significant than the first. Since it was written by Sophocles when he was an old man of 89, we can suppose it contains the wisdom of his old age as well.

One theme we find in old Oedipus' meditation at Colonus is *guilt*—the difficult problem of the relation of ethical responsibility to self-consciousness. Is a person guilty if the act was unpremeditated, done unknowingly? In the course of his probing, old Oedipus has come to terms with his guilt. He defends himself indignantly against the brash accusations of Creon:

---

* Note: All Sophocles quotes here and to follow are from the 1949 edition of *The Oedipus Cycle*, "Oedipus at Colonus," D. Fitts & R. Fitzgerald, Trans., published by Harcourt Brace Jovanovich.

If then I came into the world—as I did come—
In wretchedness, and met my father in fight,
And knocked him down, not knowing that I killed him
Nor whom I killed—again, how could you find
Guilt in that unmeditated act? . . .
As for my mother—damn you, you have no shame,
Though you are her own brother,—
But neither of us knew the truth; and she
Bore my children also— . . .
While I would not have married her willingly
Nor willingly would I ever speak of it.

Again, about his father he cries out that he has

A just extenuation.
                    This:
I did not know him; and he wished to murder me.
Before the law—before God—I am innocent!

Thus Oedipus accepts and bears his responsibility, but he insists that the delicate, subtle interplay of conscious and unconscious factors (as we could call them) always makes any legalistic or pharisaic imputation of guilt inaccurate and wrong. Since Freud, it has been a truism that the problem of guilt is as much within the heart as within the act. The play holds that the sins of meanness, of avarice and irreverence of Creon and Polyneices are "no less grave than those sins of passion for which Oedipus was punished; that in condemning them to the merciless justice soon to descend, Oedipus acts thoroughly in accord with a moral order which his own experience has enabled him to understand."

The play points toward a conclusion emphasized by modern existential psychologists: because of the interplay of conscious and unconscious factors in guilt and the impossibility of legalistic blame, we are forced into an attitude of acceptance of the universal human situation, a recognition of the participation of every one of us in human beings' inhumanity to others. The words to Oedipus from the hero,

King Theseus, who exhibits no inner conflict at all, are nevertheless very poignant. Theseus says,

. . . for I
Too was an exile. . .
I know I'm only a man; I have no more
To hope for in the end than you have.

Another theme in this reflection about the meaning of the terrible tragedy Oedipus has participated in is *presence*. Theseus says to him, "Your presence, as you say, is a great blessing." This capacity to be completely present with somebody else is a tremendously important thing in all therapy, and it is especially emphasized in existential therapy. Oedipus goes on to say,

One soul, I think, can often make atonement
For many others, if it be devoted. . . .

There is a clear symbolic element to make the point in this presence; namely, wherever his body may lie after he is dead, that country will have peace.

The concept of presence is exceedingly important in existential psychotherapy. Karl Jaspers, originally a psychiatrist and then an existential philosopher, remarked, "What we are missing! What opportunities of understanding we let pass by because at a single decisive moment we were, with all of our knowledge, lacking in the simple virtue of a *full human presence*" (Sonnemann, 1954, p. 343).

Presence is not to be confused with a sentimental attitude toward the client. Presence depends firmly and consistently on how the therapist conceives of human beings. Any therapist is existential to the extent that, with all the technical training and knowledge of transference and dynamisms, he or she is still able to relate to the client as "one existence communicating with another," to use Binswanger's phrase (May, 1983, p. 158). In my own experience, Frieda Fromm-Riechman particularly had this power in a given therapeutic hour. She would say, "The patient needs an experience not an explanation" (personal communication).

Nor does presence mean the burdening of the client with your own problems as therapist. He has enough problems without having yours too. Presence is shown in empathy and by the sensitivity with which you listen to him, the other person.

This does not at all leave out Freud's tremendously important insights about transference. But we must remember that a relationship is never *just* transference. To use that term in psychotherapy seems to me, generally, to avoid the real relationship. Transference is certainly a valuable concept and is present probably in all communication. But the existentialists are careful not to use the term transference as an excuse for something which is too confusing to talk about.

The concept of presence is what Socrates named the *midwife*—completely real in being there, but being there with the specific purpose of helping the other person bring to birth some new life from within himself or herself.

A last emphasis I wish to mention in the out-working of the myth is love. The messenger who came back to the people to report the marvelous manner of Oedipus' death, states that in his last words to his daughters Oedipus said,

. . . And yet one word
Frees us of all the weight and pain of life:
That word is love.

Oedipus does not at all mean love as the absence of aggression or as the strong affects of anger. His sharp and violent temper—present at the crossroads where he killed his father years before and exhibited in his sharp thrusts with Tiresias—remains unsubdued by suffering or maturity and is still much in evidence in this last drama. The fact that Sophocles does not see fit to remove or soften Oedipus' aggression and anger—the fact, that is, that the "aggression" and the "angry affects" are not the "flaws" that he has old Oedipus get over—lends support to our thesis above that the aggression involved in killing the father is not the central issue of the dramas. Oedipus' maturity is not at all a renouncing of passion to come to terms with society, not a learning to live "in accord with the reality requirements of civilization." It is a reconciliation with himself, with special persons he loves, and with meaning in his life.

Love, thus, is not the opposite of anger or aggression. Old Oedipus will love only those he chooses to love. His son, who betrayed him, asks for mercy and remarks, "Compassion limits even the power of God." But Oedipus will have none of this sentimentality. Rather, the love he bears his daughters, Antigone and Ismene, and the love they have shown him during his exiled, blind wanderings, are the kinds of love he chooses to bless.

Finally, describing Oedipus' miraculous death and burial, the messenger says,

But some attendant from the train of Heaven
Came for him; or else the underworld
Opened in love the unlit door of earth.
For he was taken without lamentation,
Illness or suffering; indeed his end
Was wonderful if mortal's ever was.

This touching and beautiful death of a great character is magnificent as presented dramatically by Sophocles. As *Oedipus Tyrannus* is the drama of the "unconscious," the struggle to confront the reality of the dark, destructive forces in man, *Oedipus in Colonus* may be said to be the drama of consciousness, the aspect of the myth which is concerned with the search for meaning and reconciliation. Both together comprise the myth of the human being confronting his own reality.

Another confrontation in existential psychotherapy is the problem of death. Death is present wherever there is life. Death is believed by many therapists, including myself, to be the ultimate source of anxiety and the feelings of isolation. Here we consider again how existential therapists get aid from the classics in help-

ing the patient deal with the ever-present threat of death—present in a little child who sees a dead bird and present as a threat all through our lives. Abe Maslow wrote me as he awaited his fatal heart attack, "I wonder if we could love, or love passionately, if we knew we'd never die."

The gods on Mount Olympus were immortal and were bored for most of their lives. They needed, in order to put zest into their experience, to fall in love with some mortal. Mortality had to be brought in to give renewal to immortality.

Jean Giraudoux wrote a drama which is a new form of the old Greek myth of Amphitryon, called *Amphitryon 38*. In this, Zeus falls in love with a mortal woman and is very much occupied in yearning for her, from his heavenly post on Mt. Olympus as he sees her down on the earth. Mercury suggests to him, "Why don't you go down and masquerade as her husband and achieve some expression of your love?" (Feifel, 1965, p. 124). When Zeus comes back to Mt. Olympus, he describes to Mercury what it is like to love a human being,

She will say, "When I was young. Or when I was old. Or when I die." This stabs me, Mercury. We miss something, Mercury. We miss the poignancy of the transient—that sweet sadness of grasping for something we know we cannot hold." (p. 124)

Passionate love arises out of our knowledge that we will die. Within this loneliness, we need each other. And out of this loneliness human beings are bonded in community. We love because we die, and death has meaning because we can love—we know we will lose each other some day in death.

PART IV

Predicting the future is always dangerous but always necessary. We need to exercise our imaginations by positing a future, whether we turn out to be right or wrong.

I propose two scenarios. The first is that therapy is a learning to help each other. In some parts of California there are so many therapists that the client who comes to you may also be the therapist for someone else who may in turn be supervising a third client who in turn may be your therapist when you need some consultation.

This could mean we will all learn to help each other. I do not believe this scenario is probable.

The other scenario requires that we bring society into our picture. I look forward to a society which will have mastered the nuclear threat, a society which will be a *planetism*. All countries will realize that there can be no country outside the United Nations of the World; that society must regard races and genders as equal, though each will bring its special contributions to make to the whole; that a society must have the computers as its slaves so that we human beings can spend our time with the richness of the humanities.

I look forward with hope to a new renaissance, which will reunite our passions in the great arts.

In short, I look forward to a society that will have little need for therapists of any sort.

REFERENCES

Bettelheim, B. (1977). *The uses of enchantment.* New York: Vintage Books.

Bettelheim, B. (1983). *Freud and the soul.* New York: Random House.

Feifel, H. (Ed.). (1965). *The meaning of death.* New York: McGraw Hill.

Lasch, C. (1979). *The culture of narcissism.* New York: W.W. Norton.

Lucretius. (1951). *The nature of the universe.* London: Penguin Books.

MacLeish, A. (1958). *J.B.* Boston: Houghton Miflin.

May, R. (1983). *The discovery of being.* New York: W.W. Norton.

Sonnemann, U. (1954). *Existence and therapy.* New York: Grune & Stratton.

Sophocles. (1949). "Oedipus at Colonus." In *The Oedipus cycle.* (D. Fitts & R. Fitzgerald, Trans.) New York: Harcourt Brace.

Tuchman, B. (1978). *A distant mirror.* New York: Knopf.

Whyte, W. (1972). *The organization man.* New York: Touchstone.

Yeats, W.B. (1950). "The second coming." In *The collected poems.* New York: Macmillan.

Discussion by Bruno Bettelheim, Ph.D.

We were all privileged to hear one of the best papers given in this conference. So, I want you to view everything I am going to say now under that perspective, that I think this was one of the best pa-

---

Ed. Note: As was true of a number of presenters, Dr. Bettelheim received the paper to be discussed only the day before it was presented. It is important to bring this fact to the reader's attention because it illuminates the depth of Bettelheim's intimate knowledge of literature and the classics.

pers. If you don't accept that, I couldn't say the things I am now intending to say.

Dr. May has painted for us a very beautiful picture of the future. He talked a great deal about Sophocles, but he didn't give us the entire Sophocles. Firstly, there are not only two, but three Theban plays: *Oedipus Tyrannus, Oedipus in Colonus,* and *Antigone.* He described Oedipus in Colonus as a wise old man. What he didn't tell us was that this wise old man cursed his sons. As he had been destroyed by his father, as he had destroyed his father, so he in turn destroyed his sons. And in *Antigone*, we learned that they killed each other. For more reasons than his Oedipal curse, his sons destroyed each other. Also, his beloved daughter, Antigone, got destroyed. So you see the curse of Oedipus, the generational conflict about which Dr. May did not talk. In this generational conflict, the father is subconsciously jealous of the fact that while he is declining, his sons are coming into the full bloom of their power. Out of this parental jealousy arises destructive tendencies in the father's unconscious against his sons, even while the sons have unconscious destructive tendencies against their parents.

Now, Dr. May also talked about the fact that death is what gives deeper significance to human life. Incidentally, the Greeks had a view of the gods similar to that of Giraudoux, a twentieth-century skeptical French writer. They didn't consider their immortality a curse; they considered it a blessing. Be this as it may, there wouldn't be any existential philosophy or existential therapy if Freud had not conceived of the concept of the death tendency of Thanatos. He said that eternal Eros is in eternal battle against Thanatos, and in individual life, Thanatos always wins in the end, since we all die. Dr. May did not mention that this all comes from Freud, that there was no existential philosophy before Freud conceived of the death drive because Heusserl got it from

Freud, Jaspers got it from Heusserl, Heidegger got it from Heusserl, and Sartre got it from Heidegger —a direct line back to Freud. That's why I cannot be as optimistic about the future. It is wishful thinking on Dr. May's part because Thanatos, the destructive tendencies in man, will not go away just because we want them to go away. They are here to stay. This is the depth of Freud's tragedy of man and his conceptual structures.

Now, this is a conference on the evolution of psychotherapy, so maybe a few words should be said about where it all evolved from, because listening here, no one would have guessed that it all came from Freud and psychoanalysis. Dr. May spoke about some predictions he made some 30 years ago. Good for him. But Freud made a prediction more than 60 years ago, wondering what would happen to psychoanalysis in the future. He especially worried about what would happen to it in the United States, where he said it would be readily accepted. Indeed, with the exception of behavior modification, that manipulative therapy of man which is an American invention, all other psychotherapies directly and indirectly come from Freud. But listening to what is said here, you wouldn't have guessed it. So the oedipal killing of the father is still going on. The solid wine of psychoanalysis has been watered down to such degree that everything of its substance and essence has been washed away and only the dregs remain.

SECTION IV

$\blacklozenge$

Psychoanalytic Therapists

The Therapeutic Milieu

◆

Bruno Bettelheim, Ph.D.

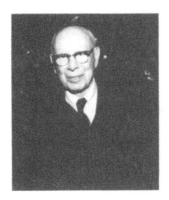

Bruno Bettelheim, Ph.D.
Currently residing in Portola Valley, California, Bruno Bettelheim is active in teaching at Stanford University and continues to conduct research on the application of psychoanalysis to child rearing, education and social problems. He is the Stella M. Rowley Distinguished Service Professor Emeritus of Education, Psychology and Psychiatry at the University of Chicago.

Bettelheim's career as one of the world's foremost psychoanalysts spans more than four decades. He worked as Director of the Orthogenic School at the University of Chicago for almost 30 years. The Orthogenic School is the University's residential treatment center for severely emotionally disturbed children.

Bettelheim has authored more than a dozen books, several of which describe his work at the Orthogenic School. He is a regular contributor to professional journals and publishes articles in The New Yorker, Scientific American, Commentary, *and* Parents Magazine.

Born in Vienna, Austria, in 1903, he received his Ph.D. in psychology and philosophy from the University of Vienna. He immigrated to the United States in 1939.

Bettelheim's moving and sensitive chapter presents tenets of his child-centered, residential treatment of severely disturbed children. The milieu is carefully devised to be consistent with psychoanalytic treatment goals of fostering autonomy and developing latent potentials.

The history of mental institutions for the insane goes back several centuries, and so does that of orphanages. By contrast, the idea that mentally disturbed children may need and could greatly benefit from a psychiatric setting designed to meet their special needs is a relatively new one. In the past, children who for some reason could not be kept within society were placed in institutions for adults. These institutions were entirely unsuitable for the needs of children.

Ann Sullivan, who gained international fame as the miracle worker who returned Helen Keller to the world of the living, was a child when she was placed in a terrible institution. Although only a child, she took the initiative to speak out for herself. She managed to save herself from oblivion by convincing a group of Massachusetts legislators, who chanced to visit the miserable place in which she had been placed, that it meant living death for a child to have to vegetate in such an unsuitable setting. The result of her courage made history, but, at that time, only for blind and deaf children, not yet for mentally disturbed children. They had to wait for more than the better part of a century, and the development which eventually led to their finding help began in another continent.

When Ann Sullivan was asked to help Helen Keller, who was not only blind and mute, but in all other respects also acted like a wild autistic child, Sullivan recognized that treating Helen Keller while she continued to live with her family was an impossible proposition. So she created a special setting, if you like, a therapeutic milieu, for her young charge. There she lived, day in and day out, all by herself with little Helen Keller, and there she cared for her in all respects. As you know, Ann Sullivan's plan of treating Helen Keller in a special milieu succeeded. By creating a totally therapeutic milieu she made it possible for the completely unrelated child to begin to relate to her. Thus, world history was made. But despite a success at which the entire world marvelled, there was no sequence to this unique, and uniquely successful, experiment. Its lessons were not yet learned and generalized.

For the continuation of our story we must move to Freud's Vienna. There, about a quarter of a century after he had created psychoanalysis, some of Freud's younger students, foremost among them his daughter, Anna, together with Siegfried Bernfeld, August Aichhorn, and a few others, tried to apply the new insights and methods of psychoanalysis to the treatment and education of children. Particularly Bernfeld, in his all-too-short-lived *Kinderheim Baumgarten* outside of Vienna, attempted to create a residential setting for war orphans of World War I—a place where they would be given a chance to overcome the traumas inflicted on them by their war experiences. Here, he and a very few collaborators tried to put into practice entirely new notions about a psychoanalytically informed living which would cure emotional disturbances. Unfortunately, the experiment lasted barely six months. Their ideas were much too radical even for the progressive and reform-minded educational establishment of the socialist city government of Vienna.

However, much was learned from this brief experiment. It resulted, among other reports, in several pioneering books which had a great influence on our thinking about the psychoanalytic education and treatment of children. They are Siegfried Bernfeld's *Sisyphus, or the Limits of Education* (1973), August Aichhorn's *Wayward Youth* (1983), and Anna Freud's *Introduction to the Technic of Child Analysis* (1975) and *Psychoanalysis for Pedagogues*.

While the idea of a psychoanalytic residential setting for children failed to come to fruition in Vienna, it did so to some degree in London during World War II in Anna Freud's Hampstead War Nurseries. However, several years before this, another experiment was conducted in Vienna which, in due time, led to the idea that only a *total* therapeutic setting could rehabilitate the most severely disturbed children.

This idea originated because of the initiative of Anna Freud. In the early 1930s an American mother brought her mute autistic child first to Sigmund and then to Anna Freud, after all peregrinations through the American continent and many parts of Europe had failed to secure a specialist willing to undertake the treatment of the child. They all declared her hopeless. Of course, nobody knew that she was an autistic child because at that time this disturbance had no name, nor had it been described or studied. This happened only a dozen years later when Leo Kanner (1943) published his first paper on the disturbance of affective contact which he named *infantile autism*.

Anna Freud immediately recognized that psychoanalytic treatment alone would not help this child. Therefore, she suggested that the child live permanently, throughout the year, in a special milieu which would meet her daily needs and her educational and treatment requirements on a psychoanalytic basis. This, combined with daily child analysis, might offer a chance to help the child. In a way, Anna Freud suggested a setting like the one Ann Sullivan had created for Helen Keller. However, at that time neither Anna Freud nor anyone else in Vienna concerned with the case of this autistic child knew how Ann Sullivan had proceeded.

My wife and I decided to devote ourselves to this experiment. We took the child into our home which we completely reorganized to meet the needs of this child as we understood them. The experiment succeeded beyond our hopes. After a year and a half, the girl began to relate and to talk, although she remained extremely disturbed for several more years. After she had lived three years in this therapeutic milieu, formal academic education could be started. She made steady, albeit slow, progress. Unfortunately, the experiment was prematurely aborted by Hitler's invasion of Austria. Full rehabilitation could have been achieved, but it probably would have required treating and guiding the girl well into her adolescence. Still, she developed considerable artistic talent which culminated in her having shows of her paintings in New York, which she returned to after the annexation of Austria. From that time to the present she has been living a fairly satisfactory, although somewhat sheltered, life in society.

Soon after this child had been repatriated to the U.S., I was imprisoned in German concentration camps for over a year. This experience, which I have discussed in some of my writings, convinced me even more than having this child live with us in our home to what extraordinary degree a total environment can alter personality: The one created for this girl in our home for the better; the one the Nazis created in the concentration camps for the worse. If a total environment is designed to help severely disturbed children get well, that is, to restructure their personalities in positive ways, it can achieve for them what had been previously declared by the best experts as unattainable. Sim-

ilarly, if a total environment is designed to disintegrate previously well-established personalities, it, too, succeeds all too well in this evil purpose.

In 1944, five years after I was fortunate enough to be able to reestablish myself professionally at the University of Chicago, I was asked to reshape and completely reorganize the University's Orthogenic School to serve the interests of children so severely disturbed that all treatment efforts had failed; hence, they were considered untreatable. This task was entrusted to me because of my Viennese experience in rehabilitating the autistic girl. By this time, infantile autism had been described and named. It was no simple task because an institution for some 30 children as the School then served, and for some 40 to 50 children as the institution soon served, was an entirely different proposition than reshaping a relatively spacious private home, in which one continued to live, to serve the rehabilitation of one or two schizophrenic youngsters. Still, I tried to do my best, based on my experience with what kind of total therapeutic environment had been conducive to the rehabilitation of the child who, as I now knew, had suffered from infantile autism.

From my experience with the child I learned what such an environment had to consist of, what features it had to contain, and on what thinking it had to be based— and also of what features it had to be entirely free. Particularly in the latter respect I took advantage of the lessons I learned in the German concentration camps where I both experienced and observed which aspects of an environment are most destructive to personality and lead to its disintegration. In all this I was helped by living intimately with the autistic child. Through this, I came to comprehend what had been so destructive in her life that her personality did not develop until she had lived with us for a few years. In retrospect, I was shaken by the parallels between the early destructive experiences to which she had been exposed and which led her to become autistic and those which destroyed the personalities of prisoners in the concentration camps.

By the time I undertook the reorganization of the Orthogenic School into a total therapeutic milieu, I could also draw on what had been learned about group work, foremost from Slavson, and also benefit from the experience of the Southard School of the Menninger Foundation and from a few other institutions which groped along parallel lines. None, however, tried to create the total therapeutic milieu I was determined to bring about. On the contrary, in these few institutions which tried to apply psychoanalysis to the treatment of children, the emphasis, as far as treatment was concerned, was on the few analytic hours; while for the rest of their days the children were kept, to use Fritz Redl's term (1966), in "cold storage." That is, the effort was to prevent further damage, whereas no attempts were made to make the rest of the children's days serve therapeutic ends.

Long before therapists knew that extremely disturbed individuals need a total therapeutic setting to get well, patients themselves were keenly aware of this need. For example, Anna Freud (1954) quotes a schizophrenic adolescent as telling her:

You analyze me all wrong. I know what you should do; you should be with me the whole day, because I am a completely different person when I am here with you, when I am in school, and when I am home with my foster family. How can you know me if you do not see me in all these places? There is not one of me; there are three.

The girl could as well have said, "How can you treat me in only one hour a day, the analytic hour, and only in one setting, when I am all in pieces?" Anna Freud, devoted to the classical method of child analysis, did not heed the advice of her patient. From my experience, I knew that if schizophrenic children are treated as this girl suggested only then is there hope for their rehabilitation.

I was not the only one who tried to create such a total therapeutic milieu for the treatment of severely disturbed children. Redl, a close friend and frequent visitor in my Viennese home, was familiar with our efforts to create such a therapeutic milieu in our home. After his emigration to the U.S. Redl tried to do the same, at least for a few summer months, for delinquents in the Fresh Air Camp which he conducted for the University of Michigan.

As soon as I began my work at the Orthogenic School, Redl took a lively interest in my efforts, encouraging me with support and advice. Possibly because of what he saw developing at the Orthogenic School, as well as on the basis of his own experience in the Fresh Air Camp, he decided to create Pioneer House in Detroit. There he put into practice, among other things, the principle that therapeutic intervention best takes place in the here and now of the patient's life, rather than in the security and isolation of the therapeutic hour. Part of the practice he developed at Pioneer House and we developed at the Orthogenic School, he described in his concept of the life-space interview. He wrote (1966):

In contrast to interviewing in considerable detachment from the "here and now" of Johnny's life like the psychoanalytic play-therapy interview, the life-space interview is closely built around the child's direct life experience in connection with the issues that become the interview focus. Most of the time, it is held by a person who is perceived by the child as part of his "natural habitat, or life space," with some pretty clear role and power in his daily living, as contrasted to the therapist to whom he is sent for "long-range treatment." One of the great advantages of the life-space interview is the very flexibility in timing that it offers us. We don't have to hope that the child will remember from Friday noon until his therapy hour next Wednesday what was happening just now. Or having watched the event that led to a messy incident, we can quite carefully calculate how long it will take the youngster to

cool off enough to be accessible to some reasonable communication with him, and we can
move in on him at that very calculated time.

Redl, working mainly with delinquents,
many of whom are quite verbal, stressed
the importance of talking with his patients
in the here and now. We who worked
mainly with schizophrenics—although
some of them were also quite delinquent
in their behavior—and with mute or
mainly nonverbal children had to use many
other nonverbal methods of therapeutic
interferences, and not only the method of
life-space interviews.

To stress some of the most essential
features of such a total therapeutic milieu,
it must instill in the patient a desire to
live—a desire which his past experiences
had either never created or had destroyed
at an early age—a feeling that he is considered very important and that all hu-
manly possible efforts are being made to
make him feel desired and desirable. To
achieve this, his ways of responding to
his environment must be respected and
accepted, as outlandish as they may seem
to most people. And he must know that
all efforts are made to give him the feeling
that he now can be in charge of how his
life will be arranged and how it will proceed.

Just as the first life activities of the
infant are to be fed, cleaned, and permitted to sleep as he desires, initially the
therapeutic milieu will try to show the
child that within it he can eat when and
what he wants, in whatever manner he
wants; that he can sleep and rest when
and how long he wants; and that bathing
is not intended to make him clean in line
with our standards, but is only to give
him comfort in line with his desires. Since
it is readily understandable what is involved in arranging for a child to eat what
he wants and when he wants, and sleep
as he wishes, perhaps an example concerning being bathed will be illustrative.

One ten-year-old girl had not moved her
bowels on her own since the age of two
and a half. From this age on she had been
given enemas at regular and frequent intervals—a procedure she fought strenuously for years, until she finally let them
be inflicted on her passively, as she with-
drew ever more into utter passivity in all
respects.

When she entered the Orthogenic School,
we promised her that no enemas would
be used, that when and where she would
move her bowels would be strictly her
decision, although we hoped she would do
so, since we knew that holding on to her
stools for prolonged time was uncomfortable to her. She tested our promise by not
emptying her bowels for a considerably
longer time than she had previously been
permitted to hold on to her stools, since
she had been given enemas about every
three or four days. For most of the first
two weeks, she was completely unrespon-
sive to our efforts to make her comfortable
and to reach her emotionally. But after
ten days she gave a slight indication that
she liked her long warm baths where we
sat with her, tried to play with her, using
ourselves and various bath toys, including
some which expelled water and some specially selected ones which expelled tiny
rubber balls, to make the process of ex-
pulsion enjoyable.

After two weeks we became worried
whether we would be able to keep our
promise; yet, remained firm. Fortunately,
our encouragement to release her bowels,
as suggested by the toy, became effective—she began to eliminate in the water
of the bathtub. You can well imagine our
pleasure and our relief as she relieved
herself into the water of the tub. We were
glad that she took the initiative in respect
to her own body functions by making her
bowels function appropriately. Until then
she had refused to let them function. She
responded with a little smile—the first one
since she had been a baby—and this rewarded our expressions of delight.

For several more weeks she eliminated
only in the bathtub, accompanied by our
praise and our pleasure in her achievement; and she did so ever more frequently
and easily until one day she decided to

go on the toilet, without our having suggested this in any way. What had been a determined rejection of the world and an obstinate holding back from it became a first giving of her self—her stools—to the world and a way of relating to significant others. For several months she would eliminate only when her favorite caretaker held her hand and spoke gently and lovingly to her as she sat on the toilet. Then one day she decided to flush the toilet herself, which before this could be done only after she had left the toilet stall. From then on she went to the toilet herself, when she felt like it, and no longer needed any special help in doing so.

As a conscious act, eating is perhaps even more primitive and an experience which the infant is aware of even earlier than the act of elimination, although one cannot be certain about this. In any case, our acceptance of when, how, and what they want to eat was the beginning of the rehabilitation of some severely anorexic children. In one case, the child defended herself against anything reaching her from the outside by closing her ears with her hands. This interfered with her being able to feed herself. The rudiments of a relation were established with her when her caretaker offered to close the girl's ears with her own hands so that the girl's hands would be free to put food into her mouth. As this evolved into a game, she began to enjoy eating.

A boy slowly returned to the world of the living and feeling when his caretaker—following some of the boy's acts— let him spread food on her bare arms, from which he then ate. Just as the infant feeds from the mother's breast, he had to return to feeding from the body of a mother substitute before he could begin to enjoy eating, and in slow steps, relating to and becoming a cherished part of this world.

Even though I discussed here a total therapeutic milieu, when we began our work at the Orthogenic School along the lines just suggested, what we did had no name. When I first decided to report on it, I had to find a name for it, just as I had a few years previously when I published the first report on the psychologically disintegrating effects of the concentration camps. For this I invented the term *extreme situation,* which has since become a current concept in psychology. In contradistinction, I toyed with the idea of calling it an extremely accepting situation, or an utterly benign environment. But since the purpose of our endeavor was therapeutic, I decided on the name *therapeutic milieu,* suggesting a setting in which everything is designed to promote the goals of therapy.

By this name I tried to suggest that what was of paramount importance was that every, even the most minute, aspect of the environment had to serve its therapeutic goals, and that every single aspect of the patient's life needed to be planned and organized to further the integration of his personality, in ways and at a speed he chose. This meant that from the moment he entered the institution all efforts were made to convince him that the milieu was there for him, and in no respect would he be required to conduct his life in line with the convenience or the preconceived notions of the institution and its staff. Everything had to give way to the all important task of providing him with the opportunity to reintegrate his personality in ways that he thought best. This had to begin with the moment he entered the institution and continue every single morning with the way he met the day on awakening: how he was dressed or helped in getting dressed; how he was fed what he preferred to eat; how he was played with; how he was educated academically, when the time was ripe for it, and ripe in *his* and not in our opinion; how he was bathed, when and how he desired; and how at the day's end he was put to bed and things arranged so that he would feel safe during the night. All these things had to be carefully thought out and arranged so as to foster his therapeutic progress— a progress which often consisted for some time in his regressing, a regression which, to be effective, also had to be viewed as necessary progress in finding himself.

When we first felt ready to present our

work to the profession, we felt overwhelmed by the task of how to give others some idea of what we had tried to do. Finally, we decided that we could do so only by indicating how we had to serve the children in ways they would feel are good, from early in the morning until way past midnight (because it took them so long to be able to fall safely asleep) and how we had to be ready when needed to be there for them all through the night.

Following the success of such a presentation, I used the same manner of presentation when I first described the working of the Orthogenic School in my *Love is not Enough* (1950). Here I suggested that while love is certainly important, careful planning and thorough thinking along psychoanalytic lines are also required if the goal is the rehabilitation of children so severely disturbed that other treatment efforts, such as child psychoanalysis or residential placement plus psychiatric treatment, had failed and the children had been diagnosed as untreatable.

With these children, the way they are tucked in or handed their favorite stuffed animals as their protectors during the night can often restore their shaken trust in the world better than the best chosen verbal statements. For many of these children, once they become accessible to our words, the main battle is already won. Hence we have to reach them through actions rather than through words. A baby bottle given in the right manner or the child being held in the right way can be much more effective in giving a previously unknown feeling of security and well-being than the words which accompany the action.

Just as the infant responds to what he sees in his mother's face, both negatively and positively, so these disintegrated children often respond first to what they discover about us from watching our faces and our body tonus, and what they deduce from that about our intentions. This they are able to trust much more than our words. Bateson (1956) has pointed out how utterly destructive double-bind messages are to children who, because of them, come to distrust everything they are told.

From their unhappy experiences with words, these children become convinced that they cannot trust what people tell them. They are much more ready to trust our actions when they can observe them at their leisure and in safe situations. Because they have such distrust of what adults tell them, nonverbal messages are much more readily received and much more meaningful to them. They trust only what they themselves observe and on this basis decide what it all means. This is why nonverbal messages within the life-space are so all-important for their learning to trust, for restoring to them that basic trust which Erik Erikson (1959) believes has to stand at the beginning of a successful life, and which we hence have to convey to those who have never before experienced it.

Since double-bind messages are utterly destructive when they spring from those persons in the child's life such as his parents, who are the most important people to him, it would be counterproductive to the effectiveness of a therapeutic milieu if double-bind messages originated from persons important to the child there. Others have described how destructive it is to patients in mental institutions when staff members disagree either openly or in hidden ways—so destructive that some patients may commit suicide or engage in violent actions, so much so that the institution itself may flounder, as Stotland and Kobler described in *Life and Death of a Mental Hospital*.

Therefore, true consensus based on the inner convictions of the staff is of paramount importance if the institution is to form a total therapeutic milieu. Staff consensus on all essentials and, as far as possible, on nonessential matters must be the basis for all workings of the institution. It is so important that the children will often test it to make sure of it.

Such staff consensus can spring only from a common philosophy—namely, the psychoanalytic understanding of man and of the origin and nature of functional disturbances, of child development, of the importance of the unconscious and of need satisfaction, and in regard to other innumerable aspects of daily living. For it to work, even under difficult circumstances, it has to become a common way of life for all who work at the institution.

And this is true not only for those usually considered to be the professional staff caring for the children, but it must also extend to everyone working there—maids, janitors, office staff, in short, *everybody* who works at the institution. If the children are free to move about the institution however they want, they will come into contact with everybody who works there. And if they cannot do so, they will always fear that some dangerous secrets are hidden from them and hence they cannot trust the institution or what goes on in it.

If the office staff resents the children's intrusion into their working area, the children will not believe that they are really welcome within the institution, that they are welcome to explore everything they want. And if we do not want them to explore what the office staff, the maids, the cooks, the janitors are up to, how can the children believe we want them to explore what goes on in their unconscious, which is so much more hidden, so much more difficult to understand? If we handle their favorite, or even not so favorite, stuffed animals and toys with loving care, but the maids who make their beds and clean their rooms do not, the children will not feel really welcome in the institution. If the maids or the cooks who serve them their food resent that they mess with it and waste it, the children will not be able to feel that they are being given to unconditionally.

Obviously we cannot expect typists, cooks, maids, and janitors to be well-versed in psychoanalytic thinking and hence understand readily why the children act as they do and why being able to do so is so important for their rehabilitation. So the staff must be made part of the therapeutic venture, which a total therapeutic milieu is, on some other basis than an understanding of unconscious motives on a psychoanalytic basis. This can be done, but it is not easy.

It can be achieved only through daily formal and, even more important, many informal exchanges of views among the staff on their various levels of understanding. At the Orthogenic School, we found that it required that the staff discuss matters with each other not just daily, but, if at all possible, several times during the day. Once a consensus has been established there need not be long discussions, a few words can then suffice, but only after a consensus in regard to the main viewpoints has been established. When this has been achieved, then the patient does not need to be a different person in different settings, and with different staff members. Then the split in personality similar to that objected to by the patient whom Anna Freud quoted is avoided. While treatment only in the seclusion of the treatment hour tends to split the personality into many disparate pieces (and this even more so for a patient who already suffers from a split personality), the total therapeutic milieu heals this split.

If the children in such a therapeutic milieu are to feel it is truly theirs, that it is here for them, then they must have their say about all aspects of the institution's operation—and so must the staff. William Gibson, basing his novel *The Cobweb* (1979) on his experiences at the Menninger Hospital, imaginatively describes the havoc created in a psychiatric hospital when curtains were replaced by others which a staff member thought preferable. Not that the new curtains were not serviceable; they were, but the patients and the staff had had no say in the selection and hence resented the curtains as a demonstration that they were manipulated. Thus, as far as the meals that are served, as far as the china on which they are served, as far as the furniture is selected and arranged, as far as curtains and bedspreads are chosen, as far as the colors which the walls are painted—in regard to all these, patients and staff, in cooperation, have to make the decisions. This is by no means as difficult as it sounds. I have described the selection process in some detail in some of my writings (1974); and the slides, which illustrate at least the outer appearance of things, will show that the results can be quite harmonious.

To restate here the bare outline of the process and how it can work: Either the head of the institution or a staff committee presents to the children and the rest of the staff about five selections of, let's say, china dishes. From these the children select one which pleases them. And if they cannot get together, then five different selections are presented to them, and so forth, until they can get together on one pattern. Since the committee wisely presents to children and staff only patterns which it likes, there is no chance that the committee will not like the children's choices. With dishes, which are common to all members of the institution, all staff and all children, it may take a while until consensus is reached. Where the children's dormitories are concerned things are much easier, since not more than eight children and three or four staff members are involved. Here consensus on curtains or furniture or wall colors can be reached more easily.

That one is much more comfortable with furniture one has selected oneself goes without saying, and so does that one is much more careful with objects one has chosen for one's own use. As an example: Whereas before the children and staff chose the dishes, very sturdy china was used to reduce breakage; while after the children and staff made their own choice from among very nice and expensive china patterns, breakage was immediately reduced to a minimum. And the same went for other furnishings used in the institution.

But since, as the saying goes, a picture can tell more than a thousand words, slides may illustrate at least the outer appearance of one example of a total therapeutic milieu for children—an appearance which contains a silent message to the children who live there, a message whose meaning they can evaluate all on their own, since nobody tells them what to make of it. For this reason I shall avoid telling you what you should make of it, but will let you form your own opinions whether you think this external experience conveys a feeling for what I have been trying to tell you about the nature of a therapeutic milieu.

REFERENCES

Aichhorn, A. (1983). *Wayward youth*. Evanston, IL: Northwestern University Press.

Bateson, G., Jackson, D. D., Haley, J., & Weakland, J. (1956). Toward a theory of schizophrenia. *Behavioral Science, 1*.

Bernfeld, S. (1973). *Sisyphus, or the limits of education*. Berkeley: University of California Press.

Bettelheim, B. (1950). *Love is not enough*. New York: Free Press-Macmillan.

Bettelheim, B. (1974). *A home for the heart*. New York: Alfred A. Knopf.

Erikson, E. (1959). *Identity and the life cycle*. New York: International Universities Press.

Freud, A. (1954). The widening scope of indications for psychoanalysis. *Journal of the American Psychoanalytic Association, 2*.

Freud, A. (1975). *Introduction to the technic of child analysis*. Salem, N.H.: Ayer Company Publications.

Gibson, W. (1979). *The Cobweb*. New York: Atheneum.

Kanner, L. (1943). Autistic disturbances of affective contact. *The Nervous Child, 2*.

Redl, F. (1966). *When we deal with children*. New York: Free Press-Macmillan.

Discussion by R. D. Laing, M.D.

It is one of the very sad things in this world that Dr. Bettelheim's efforts have found so few people to follow them and to emulate them. I think everything he has written and exemplified about total therapeutic environment, about the features that it has to contain and those that it must not contain, are true—not only about total therapeutic environment for autistic children, but for the total therapeutic environment for the human race.

I have one or two minor reservations about Dr. Bettelheim's manner of putting into words his nonverbal message (without, I hope, detracting from the importance of, and the honor that is due to, Sigmund Freud and his daughter, Anna Freud). I feel that there are passages here that have a touch of bathos, for instance, when talking about the fact that "staff consensus can only spring from a common philosophy, namely, that of the psychoanalytic understanding of man and the original nature of functional disturbance." Surely, we have a perennial philosophy of communion, compassion, whatever you call it, in different languages and different traditions, of which psychoanalysis at its best is an application and a derivation.

I also have reservations about the way the message about basic trust is put forward. When a child listens to what we say and watches what we do, the two don't necessarily coincide. When I say, "Do you love me as I love you? Then, if you love me, believe me," I'm doing extreme violence to a child, especially if I love that child. I never ask a child to believe me—never ask, if I love a child, for that child to trust me. The request to be loved is a request to see me as I am and take me as I am, as I hope I'm able to do with you, not because you love me, believe me or trust me. As William Blake

said, "Child born of joy and mirth, go live without the help of anything on earth."

We can't rely on being loved. We must not fall into what I think is the extreme pitfall of asking children to believe us, especially if they love us. And especially if we love them.

Nevertheless, these are small points of nuance, of a double message which is, as Dr. Bettelheim says, "Pictures tell, speak louder a thousand times more than words, and actions speak a thousand times more than pictures." So, I would say that if there's anyone among our company, at this conference and in our generation, who deserves a Nobel Prize for what we've done in our field, it is Dr. Bettelheim.

QUESTIONS AND ANSWERS

Bettelheim: Fortunately, we still have some time for questions from the audience and of course, I'm very much interested in what your questions might be. I hate to take time away from this, but I would like a moment to thank Dr. Laing for his very kind remarks. Most of all, I would like to thank him for correcting me on a very important point. Consensus can be reached on many different levels; of course, psychoanalysis is by no means the only area by which consensus can be reached. What I meant to say, and I'm glad that Dr. Laing's remarks offer me this opportunity to correct myself, is that I started a therapeutic institution that is based on psychoanalytic thinking; the consensus has to be on that basis. Of course, there are many other bases on which this consensus can be reached. And you know, different religions base their very last decree, their claim of helping man, on the consensus they reach on the basis of their common religion. My only reservation is that on the basis of this religious consensus, too many people have been burned like sticks. But it is true that there are many ways in which consensus can be reached. And not just for psychoanalysts. As for the rest, you heard what Dr. Laing has to say and I'm very happy with his remarks. However, he grossly overrated my importance with the last thing he said. Thank you.

Question: Dr. Bettelheim, I was struck with the empathy and the care and respect you showed for the children in your charge. I'm wondering, however, in addition to the nurturing and the caring, isn't the setting of some limits on the children's behavior ultimately perceived by the children as a sign of caring and consistency?

Bettelheim: Whenever a limitation was placed on me as a child, I hated it. Maybe you felt differently as a child, but I've never yet found a child who didn't hate it, when limitations are put on his behavior. Most of all, who has the right to put limitations on me? We resent it when limitations are put on us. So do children, so do insane people. The only limitations which are acceptable are limitations we put on ourselves. And I certainly would hope, with the right treatment, the right handling, children will eventually grow up to put limitations on themselves. I don't think you have any right to put any limitations on anybody. Thank God, I wouldn't know how to do it.

Question: Dr. Bettelheim, could you address what criteria you use for choosing the childcare workers whom you employ?

Bettelheim: I have to like them, because otherwise I couldn't work very well with them. They have to be good people, or at least want to become good people. They have to be intelligent. They have to be flexible. And they have to have a great desire to serve others, out of their own needs, out of their own convictions, what-

ever they may be. Does that answer your question?

Question: Yes, sir. Can you also tell me how you recruit them?

Bettelheim: We always have 20 times as many applications as we have positions. For example, in one of my presentations at this meeting, you saw a film featuring Dr. Sarah Wheelen, who is now in private practice. She came to me as a music major and she applied for an office job as a typist. I talked to Sarah for awhile and said, "You don't want to be a typist." "Yes," she said, "I just wanted to work here, but I didn't think that I'm good enough to work as a staff member with the children." I said, "That convinces me that you're more than good enough to work with the children." She became one of the best workers I ever had.

Question: Dr. Bettelheim, I have the privilege of working in a facility very much like the one you're describing. Now I live in Miami and I've worked in the same psychiatric hospital for five years. It's been sold and resold three times in that period. We're now owned by something similar to a fast food chain. One of the things I've seen happen is that our staff to patient ratio went from 4 to 1 to 2 to 1. I wonder if you know what your staff to patient ratio is, including everyone working in the facility. And I'm also asking, do you think that facilities should be taken out of the hands of private enterprise?

Bettelheim: When I need surgery, I'm not concerned about the cost. I want the best surgery available. I'm biased that way. I found that most people, when they are themselves concerned, when the chips are down and it's something very important, don't worry about the cost, if they can afford it, of course. They worry that it should be the very best available to them.

Question: Our facility costs more than $10,000 a month. People cannot afford that for more than a month. I mean, most people can't afford it at all. It has to be covered by insurance.

Bettelheim: Well, that's where the evil starts, because the insurance decides on how long the person is treated, not on the needs of the patient. This is the terrible thing that happened when I was on Medicare. Treatment is based on what the state or the government pays. It's no longer based on what the patient needs. Now what kind of thinking this is, I don't have to describe to you.

Now, I can be more specific on the staff/ child ratio. In general, we have two professional staff members for three children; in addition, there are three staff members for two children. So, there are more staff than children.

Question: I work in a psychiatric residential rehabilitation center and our program has three tiers: a halfway house which is a supervised setting, apartments with intensive support, and supportive settings. Currently, the way clients move through our program is to go from one setting to the other as they improve and need less supervision. But there is a notion that instead of moving the client, one might move staff and decrease the supervisional structure while maintaining the setting for the client. One simple difference that I see is the difference between putting the client through changes and putting the staff through changes. I'd like to know your comments.

Bettelheim: I'm a little bit perturbed by the concept of supervision, you know. Who has a right to supervise somebody else? I'm much more in favor of the concept of service. I think we're not here to supervise, I think we're here to serve. According to some of the presentations here, we are called the supervising profession. I thought we are the serving or helping profession. The things I hear give the impression I'm all wrong and that there are tendencies to consider ourselves as a ruling and determining and supervising profession. It doesn't agree with me. I had more than enough supervision from the Nazis to serve my supervisory needs for the rest of my life. So, I'm very sensitive to it, you know. On the other hand, if you believe that permanent human relations are very important and that it is important to form attachments, then you have the answer about the moving, and who should be moved, and how.

Question: Dr. Bettelheim, I work in a longterm residential setting for severely disturbed young children and young adolescents where our milieu is considered our central focus and our main therapeutic thrust. How do you deal with the issue of confidentiality between individual therapists or group therapists and our direct care, front-line staff in the milieu which we view as the most important focus?

Bettelheim: Well, if we assume for a moment that in some degree the staff is in loco parentis—of course, in the place of a very good parent—wouldn't you think that the parents talk with each other about what goes on with the child?

"Yes, absolutely."

Alright, so I don't understand where the concept of confidentiality comes in. From whom do we keep things secret?

"In our agency, it comes up among the adolescent population, where some therapists feel that it's very important and significant for the adolescent to have someone they might bare their soul to, and that it should be kept from the caretakers, just as a child in the family might seek out an aunt or an uncle in the extended family to seek help when they can't deal with something with mom or dad."

Well, I would be very suspicious of an auntie who makes such promises.

Question: I would like it if you could address a few comments to the difference between working with adolescent populations in this kind of milieu as opposed to working with younger children.

Bettelheim: None whatsoever, with youngsters from four to 20. Does that answer your question? What could be the difference? We all want to be well taken care of, we all want to develop our own personalities. Some of the residents are babies and some children are quite mature for their age. Isn't that true? What's good for the goose is good for the gander.

Question: Dr. Bettelheim, the residential treatment program for which I am responsible has adults from 30 to 60 years of age, all of whom have an average length of state hospitalization experience of 15 or 20 years. All have been considered untreatable. We're in our eighth month, and so far we've been able to create a milieu of love and kindness, trying to develop trust and attachments. Somehow or other, I have been very fortunate in picking staff who all respond to my attempts to try to maintain that milieu at all times. But the whole time I'm sitting here, I'm wishing that you could tell me where in your literature, and maybe in that of others, I could find some more direct, succinct help to use in training my staff to reinforce the ideas that I've been trying to express, but not so well as I've heard here. I'm also overcome by what you have said here, because I feel it everyday where I live with my patients.

Bettelheim: Well, first let me tell you that it takes a great deal of time to create such an institution. You have to give yourself time, you have to give your staff time. Rome wasn't built overnight, nor are residential treatment institutions built overnight. It takes time, it takes learning—learning from one's experience, learning from one's mistakes. We all make mistakes. We shouldn't expect to be perfect. Perfection is deadly. It's human to err, but I also think it's human to learn from one's errors. Most people have to learn by doing. Be sure to learn from your mistakes. That's the most important learning.

The Evolution of the Developmental Object Relations Approach to Psychotherapy

James F. Masterson, M.D.

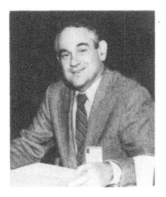

James F. Masterson, M.D.
James F. Masterson (M.D., Jefferson Medical School, 1951) is Director of the Masterson Group, P.C., which specializes in the treatment of adolescent and adult character disorders. Additionally, he is Director of the Masterson Institute (formerly Character Disorder Foundation); attending psychiatrist at New York Hospital, Payne Whitney Clinic; and Adjunct Clinical Professor of Psychiatry at Cornell University Medical College. Masterson has authored seven books and edited two volumes, mostly on the topic of psychoanalytic approaches to character disorders and adolescents. His seminal work on the borderline personality has made him one of the most influential and studied practitioners of modern psychoanalytic methods.
Writing about both personal and professional struggles, Masterson allows us to be privy to the development of his important approach to character disorders. We can trace the growth of both the psychoanalytic concepts that influenced him, and those that he courageously and insightfully developed.

INTRODUCTION

The developmental approach is not "revealed knowledge" and did not spring full-grown like Athena from the head of Zeus. It emerged from a long, slow, often laborious and tedious professional struggle which required the grappling with and resolution of both personal conflicts and professional challenges.

The prospect of describing this struggle evoked my anxiety about my own self-expression. This was brought to my attention one morning when I drove into the garage of my office and misread a sign to say, "Don't blow *your* horn." I laughed as

I realized that the sign actually said "Don't blow *the* horn."

I had misread the sign as a reproof to myself for any temptation to use this occasion to gratify my own infantile grandiosity rather than to perform the task of describing the struggle.

In thinking the matter through, I realized I was not so concerned about my own grandiosity; rather, the misperception referred to an ancient conflict with my exhibitionistic father who resented anyone attempting to occupy some of his space. I was admonishing myself for attempting such an effort.

This vignette illustrates one of the ways

in which we as adults have dormant residuals of early infantile grandiosity which certain life situations can reinforce and bring out of hiding. However, awareness of infantile grandiosity allows one to keep it within limits so that it does not intrude on the present-day reality task.

The evolution of the developmental, object relations approach after my psychiatric training can be divided into three stages, each of which had a central preoccupation which resulted in a book. The first, or psychiatric, descriptive stage (ages 30–42, years 1956–1968) resulted in the *Psychiatric Dilemma of Adolescence* (1967, 1984). A second, or developmental, stage (ages 42–48, 1968–1974) produced *Treatment of the Borderline Adolescent, A Developmental Approach* (1972, 1984). The third stage, the developmental object relations theory stage (ages 48–56 and up, 1974 plus), began with the *Psychotherapy of the Borderline Adult* (1976), which was followed by several other books on the same theme (1980, 1982, 1983, 1985). The progression was from a clinical psychiatric descriptive perspective to a psychoanalytic developmental perspective to a final integration of the descriptive, developmental and object relations theory.

FIRST STAGE
Psychiatric Dilemma of Adolescence
(Ages 30–42, 1956–1968)

I was looking for a subject for a required research project during my residency. I began to notice at case conferences that whenever an adolescent was presented someone would inevitably say that one had to be careful about diagnosis because "He may well grow out of it." I checked the literature for research on adolescents who had "grown out of it" and found next to nothing. This began a central preoccupation about "what happens" that was to dominate my professional life for 20 years and involve three follow-up studies. During my last year as a resident and a postgraduate year as chief resident, I finished and published a follow-up study

on what happens to hospitalized adolescent patients.

I then began practice half time, started personal analysis, and organized and ran half-time an adolescent outpatient clinic. At the same time, dissatisfied with the methodological limitations of the inpatient follow-up study which was retrospective, I wanted to do a prospective study that would eliminate as many of the methodological loopholes as possible. What I didn't realize at the time was that (a) I was now flirting with becoming a methodological researcher and relegating the intrapsychic and psychodynamic to the background as a means of dealing with my own intrapsychic problems, (b) I had made a decision to undertake a project that would take 12 years from 1956–1968 to extricate myself from, and (c) when I emerged, the temptation to use work as a resistance to understanding my own intrapsychic problems would have been resolved with the crystallization of a unified, harmonious perspective on both the inner and the outer, on both my self and my work.

Those years entailed a dramatic Devil and Daniel Webster personal conflict as to what perspective I would adopt on clinical material, as well as inferentially on my own emotional problems and, consequently, of course, on what direction my career would eventually take. For the follow-up study, I had obtained a large research grant which provided two complete research staffs, each comprised of two psychiatrists, a social worker, a secretary, a statistical assistant, and a statistical advisor. The size and the momentum of the research accelerated like a snowball rolling downhill. I now began to wonder if my reach had exceeded my grasp. It became necessary to drop my clinical duties in order to accommodate the research.

This was the post-Sputnik time in science. The physical sciences, spurred on by the Russians' initial success with Sputnik, were beginning their ascendancy. Psychiatrists were feeling quite bad about the inadequacy of their own research methodology compared to that of the physical sciences. At this point the social scientists came to the fore with an "objective" research methodology focusing on such matters as "defining variables, validity, reliability and statistical analyses."

I came under the influence at that time of an extraordinarily talented social psychiatrist researcher by the name of Alexander Leighton, M.D., who was engaged in what is now the well-known Sterling County Midtown Mental Health studies of the prevalence of psychiatric illness in the population. He made his methodology and his statisticians available to me. Burying my reservations as to how appropriate this approach was to clinical work, I plunged in.

A conflict began to rage in me between the social-science methodological point of view and the clinical point of view which emphasizes the importance of considering all variables at one time, with clinical judgment as the only final instrument of observation and decision. At the same time, in analysis five days a week I was delving deeper and deeper into my own psyche. I would spend three hours a day at the clinic trying to refine methodology, for example, reliability studies or various statistical approaches to clinical material. Then I would go to an analytic session which would again and again demonstrate how these activities served to reinforce my resistance to facing my own emotions.

I will never forget the day this conflict was finally resolved. It happened at a conference with both staffs and all statistical advisors and consultants. The entire assemblage sat around all day listening to the statisticians debate various microscopically different statistical ways of approaching clinical material. I became impatient and exasperated. That day I settled the matter in favor of the clinical point of view.

I felt that the statistical-methodological approach had serious limitations in clinical work, and I became committed to the clinical point of view in research and to basically a psychoanalytic point of view. At the same time, my use of work as a

resistance to my own intrapsychic problems diminished dramatically.

The findings of this project were published in a book entitled *The Psychiatric Dilemma of Adolescence* (1967). We found the adolescent "did not grow out of it." Five years later, more than 50 percent of the adolescents were still severely impaired. At that time we called them personality disorders rather than borderline, and we found on review of their treatment records that if they and their parents were treated once a week over the course of a year, their symptoms, such as anxiety, depression, acting-out, did indeed diminish. But what was giving them so much trouble five years later was their pathologic character traits which had not been touched upon in the treatment at all.

At this time the chairman of the Department of Psychiatry at Cornell-New York Hospital retired. The change created turmoil in the department. I needed additional time to write the book, so I left the Department and began to ponder how to pursue the questions the study had raised. What are these pathologic character traits? Where do they come from? How can we identify them and how can we devise better methods of treatment? I then got a call from the new chairman asking if I would come back to take charge of the adolescent inpatients who in the last six months had kicked out some 50 door panels. This presented an ideal opportunity to pursue these questions in an inpatient setting over the long term where we would have a chance to carefully monitor and correlate the interviews with the adolescents' behavior.

STAGE TWO
Treatment of the Borderline Adolescent: A Developmental Approach
(Ages 42–48, 1968–1974)

I designed a research unit for the intensive psychoanalytic psychotherapy of personality disorders in adolescents. I received the necessary commitments for a staff and residents from the chairman who was willing to do almost anything within reason to get the nettlesome adolescent problem off his back. He agreed to allow patients to stay at least a year and the resident to remain on the service for that period of time. Those next six years were extraordinarily fruitful for the development of my own thinking; in retrospect, they came to provide the bedrock of what later became my point of view on the psychotherapy of the Borderline and Narcissistic Personality Disorders.

The adolescents who were admitted had behavioral difficulties such as not attending school, taking drugs, and other forms of socially unacceptable behavior. The principal clinical symptom was acting-out. In order for the unit to survive, we realized we had to find means to set limits to this acting-out. Having to deal with acting-out adolescents in a structured setting presented an absolutely unparalleled opportunity to learn how to understand and manage this defense mechanism. The adolescents were forever putting the residents' and sometimes my own "feet to the fire" to test our competence and trustworthiness. The successful survival of these adolescents' "trials by fire" taught us the therapeutic management of acting-out. Today, in supervision, as I see the problems most therapists have in understanding and managing acting-out, I only wish they could have had that experience in that unique crucible. Only after we had become professionals at setting limits in order to survive did we later learn that it had a far more important and profound psychodynamic effect. We saw the adolescents become depressed as they controlled their behavior—the first link between affect and defense.

It was now clear to us that the acting-out was a defense against the depression. However, the source of the depression remained unclear. We speculated it might have to do with adolescent conflicts over emancipation. In trying to puzzle it out I had exhausted all known resources, including Anna Freud's writings (1965) and conversations with her and Peter Blos (1962).

Another day which I shall never forget is the one in which the breakthrough came in understanding the sources of the depression. I was browsing through journals in the library when I ran across an article by Margaret Mahler (1958) on her study of psychotic children entitled "Autism and Symbiosis: Two Disturbances in the Sense of Entity and Identity." This article led me to investigate further her reports of her child observation studies of the development of the normal self through the stages of separation/individuation.

I stayed like a bloodhound on the track she outlined and began to follow her work closely. At the same time, our depressed adolescents began talking not about conflicts with their parents in the here and now, but about earlier and earlier separation experiences, and finally about the mothers' inability to acknowledge their children's emerging self.

It dawned on me that serendipitously I was in the midst of two complementary research experiments. In other words, Mahler's work (1958, 1968, 1975) educated me about the early development of the normal self while my own adolescent patients were describing and demonstrating dramatically the failures of that same normal process, namely, the developmental arrest of the Borderline Personality Disorder.

I put the two together, which led to a point of view that the Borderline Personality Disorder was a developmental problem—a failure in separation/individuation.

This was the initial opening of the doors to some of the mysteries of the Borderline Personality Disorder: to the concept of maternal unavailability for acknowledgment of the self and the resultant abandonment depression and the developmental arrest of the ego. It also led to the design of a treatment to deal with this developmental failure: confrontation of the adolescent's defenses against his abandonment depression leading to the working through of the depression, which attenuated or removed the anchor from his developing, activating self and allowed it to resume its development.

These findings were published in *Treatment of the Borderline Adolescent: A Developmental Approach* (1972, 1984). This book, in retrospect, must have been far ahead of its time as its appearance was greeted with thundering silence. I felt as if it had been dropped down a bottomless well. It was only after the second book, *Psychotherapy of the Borderline Adult* (1976), was published that this adolescent book finally came into its own.

STAGE THREE
Psychotherapy of the Borderline Adult: A Developmental Object Relations Approach
(Ages 48–56 plus, 1974–   )

A key question remained: What was the link between maternal libidinal unavailability and the developmental arrest? Object relations theory (Jacobson, 1964; Kernberg, 1967; Rinsley, 1968, 1982) supplied the link I had been looking for and was an enormous catalyst to my own thoughts about the role of maternal acknowledgment in the development of the self and of intrapsychic structure.

After the adolescent book was published (1972, 1984), I was asked to present a paper on the treatment of the Borderline Adolescent at a symposium in Philadelphia honoring Margaret Mahler. I suggested presenting another paper I was preparing with Donald Rinsley on integrating object relations theory with separation-individuation developmental theory. In this paper (Masterson & Rinsley, 1975), we combined four ideas: (1) the developmental point of view about separation-individuation and maternal libidinal availability and acknowledgment (Masterson, 1972, 1984); (2) object relations theory of the development of intrapsychic structure

(Jacobson, 1964); (3) an early paper of Freud's (1911) on the two principles of mental functioning, and (4) my own clinical observation that as Borderline adolescents improved and became more adaptive—in other words, as they separated and individuated—they felt worse not better—more depressed. The day I gave the paper at the meeting I felt confident that I had made a breakthrough—at least for myself—and that a whole new perceptual world lay before me. I realized, also, that I would have to move out of adolescent psychiatry and into the broader world of the psychoanalytic developmental object relations approach to the character disorders.

I immediately applied these new ideas to adults in my own private practice. This work with adults was presented in *Psychotherapy of the Borderline Adult, A Developmental Approach* (1976). This text modified, crystallized and consolidated my developmental object-relations point of view of the Borderline, as well as my image of myself which changed from adolescent psychiatrist to psychoanalytic psychiatrist with an interest in the developmental object relations approach to the character disorders in adolescents and adults.

This change, of course, led to another identity crisis. It was one thing for me to feel inside that I was no longer primarily an adolescent psychiatrist, but rather an expert on psychoanalytic psychotherapy of character disorders. It was quite another to get my peers in the field to accept this change. For example, although I had had a thorough personal psychoanalysis, I had not attended a formal psychoanalytic institute and was not therefore a card-carrying psychoanalyst. In addition, the chairmanship of the Department of Psychiatry at Cornell had again changed, my long-term unit had to be closed—a victim to finances and the tidal wave of interest in quick cures, I had to find something else to do.

My reputation up to that point was based on adolescent psychiatry, but I was no longer interested in doing principally that kind of work. On the other hand, the book (1976) had not yet been published so I could present no evidence on which to base an effort to get the kind of work that I wanted. I couldn't accept what was offered nor could I reasonably expect to get what I wanted.

I sent the book to my publisher with some misgivings, knowing full well that the adolescent book hadn't done that well. The editor sent the book out for review and several very long months later called me in for what was the briefest and most depressing interview of my life. He turned the book down flat, quoting his reviewer as saying, "People interested in development read Mahler and there is much written on the Borderline. There is no place for your book." He then asked if I would like him to send it out to another reviewer. I said, "No thanks, with your talent for picking reviewers, I already know what will happen." I left dismayed and despondent. I had anticipated trouble but not that much. Nevertheless, my conviction about the value of the work itself was not in the least shaken.

Luckily, through the good offices of another publisher, I was referred to Brunner/Mazel, who accepted the book immediately. One hurdle accomplished, I now had to await the book's reception. While the book was being prepared for publication, a good sign occurred: It was accepted as a selection by most of the psychiatric book clubs. But a feeling of doubt remained in the air. I couldn't help remembering the awful silence that had followed publication of *Psychotherapy of the Borderline Adolescent*.

A good sale of a featured book for a psychiatric book club is several thousand copies. Several months after the book was published (1976), I returned to my office to see a note my secretary had left on my desk. It read simply, "Psychiatric Book Club—13,000." I knew immediately the comma had been misplaced and that the figure was 1,300 not 13,000. And, that wasn't too bad. When I brought the error

to my secretary's attention, she assured me I was wrong as she had checked carefully and the number was 13,000. I cannot adequately describe the feelings of both relief and fulfillment that flooded me at the realization that the identity crisis was over. My own inner image of my self was now being accepted and reinforced by my peers.

That book had and continues to have an extraordinary outreach. It opened a whole new and exciting world for me. I received numbers of spontaneous letters from therapists across the country describing how exactly it explained their problem with the treatment of the Borderline patient and how helpful it had been. I also received a number of similar letters from Borderline patients. I was inundated with requests for lectures from all over the country. The lectures were crowded with enthusiastic and responsive audiences. Concurrently, I found that my own integration of this developmental object relations point of view had greatly expanded my own grasp and perception of clinical problems, as well as my ability to manage them. It was as if my mind had literally expanded.

This momentous development also helped me decide to leave Cornell which had been my professional home ever since I became a psychiatrist. We were unable to agree on suitable work. I set up my own organizations, The Masterson Group for the treatment of character disorders, and The Character Disorder Foundation, a nonprofit organization for teaching and research on the character disorders. This decision expanded my teaching from one institution to many institutions. The Masterson Group had its inaugural public conference on the Borderline in October of 1977 at Hunter College where we planned for several hundred people. We were inundated by 2,200 people. The identity crisis was now further resolved by further reinforcement and the clarification of my own self-image.

In 1976 I received a call from a young woman finishing her Ph.D. studies at Smith

College who wanted to know if I would allow her to use the adolescents from our unit to do a follow-up study. I was appalled that anybody would think I would turn over these "jewels" to anyone else, since I had long planned to do the follow-up myself. I asked for an interview, curious to know what a person with so much gall looked like. It turned out that she was sound in every respect. We ended up doing a joint follow-up study of the Borderline adolescents treated in our unit which was published as *From Borderline Adolescent to Functioning Adult: The Test of Time* (1980).

This study demonstrated the results of the treatment, results whose effectiveness could be predicted by the degree to which the patients' treatment course followed the hypothetical model.

I then extended the clinical application of the theory in two other books: *The Narcissistic and Borderline Disorders: An Integrated Developmental Approach* (1982) and *Countertransference and Psychotherapeutic Technique* (1983).

In these books a developmental object relations approach to narcissism and the narcissistic Personality Disorder was spelled out and the concept of the underlying etiology of the Borderline Personality Disorder was extended as follows:

There were three inputs into etiology, namely, nature, nurture, and fate, and the therapist would have to make a clinical decision how much each contributed to his patient's disorder. Nature consisted of organic problems, constitutional defects, or genetic defects. Nurture referred to maternal libidinal unavailability regardless of the cause. Fate referred to those accidents of life that might affect either track of the two-track separation-individuation process—namely, any event that diminished mother's libidinal availability or interfered with the child's individuation in the first three years of life.

By 1983 with the publication of the *Countertransference* book I thought that my writing days might be over. However, I felt that the developmental object-rela-

tions theory as outlined still did not give adequate consideration to the self, and the concepts of the self offered by others seemed to lack something. I found myself without intention or plan focusing more and more in my clinical work on the patient's self to the point of spontaneously developing symbols, for example, "S" when the patient was activating his real self in the session and "O" for his relationship with objects. I began thinking and talking more and more in terms of a real and defensive self as it became clearer in the clinical material. Only after I had been using this concept of the self in psychotherapy for several years did I finally decide I had to think it through further, organize it and write it up if only to clarify it myself and to get it out of my system. This became *The Real Self: A Developmental, Self, and Object Relations Approach* (1985).

This theory of the self now seems to bring the Developmental Object Relations approach to a kind of fullness or completeness appropriate to the demands of the clinical material. At least it is probably as full or complete as I can make it.

It has been extremely exciting and gratifying to have been fortunate enough to be involved in the veritable explosion of knowledge that has taken place in this field in the last 30 years . . . to see the gaps being filled and the pieces of the puzzle coming together. I had worked with Borderline and Narcissistic Disorder patients for years without being able to help them with their struggles. To finally have the tools to do the job with many patients as well as to teach others to do the job— to have mastered this task as much as it can be mastered—has provided the ultimate fulfillment and satisfaction in the work.

REFERENCES

Blos, P. (1962). *On adolescence.* Glencoe, IL: Free Press.

Freud, A. (1965). *Normality and pathology in childhood—Assessments of development.* New York: International Universities Press.

Freud, S. (1911). *Formulations on the two principles of mental functioning.* Standard edition 12:218–226. London: Hogarth Press.

Jacobson, E. (1964). *The self and the object world.* New York: International Universities Press.

Kernberg, O. (1967). Borderline personality organization. *Jnl. Amer. Psychoanalytical Ass., 15:*641–685.

Mahler, M. (1958). Autism and symbiosis: Two extreme disturbances of identity. *Int. Jnl. Psa., 39:*77–83.

Mahler, M. (1968). *On human symbiosis and the vicissitudes of individuation.* New York: International Universities Press.

Mahler, M. (1975). *The psychological birth of the human infant.* New York: Basic Books.

Masterson, J.F. (1967). *The psychiatric dilemma of adolescence.* Boston: Little Brown & Co. (Reprint 1984, New York: Brunner/Mazel)

Masterson, J.F. (1972). *Treatment of the borderline adolescent: A developmental approach.* New York: John Wiley & Sons. (Reprint 1984, New York: Brunner/Mazel)

Masterson, J.F. (1976). *Psychotherapy of the borderline adult: A developmental approach.* New York: Brunner/Mazel.

Masterson, J.F., with Costello, J.L. (1980). *The test of time: From borderline adolescent to functioning adult.* New York: Brunner/Mazel.

Masterson, J.F. (1982). *The narcissistic and borderline disorders: An integrated developmental approach.* New York: Brunner/Mazel.

Masterson, J.F. (1983). *Countertransference and psychotherapeutic technique.* New York: Brunner/Mazel.

Masterson, J.F. (1985). *The real self: A developmental, self, and object relations approach.* New York: Brunner/Mazel.

Masterson, J.F., & Rinsley, D.B. (1975). The borderline syndrome: The role of the mother in the genesis and psychic structure of the borderline personality. *Int. Jnl. Psa., 56:*163–178.

Rinsley, D.B. (1968). Economic aspects of object relations. *Int. Jnl. Psa., 49:*38–48.

Rinsley, D.B. (1982). *Borderline and other self disorders.* New York: Jason Aronson.

Discussion by Jay Haley

I am glad to know that Dr. Masterson has had a successful career and that he progressed through different stages and produced a book at the end of each stage, which I think is an example he has set for us all. My problem in discussing this is that I am not sure how that is relevant to the subject of this meeting; I will try to make it relevant in some brief comments.

I think one of the purposes of this meeting is to present divergent views. There is a lot of variety in the field of therapy. We have different points of view and I think it is our obligation to state our own position, even if it disagrees with someone else's. If I offend anybody in what I say, you should understand I am only doing it out of my duty not because I enjoy it.

But I think Dr. Masterson's paper and this meeting illustrate a remarkable situation. Many of us have worked in the field and done research and therapy for many years, particularly in the area of adolescence, and yet we can function in the same field while having no similarities whatever in our ways of thinking or doing therapy. I think that is remarkable. This is supposed to be a meeting bringing together a faculty which has in common the ability to change things, yet the differences are so marked that you wonder if it is the same field. I was reluctant to discuss this paper when I heard the subject matter. Moreover, I didn't receive the paper in advance and when I finally read it I was even more reluctant to discuss it.* One reason is that I really don't have much interest in the psychoanalytic point of view and I gave up debating psychoanalysis many years ago. As a force in the world of ideas, psychoanalysis died in 1957 and the funeral goes on in the large cities, but I don't think it is an effective force anymore. So talking about psychoanalytic ideas really just doesn't appeal to me.

In addition, I have never met a borderline personality and when I realized I was going to be on this program, I went out in the waiting room and started looking for a borderline personality and I couldn't find one. (I have a very busy clinic and training program with lots of patients of all ages. We don't turn anybody down so we have great variety.) And I asked our staff, "Do you have a borderline personality whom I could talk with?" They didn't have any so I had to conclude that they must go elsewhere. They don't come to us, at any rate.

So it is something of an effort for me to take myself into that kind of thinking which is to me going back in time. However, since I am here, let me try to say something sensible about the differences.

I think that Dr. Masterson and I both participated in the explosion of knowledge that he mentioned, the explosion that has taken place in the last 30 years, but I think that we exploded in different directions. Let me tell about something that had a large influence on me. Beginning in the 1950s, there was a new trend in the social science research: There was extensive study of the birds of the air and the beasts of the field, particularly in their natural settings. The biologists taught us about the personal lives of our fellow crea-

tures. And today there is probably not a primate out there without someone watching him with binoculars, because this study goes on. I recall a study in the 1950s which impressed many of us, especially those of us doing therapy in hospitals. (I had been working on a research project in a hospital for ten years so I was familiar with hospitals.)

There was a woman known as the goat woman. This was because her specialty was observing goats. Everybody had a special animal they observed; for example, there was a buffalo woman who followed buffaloes across Colorado. This was the goat woman. And she did some experimentation with these animals. She reported that if you take a young kid, a small goat, away from its mother and from the group, and then in a couple of days you return that kid to the group and its family, it will be shunned as if it is not normal. The other goats treat it like a strange goat. And that becomes the career it has, it doesn't grow out of this. Now this woman was not sure if it is the absence of the group or the smell of human beings that might cause this problem, but there was a general recognition that taking a creature out of its natural setting and then putting it back had a marked effect on it. This woman and other ecologists at that time were saying that our understanding of animals for many years had been too long perverted by our studying animals in the zoo. Animals in captivity, animals in a zoo, exhibit really quite unnatural behavior. They have perverse sexual behavior, they seem depressed, they often behave in bizarre ways. And no one knew this until they began to observe them in their natural settings. When animals are blocked off from their natural behavior appropriate to a social context, they begin to behave in rather abnormal ways.

This argument began to be applied to human beings. It was said they should be observed not in artificial settings but in their natural environment. That is when studies of the family developed, in that same period, as well as studies of the

---

* Masterson submitted his paper to the conference office in good time. It was a clerical oversight that a copy was not sent to Haley.

community. We wanted to see a person responding in his natural situation, the family, believing that we could thus understand why he behaved the way he did. We also developed the idea that it was an error to pluck somebody out of his family, put the person in a hospital isolated from his family, and assume that this was a sensible therapeutic procedure. Instead, it could be expected that the person would behave abnormally when he returned to the community.

When we studied adolescents, we didn't want to study them in a zoo, but rather in the community with their friends and family. And we didn't want to do therapy with them in a zoo like a psychiatric hospital, but in their natural setting. That is where they have to succeed in life and that is where they belong. Now, granting that some people have to be locked up for the protection of the community because they are menaces, we attempted to differentiate the idea of social control from therapy. For a young person to return to the community with the stigma of the hospital upon him was to set him off on an abnormal path and I think that should be done only with great reluctance. In the hospital they are often taught to think in strange ways. They live with marginal people. They are infantilized by having to be taken care of in there; they don't have to go to work. If they are hospitalized for a long period, they miss the whole fashion of the times, the whole drug scene, or whatever might be current. Things change very fast among young people, so that when they come out they are behind everybody. Also, I don't think it is good for them to spend their time and make their friends with people with problems.

You know, the other day I was talking with somebody who said she had a depressed patient and thought she would find a depressed group and put him in it. It is a strange thing to do with a depressed person. You would think one would find a cheerful group and put him in it.

If you have a young person in trouble and marginal and having difficulty, I think that putting him in with a group of young people who are marginal and having difficulty doesn't make a great deal of sense. But it took some time to get to that point of view. As a result of studies like these and a shift in everyone's thinking, there began to be appreciated a discovery that the social context can be an explanation of why people behave as they do. Thus, it is very different to explain why people do what they do in terms of their social milieu than to do so in terms of some inner conflict or past programming. And that new explanation, I think, was revolutionary for many of us. It led to family therapy for many problems. It led to new explanations of human beings. My objections to these ideas about borderline personalities are that they take us back to a period where it was assumed that an individual was autonomous and independent of any social influences, except possibly some past maternal influence in infancy. Many of us made an effort to get out of that way of thinking, which is a very seductive one.

I recall that Don Jackson suggested that object relations theory was very helpful to some people in getting out of the individual way of thinking. If at first they could put the idea of this object in their head in relation to each other, then they could move objects outside and make them real people in relation to each other. So that point of view was helpful but everybody found a different way to get out of that individual point of view. Many went through Sullivan. Sullivan had a very large influence on almost every family therapist. They had some connection with him because he, despite his turgid style of language, was making a change out of that individual sort of orientation.

Many of us made a transition from thinking of the individual to thinking of dyads and triads when doing therapy. That is, the idea that an adolescent misbehaved because of an inner impulse was very different from thinking of this same behavior as caused by that adolescent's father, for example, encouraging him to behave that way. And that was different from explaining the same behavior, occurring when the family became unstable, as a way of stabilizing the family. Thus, there seem to be young people who make trouble at the moment the parents are about to separate and the family is going unstable. Then the family would pull together to deal with this pain and stabilize. Now, each of these are different ways of explaining exactly the same adolescent. It is just a matter of the point of view and unit you think in when you explain it. The problem is that if you shift from an individual to a dyadic to a triadic view, it looks as if you take discontinuous steps, as if you really can't bridge from one to the other. There are different ways of thinking.

I think that this shift in the universe has done more than any other factor, except the economics of therapy, to differentiate therapists into different camps. By the economics of therapy I mean the question of what insurance will pay for and what it won't, as well as what theories one should have if one is in private practice or if one is in an agency. A result of these differences is that if an adolescent exhibits some kind of problem behavior, like dropping out of school or taking drugs, there are now over 100 schools of therapy with different ways of treating that. There are also quite different explanations of why the adolescent does what he does. Some like Dr. Masterson would place the cause in the past, at the stage of maternal influence, in infancy. Others would put it in the present with a focus on what is happening with the adolescent right now. To emphasize a past program would emphasize an adolescent making trouble as a way of helping his family in the present; this is such a different point of view that I don't know how there can be a bridge across that gulf.

I obtained three of Dr. Masterson's books and took a look at them in preparation for this meeting. Some years ago I gave up reading books with "personality" in the title. I felt every time I read one

that I had read it before. And every once in a while over the years I would pick one up and read it and have a kind of déjà vu feeling I had read this before. That is, I think the area of the personality has been mined for 2000 years, really. The ideas are a bit redundant.

I find it very difficult to find out what happened to an adolescent in the inpatient treatment program on one of Dr. Masterson's wards because the descriptions tended to be so internal. However, there is a preface to one of his books which was considered to be good enough to be put out in the second edition and I was appalled by this preface. It is presumably considered important since it was put right at the front of the book (J.F. Masterson, *Treatment of the Borderline Adolescent*, Wiley, 1972; Brunner/Mazel, 1984). Let me read it to you, "The distraught and doting mother of a two-year-old calls her pediatrician to complain that her toddler follows her around the house and will not leave her side. The angry, depressed and frightened mother of a 15-year-old calls the pediatrician in despair about her son's dropping out of school and taking drugs. These two children, examples of the borderline syndrome at different ages, suffer from the same developmental failure—the failure of separation individuation."

Now I think this is an extraordinary kind of statement from two or three different points of view. A pediatrician reports this behavior of a two-year-old and a 15-year-old, and apparently Dr. Masterson diagnoses them from that report. You know, what I am reminded of, and why I am interested in that point of view, is that I just had a visit from a family from India with a kid in trouble and I found out how, in that section of India, a psychiatrist diagnoses. What happens is that the parents take their kid to their regular physician. They describe how the kid behaves. The physician calls the psychiatrist and tells them how the kid behaves. The psychiatrist prescribes on the phone medication which the physician then gives the kid; that is psychiatric treatment. The kid is an 18-year-old who already has some tardive dyskenisia from this treatment. I think that in India they could at least do what psychiatrists in this country do and see the kid for five or ten minutes before they medicate him.

At any rate, I think the main issue is that there is kind of a fixity of ideas when you get into the individual diagnosis and you are so sure of the origins of behavior. I think you really couldn't diagnose a two-year-old who follows his mother around as a borderline personality. I think you would have to find such personalities behind every bush to make such a statement. Granted the two-year-old might be unsociable and not have many friends and he might even refuse to go to nursery school. The fact that children cling to their mothers at two years of age doesn't seem to me to be an indication of a type of personality that is pathological. But if it is so, then there is a lot of business for all of us for many years because there are a lot of two-year-olds clinging to their mothers and following them around.

When we turn to the 15-year-old who drops out of school and takes drugs and therefore is a borderline personality, that also is a remarkable diagnosis. It is also good for business since there are hundreds of thousands of kids who take drugs and drop out of school. It is the fashion to take dope these days among young people in the community. At any rate, I would hope that these two-year-olds and these 15-year-olds don't end up on a psychiatric ward being confronted with their separation/individuation problems. There are so many ways of doing therapy today and so many techniques that are effective as a result of the therapeutic revolution in the last 30 years that I think a therapist is obligated to learn about them, that he or she is obligated to try out those procedures if the case merits it. To force adolescents into one method of therapy and to have one way of thinking about them, I don't think is revolutionary. I think it is naive.

RESPONSE BY DR. MASTERSON

Mr. Haley, are you sure you are not one of those guys who reviewed one of my original books when it came out? Now you have had a field day at my expense and the expense of my point of view; but in my judgment, in the direction and course of your field day, you have revealed, I feel, what is wrong with your perspective. Yesterday, in discussing Dr. Bowen's paper, I mentioned, following his line of thought, that human beings have to develop theories. It is our way of dealing with our perception of ourselves and the world and trying to manage both. Every theory designed for this has two purposes: to maintain a sense of inner comfort and inner equilibrium as well as to try to apprehend the external truth. Once we have achieved a stable sense of inner comfort, then so often we are unwilling to sacrifice it even to search for an external truth. In order to maintain that comfort, I think Mr. Haley is approaching this material not from a reflective or critical and thoughtful point of view, but to derogate it and put it down prima facie.

In taking up the issue of how you approached it—that psychoanalysis died in the 1950s—I am not presenting the classical psychoanalytic point of view. It is a modification of it. If it died, what is going on here at this meeting? Maybe it is an example of denial on your part. Now the best illustration, as I see it, of how your comfort in your family therapy point of view makes it very difficult for you to open your mind to other possible stimuli is the example you used from the preface of that book to imply in a derogatory and pejorative way that I make a diagnosis on one symptom or one history and so forth, not letting the audience in on the fact that that preface obviously was an effort to gain the reader's attention for the entire book. Remember that it is a preface to a book which exhaustively and in detail outlines the careful attention we pay to *all* the factors present, including the family. There are whole sections in that book on family treatment, along with those on the adolescent. Moreover, our perspective is not to "delve" into the past. *Our experience has been that if you deal with the present in a competent and adequate fashion therapeutically, the past emerges and forces itself on you to be dealt with.*

I also found that your rationalization for ignoring, basically, the content of my paper in order to present your own points of view unfortunate, since you had two other options, it seems to me. You could have taken the one I took with Dr. Bowen yesterday. I am not a subscriber to family therapy. I was discussing a paper by a family therapist, and what I did was stretch myself a bit to see what I could find to contribute to his point of view. I am only sorry that you couldn't find it within yourself to stretch yourself to do the same for me. I strongly suggest that the reason you didn't was that it would disturb the comfort you have found in your family theory approach; that left you no other alternative than to more or less offhandedly dismiss my point of view.

You made a number of negative comments about hospitalization, as if relating it to the holocaust. I think I would agree with you that hospitalization should never be undertaken lightly, that it does have some of those effects that you mentioned. On the other hand, there are adolescents around who cannot manage themselves, who do not have the capacity to manage themselves, and not only will be a danger to others but might kill themselves. It is next to impossible to have these adolescents treated on an outpatient setting, and so, with careful and thoughtful evaluation of all the features involved, you have to take the handicap of putting them in a hospital to provide them with the help that they need.

Now, if you don't use a personality approach, a diagnostic approach, obviously you are not going to find borderline personality disorders. In the world in which I come from, in which I live, which I gather you feel is some sort of ancient, dinosauric, northeastern culture, these concepts are taken as commonplace. But I must also emphasize here—since you seem to see an almost mutually exclusive quality to individual versus family versus the other members of the family—that I think one of the great contributions of family therapy has been to teach us that we must include adequate consideration of the family in our work with our patients, which is what we all do.

However, I want to say that, with all the advantages of family therapy and all its contributions, yet to me, intellectually, the one Achilles' heel in your argument against the kind of work that I am putting forward is, I think, that family therapy does not adequately understand the consequences of internalization and fixation, which is what we are dealing with in (pardon the term) borderline personality organization. I cannot conceive that these structures, once they are set, are fixed. And in order to be able to unset them in an intrapsychic way, you must have a certain amount and kind of therapeutic input. And I don't think they can be unset in another way.

Now, you raised the question, "There are so many therapeutic approaches." Yes, there are. Human beings are extraordinarily plastic. Particularly needy patients. Therapists have enormous needs for comfort, as well as searching for truth. You put these together and you get a tremendous variety of combinations, you get therapeutic results which, if you look at them on the surface, seem quite comparable; if you study them in detail, not so comparable. So I hope that in the future the question of whether it is your point of view or my point of view which is most useful, and where, will not have to come out of debates at meetings, but will come out of research studies demonstrating where and in which way each is most beneficial.

Canter (Moderator): As moderator and one of the members of the steering committee for this meeting, I hope that as we view the evolution of psychotherapy, we can see our divergent viewpoints and begin the effort, if you will, to once again converge. You know, the old notion of thesis, antithesis and finally the synthesis. Or perhaps, this is what we are witnessing here—the divergent aspects or approaches to psychotherapy. Yes, we do disagree, but out of that disagreement can indeed come an evolution, a convergence once again.

The Evolution of Psychotherapy: Future Trends

Lewis R. Wolberg, M.D.

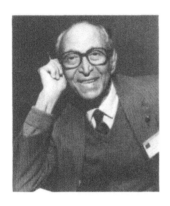

Lewis R. Wolberg, M.D.

Lewis Wolberg has practiced psychiatry and psychotherapy for more than 50 years. He received his M.D. from Tufts College Medical School in 1930.

He is the author, co-author or editor of 26 books and has authored 35 book chapters and numerous papers. He is Founder of the Postgraduate Center for Mental Health in New York, with which he has been associated since 1945, and a Founding Fellow of the American Academy of Psychoanalysis.

Wolberg reminds us of the important contributions and place of psychoanalysis. Arguing against parochialism in analytic and nonanalytic schools, he elevates eclectic approaches: Eclecticism facilitates analytic goals; it does not water them down. Wolberg speaks to the importance of resistance—not only resistance of patients but also resistance of psychotherapists who remain doctrinaire in the quest for dogmatic purity.

The title of this conference is "The Evolution of Psychotherapy." Therefore, it seems fitting to say something about the contemporary events that are shaping evolutionary forces and to venture some guesses about the future. The latter I do with some trepidation because historically, prophesies about the future, from Isaiah to H.G. Wells, have proven to be of a dismal order of accuracy.

Carloads of statistics can be juggled about, but they must also be interpreted and the possibilities of miscalculation are high because many of the variables underlying change are fleeting and beyond our control. The experience of American business is an example. Projections beyond five years are tricky because financial, political, social, and entrepreneurial factors tend to interfere with accurate prognostications (*Newsweek*, November 26, 1973, p. 101). However, not long ago, a group of blue chip companies organized an "Institute of the Future," devoted to comprehensive studies of the future. In addition to making such casual forecasts as the extinction of underpants and pajamas, "Project Aware" predicted an increase in crimes of violence and, striking terror into the heart of the American Medical Association, the eventual complete socialization of medicine. Apart from the Institute's computerized calculations, a few lonely prophets among psychopharmacologists foresaw a psychological millennium within 10 or 20 years, brought about by new wonder drugs and cranial electrodes that guaranteed an era of eternal bliss for all people on earth. This augury has proven to be grossly overoptimistic, having been hampered by some stark realities that are bleeding over onto the future of psychotherapy. We must admit that what happens in mental health in times to come must not be dissociated from unforeseen happenings in the real world, whether these be geopolitical or economic. Such happenings are not always to the good.

In 1932 when I was assistant executive officer at the Boston Psychopathic Hospital (now the Massachusetts Mental Health Center), Karl Bowman, the clinical director, said during ward rounds one morning, "It will be a sad day if economics ever becomes the dominant influence of how we treat our patients." Well, sad times seem to be upon us with the current proposals of payment for services in terms of diagnosis-related groupings (DRGs), with the encouragement of marketplace competition by preferred provider organizations, and with the entry into the field of corporate-controlled health combines. Even though the current proposed plans are not carried to extremes, changes in our mode of delivering services are inevitable. For example, restriction of the number of sessions allotted to patients will necessitate a limitation of therapeutic goals. This will necessitate more thorough treatment planning to achieve selective objectives and will require the use of a broad range of interventions that have proven of value in special syndromes and for designated symptoms.

As payments for mental health services have escalated, cost containment has become an important issue in fund allocation. Questions have arisen regarding the effectiveness of psychotherapy and severe limitations have been placed on reimburse-ment. Many paying agencies consider that the most suitable objective in psychiatric treatment is a reasonably adequate work and social adjustment. This has shifted psychotherapeutic interventions toward supportive and educational techniques with emphasis on crisis intervention, stress reduction, and a wellness rather than a sickness model. The chief casualty has been long-term therapy aimed at personality reconstruction; the specific targets have been psychoanalysis and reconstructive psychotherapies in general.

It is no exaggeration to say that psychoanalysis has come upon some hard times. Internecine warfare, challenges of the validity of its metapsychology, questioning of its cost effectiveness, invasion of useful short-term approaches, shrinking of the health dollar, and competition with lesser-trained providers have shaken up what was once considered the paragon of psychotherapies. Its detractors irreverently regard psychoanalysis as a mosaic of turgid precepts and metapsychological slogans, and they insist there is little we can salvage from its wreckage. Its loyal devotees point out that its essential truths more than balance off its blunders. Whatever its shortcomings, they insist, psychoanalysis has penetrated every crevice of the mental health field and there is little doubt about its utility and survival. We may legitimately ask the question, what does the future hold for this aristocrat of the psychotherapeutic families?

Some years ago I asked Franz Alexander where he thought psychoanalysis was headed. Alexander then revealed to me a conversation he had had with Freud in London, several years before the founder of psychoanalysis passed away. In response to Alexander's query about his speculations on the future of analysis, the venerable genius replied, "Franz, I am not worried about the enemies of psychoanalysis, I am worried about its supporters and friends."

Freud was probably referring to the response of some of his devotees to changes in his ideas about analysis. In his last, and perhaps most important, clinical paper, "Analysis: Terminable and Interminable," Freud stated that psychoanalysis was a lengthy business with an uncertain outcome. This statement was amplified and interpreted as the obituary of psychoanalysis by its critics. Many of the supporters of analysis felt that Freud had let them down by expressing a loss of faith in his own canonical teachings. They were also disturbed by Freud's dalliance with such apostasies as short-term therapy and with other deviations from the classical technique. Alexander told me that during the conversation Freud remarked impishly, "Franz, if I were writing my observations today there are many things that I would change, but I am afraid to do this because the New York group wouldn't like it."

What Freud passed off as a joke has some serious implications for the future not only of psychoanalysis but also for the future of psychotherapy in general. Many professionals are hostages to their early training rigidities. Consequently, the field of mental health has been and is still burdened by enclaves of warring factions marching to the drums of their hardened theoretical imperatives. A plethora of competing models exists, each claiming psychotherapy as its sovereign possession and purporting to explain in its own philosophic and linguistic terms, how people become neurotic and get cured.

Fifty years ago, I was in the middle of a historic controversy that painfully illustrates this point. I was a candidate in psychoanalytic training at the New York Psychoanalytic Institute when Karen Horney hoisted her sails and scudded away from classical theory. Her ideas were published in *The Neurotic Personality of Our Time* (1937), which created enthusiastic excitement among the students and consternation among the faculty. The Oedipus complex was no longer the center of the psychopathological universe. Instead, the vicissitudes of the character structure were presumed to be the hub of man's basic

conflicts. Arguments raged back and forth; and in the end, Horney left the Institute or was thrown out, depending on who told the tale of her defection. Thus, Horney joined the long list of renegades whose disloyalty to Freud, in the opinion of the faithful, qualified them for a place among those who were retarding scientific progress.

There were some among the faculty who did not exactly subscribe to the formulations proposed by Horney, but who nevertheless upheld her right to maintain them. They, too, experienced the fiery brand of disapproval; and on one fateful evening while classes were going on, we followed Horney out of the Institute door onto the New York sidewalks of West Eighty-sixth Street to our favorite delicatessen on Broadway, the Tip-Toe-Inn. Now I have always felt that in the history of the psychoanalytic movement not enough credit has been given to the local delicatessen. At the Tip-Toe-Inn, the level of innovative debate and disputation was at least as spicy as the pastrami. It was here that a new organization was born, dedicated to the tolerance of deviant opinions in psychoanalysis. Aptly, it was titled "The Society for the Advancement of Psychoanalysis." There were about 20 of us then and our enthusiasm was high. Fresh breezes of empiricism were blowing; we could no longer be accused of being custodians of fossilized psychological theories.

At the time I was on the staff of the New York Medical College, Flower-Fifth Avenue Hospital, and my wife was the chief social worker there. The thought occurred to me that the medical school would be a good locus for this scientific society. Sharing my fervor, my wife suggested that I talk to the Professor and Chairman of the Department of Psychiatry, Dr. Stephen P. Jewett, who was partial to psychoanalysis, having been an analysand of Sandor Ferenczi. Jewett agreed to let us bring the new group into the New York Medical College. However, soon the fresh breezes died down and new dogmatisms developed, causing a number of splinter groups, each again brandishing its own orthodoxy. The old adage that history repeats itself was confirmed.

Psychoanalysis had its heyday in the United States from 1940 to 1960, when it was hailed as the inspired hope for most, if not all, of the problems in mental health. Although it scarcely lived up to this grandiose promise, it did spawn the development of a number of methods that drew their rationale from Freud's emphasis on intrapsychic conflict and unconscious ideation. It became apparent that classical psychoanalytic theory had many shortcomings as a consummate understructure for therapeutic process. This prompted a search for more clinically relevant dynamic theories and diverted interest from the vagaries of instinct to defenses of the ego (Anna Freud, 1937; Hartman, 1958), the complexities of character structure in formation and operation (Horney, 1937, 1939; Reich, 1949; Fromm, 1941, 1959; Sullivan, 1947, 1953), and the consequences of distortions in the early development of the child in relation to the original caretaking agencies (Melanie Klein, 1948, 1957; Jacobson, 1964, 1971; Mahler, 1967, 1975; Fairbairn, 1954; Winnicott, 1965; Guntrip, 1968, 1971; Bion, 1959; 1970).

From these studies an attempt was made to extend the usefulness of psychoanalysis beyond its traditional focus on the neuroses. More recently, elaborations of object relations theory (Kernberg, 1976, 1980) and self-psychology (Kohut, 1971, 1977) have been applied to the therapy of borderline and narcissistic personality problems. The many theoretical diversions have led to disagreements within the analytic movement that continue in spite of efforts toward reconciliation of differences (Gedo, 1980). As with most theories, a good deal of fanciful surmise has gone into their organization; but attempts are being made to subject visionary ideas to empirical testing and structured research.

Hopefully, this will resolve some of the misconceptions fostered by the teachings of clashing individual personalities fired by differing perspectives and priorities.

Research, however, will not resolve some of the basic problems in our field which are oriented around the need to cling to obsolescent traditional forms. Tradition is a compelling force that can triumph over education and even over common sense. At its best, it attempts to justify itself by putting the reins on unbridled speculation. At its worst, it can shackle or destroy creativity and innovation. It must, therefore, be constantly checked to avoid a hampering effect on experiment and change. An example of this is the doctrinal idea that a focus on symptom removal is antagonistic to character change. Symptoms are, according to this surviving concept, always manifestations of unconscious conflict. They are the smoke that arises from hidden fires within. Remove the smoke and the causative conflagration continues. Quench the fire and the smoke disappears. Many attempts have been made to correct this mistaken idea; but it persists nevertheless, even among some young professionals who should know better.

Both beginning and graduate therapists often have a curious investment in maintaining theoretical purity. I remember one graduate, at a graduation dinner party of the psychoanalytic division of the school where I was teaching, who asked my advice on how to deal with a particularly resistive, seriously depressed patient. "Why don't you try a supportive symptom-oriented approach?" I suggested. The shocked expression of the trainee could not have exceeded mine when she retorted, "Dr. Wolberg, how come a psychoanalyst like you still uses supportive therapy?" Legends have long legs, and even though we may try to be more liberal and eclectic in training, many young graduates still maintain a legendary orthodoxy. Our hope is that in the future eclectic open-mindedness will encourage experimentation with tactics other than those taught by conservative instructors and supervisors wedded to monolithic approaches. There are still many paladins, particularly in the analytic field. The focus, it is contended, should be on resistances not symptoms.

Admitting that a primary concern in analysis is the working through of resistance, we may ask ourselves, how can a man deal with his oedipal fantasies when he is so depressed in the morning that he can hardly get his shoes on? How can a woman delve into the discordance of archaic introjects when she is beaten up regularly by an alcoholic husband? How can a rebellious adolescent whose brain is befogged with marijuana mediate issues of separation-individuation? How can a patient in the manic phase of a bipolar disorder lay quietly on a couch to associate freely about his past? How can a phobic individual arrive at the 20th floor of an analyst's office when he cannot even get into an elevator? These are examples of practical issues that are never taught in analytic school. They are not as exciting as learning about object- and self-representations, but they surely will come up to plague even the most dedicated analyst.

What I am referring to are symptomatic resistances to analytic process. Among the obstructions that impede the effectiveness of psychoanalysis, the resolution of symptoms may be a most important factor in getting a patient to concentrate attention on underlying personality distortions and their genetic origins. Otherwise anxieties and pain may prevent utilization of what analysis has to offer.

In order to get the patient to a point where he will be susceptible to analysis, it may be necessary to employ some non-analytic techniques. Here is where some analysts manifest their own resistances. I remember chairing a symposium in Sweden on psychotherapy which included a distinguished classical psychoanalyst from West Germany. After giving his presentation of a case, he was asked by a member of the audience whether he ever employed

group psychotherapy. Stunned, he replied, "Group psychotherapy? If you put a revolver to my head I wouldn't do it."

I have personally had my share of disapprobation and censure for using hypnosis as an adjunct in psychoanalysis. I recall a visit some years ago to a prominent authority on psychoanalytic theory who sat majestically in a chair at his desk under a gloomy lithograph of Sigmund Freud. While he proceeded to chide me for polluting the transference with hypnotic hanky-panky, Freud glowered at me with redolent disapproval. I must have defended my position well because at the end of our visit the good doctor asked if he could refer to me a recalcitrant patient whose unconscious he had found hard to penetrate. And even Freud seemed to have a more accepting expression on his face.

Psychoanalysts are not the only practitioners who rigidly cling to dogma. There are many biological, behavioral, experiential and other therapists who adhere to their credos with an unwonted ferocity, being loath to accept doctrines other than their own. Most of the prejudice is extended toward psychoanalysis and intrapsychic approaches in general. Such rejection cannot help but leave a therapeutic program denuded. Admittedly, psychoanalysis has periodically been burdened by metapsychological absurdities that have little clinical relevance. However, it has also introduced a dynamic dimension that is fundamental to an understanding of human nature. It is difficult to see how anyone can do good psychotherapy of any kind without recognizing the interplay of forces in the unconscious, the defenses and compromise formations that are developed to subdue anxiety, the symbolic representations of conflict that express themselves in symptoms, the determining influence of early development on character structure, the understanding of dreams, and the operation of transference and resistance in expediting or retarding the therapeutic process.

One does not have to be a psychoanalyst to acknowledge the tremendous debt that humanity owes to Freud for introducing these and other fundamental concepts that have revolutionized our knowledge of how the mind operates in illness and health. Even though some of his enemies have succeeded in burning Freud at the stake, they have not been able to dispose of the ashes which continue to influence the mental health field in a determining way. I do not see how it is possible, without a reasonable psychoanalytic perspective, to divest psychotherapy of its present-day ambiguities; to make it less of an art dependent upon faith and the profits of placebo and more of a scientific discipline; to accomplish outcomes not only of symptom relief, problem solving, and behavioral betterment, but also of the permanent correction of deficits brought about by faulty rearing; and to achieve the objective of at least some reconstruction of the personality organization.

By the same token, if we are to go about with the planning of training programs in the future, we must also concern ourselves with other than intrapsychic processes. The problem with present-day models of psychotherapy is that they are too limited to deal with more than a few circumscribed areas of pathology. Human behavior is an integration of many complex systems. Attempts to explain any aspect of behavior in terms of one or another system and to search for common denominators among the different systems usually lead to a blind alley. Yet this is precisely what we try to do when we compare such therapies as psychopharmacology with existential therapy, or behavior therapy with psychoanalysis. We are reminded of the conundrum, what does the Titanic have in common with a martini? The answer, of course, is ice. But ice tells us nothing about the Titanic and little about a martini. To explore our martini a bit further, we can describe it in terms of its constituent physical ingredients—the gin or vodka, the vermouth, the olive or onion, the glass that holds it—or we can talk and become sentimental about the taste, or delineate the effect of the martini on

our behavior, or explore the motivations that inspire the drinker to inbibe it, or describe the physical, social, psychological, or moral consequences of its alcoholic content.

The models of explanation will have little in common with each other; however, we can "scientifically" try to torture them into some kind of conformity. The result will be as absurd as the effort of a boy who, asked to define a cow, replied,

A cow is a completely automatic milk manufacturing machine. It is encased in untanned leather and mounted on four vertical, movable supports, one on each corner.

The front end contains the cutting and grinding mechanism as well as the headlights, air inlet and exhaust, a bumper and foghorn.

At the rear is the dispensing apparatus and an automatic fly swatter.

The central portion houses a hydrochemical conversion plant. This consists of four fermentation and storage tanks connected in series by an intricate network of flexible plumbing. This section also contains the heating plant complete with automatic temperature controls, pumping station and main ventilating system. The waste disposal apparatus is located at the rear of this central section.

In brief, the externally visible features are: two lookers, two hookers, four stand-uppers, four hanger-downers, and a swishy-wishy.

There is also a similar machine known as a bull, which should not be confused with a cow. It produces no milk, but has other interesting uses. (Author unknown, *Delaware County Farm & Home News*)

The search for a single theory of emotional illness has inevitably led into similar jumbled language. Because in behavior we are dealing with multiple constituents, from biological to spiritual, we must utilize a variety of explanatory models, biochemical, physiological, learning, psychoanalytic, dynamic, role, sociological, philosophical and others, each of which contains clusters of theories.

Naturally, the question is whether such diverse theories can be mixed in the hope of achieving an effective integration. Some attempts have been made to do this. For example, we find this in the writings of a few theorists who, while oriented toward biological or relationship paradigms, adhere to the principles of classical metapsychology. The result is that they get into the same position as the boy describing the cow. An outburst of vertiginous linguistics indicates, one suspects, that the followers of these ideas are too embarrassed to admit that they do not understand what they mean.

The task for the future is to determine how the interfaces of the different models relate to each other. We still do not possess the template that will permit us to do this now. This does not mean that we cannot try to evolve one without getting bogged down in contradictions. As a result of experience in the past few decades, we have come to realize that no one model (medical, behavioral, sociological, ecological, etc.) suffices in understanding and treating all emotional problems. A direction is now being suggested by the increased use of multimodal therapy (Lazarus, 1976) and differential therapeutics (Frances, Clarkin & Perry, 1984). Differential therapeutics is metaphorically old wine in a new bottle.

For many years, clinicians have emphasized the need for a systems approach that recognizes that in any emotional or mental illness we are dealing with multiple variables requiring a broad eclectic orientation. One of the pioneers of this idea was Adolph Meyer of Johns Hopkins Medical School. Many therapists are only now coming around to accepting the wisdom of Meyer's thinking. Pathology never restricts itself to one region. Rather through the process of feedback, any emotional problem implicates all adaptational systems.

The symptomatic consequence of disruption of any one of these systems, as has been mentioned before, is that it tends to concentrate so much of the patient's attention and coping energies on alleviating distress that it interferes not only with analysis but also with any kind of psychotherapy. For instance, obsessive-compulsive syndromes are peculiarly resistive to analytic, cognitive and other therapies, and patients may be in treatment for many years without benefitting. However, dealing with the biological component of this disorder may prove rewarding. Recently we have chanced upon a medication (clomipramine) that has given us a new outlook on this obstinate disorder. In the past few months I have treated some obsessive cases that had been resistive to psychotherapy for 30 years or more. Within a few weeks, the drug had cut down on the symptoms so effectively that my patients were able to utilize dynamic insights for the first time. Interpersonal disorders often respond better to individual therapy when family or couples therapy are conjointly employed to resolve interfering tensions. There are many other examples of how the combined employment of therapies catalyzes treatment.

A systems approach recognizes that no unit of psychopathology exists in isolation, but rather it is part of an aggregate of interrelated units. These consist of interacting biochemical, neurophysiological, developmental-conditioning, intrapsychic, interpersonal, and spiritual-philosophic systems that determine how a person thinks, feels, and behaves. Obviously some of the systems are more intimately connected than others with the complaint factor from which an individual seeks relief. The most immediate help will be rendered by diagnosing and targeting initial treatment on the system area most importantly implicated. Dealing with the other systems may, of course, be necessary, coordinately or in timed sequence. A *behavioral chain* chart, as it is described in another work of mine (Wolberg, 1980), may serve as a convenient means of organizing the complex data that such a practice entails.

The different systems are so amalgamated that a feedback up and down the chain occurs when any one system is functionally disturbed. Actually what may most concern an individual is an end product of such a feedback. In therapy we would have to deal with both the consequences and the sources of this feedback. Thus a man who seeks relief for depression and anxiety may only indirectly refer to his marital discord. This, in turn, is inspired by unsatisfied dependency needs that promote hostility to his wife and stir up hopelessness and depression. If we merely focus on the symptoms that disrupt his well-being, namely, depression and anxiety, and treat only the involved biological system with an antidepressant anxiolytic like alprazolam (Xanax), we may expect a rapid diminution of symptoms. But the intrapsychic and interpersonal systems in turmoil will not be influenced greatly and will continue to give the patient trouble. It would be appropriate, then, to consider marital therapy and individual dynamic psychotherapy, in addition to psychopharmacologic treatment, even though through feedback the marital situation is temporarily benefited when the patient is quieted down by medication. It may be expedient when first utilizing multiple therapies to treat the system that the patient feels most motivated to change and that is most amenable to alteration. This may be a holding pattern while we work on educating and motivating the patient to accept more extensive help than he is willing to countenance at the beginning.

Multimodal therapy and differential therapeutics are predicated on the principle that combinations of therapies are better than the exclusive use of one modality alone. The evolution of psychotherapy is linked to empirical studies of how such combinations can best work. Psychopharmacological research has already yielded medications of value in depression, mania, psychoses, anxiety, panic, phobic disorders, obsessional neurosis, hyperactivity and bulimia. Dealing with the biochemical link in the adaptational chain has revolutionized the short-term management of these ailments.

Understandably, drugs have not brought about a millennium because difficulties related to other than biological areas cannot be eradicated by medications; and when these difficulties are troublesome, they will require other kinds of intervention suited to their nature. Thus, anxieties originating in past conditionings may be approached by behavior therapy. Intrapsychic problems brought about by unconscious conflicts and faulty psychological defenses will invite psychoanalysis or dynamic psychotherapy as a principal therapy. Interpersonal problems bring to mind group therapy, couples therapy, or family therapy as preferred interventions. Troubles rooted in environmental, social, and cultural factors are targets for counseling and milieu therapy. Distortions in adjustment encouraged by faulty self-statements, values, standards, and beliefs may be helped by reeducational promptings and, in their severe form, by cognitive therapy. Through differential therapeutics, we may zero in on the systems most directly affected by an illness; and this may be a boon, especially in short-term therapy. More often than not, several systems are simultaneously malfunctioning; and here, as I have mentioned before, combinations of therapies may be required to obtain the most rewarding results.

The accusation has been made that differential therapeutics tends to deal with superficial symptomatic and problem-solving issues and therefore may by-pass the deeper fundamental psychodynamic constituents of a problem. Experience does not substantiate this. No matter what techniques are being employed, the individual will react to these with his usual defensive ploys and evasions. Inherent dependencies, hostilities, oppositional behaviors, resistances, and transference reactions will precipitate out, manifested in the way the individual responds to the therapist and his techniques, either directly during the transference or symbolically in dreams or acting-out.

If a therapist is trained to recognize dynamic interactions he will be in a better position to deal with them, particularly when they arise as resistance to any technique that is currently being employed. In this way, any form of therapy may serve as an entry wedge into the patient's inner life; and if the patient's reactions are handled expertly by clarification and interpretation, and if the therapeutic relationship is a good one, the patient will benefit personality-wise as well as being relieved symptomatically. Thus, every therapeutic enterprise, even pharmacotherapy, may potentially become a psychoanalytically oriented venture geared toward some character change. I believe the future of psychotherapy is tied to this kind of orientation.

Because of highly specialized training, many of us are brought up to consider our own brand of therapy as paramount and the others as tangential and unimportant. Accordingly, our skills become too restricted and put us in a straightjacket when we are confronted with a pathology that calls for techniques outside of our specialty. Thus, if we are pure behavior therapists, we may not be able to deal effectively with a dangerous depression where the threat of suicide necessitates immediate pharmacological or electrical convulsive interventions. Alternately, if we are orthodox psychoanalysts, we will be stymied by an acting-out adolescent with whom family-oriented crisis therapy will be needed. Whenever therapists grounded in a monolithic approach recognize and accept their limitations, and are willing to refer problems outside of their domain to colleagues trained to manage the referral, their patients have a better chance of being helped. But due to overconfidence, the exigencies of economics, or simply narcissism, some therapists fail to listen to the voice of reason and try to squeeze all problems into their specialized approach, with none too outstanding results. As a consequence, the vast majority of patients do not receive the optimal kind of therapy.

Assuming that a therapist is sufficiently astute in diagnosis to recognize that an immediate problem is beyond his competence and that referral to a specialist is necessary, and assuming that he is willing to make such a referral, what happens if there is no such specialist within a reasonable range to whom he can send his patient? This is not an unusual situation, and apart from a few cities in this country, sophisticated resources are limited. It seems to me that in any planning for the future in psychotherapy the educational programs must take congnizance of this fact. Training in a broad range of techniques should be required; and ideally this training should include psychoanalysis, behavior therapy, cognitive therapy, hypnosis, strategic therapy, milieu therapy, group therapy, family therapy, couples therapy and pharmacotherapy. Training should embody when and how to implement these techniques and the effective integration of the techniques aimed at the most extensive objective of personality reconstruction, to the maximum benefit of the patient.

As stress mounts, due to economic dislocations and continued unrest the world over, national, community, family, and personal instabilities will create more candidates for psychotherapy. We will be forced more and more to open our minds to new modes of operation. This is particularly demanded of us as psychotherapists—whether we be classical analysts tracking the unconscious, seeking to wring the secrets of infantile neurosis out of our patients through pushing them into a transference neurosis; or neo-Freudians striving to provide a corrective emotional experience for our patients within the therapeutic interpersonal relationship; or behavior therapists attempting to correct behavioral deficits or to expand the constructive repertoire by manipulating the independent variables of which behavior is a function; or even drug therapists waging chemical warfare on the neuroses.

We must liberate ourselves from the frightening spectre of men so committed to our beliefs that we refuse to relinquish them even when circumstances prove that we are wrong. If we countenance the right of others to maintain heretical opinions and even to practice methods that we hold in disdain (always, of course, with the experimental attitude of distilling from these experiences hypotheses that might lend themselves to testing), we will no longer be prisoners of our own conceptual models. Tolerance for points of view other than our own is then the keynote—no matter what labels we pin on ourselves as therapists—to realizing that other therapists may not pursue the same paths that we do. By abandoning our parochial attitudes toward each other and toward our special techniques, we will help bring psychotherapy out of the deep pessimism that periodically envelops its evolution. We may even lift it out of its isolated orbit in the sky to fulfill its ultimate evolution by taking its rightful place in the solar system of the other sciences.

REFERENCES

Bion, W. (1959). *Experiences in groups.* London: Tavistock.

Bion, W. (1970). *Attention and interpretation.* London: Heinemann.

Fairbairn, W.R.D. (1954). *An object-relations theory of the personality.* New York: Basic Books.

Frances, A., Clarkin, J.F., & Perry, S. (1984). *Differential therapeutics in psychiatry.* New York: Brunner/Mazel.

Freud, A. (1937). *The ego and the mechanisms of defense.* London: Hogarth.

Fromm, E. (1941). *Escape from freedom.* New York: Holt, Rinehart & Winston.

Fromm, E. (1959). *Sigmund Freud's mission.* New York: Harper & Row.

Gedo, J. (1980). Reflection of some controversy in psychoanalysis. *Journal of the American Psychological Association, 28,* 363–383.

Guntrip, H.J. (1968). *Schizoid phenomenon, object relations and the self.* New York: International Universities Press.

Guntrip, H.J. (1971). *Psychoanalytic theory,* *therapy and the self.* New York: Basic Books.

Hartmann, H. (1958). *Ego psychology and the problem of adaptation.* New York: International Universities Press.

Horney, K. (1937). *The neurotic personality of our time.* New York: W.W. Norton.

Horney, K. (1939). *New ways in psychoanalysis.* New York: W.W. Norton.

Jacobson, E. (1964). *The self and the object world.* New York: International Universities Press.

Jacobson, E. (1971). *Depression: comparative studies of normal, neurotic and psychotic conditions.* New York: International Universities Press.

Kernberg, O. (1976). *Object relations: theory and clinical psychoanalysis.* New York: Jason Aronson.

Kernberg, O. (1980). *Internal world and external reality.* New York: Jason Aronson.

Klein, M. (1948). *Contributions to psychoanalysis, 1921–1948.* London: Hogarth.

Klein, M. (1957). *Directions in psychoanalysis.* New York: Basic Books.

Kohut, H. (1971). *The analysis of the self.* New York: International Universities Press.

Kohut, H. (1977). *The restoration of the self.* New York: International Universities Press.

Lazarus, A.A. (1976). *Multimodal behavior therapy.* New York: Springer.

Mahler, M.S. (1967). On human symbiosis and the vicissitudes of individuation. *Journal of the American Psychoanalytical Association, 15,* 740–763.

Mahler, M.S. (1975). *The selected papers of Margaret S. Mahler.* New York: Jason Aronson.

Reich, W. (1949). *Character and analysis* (3rd ed.). New York: Orgone Institute Press.

Sullivan, H.S. (1947). *Conceptions in modern psychiatry.* Washington, D.C.: William Alanson White Psychiatric Foundation.

Sullivan, H.S. (1953). *The interpersonal theory of psychiatry.* New York: W.W. Norton.

Winnicott, D. (1965). *The maturational process and the facilitating environment.* New York: International Universities Press.

Wolberg, L.R. (1980). *The handbook of short-term psychotherapy.* New York: Thieme-Stratton, Inc.

Discussion by Arnold A. Lazarus, Ph.D.

◆

One of the main reasons I entered into the field of psychotherapy is coming across a book Dr. Wolberg had written in the 50s called *The Techniques of Psychotherapy* (Orlando, FL: Grune & Stratton, 1977). At the time I was an undergraduate at the University in Johannesburg, thinking of going for an English major. I happened upon that book, which was a big, thick brown book, very impressive. I started to read with my eyeballs hanging out and said, "This is what I want to be doing." So I blame Larry for my being here today, not knowing as I was reading that some 30 years later I would be sitting in Phoenix, Arizona, discussing Dr. Wolberg's paper. What struck me all these years is the encyclopedic breadth of Dr. Wolberg. His book on *Medical Hypnoanalysis* underscored many points that people are only beginning to discover now. One of the things that strikes me in our field is how our colleagues are continuously reinventing the wheel. It is an amazing phenomenon.

Now what does one say when one is dealing with a man who writes so superbly? As I was reading his paper for this discussion, my first thought was, "I wish I could write like this." And I want to read just one paragraph to show you what I mean. Then I will have the audacity, as it were, to start doing battle. After all, if we don't do battle, what is the fun of this conference?

I loved this particular paragraph for many reasons. "Many professionals," says Dr. Wolberg, "are hostages to their early training rigidities." Now I am going to attack Larry for being somewhat of a hostage to his early training rigidities and he can defend himself, as I am sure he will. "Consequently," says he, "the field of mental health has been and is still bur-dened by enclaves of warring factions marching to the drums of their hardened theoretical imperatives." That's a beautiful turn of phrase. "A plethora of competing models exists, each claiming psychotherapy as its sovereign possession and purporting to explain in its own philosophic and linguistic terms, how people become neurotic and get cured." And that is, indeed, I think, one of the main impediments to growth in our field, that people do have a sort of a unimodal, bimodal frame and are not open to the many different influences. Throughout his paper, Dr. Wolberg was underscoring the range of models that has to be incorporated into any kind of comprehensive understanding of human functioning.

I don't know whether Dr. Wolberg makes the same distinction that I do about the incredible dangers of theoretical eclecticism as opposed to the merits of technical eclecticism. As you talk about combining psychoanalysis and behavior therapy (and there are many people who are into this kind of integration), if you take a good hard look at the fundamental models, at the epistemological foundations of the understanding of these different disciplines, you would see that they are totally incompatible in their final analysis. This is not to gainsay the use of techniques derived from either discipline. But to say, "Let's combine psychoanalysis and behavior therapy, let's take the best of both," is one of the dangers that can result only in simplistic models. This is not the place to really underscore the virtues of technical eclecticism. I did so in my workshop that some of you attended.

But here is what I want to take some issue with, when I said I think to some extent Dr. Wolberg is also a hostage to his early training rigidity. He is very eclectic and he was one of the first analysts back in my days when I was still an arch-behavioralist who said something to the effect that what was then called "symptom removal" was not inevitably going to result in relapse symptom substitution and horrendous breakdowns into psychosis, that in fact symptom removal realigned the psychic forces. This was a breath of tremendous fresh air at that particular juncture. He has continued to espouse a very eclectic view, but it might be theoretically eclectic, in which case we have to cross swords.

A statement that Dr. Wolberg made earlier reminded me of something that happened to me years ago when I made an archenemy, inadvertently, of a psychoanalyst who had referred a patient to me. The statement was, "In order to get the patient to a point where he can be susceptible to analysis, it may be necessary to employ some nonanalytic techniques." So you see, the concept is that the final and most refined procedure is still psychoanalysis and these other things get the person to the point where he or she can benefit from real therapy. That is what it sounds like.

So what happened in this case? The analyst referred to me this patient who was giving her an incredibly hard time because he had read stuff on rapid therapy and was very phobic, very hypersensitive, very anxious. The analyst said, "OK, I will refer you to Lazarus who can clear up this nonsense, thereby rendering you susceptible to the real working through of unconscious factors." So the patient was referred to me with the understanding that I would trim away these trivial symptoms and then return the patient for the real work. I got stuck in my multimodal mishmash and proceeded to do a number of things like assertiveness training and social skills training, getting into a number of dysfunctional beliefs, dealing with dyadic problems, bringing in the wife, and so on. After six or seven months this individual was functioning very nicely. That is to say, the anxieties, the phobias, the

sensitivities had been dispelled and this individual was now quite happy. Now came the ethical understanding that the patient must go back to the analyst. And the patient said, "For what?" And I said, "For analysis." "Why?" "Well, this is apparently what is needed." He didn't go back to the analyst and the analyst thinks that I poisoned his mind and unethically seduced him away. Therefore, they said that Lazarus was a bad psychotherapist.

I want to hear a little bit more, perhaps in Dr. Wolberg's rebuttal, about this business of getting the patient to the point where he is susceptible to analysis, when the nonanalytic method might suffice.

Now we turn to another aspect that I find most interesting. What has happened, and I think the differential therapeutics orientation is pointing in this direction, is that treatments of choice have become more and more viable in our field. That is, there are specific treatments of choice. If you take, for example, phobic individuals, what is the treatment of choice? Freud said it himself: "Exposure." Freud said that unless you expose the phobic patient to the phobic stimuli, you will hardly ever enable the person to give up the phobia. Freud's notion was that the exposure would produce rich associations which could be analyzed and dealt with. He didn't run the control, which would be just doing the exposure without free association or analysis. However, exposure is a sine qua non, and the therapist who thinks he or she can interpret away a phobia will generally not succeed.

Many textbooks will tell you that obsessive-compulsives are often intractible, very difficult patients, as indeed they are. But let us take a look at the outcome to see what works. If you are confronted by an obsessive-compulsive with encrusted rituals, malignant obsessions, let me tell you that tender loving care will not get you anywhere. As for desensitization, hypnosis, and meditation, forget it. These will not touch most of these obsessive-compulsives. But what will?

What will touch them is response prevention, participant modeling, and flooding. Now some people might not know what response prevention means. It was brought out some years ago by Mel Brooks in his comedy routine on the 2,000-year-old man. This man had a compulsion—he was always tearing paper. And he had gone to all kinds of therapists for help. He'd been analyzed, he'd been hypnotized, and nothing helped. Finally somebody said to him, "Don't tear paper." And he said, "Wow, nobody ever said that." That is response prevention.

Looking at an actual clinical situation, some years ago my colleagues and I were confronted with an individual who displayed many obsessive and compulsive elements, including weird rituals where he would make circles with his hands. He was apparently not psychotic, but he was doing some very bizarre things, including hand-washing compulsions and germ phobia, circles with his hands, and a semi-delusion that if anyone who was obese touched him, he might contract obesity. Therefore, he would avoid like the plague anyone who was overweight.

This poor chap had suffered incredibly, so we proceeded, first, to use response prevention to stop what he was doing. We had him under 24-hour surveillance. He was not to do the circles. We even put mittens on his hands. Second, in terms of the germ phobia and the flooding, we got him to handle all of the dirty laundry in the hospital and he was not allowed to wash his hands for a week. He had to eat his food everyday without even washing his hands once. I was terrified that, with my luck, he would come down with the flu or a cold, and that would be the end of the therapy. Luck does play a great part. However, he was fine and of course he was flooded with anxiety. As for the obesity, we got everybody who was fat to sit on him, to roll him, to touch him; this was the flooding technique. Some people said to me, I hope you get a good EKG before you start these things. But the point is that sometimes these heroic methods are essential or else you are not going to get anywhere with these kinds of encrusted problems.

However, if this is all you do, if breaking the web of obsessive-compulsive rituals is all you do, my prediction is that relapse will be pretty rapid. But having broken through with response prevention and participant modeling and flooding, in my approach you proceed to work on the other residual problems; sensation, imagery, cognition, and personal and biological malfunctions have to be looked at as well. That is the multimodal concept.

However, if you look at the outcome research, you would see that one of the main factors in this is performance-based methods, which are generally the most effective. The performance-based method will always win out over any sort of pure cognitive intervention. That is to say, if you can persuade somebody to do something different, to do it differently, then you can proceed to go places. Dr. Wolberg was one of the first analysts to say that there is a two-way street, that a change in behavior often produces an insight. It doesn't have to be the other way around, that the insight must always proceed the behavior change; it is a two-way street.

That concludes my discussion. I just want to say that I think that one of the fundamental points that Dr. Wolberg has represented that has influenced me throughout my career is the breadth of his flexibility. This is what I said struck me back in the 50s as an undergraduate when I first read *The Techniques of Psychotherapy*—that breadth of understanding rather than depth, in my vernacular, is the significant thing to look for across many modalities. In this sense, Dr. Wolberg has been one of my heroes, one of my stimulators, one of my influences, and is obviously my favorite analyst.

COMMENT BY DR. WOLBERG

I want to talk a bit about the comment that Dr. Lazarus made about symptom removal. Sometimes, symptom removal may be the most indicated kind of therapy. Certainly in short-term therapy it is the preferred goal. I remember the case of a three-year-old boy who was virtually starving himself to death. They took him to all sorts of clinics. They had given him everything and the little boy was just refusing to take food. When they forced it on him, he would vomit it up. They had him in a hospital, they tube-fed him for three weeks and he gained weight. When they came home, he lost it all. They were beside themselves. The doctor called me and said, "Would you consent to hypnotizing this boy to see if you could get him to eat?" So I said, "Well, that is a peculiar thing to do, but I will be very glad to talk to the family." On the appointed day the mother was in the waiting room and this little boy, virtually a skeleton, walked into my office. We talked for a while and then I utilized hypnosis. When the session was over, he walked out of the room, his mother grabbed him by his hand, and they just scurried out. I never saw them again. I was extremely busy so I never followed up on this. I figured nothing had happened.

They never came back, but about six years later I got a telephone call from the same doctor and he said, "Dr. Wolberg, you did so well with this boy that I am going to send you another patient. She is a girl from Switzerland who is plucking out her eyebrows and eyelashes." I said, "By the way, what case was it?" I had forgotten about the patient. He told me and I remembered. "Do you mind giving me the address if you have the most recent address? I would like to write to the mother and find out what happened." And he did and I wrote to the mother and said that I would very much like to know what happened after I had seen the boy. Well, I got a letter from the lady with a picture of a nine-year-old boy who was quite plump. In the letter she said, "Doctor, it was marvelous. The minute he came out of your room, he asked me for a potato. He never liked potatoes. And after that he started eating." She said, "I have a secret I have to tell you. While you were

in the office, I was getting very nervous so I walked over and put my ear against the door and I heard you say, 'You will want to eat. You will want to eat. You will want to eat.' And Doctor, I gained 15 pounds." Which proves either that suggestion is powerful even through a closed door or that there is something in symptom removal that can be extremely effective so that one may need no further therapy.

Unfortunately I think this is the rarity and that people, in addition to having their symptoms removed, do need some sort of direction, some sort of guidance, some sort of understanding that will enable them to adapt themselves to the stresses of life without collapsing into some form of symptom or problem.

QUESTIONS AND ANSWERS

Question: I would like to address a question to both Dr. Wolberg and Dr. Lazarus. It seems as if you talked about symptom removal as the end of the role of the therapist. I am curious as to what you see as the role of growth and fulfillment—the human potential concept—in either of your styles.

Wolberg: I thought I had emphasized that even symptom removal can eventuate in growth and better self-understanding, but that sometimes this does not occur spontaneously. It may be necessary to utilize other methods, other techniques different from those that remove symptoms, in order to bring a person to an awareness of some of his underlying problems and to aid him in terms of his own growth. Here is where a dynamic understanding can be so important. This doesn't mean that a person who uses psychoanalysis has to go through a rigid psychoanalytic training process. People who do not fundamentally have deep emotional problems themselves are able to relate productively, congenially and empathically to their patients and utilize themselves constructively with dynamic concepts. A moderate understanding of dreams, an understanding of transference, and mostly an understanding of one's own problems and of how these problems are elicited and can interfere with good therapeutic process can be quite fundamental. Obviously, a training analysis helps tremendously toward the subjective, but is not an absolute must.

Lazarus: In my approach, I never use the word "symptom," because symptom to me means symptomatic of something else. So I never remove symptoms. What I deal with are problems and problem removal is quite different from symptom removal. Sometimes the problem is the entire difficulty and nothing else has to be done. At other times, it is linked to other elements and so you get a whole hierarchy of removals. But growth clearly is something that comes when you do remove the problems that are impeding happiness. People are then able to capitalize on available stimuli that were previously inaccessible because they were blunted by pain. That is a quick thumbnail sketch of my ideas.

Question: Moving beyond the constraints of our profession, I would like you to comment, if possible, on what I would call a parallel force to our profession. That has to do with the instant change movement, whether we are talking about est or Hari Krishna or the tragedy in Jonestown. It seems to me that there is a borrowing of techniques utilized by people outside of the profession. I hope you will comment on our responsibility there, or give just some general impressions of that phenomenon.

Wolberg: There are no less than 250, even more, therapies that seem to be effective. Among these therapies are these movements like Krishna and the Rev. Sun Moon phenomenon. People are constantly reaching for some sort of relief of their problems. Most of the people who go in for these innovative therapies that involve a godlike figure whom they can worship are reaching for a dependence prop of some kind. They don't trust the usual authorities and they look for some sort of nebulous, magical figure who can lift them out of the morass and bring them to some sort of destiny.

Actually, many of them are projecting their own needs for grandiosity into building up a grandiose figure whom they can rely on. Many religions are dependent on this. In these movements you will find people, many of them very sick, who gain relief from these movements while they cannot seem to adapt themselves to other forms of therapy. What is peculiar about such people is difficult to say. Nevertheless, it seems to me that where a person is capable of finding relief through the interaction of some sort of a godlike figure, then there will be a continual reaching for new authority figures on whom one can rely. I would estimate that the relief that a person gets from this is merely contingent upon his ability to put the authority figure into the godlike role. When that role dissipates itself, the person will relapse into his usual illness and reach out for some other authority figure.

Question: I would like to ask Dr. Wolberg his opinion as to the advisability of psychotherapy being included as more of an educational function rather than as a medical function?

Wolberg: I think that is an excellent point. I have always felt that psychotherapy was an educational process rather than a medical process. Many therapists are wedded to the medical model. Certainly, with the upsurge of biological therapies, the medical model has gained a great deal of prominence. However, I think that psychotherapy is fundamentally an educational process.

Question: The message I am getting this morning is that eclecticism is part of the wave of the future and is necessary for the growth of the profession. This makes sense to me. I feel, and I think other people at the conference feel, that it is very difficult to maintain an open mind without getting befuddled. I am wondering if there could be some suggestions as to how to keep from getting confused by an array of possibilities?

Wolberg: I think that that too is a very important point. The conference on differential therapeutics that I have talked about previously is dedicated to exactly this point. How do you integrate all of these therapies, how do you combine them? When do you utilize them? What do they do to one's cherished approach? How does one combine his own approach to all of the tremendous numbers of modalities that are coming out? This is the future of psychotherapy. This is where we are at this particular point. We don't know too much about the interfaces of the various systems with each other but we do know that modalities, as they relate to each of these systems, have to be combined in a way that will be most productive to the patient. This is where future research lies, it seems to me.

Lazarus: There is a book coming out very soon edited by John Norcross and called, *Handbook of Eclectic Psychotherapy* (New York: Brunner/Mazel, 1986) which advocates a systematic prescriptive eclecticism. I would recommend that book very highly. Of course, I think that a lot of authors, myself included, have tried to make sense of that very important question.

Question: A question for Dr. Wolberg. The American Psychiatric Association is now in the process of wanting to publish, to the consternation of some, a handbook on therapies, on all therapies. I wonder what you think of such a development and, at the least, what kind of standards would you prescribe for such a handbook?

Wolberg: I think this is a very constructive thing to do. It does outline the essential points in each of the therapies.

However, it also can be very confusing. One has to be able to differentiate among the therapies and know when to apply them. All of us have our own prejudices about what works for us. We all have our styles of therapeutic operation and we all reach for those therapies that are most meaningful to us. Probably, they interrelate to our own personal problems.

I also believe that no matter what therapy a person is practicing and seems to be most comfortable with, whether it is behavior therapy or psychoanalysis or drug therapy, or whatever, this therapeutic process that he utilizes is an opening wedge into the inner problems of a person. The patient's self-system, personality drives, and defensive mechanisms can be revealed in the way he or she responds to a particular therapy. It makes no difference whether a person is exposed to behavior therapy, cognitive therapy or any other kind of therapy; he is going to respond with his transferences toward the therapist, with his attitudes toward what is being directed at him, and with his feelings about himself. Very often he will say, "Nothing will benefit me. I can't respond to this. Nothing is helping me." And one then has to deal with the patient's fundamental problems on a different level than the system that one initially utilized.

I am tempted to tell you the story about this man who was in therapy for a considerable period and told the therapist, "You know, you are not helping me. In fact, I am getting worse and I don't see any progress at all. It seems to be that I am never going to get well." And this went on in every session. He would barrage the therapist with complaints about how he was failing, how he wouldn't get well. The therapist would often respond by saying, "I wish I had six patients like you." Finally, the man said, "Doctor, I want to ask you a question. I know I have been giving you a hard time for a couple of years. How come you keep saying that you would like to have six patients like me?" He says, "Well, I have 12 patients like you. I wish I had six."

The Psychotherapeutic Process: Common Denominators in Diverse Approaches

◆

Judd Marmor, M.D.

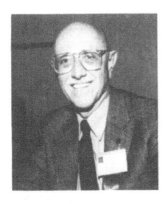

Judd Marmor, M.D.

Judd Marmor, adjunct Professor of Psychiatry at the University of California in Los Angeles, was Franz Alexander Professor of Psychiatry at the University of Southern California School of Medicine. He has practiced medicine for more than 50 years, having graduated from Columbia University College of Physicians and Surgeons in 1933. He is past president of the American Psychiatric Association, American Academy of Psychoanalysis, and The Group for the Advancement of Psychiatry. He is recipient of the Bowis Award for Outstanding Achievements in Leadership in the Field of Psychiatry from the American College of Psychiatrists and the Founders Award from the American Psychiatric Association. Dr. Marmor serves on the editorial board of 14 journals. He authored five books and co-authored one. He has written or co-written more than 300 scientific papers. Much of his writing has been on psychoanalysis and human sexuality.

Marmor outlines seven factors that are the therapeutic wellspring of all schools of psychotherapy. Personally, he advocates nondirective psychodynamic methods that foster patient autonomy. He explains the importance of taking a thorough history, indicating that the choice of therapy can be dictated by diagnostic discoveries. Therapeutic efforts should be based on promoting patient welfare rather than dogma.

My career in psychiatry began about 50 years ago, in the mid-1930s. In those days, the psychoanalytic institutes were the only places in which one could get training in how to do psychotherapy; there were no other schools of psychotherapy of any account. The mid-1930s was also a time of great ferment in the psychoanalytic movement. There were analysts of diverse persuasions, each advocating his or her particular school of thought as the only correct one. There were classical Freudians, Adlerians, and Jungians; there were adherents of the schools of Karen Horney, Eric Fromm and Harry Stack Sullivan, as well as followers of Abram Kardiner and Sandor Rado—each group with its own particular type of insight. Thus, even within the psychoanalytic movement itself, there was a great deal of diversity and conflict.

It was my good fortune at that time to

have friends who were members of all of these different groups, and I was interested to observe that they all seemed to be reporting equally good results. Their patients also seemed to be equally enthusiastic about their experiences with their diverse analysts. Another observation that intrigued me was that some patients did not do well regardless of which group they received therapy from, and the poor results seemed less dependent on the theoretical orientation of the therapist than on the experience and personal characteristics of the therapist. Those analysts who seemed to be most understanding, wise and empathic, regardless of the school to which they adhered, appeared to have the best results.

As a result, I began to ask myself how it was possible for psychoanalysts of differing theoretical orientations to achieve comparable therapeutic results. It seemed clear that inasmuch as interpretations within one theoretical framework were as effective as those within another, to account for the comparable results there had to be some therapeutic common denominators cutting across all the schools of psychotherapy.

Then, in the mid-1950s, an opportunity presented itself to explore this question in more depth. I became a participant in a collaborative three-year research study into the nature of the psychotherapeutic process, undertaken with the noted psychoanalyst Franz Alexander and a number of other colleagues. In the course of this study, the psychotherapeutic transactions between a number of experienced therapists and their patients were meticulously observed and recorded through one-way mirrors. One of the basic premises of this research was that because they were an intrinsic part of the process itself, no therapist, or patient, for that matter, could adequately describe what goes on in the psychotherapeutic process; only an outside observer could objectively perceive the totality of the transactional experience between the therapist and patient. Prior to that time, it had generally been

assumed that such external observation would drastically affect or modify the psychotherapeutic process, but we found (as is now widely recognized) that except for some initial self-consciousness on the part of both therapist and patient, the psychotherapeutic process went on as usual.

What did we discover? Perhaps the most important single awareness that emerged from this long and meticulous study was a recognition of the complexity and multiplicity of the interacting variables, both verbal and nonverbal, that enter into the psychotherapeutic process. Where once psychotherapy was thought of as something a therapist did to or for a patient, we now saw it as something that took place between them, with the therapist's "particular technique" being only one of many factors involved.

Let me try to give you some idea of what these factors are. Later in this chapter, I will also try to demonstrate how these factors play a role in other forms of psychotherapy.

The first and most important element in all psychotherapeutic transactions is the nature of the relationship between the patient and the therapist. Although this is a term that is frequently used, it is actually a very complicated matter. The patient enters into psychotherapy because of pain, suffering, maladjustment or confusion, seeking help from a therapist who is endowed, by virtue of his or her social role, with a help-giving potential. Thus, the patient brings with him not only varying degrees of motivation, but also some degree of expectancy and hope that the therapist will be able to help him. The real attributes that the patient brings to the therapy—his intelligence, his social and vocational competence, his articulateness, his value system, and his life situation—all play a part in the therapeutic transaction, along with the nature of the patient's disorder, the quality and quantity of his defenses, resistances, transference distortions, and the degree of secondary gain present.

Incidentally, some psychotherapeutic

schools tend to ridicule the concept of transference as though it was something invented by Freud that doesn't really exist. The fact is that transference was not invented by Freud; he simply gave it a name. All it means is that every individual, in an interpersonal transaction, brings to that transaction certain ways of looking at life and perceiving other people, that have been determined by his or her past life experiences. These past experiences often distort the way in which the individual perceives his current reality. Thus, based on his past experience, an individual may feel that all authority figures are rejecting, punitive, authoritarian, or condemnatory; and thus, he may react to current authorities with distorted perceptions and expectations. These unconscious distortions constitute the phenomenon of transference.

Most often, a therapist tends to be idealized because he is identified with the patient's wishes and hopes that the therapist will turn out to be a perfect parent, who can help him most effectively. Therapists also have their own backgrounds and experiences that may result in certain distortions, despite their own personal analyses. When these distortions are carried through into the therapeutic process and influence the ways in which therapists perceive their patients, or behave toward them, these distortions constitute what is meant by countertransference reactions.

Thus, the therapist also brings both conscious and unconscious attributes into the psychotherapeutic interaction. Therapists, we now know, are not interchangeable units, like razor blades. Their real attributes—their warmth, genuineness, empathy, knowledge, appearance, emotional maturity, personal style, and so forth—play a significant role in the patient-therapist interaction. Add to these the therapist's own emotional needs, ambitions and value systems, as well as any countertransference distortions that may be present, and you begin to get only a faint inkling of the complex variables that enter into the patient-therapist relationship. The way in which this patient-therapist matrix evolves and is shaped in any individual therapeutic encounter is the basic foundation on which the therapeutic process rests, and upon which a positive or negative therapeutic outcome depends.

Given this basic matrix, a number of other things also take place in the psychotherapeutic process. To begin with, the ability of the patient to confide and express feelings to a person whom he trusts and counts on as being supportive, understanding and ultimately helpful, is an important factor in reducing emotional tension. The greater the trust in the therapist, and the greater the hope and expectancy of receiving help, the greater the sense of relief.

The therapist, by virtue of his questions, confrontations and interpretations, by what he chooses to focus on or ignore, and by his verbal as well as nonverbal reactions, begins to convey to the patient a certain cognitive framework upon which their therapy is going to be based. There are some schools of therapy that deny that any cognitive teaching is involved. For example, the Gestalt school, or the behaviorists, place relatively little importance on cognitive teaching. Yet cognitive teaching, whether explicit or implicit, is an inevitable part of every psychotherapeutic process, because once a therapist tells a patient the rationale behind the process, he sets up a cognitive framework. In effect, psychodynamic therapists say to the patient, "You have developed these problems in the course of your personal development in relationship to significant people in your past. This has created certain distortions in the way you look at life and the way you perceive yourself. We are going to try to uncover those causes, and in the process of uncovering those causes, you will begin to feel better."

Gestalt therapists tell their patients that their problems are due to a failure to be sufficiently aware of their feelings, and that in the course of their work, they will learn to express their feelings better, and that this will make them feel better. This, too, is a cognitive framework. Behaviorists who tell their patients that they have acquired certain inappropriate habits as a result of faulty conditioning are also setting up a cognitive framework upon which their psychotherapeutic approach depends.

In all therapies, a certain amount of cognitive learning exists that gives the patient an intelligible, meaningful and rational framework for understanding why and how his problem has developed. Incidentally, in the course of their confrontations and interpretations, all therapists also convey both their therapeutic objectives and their value systems to the patient. Analysts sometimes assume that a meticulously neutral stance avoids such communication of values, but this is a myth. All therapists, wittingly or unwittingly, inevitably purvey their values to their patients, by what they choose to comment on or not comment on, and by what they react to as healthy or neurotic.

Actually, the therapeutic objectives of most psychotherapists in our culture are essentially similar and reflect our culture's normative ideals. All basically aim at enabling their patients to have meaningful and satisfying social and sexual relationships, to work and love effectively, and to become productive and responsible human beings.

In the course of pursuing these objectives, a certain amount of operant conditioning takes place. This occurs through the kinds of responses that the therapist makes to the patient's verbal or behavioral expressions. Certain behaviors are approved, others are disapproved. This is not always explicit. The approval may be in the shrug of a shoulder or an expression of the eyes. It may be in the interpretation of what is considered healthy or unhealthy behavior. Even behind the couch, the analyst's "aha's" and how he gives them are responses that patients are sensitive to. A number of research studies demonstrated experimentally that these minimal signals of interest or disinterest, approval or disapproval, not only influence the content of the patient's communication, but also act as a subtle operant conditioning system reinforcing approved thought and behavior and discouraging that which is disapproved.

Another kind of operant conditioning that takes place is what Franz Alexander called *the corrective emotional experience*. By virtue of the fact that the therapist responds differently, more objectively, more empathically or more realistically to the patient's emotional or behavioral expressions, the patient receives a different kind of emotional experience than he or she may have received from the significant authorities in his or her past life. These corrective emotional experiences occurring within the matrix of the patient-therapist relationship are important elements in the therapeutic process.

Still another factor that we observed in the therapeutic process was the degree to which patients, consciously or unconsciously, tended to model themselves after the therapist, gradually incorporating some of the explicit or implicit values that they were being exposed to. This kind of modelling is called *identification* by analytic psychotherapists, while learning therapists call it *social learning*. There is no doubt that it is one of the most important ways in which human beings learn from one another.

Another factor that occurs in all therapies (even though there are schools that would tend to deny it) is suggestion and persuasion. Whenever a therapist presents his rationale for his therapy, and implies or explicitly states that the patient will feel better as a result of following that therapeutic model—whether it be psychodynamic, Gestalt, or behavioral—that therapist is using suggestion. The patient's expectancy of being helped, the implicit assumption that this help will be forthcoming if he complies with the therapeutic program, and every indication received in therapy that certain patterns of behavior are more desirable or "healthy" than others, all involve implicit, if not explicit, elements of suggestion and persuasion. The greater the faith of the patient in the therapist, the greater the degree of idealization or positive transference, the greater is the impact of these suggestions on the patient.

Finally, for therapeutic change to become really consolidated, for things to be learned (note that what I am saying is that psychotherapy is essentially a learning procedure), a certain amount of rehearsal and repetition has to take place. This rehearsal can be explicit, as in certain behavioral therapies; it can be implicit, as it occurs in the so-called working-through process of dynamic psychotherapy; or, it can be deliberate, as in the giving of homework assignments. But regardless of how it is done, the things that are learned in the psychotherapeutic process have to be generalized, and the patient must be able to express these new adaptive techniques of behavior in other aspects of his life— to his boss, to his friends, or to the spouse or children.

I have likened this learning procedure to the way people learn to play golf or tennis. Cognitive insight alone is not enough to change an individual. Mere understanding alone doesn't do it. In golf or tennis lessons, the pro explains what is wrong with the stroke. You don't immediately become an expert golfer or tennis player. (Incidentally, different golfing instructors and different tennis instructors belong to different "schools" so that diverse approaches to teaching do not occur only in psychotherapy!)

The point is that when you receive a cognitive insight, you still have to learn to apply that insight by practice, and that requires work. This takes place under the benign and empathic influence of the pro, who says to you, "There you go again. You did it again. You lifted your head. You forgot to look at the ball," or whatever it is that you are doing maladaptively. After a while, you learn to introject that understanding and are able to say for yourself, "There, I did it again." Fur-

ther along the way, you begin to recognize the tendency even before you do it, and you are able to correct it. Once a new pattern of behavior has been thoroughly introjected and assimilated, you are on the road to doing things in a way that you could not do before. Just as in psychotherapy, the best golf or tennis pros are those who are noncritical and who can be supportive and empathic in the process of helping you overcome maladaptive tendencies. If the relationship to the teaching pro is a negative one, a critical one or a nonempathic one, the learning process will be impeded.

In psychotherapy there is also a difference in the directive or nondirective approach. It is possible to help patients both ways, but the ultimate goals and results may be quite different. By directing the patient as to what to do, the directive therapist tends to perpetuate the dependency and infantilism of the patient, even though the patient may feel better by following directions. The nondirective therapist aims at facilitating the autonomy of the patient, to enable him to learn to think for himself, and ultimately to function in a more mature and self-directed way.

In summary then, I have said that there are at least seven different major factors that take place in the psychotherapeutic process. The most basic of these is the patient-therapist relationship. Other factors are the release of emotional tension in the context of expectancy and hope, the acquisition of cognitive insight, operant conditioning (including corrective emotional experiences), identification with the therapist, suggestion and persuasion, and finally, rehearsal and working-through of the new adaptive patterns of behavior and thought.

After learning about these factors in the course of my research studies, I became interested in whether or not these factors were equally present in other therapeutic approaches. I spent a number of years during the 1960s and early 1970s studying the ways in which therapists from other schools operated, either through personal observation or videotapes. It is characteristic of psychotherapeutic schools to try to explain the success of their approaches by a single and unique principle that differentiates their technique from all others and, presumably, makes it superior. Analytically oriented psychiatrists attribute their success to their particular cognitive insights and transference interpretations; Rogerians believe that their technique uniquely releases the patient's own self-actualizing mechanisms; behavior therapists are convinced that the specific conditioning technique that they employ is the essential factor in their achieved therapeutic results; Gestalt therapists place their emphasis on the release of repressed emotions; transactional analysts, on bringing into awareness the game patterns employed by patients in their interpersonal relationships, and so on.

As a result of my subsequent studies, I became firmly convinced that in no instance are the therapeutic results of any of these schools attributable to any such presumptive unitary factor. I believe that the substantial weight of evidence is that the same factors I outlined as common denominators in dynamic psychotherapy are also operative in these other approaches, although different therapies differ in the emphasis they put on one or another of these factors.

Let us review how this works in several of the different approaches. The Rogerian client-centered approach places its emphasis on creating a good client-counselor relationship and assumes that no interpretive interventions are involved. Instead of making interpretations, the counselor simply and empathically reflects back to the patient his own statements from time to time. Within the context of this benign relationship, it is assumed that the patient begins to reconstitute himself by virtue of his own innate self-actualizing tendencies. However, in observing Rogerian therapy, it can be noted that the Rogerian therapist encourages and reinforces certain patterns of communication and behavior in preference to others, by means of the tone of his voice, the expressions on his face, the material that he chooses to reflect back in contrast to that on which he makes no comment at all. He thus implicitly communicates to the patient his values and therapeutic objectives. He inevitably becomes a model for identification, and implicit suggestion and persuasion are inevitably involved. Cognitive insight is deemphasized, and whatever cognitive learning takes place is more apt to result from implicit rather than explicit communication. Thus, most, if not all, of the psychotherapeutic variables that I listed for dynamic psychotherapy also are present, albeit in modified form, in Rogerian therapy.

I then went on to study the different kinds of behavior therapy. Dr. Wolpe's technique of *reciprocal inhibition* is an excellent paradigm of this approach. If you observe the way he works, it is quite clear that a great deal more is going on in his therapeutic process than simply his technique of reciprocal inhibition. His relationship with the patient is warm and empathic; he takes a careful history; he makes interpretations; he communicates values; he uses suggestion and persuasion by telling the patient that if he goes through his series of hierarchical relaxations, he will begin to feel better. This is not only suggestion; it is also a cognitive interpretation, because it says in effect, "This is how your problem started—as a result of faulty conditioning and faulty habit formation. And in the process of deconditioning these habits by our technique, you will begin to feel better." So that here, too, the quality of the relationship, the cognitive learning, corrective emotional experiences, the empathic nature of the therapist-patient relationship, the modeling, the rehearsal—all of these are present.

The Gestalt approach places great emphasis on emotional release and purports to downgrade cognitive awareness. The emphasis is on uncompromising emotional honesty and expressiveness, an important emphasis that also is shared by most of the psychodynamic schools. But there is a cognitive element, because the patient is taught, either explicitly or implicitly, that his illness is the result of a failure to properly recognize and express his true feelings, and that the path to cure lies in being able to do so. Obviously there is also a strong element of suggestion in stating this rationale. Here, too, we see the same basic variables in operation, albeit in a different mix. The basic factors in the patient-therapist relationship are all present and demonstrable in Gestalt therapy—the initial discharge of emotional tension in a setting of hope and expectancy; the powerful operation of suggestion by the assurance that if the therapist's program is followed, improvement will ensue; operant reconditioning by covert or overt indications of approval or disapproval from the therapist; the therapist's implicitly or explicitly offering himself as an identification model; and explicit techniques of rehearsal.

Incidentally, Gestalt therapies, as you know, often are held in group settings, where the impact of suggestion and persuasion is powerfully enhanced by the group process. Group therapies fall into just as many different kinds of "schools" as individual therapies. In groups, too, the particular ideology that is employed lends support to the relationship and the process. Groups do offer a wider variety of transference possibilities than occur in one-to-one therapies and also offer the potential for multiple corrective experiences. In addition, new adaptive techniques often are openly rehearsed in the group situation, generally more than in individual one-to-one therapy.

The fact is that psychotherapy can take numerous forms. There are at least 300 different forms of therapy taking place in America today. In the past quarter century we have seen an explosion of new therapies. Cognitive, abreactive, behavioral, individual, conjoint, family and group therapies, as well as any combination of these. There are poetry therapies, bibliotherapies, art therapies, and many oth-

ers. However, I have yet to encounter any psychotherapeutic approach in which the basic elements of a trusting and empathic patient-therapist relationship, suggestion, persuasion, identification, emotional support, cognitive learning, emotional release and reality testing were not major factors in the therapeutic process and in the progress made by the patient.

Despite all we have learned, there is no room for complacency in the field of psychotherapy. There are numerous unsolved research questions, and you must be cautious when someone tells you all of the answers are in. One of the important challenges we are faced with is to decide with some degree of assurance which specific form of psychotherapy is best suited for any particular patient. Although it is probably true that there are some patients who could be helped equally by a variety of approaches, it is also true that some forms of psychotherapy are probably more suitable than others for some patients and some conditions. Just as there is no single best way of teaching all subjects to all people, there is almost certainly no single best way of treating all patients and all conditions.

Let me now introduce my own bias. The best way that I know of to introduce some degree of rationality into what otherwise might become a blind or haphazard choice is a sound knowledge of psychodynamic principles. By that I don't mean just an analysis of intrapsychic factors; I mean an awareness of all of the variables that are playing a part in contributing to the patient's psychopathology, including biological factors, intrapsychic factors, interpersonal processes, and socio-economic conditions. In order to have that kind of understanding, a therapist needs to take a sound history. We have to know not only what is going on in the present, but also what the background of the individual is.

A careful history serves at least four vitally important purposes in the initial evaluation of any psychotherapeutic problem. First, it sheds light on the onset of the disorder. Was the onset acute, or insidious? Were the precipitating factors massive or minimal? Crucial or trivial? Were they mainly intrapsychic, interpersonal, or environmental? Second, a developmental history provides an idea of what kind of strengths the patient brings to the therapeutic process. This can be determined by evaluating the intelligence of the patient, his educational background, how he has dealt with the demands of sexuality, marriage, or interpersonal relationships, social and vocational adjustments. Third, a careful history facilitates an assessment of the relative balance between the stresses in the patient's life and the capacity of the patient to deal with those stresses. This helps determine the placement of major therapeutic emphasis. Fourth, a good history tells which environmental supports can be counted on in the efforts to help the patient, because those supports do make a difference. Does the patient have financial resources? Does he have vocational skills? The best of therapies can run aground if a patient is surrounded with inordinate adversity.

In short, the process of taking a careful history and of doing a careful evaluation at the onset of therapy helps therapists make certain fundamental decisions concerning the type of treatment technique that is best indicated for a particular patient. If the history reveals an acute disorder of recent onset, with a significant degree of triggering stress in a patient with previously good coping capacities, it is reasonably certain that the patient's difficulties will respond to any one of, or a combination of, a variety of relatively benign tools of interventions, such as modification or removal of the stress factor (perhaps by simple environmental manipulation), by short term psychotherapy, by hypnotherapy, or by various behavioral techniques aimed at the alleviation of the acute anxiety or other symptoms.

On the other hand, if initial evaluation points to a long history of deficient coping techniques with a gradually progressive development of disturbed interpersonal relationships, impaired self-esteem and self-image, and all kinds of associated symptomatic disturbances, then therapeutic emphasis has to be an effort to help the patient achieve some basic personality changes and learn to cope more effectively with life. For such a patient, a more cognitive type of approach that will go on for a somewhat longer period of time is needed. The patient may also have deficiencies in social learning; some people just don't do well because they haven't learned social skills. Not everything that disturbs people is based on intrapsychic conflict.

Again, if the history shows that the major stress factor is in a certain kind of intrafamilial situation, such as a marital problem, conjoint marital therapy may be the best approach to this problem. Or, if one is dealing with an adolescent whose family dynamics are chaotic, a family approach may work the best. I have long believed that, in general, with childhood disturbances, family therapy is the best way to work rather than individual therapy with a child, although there may well be circumstances in which both may be indicated simultaneously.

By the same token, a psychodynamic understanding of the inner structure of the patient's personality adds further refinement to the therapist's ability to plan treatment intelligently and meaningfully. For example, does the patient suffer from a basic inability to trust others? Does he have poor impulse control, or what analysts call a poor *superego*? Or is he a victim of an overstrict and tyrannical superego that is constantly punishing him for things that other people take for granted? Is he immature, passive dependent, suffering from low self-esteem? Or is he rigid, overcontrolled, compulsive, and defensively distant? The better we understand these specific personality dynamics, the more effectively and meaningfully we are able to target our therapeutic efforts. *It is precisely this ability to evaluate both the inner and outer dynamics of a patient's personality and life situation that distinguishes the focused efforts of a trained psychotherapist from the simple empathy of well-meaning friends, or the blind gimmickry of unqualified and unprincipled purveyors of psychotherapeutic services.*

In closing, I hope I have succeeded in providing some understanding of the nature of the psychotherapeutic process, and of the common denominators that underlie the wide profusion of therapeutic approaches that have blossomed in the past few decades. I would hope that some day we may see an end to the passionate and partisan proclamations of the superiority of one particular technique over others, and that we can devote ourselves to the fundamental and basically more promising task of developing a unified science of psychotherapy that will enable us to fit the patient, the therapist and the technique together in a way that will most effectively, economically and humanely achieve the desired objective of mental health.

Finally, to highlight an attitude that I would like to promote with regard to the various schools of psychotherapy, I would like to share one of my favorite James Thurber fables. Thurber tells about the barnyard rooster who found a gilded goose egg, and who insisted, in spite of the skepticism of the hens, that it would eventually hatch into a golden goose of priceless value. So the rooster stubbornly sat on it, until one day the egg broke, and that was the end of his dream. Thurber's moral, which is as applicable to the field of psychotherapy as it is to all of science, is that it is wiser to be hendubious than cocksure!

Discussion by Aaron T. Beck, M.D.

◆

I enjoyed reading Dr. Marmor's paper and thought I would do a kind of secondary elaboration and repetition in working through so that his message would really get across. Then I had some additional ideas.

I, personally, have been greatly influenced by Franz Alexander and also by T. M. French, who I think is one of the great psychiatrists. Alexander himself, I would say, was the first cognitive therapist. Although he didn't use that word, he wrote a fine paper called *Psychotherapy as a Learning Process.* (Alexander, F. (1964) Dynamics of psychotherapy in the light of learning theory. *Bulletin of Phil. Asso. of Psychoanalysis,* 14.) Learning, of course, is a cognitive process.

French was extremely influential in his work on cognitive patterns, both in dreams and ideational material. He influenced me at an early stage in my career to do dream studies which were designed to test various psychoanalytic hypotheses regarding the nature of depression. Eventually, I ended up with a more cognitive and less motivational model than I had started out with. I did want to take this opportunity to show my high regard for the Chicago school in general and in terms of my own development.

I thought I might give you just a little more historical data so you can get some kind of backdrop by which you might evaluate what I have to say. I was trained in Philadelphia, but my two most influential teachers were trained in Chicago and so I got a strong feeling for the corrective emotional experience that Alexander exposed so well. I also gained a healthy respect for transference reactions. One conclusion that I reached, and this was where I'd say I evolved rather than diverged from psychoanalysis, was that transferences were extremely important for many reasons, but psychoanalysis was a relatively ineffective way of utilizing transference. I'll show you exactly what I mean by this apparently paradoxical statement.

I had been doing formal analysis for a long time. The patients were following the fundamental rule of bringing up associations and the analyses were taking quite a long time according to the standards of that day. One day I was analyzing a patient who was depressed. He had spent the entire hour attacking me and at the end of the session I said, "Well, Mac, you must feel much better now," thinking that depression is a form of repressed hostility. Since he was getting the hostility out, he should really feel good. He said, "No, I don't feel good at all. I feel much worse." I said, "Well, that's really odd. Do you have any idea why you feel worse?" And then he said, "Well, the whole time I was tearing you apart, I kept thinking, 'Oh I'm so awful. I'm such a bad person to be attacking poor Dr. Beck this way. I'm such a terrible person, I'm evil, I'm nasty, I'm mean . . .' " And he kept on like that. I said, "This is strange. You've been in analysis for a year and you've never told me this before and I've asked you many times what you felt about me and you've only come out with hostile statements?" He said, "You know that's strange. I've never thought to tell you that." And I said, "Well what are these thoughts that you get?" He said, "They just pop into my mind and pop out, they pop in, they pop out, and unless I particularly pay attention to them, I just forget about them. I don't think to report it."

So this gave me an idea and the next session was with a woman who in those days was diagnosed as hysterical, which I think is not a good diagnosis. She was very dramatic in all her presentations and spent the entire session regaling me with stories of her various sexual escapades. At the end of this session, I asked her how she felt and she said, "I feel terribly anxious." And I thought that I was being very accepting and so on, so I said, "Why are you feeling anxious? Here I've been accepting everything you've said. I haven't been critical, you know. I'm not critical of that." She said, "I don't know, maybe I still think you're going to disapprove of my sexual escapades. You're my superego figure. My parents would have disapproved, and I'm just afraid of disapproval." So I said, "Are you really afraid of my disapproval?" She said, "Yes." So I said, "Tell me, did you have any other thoughts that were going through your mind while you were telling me all this?" And she said, "Yeah, I was afraid that I was boring you." And I said, "Boring me?" And she said, "Yes, I'm always afraid that I'm going to bore you." And I said, "Oh, so what does that have to do with telling me about your sexual experiences?" She said, "Well I'm trying to entertain you so you won't be bored." I said, "Is this the kind of thing that happens in your life elsewhere? Do you find that you have to entertain people?" She said, "Oh yes, I think I'm a very boring person and I think that people are going to reject me unless I dominate the conversation." It turned out that what was happening in the therapeutic session, of course, was pointed out by Dr. Marmor. It was a biopsy of her life in general and of her fears of being judged by other people as socially undesirable. So she would compensate with this type of dramatic behavior.

From that time on, whenever patients had any unpleasant feeling, I would ask them what thoughts they had just before that feeling. I found that these types of thoughts, these pinpoint probes, produced material that was quite different from what I was getting in the ordinary psychoanalytic session. I did this with all patients. Even though those patients had been in therapy for many months and, according to my supervisors, I was conducting psychoanalysis in the appropriate way, I was now getting at material which was not unconscious but what would have been called preconscious. It was quite accessible if one focused on it.

As a result, I changed my whole therapeutic approach. It is interesting that several years later Albert Ellis and I found out that we had quite independently gone through a similar experience of finding that there was a stratum of thinking that the person was experiencing but was not being made accessible. I changed my tactics and started getting people to report the thoughts they had prior to particular feelings. I found out that when they would report a sad or depressed feeling, they were often down on themselves or they would see the future negatively or they would be interpreting their experiences in a highly negative way. And if they were anxious, they were anticipating something bad happening to them. If they had an angry feeling, it was usually preceded by some thought of abuse transgression. If they had a manic feeling, it was preceded by thoughts of expansiveness, and so on.

I'd like to illustrate how I was able to use that. I started my transference analyses before the patient even entered the room. The patient has already developed a transference so I'm prepared to ask certain probing questions. Let's say the patient looks apprehensive or sad. I say, "What were you thinking when you were sitting in the waiting room?" And they will almost always come out with a statement like, "Well, I thought that you would reject me. You wouldn't want to take me on as a patient." I say, "Why was that?" The patient would say, "Well, you kept me waiting for five minutes so it seemed to me that you probably didn't want to see me." Or, "I noticed that you took me early so you must think that I'm very sick and won't take me on for that reason." Or, "You took me right on time. You operate this thing like a factory. Everything is clockwork and you really don't care about the patients." So that's one aspect of how I do it.

The second way in which I used these probes is by looking at the patient's affect. For example, a patient was giving me some interesting material and I made what I thought was an accurate interpretation regarding some of the feelings she was having. I saw a cloud go over her face and she said, "You know you're right." But I saw this cloud anyhow and I asked, "What was going through your mind just them?" And she said, "Oh, I had the thought I must be pretty stupid not to have thought of that myself."

By pinpointing your question right on the spot, you can rapidly get at material that is very relevant. It turned out that a major issue in her life was that she believed she was stupid. So I didn't have to wait for everything to unravel because we were able to get that material. Then I could ask, "Do you ever get these thoughts outside the session? Keep track of them by writing them down. There are lots of ways to document that type of thing." So that's the second point I want to make about transference. I certainly believe one should be aware of it as much as possible. It plays an important role in understanding the patient.

There is another thing we should keep in mind about transference reactions. It is also illustrated by the woman described above. If you're not aware of the way the patient reacts toward you, the whole therapy can become counterproductive. If I had kept on with my brilliant interpretations, correct though they might have been, I'm sure it would have made her feel much worse. So one does have to be quite alert to these possibilities. Even if you're doing an active type of therapy, you can still be quite aware of the transaction between you and the patient.

Now there's a book that was written on the commonalities among the various psychotherapies, *The Self: Cognitive Psychotherapy and the Misconception of Hypothesis* (2 vols.) by Victor Raimy (San Francisco: Jossey-Bass, 1975). He analyzed every therapy, as Dr. Marmor did, and demonstrated that every one, particularly Rogerian therapy which he was skilled at, had an underlying cognitive understructure. Even operant conditioning contains cognitive components. When the therapist approves of what you say, that has a particular meaning. Now the meaning is not always a good one. The meaning to the patient may be that the therapist is approving of this just because I'm saying what he wants. He's trying to enforce compliance. It may be coming up with a negative meaning but it's going to have a meaning and it is going to be the meaning that will be determinant of the patient's feelings and future behavior. So we always have to look at meanings and I'm sure that Dr. Marmor was getting that across to you when he was talking about learning. Meanings are critical in everything the therapist does.

The next phase of my discussion covers what I consider three major points. One is the "Corrective Emotional Experience." The second I label, "Input, Output, and the Black Box." The third is "The Final Solution." By that I mean, how are we going to solve the problem of why so many therapies work when they do work and what could be the explanation of why they work when they do work? This will be an extension of what Dr. Marmor said.

When we talk about the Corrective Emotional Experience, we want to ask a question, "What are we correcting?" I think that's a really crucial point. The emotional experience is also important and we want to be able to define what we mean by it. What I think is corrected is some type of cognitive constellation which involves all kinds of distortions. This does come up in the transference during psychoanalysis, but I believe we can get to it more rapidly through the probes I mentioned earlier.

Now what do I mean by Input, Output? The only thing we really know in transactions with patients is what is being put in and what is coming out. We can videotape interviews, we can have observations, as Dr. Marmor had in his experimental work. But they can only observe the therapist's behavior and the patient's behavior. From that they can draw certain

conclusions about the relationship between the input and the output. Among the important things in the input are so-called nonspecific factors, the Rogerian triad of empathy and wants. These are not easily measurable, but they are observable.

Another aspect of the input that I consider extremely important is the technical one. I think techniques are very important. Within the context of a good relationship, success or failure of the therapy will depend on therapeutic techniques. Dr. Lazarus made a good point about this when he mentioned that communication is the soil, but it is the technique that will cause the growth of the change. Technically, if you get a really bad obsessive-compulsive who is spending his entire day ruminating or washing his hands, if you don't apply the right technique, the most wonderful therapeutic relationship in the world is not going to get you anywhere. Thus, within the relationship, the technical interventions are crucial. As Dr. Marmor mentioned, the problem is to utilize the appropriate interventions for the appropriate individual or the appropriate problem.

Another important aspect of the therapist's input is the way he structures the therapy. To some degree, I think there is an optimum structure for a therapy which may vary from one person to another. For example, an autonomous person may do better with somewhat less structure. If he's a self-starter, it may be sufficient to just get him started and point the way; he will probably go in the appropriate directions. A dependent person may need to be structured much more. The dependent person will spend the entire session, or the entire therapy, trying to fulfill the dependency needs instead of trying to utilize the insights or integrate whatever other types of therapeutic intervention are being employed. So structure is important.

As Dr. Marmor mentioned, the rationale that is given the patient is also very important, even if the rationale is incorrect. (I hate to say that, because I don't like incorrect rationales.) A rationale that will enable the patient to integrate the information in the directions he is getting can act as kind of a road map or template. Simply by reorganizing the patient's experience in a somewhat different way, it can make the patient much more susceptible to the therapeutic interventions and help him to conquer the problem. For example, the old rationale of behavior therapy—the idea that a person with anxiety had an unsatisfactory pairing of conditioned reflex and unconditioned reflex, that this could be undone by relaxation techniques that would break the bond between the conditioned and the unconditioned stimuli, and that the patient would then get better out of this relaxation intervention—made sense to patients. Thus, they could respond nicely to a relaxation technique. I personally don't think that's what happens in the systematic desensitization, but it's something the patient can buy into so as to benefit much more.

The type of rationale offered and the type of promises the therapist makes are very important. Some therapists, for example, use carbon dioxide (CO_2) as a way of inducing relaxation in patients. (Wolpe, J. [1973]. The use of drugs in behavior therapy. In *The practice of behavior therapy* [pp. 180–191]. New York: Pergamon Press.) That always surprised me because CO_2 physiologically causes arousal and it was surprising to me that it could produce relaxation. Then I read a study in Holland in which one group of patients was given a mixture of 40 percent carbon dioxide and 60 percent oxygen and was told that this would make them less anxious. Indeed, they became less anxious in all physiological recordings. Another group was told that this might get them aroused in some way and each patient showed an increase in physiological arousal. So, taking off from what Dr. Marmor said, there is an effect caused by the patient's expectancy; what you tell the patient regarding what your intervention is going to do, is going to have an effect on what actually does happen.

So that's the Input. The Output simply refers to the observable behaviors—how the patient looks to you and also the patient's verbal reports, if you can rely on them. I'm a believer that the consumer is always right. If the patient says he feels worse, believe him. If he thinks that he feels better and shows all the signs that his depression, for example, or anxiety is lifted, then I would think that would qualify as an output measure.

The big question now is what goes on inside the head, the mind, the brain, the Black Box. To really answer that question, we ought to see what commonalities among all the therapies seem to work. By looking at the commonalities, we may be able to elicit some general principles which will explain why people do get better. This is something Dr. Marmor covered in his talk.

Probably the most crucial factor in terms of what goes on internally is the affect arousal. If change is going to take place, it has to take place when the person is in some type of heightened state. In fact, Jerome Frank once did an experiment in which he gave patients insight interventions when they received a placebo injection of adrenalin. (Frank, J.D. (1961). Experimental studies in persuasion. In *Persuasion and healing: A comparative study of psychotherapy* (pp. 106–135). Baltimore: Johns Hopkins University Press.) After the adrenalin injection, when they were in a state of arousal, they were far more susceptible to the interventions. We'll come to the question of accessibility in a minute, but let us look at some of the things we can observe as clinicians that seem to differ among the various schools.

First, the abreaction in catharsis was observed by Freud to be very powerful (I believe it was the case of Anna O). In the course of therapy, this young woman with hysterical paralysis uncovered memories of a previous experience when she was nursing her father and apparently had sexual wishes toward him. She eventually developed a whole variety of symptoms which seemed to be related to this particular nursing experience. When this memory was uncovered and she had the catharsis—not just the sterile recovery of the memory, but the emotional output—then some change started to take place. It was obvious in her case that change was taking place because she lost her hysterical symptoms.

In behavior therapy, the most powerful weapons are exposure, flooding, response prevention, and so on. These all involve a much heightened state of reactivity. Systematic desensitization, which consists of taking the person up a hierarchy, also involves affective reaction. One doesn't go up to the next step in the hierarchy until one has a particular affective response which gets extinguished over time. Then you go up the next step in the hierarchy. So even systematic desensitization, which would seem to be at the other end of the spectrum from flooding, does involve affective production.

Peter Sifneos has been effective in the short-term treatment of a variety of conditions. What does he call his type of therapy? It is Short-Term Anxiety Provocative Therapy. He deliberately attempts to provoke the anxiety and apparently does get good results using this short-term type of intervention. Yesterday, I had the privilege of watching Masterson's tape on the juvenile patient. He was also trying to mobilize the patient's affect by continuously confronting him. I believe Masterson must be working on a thesis that if the affect is not aroused, he is not going to get anywhere in therapy.

Psychodrama and Gestalt are experiential models. When we say experience, we must mean that there is feeling involved. It's not just a sterile, intellectual experience, obviously. Again, the whole concept of affective arousal is involved.

Now how about cognitive therapy which is supposed to be so rational and intellectual? A depressed patient comes in and right away we start testing his reality. Where is the affective arousal in cognitive therapy? Where I got started, you don't have to arouse the affect. The depressed patient is already aroused. He already

comes in feeling sad. If anything, you want to make him less sad by the time he leaves the office. So you can get at the cognitive structures immediately. You don't have to worry about the affect because it's there.

That isn't true when we treat anxiety patients. Many anxiety patients are so delighted to have the supportive figure that they are not anxious in the therapy sessions. So what do we do? We use some of the techniques from the other schools to arouse the person's anxiety so that we can make some headway. We use role-playing, we use psychodramatic techniques, we certainly use confrontation, we get the person to focus on unpleasant experiences. If he's afraid of particular situations, we go out with him to the situation so that he can have the true experience, activating the true problem in that particular situation. We can then make our intervention. Intervention is useless unless the person's affect is up.

The next stage has to do with what is made more accessible. I don't beleive that arousing the affect and then intervening at the affect is what produces the change. When the affect is aroused, I believe what you're getting is an activation of some underlying constellation. A person goes into a social situation and feels anxious. What is activated as he becomes anxious is his fear of, say, disapproval, of looking like a jerk, of being rejected by these people, of being treated like a nonentity. Once the affect is aroused and he has these thoughts of being socially undesirable, then you can start to get him to my phase III, the reality test—to reappraise the thinking that is now made accessible. The patient starts to test reality through a wide variety of methods that Ellis and we have developed. When the patient starts to explicitly reality test this, he begins to recognize at an experiential level, not at a sterile, intellectual level, that he has somehow misconstrued the situation.

So the mechanism of change, at least with many patients who do respond to therapy, seems to me to have to do with making accessible those constellations which are producing the nonadaptive behavior or the accessive symptomatology.

To get to the solution to the question as to why a wide variety of apparently disparate therapies can work, I'd like to say that they work because ultimately they affect the information processing of the individual. I hope I'll be able to explain that as I go along. But first I want to tell you what I mean by information processing. The current notion of this is that if we did not appropriately extract information from the environment and appropriately synthesize it and appropriately act on it, we wouldn't live very long. We'd go about like blind men and would die or get killed. So we have to be tuned into the environment, we have to make the appropriate inferences, and we have to act appropriately on them. However, in cases of psychopathology, the information processing is skewed for some reason. Sometimes, we see people with really profound depressions who develop these after having taken antihypertensive drugs. Their whole information processing gets screwed up and they come in highly depressed. What's interesting is you don't need to give them another drug to unscramble this bad information processing. You can do it through other methods. The psychological antidepressant can be a very powerful way of getting the cognitive shift or the information shift into the appropriate channels.

I believe that different methods do work because they can ultimately affect the information processing. There have been some studies in which cognitive therapy has been compared with the prescription of antidepressant drugs in the treatment of depression. By and large, cognitive therapy has been as effective as drug therapy, in some studies even more effective. If you take just those cases that improved, either with cognitive therapy or with drug therapy, and you see what happens to the patient's thinking throughout the course of therapy, you find that there's been a marked shift with people who are getting cognitive therapy in the way they perceive themselves, the way they perceive their futures, and the way they perceive their own personal world. What is interesting is that the drug therapy subjects react exactly the same way. The various investigators who have tried to understand this say this may mean that all therapies are nonspecific or that all changes are nonspecific, but I think a specific change does take place. There is a change in the way an individual processes information. The individual, initially, is processing all information in a negative way. Then, as a result of a cognitive intervention or a biochemical intervention, he starts to process the information differently.

Now why should two procedures that are so far apart—one getting a particular molecule into your mouth and then through your system and the other getting some type of statement from a therapist which goes through the ears, maybe his facial expressions go through your eyes, or some other sensory system is involved—produce the same change? My notion is that the various therapies work because they may be affecting different systems which are all related to one another. There's a kind of internal circuitry, or synchronicity, or feedback loops so that it is impossible to intervene at one system without affecting any other system. All the systems work together just as the heart and lungs work together. A therapy that is therapeutic (as opposed to a psychonoxious therapy or therapist that can make a person worse through affecting one system which then will affect the other systems) can work through pinpointing one system, producing a reverberation throughout all the other systems. Thus, you can affect the neurochemical system through drugs, the cognitive systems through cognitive therapy, the neuromuscular system through relaxation and other interventions, and bring about a reverberation or ripple effect through all the systems. So to me it's not such a great mystery anymore as to why therapies that are so different can all be effective.

Next, we would like to do two things. One that Dr. Marmor mentioned is to try to determine which therapeutic interventions are going to be the appropriate ones for the particular patients, to try to get a better fit. In addition, we want to improve our therapies, to use theoretical understanding so that we can make the therapies more economical. I think the day is long past when we can just experiment with our patients and go from one therapy to another until we find something that works. We have to be more efficient or the consumer is not going to be able to put up with it.

The endpoint of the therapy and of my talk is that we do have to target the internal black box. We can't think just of technique. We have to think in terms of what is going on inside the patient and what is necessary to modify whatever pathogenic influences there are in the black box.

RESPONSE BY DR. MARMOR

I'm most appreciative to Dr. Beck because I think he has extended and elaborated on my thesis and done so brilliantly. There is nothing I would contradict in what he has said.

I just want to elaborate on one or two minor matters. I think one of the significant things that has developed in the last 20 years in terms of psychotherapeutic technique is an increased understanding of the importance of the activity of the therapist. The early years of psychotherapy in this country were dominated by the analytic model, which imposed a passive stance on the therapist. This was a good research model, but it is not a good therapeutic model, at least as far as efficiency goes. I think one of the things that distinguishes all of the different methods that have been presented here is that they are all very active models. They involve a planned and rational activity on the part of the therapist that does two things: It is not only a technical intervention, it is also a communication to the patient at an unconscious level that you care, that you're trying, that you're making a genuine effort

at giving. That in itself is an important therapeutic maneuver.

The problem of cognitive learning that Dr. Beck mentioned is certainly true. I think some cognitive element is present in every therapeutic approach. What I want to underline is that cognitive learning is not a comprehensive thing if you're dealing with rational and well-trained therapists. Even though they may put their cognitive model in a different framework, they're all dealing with the same thing, they're all aiming at the same goal, and they're all saying essentially the same thing to patients, but within a different model. They're all trying to get a rationale for moving the patient along toward more mature and effective coping behavior. Technique is, therefore, important. The message I am leaving you with is that any specific technique is not necessarily, in and of itself, what we call absolutely essential and specific in therapy. Other techniques may achieve the same result. But some technique is necessary. To proceed in therapy without a rationale in your own mind is to allow your therapy to become diffuse, meaningless, and ultimately ineffective.

I think the point that Dr. Beck made about structuring therapy is important. A famous experiment was done some years ago with reciprocal inhibition in which two groups of college students who had snake phobias were separated. One group was told they were just going to get an experiment in learning how to form fantasies more effectively. They were asked to form fantasies at a hierarchical level of things that they were afraid of. The other group was told that they would do the same thing, but that the purpose of doing it was therapeutic to enable them to get over their snake phobia. As you can guess, the first group learned how to do fantasies but didn't overcome their snake phobia, while the second group doing the identical thing but with the expectation of it being therapeutic did get over their snake phobia.

The importance of cognitive input making sense to the patient is very true and usually this is a selective process. People who come to a particular school of therapy are coming because they are already sympathetic to that school of therapy in one way or another. People who are looking for an expressive type of therapy are not going to go to a cognitive-analytic type. There is a selective process that goes on in the beginning. It's what Jerome Frank calls the "Shared Mythology" that both patient and therapist have to have for therapy to move ahead. But it is important that the cognitive input make sense to the patient and, in so doing, offer a meaningful rationale for understanding what's going on in his life and enabling him to change.

I think Dr. Beck's point about the importance of affect arousal as a medium within which change takes place is absolutely vital and all of the current therapists are recognizing that more and more. The short-term dynamic therapists working within the analytic model are placing great emphasis on affect arousal.

One final point that I think I must make to underline one of the important elements involved is that the patient must bring to therapy a high level of motivation. I think all therapists recognize that unless that level of motivation is present the therapeutic task is a much more difficult one.

QUESTIONS AND ANSWERS

Question: Dr. Marmor, I'd like to ask you about the issue of extinction and time in therapy. I know that you're going to be on the panel on brief versus long-term therapy, so probably you don't need to go into it at too much length, but I noticed you omitted it in your list of significant factors in therapy. I believe that time is a very relevant issue, that if someone has walked along a path that's not very useful to him or her he not only has to see that he can overcome the anxiety associated with walking along alternative paths but he also has to allow those feelings and fears to extinguish over a time in that supportive environment. It raises the issue of brief versus long-term therapy and how you would approach assessing that difference in targeting the time period.

Marmor: That's a long issue in and of itself as to how you assess the differences between patients whom you think you might be able to help in a brief time and those you might be able to help over a longer period. I think that's one of the things you try to determine in your assessment of the ego-adaptive capacity, the coping capacities of the patient. But I do want to say one word about time as an important factor in therapy. It is something that is happening in the history of the psychotherapeutic movement, in the evolution of psychotherapy, if you will. We are learning that time is a significant variable and that where we do not give the impression to patients that the time therapy is going to take is open-ended and possibly endless, we subtly influence the course of therapy. One of the things we are learning in short-term therapy is that when our technique is appropriate, when we feel the patients have the strength to benefit from a shorter-term technique by setting a time limit to the therapy, we color the entire therapeutic process and it makes a difference.

SECTION V

Group Approaches:
TA, Gestalt, Psychodrama

Transactional Analysis and
Redecision Therapy

◆

Mary McClure Goulding, M.S.W.

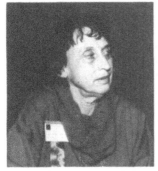

Mary McClure Goulding, M.S.W.
Mary McClure Goulding is one of the leading exponents of Transactional Analysis. Along with her husband Robert Goulding, she developed an approach called Redecision therapy which synthesizes Transactional Analysis and Gestalt. Together they founded the Western Institute for Group and Family Therapy in Watsonville, California, and co-authored two professional books about their approach. There is also an edited volume about the Redecision model. Mary Goulding has served as a member of the Board of Trustees of the International Transactional Analysis Association and is a Teaching Member of that organization. Her M.S.W. was granted in 1960 from the School of Social Welfare, University of California, Berkeley.
Mary Goulding responds to the questions sent to speakers and describes the important tenets of Redecision therapy. Change occurs when patients reexperience old impasses and "redecide" emotionally and cognitively. Mental health should not be defined solely in relationship to the individual; it must include social commitment beyond the self and family.

I have the dual assignment of presenting Transactional analysis (TA) and Redecision therapy. Transactional analysis is primarily a theory, and we use the theory in our practice of Redecision therapy. We use Eric Berne's concept of contractual therapy, which I will explain below; his Game theory, which we have modified; and the TA concept of injunctions and early decisions, which forms the basis of our Redecision work. We also use other aspects of TA theory, which I won't be discussing here.

By the way, Mark Twain said that the only people who could legitimately use the word "we" were the Queen of England and anyone with a tape worm. I do not qualify on either count. When I use "we" I mean my husband, Bob Goulding, myself, and the hundreds of Redecision therapists all over the world.

Also, I use the words "she" and "her" to mean both male and female, singular, in the so-called generic sense. In another two thousand years, it will be time again to use "he" and "him" in the so-called generic sense.

Following are the questions all presen-

285

ters at this conference have been asked to address.

HOW DO YOU DEFINE PSYCHOTHERAPY?

Psychotherapy is an art through which clients are enabled to change their lives. Psychotherapy is an art—like writing or painting or photography. It is an interesting, unique art that must involve the cooperative work of at least two active people. Mona Lisa has to do much more than just sit there. She is the model and the artist. What is the therapist? In an eerie, beautiful way, the therapist is also the model and the artist. The art of psychotherapy is the coming together of therapist and client, so that the client may change her thinking, feeling, believing, and/or behaving, in whatever ways she wants to change.

Is psychotherapy also a science? Perhaps. I know intimately the art and I know that the art is based on knowledge. The art of psychotherapy can be taught to those with any talent for it. I do not know if psychotherapy is a science, since I do not think in those terms.

WHAT ARE THE GOALS OF PSYCHOTHERAPY?

Contractual therapy was one of Eric Berne's contributions to the art of therapy. The therapist and client, working together, establish the goal of the client's therapy, which Berne called *the treatment contract*. A contract must be clear, understandable, attainable, and must have within it some reward for the Child part of the client. A Parent contract (or *should* contract) is acceptable only if the client wants to make the *should* change. The chief advantage of contractual therapy is

that the client writes the novel and paints the picture with you!

Contractual therapy works beautifully with the cooperative client, the one who comes because she wants to grow and change and has intelligent, questioning trust in the therapist she hires to treat her. The situation is more complicated if she is a person who either trusts blindly or rebels blindly. If she trusts blindly, the therapist must be extraordinarily careful not to be lulled by the thrill of being so adored, and she must immediately address the issue of blind trust. Because the client is accustomed to others thinking for her, it is especially important in her therapy that she be stroked for making independent choices.

With the rebellious client, paradoxical interventions are certainly appealing. However, paradoxical interventions simply do not fit my own therapeutic style. What fits for me is openness, candor, and cooperation with my client which result from all work being aboveboard. Therefore, I don't use paradox. When a client is blindly rebellious, I will talk directly to the client about her rebelliousness, and I will look at what the positives and negatives of rebellion are and have been for her. Then I may ask, "How about a subcontract? Are you willing to get what you want here with me, even if that means you'll change in ways that are pleasing to your mother, your father, and to me?" Many Redecision therapists do use paradoxical approaches with rebellious clients.

I hope that those who are studying the many ways of practicing the art of psychotherapy will develop a new appreciation of the vastly different psychotherapeutic methods available. I hope you will give yourselves permission to practice new ways in order to discover which therapy fits best for you.

What are the goals of psychotherapy? Ask your client! One client simply wants to stop being afraid of driving over bridges. She is not interested in any other changes. Another client, and this is especially true of therapist-clients, loves the process of change and wants to spend her years on earth changing, evolving, growing, and becoming new and different. She also loves her relationship with her therapist and her group. For years, I considered this pathology and would say to clients, "You mean, you have actually spent $10,000 on your therapist! You could take a year traveling around the world for that!" Then I realized that some people are not as interested in going around the world as I am. Such a client, considering psychotherapy an affordable and wonderful luxury, would rather buy therapy than an expensive car or a trip to China. She will make serial contracts over long periods of her life.

Another client, in order to function even marginally, in order to work and maintain social relationships, will need long-term work. She may come into therapy so confused or so hopeless that the very process of determining her own needs and wants will take a long time. Many of my Redecision colleagues believe that borderline clients cannot make contracts. I have experienced that they can and that the process is extremely helpful to them, when done slowly, humorously perhaps, and always respectfully.

During the contract-setting stage of therapy, the therapist may give feedback and may also suggest contracts. For example, if a client wants only to stop being afraid of public speaking, the therapist will, nevertheless, ask about her work and her private life. The therapist may then offer additional contracts. Whenever a client is in danger of hurting or killing self or others, the therapist must work with the client to achieve a no-suicide and/or no-homicide contract. The therapy will then focus on a no-suicide or no-homicide redecision.

In all Redecision therapy, the essence of the work will be contractual change. As the client makes the changes she desires, I expect that she will also learn a self-awe, a respect for the miracle of her own being, and that as a result, she will find a way to feel this same awe and respect for other beings.

HOW DO PEOPLE CHANGE IN THERAPY? WHAT ARE THE BASIC PREMISES AND UNDERLYING ASSUMPTIONS IN YOUR APPROACH TO FACILITATE CHANGE?

We Redecision therapists believe that human beings are autonomous. We believe that each person is in charge of her own thoughts. No one makes her think. No thought "crosses her mind." Her thoughts are accessible; and if there is an unconscious, she is ultimately in charge of her own unconscious. Each person is able to think and to plan her own life. Each person is or can be smarter about herself than any therapist she can hire.

Each person is in charge of her own beliefs. An important part of therapy is the untangling of beliefs from thoughts and the freeing of the individual to choose her own beliefs.

Each person is in charge of her own feelings. No one makes anyone else feel. People feel in response to their own thoughts and beliefs.

Each person is in charge of her own behavior. Behavior is important! One of the pitfalls of psychotherapy is the underemphasis on action and the overemphasis on feelings. The client is responsible for *doing something new and constructive* to cement any gain made in the therapist's office.

This concept of personal autonomy—the concept that I alone am responsible for my thoughts, beliefs, emotions, and actions—is crucial to change. As long as an individual blames others for her fate and spends her energy attempting to change others, she simply cannot make the desired changes in her own life. Formerly, we spent much energy teaching this concept of autonomy, but nowadays many people are writing books for therapists and laypersons that expound the importance of autonomy. I am delighted! More and more psychotherapists are agreeing that the first and most important grounding for client change is the client agreeing that she is in charge of herself.

We believe that people change in response to being stroked positively for changing. Although we are confrontive, we are also eager to praise and to teach people to praise themselves for growth and change.

We help clients learn self-nurturing. We teach delightful ways to overcome punitive self-criticism. If you are interested, read my booklet, *Who's Been Living in Your Head?* We encourage clients to enrich their nurturing of self and others.

Our Redecision work is grounded in the TA concepts of injunctions and early decisions. Bob Goulding and I were awarded the Eric Berne Scientific Award from the International Transactional Analysis Association for our classification of Injunctions and Decisions. Parents, out of their own pathology, give injunctions: don't be, don't be separate from me, don't be the sex you are, don't want, don't need, don't think, don't feel, don't grow up, don't be a child, don't succeed, don't be important, don't belong, don't be well, don't be sane. Children decide either to fight against these messages or to accept them. If they decide to accept them, they decide quite precisely how to accept them. Then, unfortunately, they make these early decisions a part of their permanent character structure.

For example, a girl may receive the message that she should have been born male, either because the family wanted a son or because she looks around her family and recognizes that boys have all the privileges. She may decide, "My family is nuts. I'm a girl and I like being a girl," and she may find herself a good role model in a favorite aunt or female teacher. She may decide, "I'm not really a girl. I am a boy trapped in a girl's body." She may decide, "I'll keep fighting until I prove I'm better than any boy anywhere." She may

decide, "I'm worthless and no one can ever love me because I'm only a girl."

People make childhood decisions about themselves for numerous reasons including, to be loved, to avoid being hurt, to allay their terrible fears of abandonment or engulfment, to make sense out of their situations, to simply survive. They accept attributes such as smart, dumb, pretty, ugly, awkward, athletic, nice, bad, and so forth. They decide which emotions are acceptable or unacceptable, and then they suppress certain feelings and overuse others. They decide what to do in life: "I'll never grow up," "I'll kill myself and then they'll be sorry," "I'll never need anybody," "I'm only important when I take care of others." In our therapy, we focus on these early decisions and then help our clients redecide so that they can free themselves to change in the present.

One way our clients make redecisions is to return to an early scene where the original decision was made. Bob and I do not use hypnosis; some Redecision therapists do. We may simply say, "Does this remind you of any time when you were young?" Or, "Hey, exaggerate the way you are sitting. How old do you feel? What's the scene?" Or, "You say you are sad and you are thinking, 'My wife doesn't love me or she wouldn't do that,' and you feel like running away. Let yourself feel your sadness and say again your words, and see how they fit when you are little." There are lots of easy ways to return to the past. Once there, the client reexperiences the scene; and then she relives it in fantasy in some new way that allows her to reject old decisions.

To demonstrate what I am talking about, here is an exercise from the book *Redecision Therapy: Expanded Perspectives* (Kadis, 1985). In this exercise, if you let yourself get into the swing of it, you will discover what is involved in Redecision work.

The exercise: Remember a time when you experienced what I call "a piddling-awful trauma." The bombs were not dropping on your home, your mother was not threatening suicide, no one was physically abusing you. But you felt simply awful, and you've kept the awful memory alive even until today. Examples: You forgot how to finish your musical piece during your piano recital, you wet your pants in kindergarten, you were caught in sex play, the neighbor boys built a treehouse and invited everyone in the world except you to play in it. You were reading aloud in class, made a mistake, and all the kids laughed at you. Your teacher called you "smarty pants." Pick your scene. Shut your eyes if you like, or leave them open. Let yourself be in your scene. Experience yourself in your scene as you lived it back then. Take your time.

As you finish reliving your scene, what do you feel? What do you say in your head about yourself and about the others? If you like, write these statements: I feel _____ (one word only, such as angry, sad, afraid, ashamed, jealous). In a sentence or two, write what you secretly think about yourself, the others in your scene, and about life itself. He/she/they is/are _____. I am _____. Life is _____.

For those of you who let yourselves have this experience, you may notice that your feeling is the same old rackety one you experienced lots of times as a child. (A "racket" is a TA term for a chronic bad feeling that is not used constructively.) What you say about self, others, and life may be early decisions you made back then. Perhaps you've already outgrown or redecided these old decisions. Or perhaps you are still living them out.

Now, if you like, you can relive the scene in a new way and come out a winner. You won't be changing others in this scene. If the teacher is cruel in your scene, have her remain cruel. If mother is stupid in your scene, keep her stupid. One of the ways we all stay stuck in our own pathology is that we wait and wait for others to change. We want everyone else to change in order for us to feel good. And,

ultimately, this means that we want everyone to change *back then*. Don't change them and don't change what you did. If you wet your pants, you wet your pants. If you stole a piece of chalk, you stole a piece of chalk. What, then, will you change? This time you may change your feelings, thoughts, beliefs, or perceptions. You may change what you say or do after the "piddling awful" traumatic action.

This time you will be a winner! Ready? First, find yourself the perfect buddy, the perfect ally. You can choose anyone—the Pope, the president, Katharine Hepburn, Superwoman. Pick an ally who can help you emerge victorious in your scene. When you've chosen your ally, take your ally with you into your scene. Let your ally help you be a winner! Make the scene funny if you like. Laughter is a fine route to change!

Did you triumph? Are you satisfied with what you and your ally did? If so, great! If not, are you keeping yourself stuck by waiting for others to change? Or did you pick the wrong ally? If you like, pick another ally and do it again. This time let yourself enjoy your ally's way of making you a winner.

Now, figure out what attributes you gave your ally and this time give yourself these attributes. Go back into the scene without your ally but with your ally's attributes. Be your own ally! Reenter your scene and let yourself emerge a winner. That is a redecision!

If you let yourself experience a redecision in this fantasy work, the next step is to practice what you've learned. After a redecision we ask each client, "What will you do differently today to reinforce your redecision?"

Now that you have finished this exercise, I want to remind you that an exercise is not the same as an experience. In Redecision psychotherapy, the client, with the assistance of the therapist, sets up her own unique scenes in order to make the redecisions she chooses. Therapist and client work together while the client reenters her past and redecides in her own scenes. The scenes may be "piddling" or may be real traumas.

If you want to know more about the Redecision process, read our two books, *Through Redecision Therapy* (Goulding & Goulding, 1979) and *The Power Is in the Patient* (Goulding & Goulding, 1978), or read the newest book, *Redecision Therapy: Expanded Perspectives*, edited by Les Kadis (1985). If you are interested in the use of Redecision in family therapy, read McClendon & Kadis, *Chocolate Pudding* (1983).

To summarize our therapy in TA terms, the client restructures her internal self, by discarding and growing beyond her Child decisions. She eliminates her carping Critical Parent, enhances her own self-nurturing and other-nurturing, decontaminates her thinking from her beliefs, and gives herself permission to be a Free Child when that is appropriate. She frees herself from the self-restricting and self-destructive straitjackets of the past. As she changes, she takes her new self into the world to relate with others in happier and healthier ways.

WHAT ARE THE BENEFITS/ LIMITATIONS OF YOUR APPROACH?

The benefits in our approach are that people make rapid changes and usually enjoy and enrich themselves in the process. They understand what they and others did to cause their problems in the past, and they experience a wonderful new sense of being in charge of themselves today. Throughout the therapy, the client knows where she is going and can evaluate her progress all along the way. The therapist also knows where she, the therapist, is going and can evaluate the progress of the client all along the way. This is Redecision therapy at its easiest, with therapist and client working together creatively to resolve impasses and restructure the personality in ways that the client has chosen.

What are the limitations of this approach? As I have stated, some people want more and some people need more. They need more time and especially they need to experience over this longer time a healing relationship between self and therapist. They need more opportunity for reality testing; more simple discussion of the here and now; much more of the warm, close, empathic relationship that, at its best, is the hallmark of long-term psychotherapy. In long-term treatment, the client may achieve the profoundly curative experience of an intimate, nonsexualized, nonexploitative relationship. Perhaps for the first time in her life she can say what she truly thinks, believes, and feels and still know herself to be valuable and lovable. In this relationship the client learns to trust and gives herself permission to grow. Within this model of long-term therapy, the client will make many redecisions and practice them in her relationships with the therapist and with others.

HOW DO YOU TRAIN STUDENTS?

Bob and I do not train students. We train psychotherapists who are already legally able to practice psychotherapy. Many professors in graduate programs, such as Peter Madison at the University of Arizona and Gene Kerfoot and John Gladfelter at the Fielding Institute, do teach Redecision therapy to graduate students.

In our workshops and in our ongoing training program, participants learn our methods by reading our books, discussing our approach with us, watching us work, and being our clients. Our chief method of teaching, which starts the very first day, is what we call "doing and reviewing." Each therapist leads a peer group for 20 to 30 minutes and then receives supervision. We have two models of supervision. Bob supervises by means of video playback. The therapist sees herself and her client when the session is played back and discussed minute by minute. This is an especially fine method for showing body language of therapist and client.

I set up a "fishbowl," which consists of one small group in the center of the room and a second, supervisory group behind it. Each member of the "supervision group" has a specific assignment: One concentrates on the contract, another on language (particularly words that discount autonomy or assume grandiosity), another on the quality of the contact between therapist and client, another on body language, another on Games and Injunctions, another reports on group interaction, and so forth. Each member of the supervisory group is also asked to look for specific strengths in the therapist and to be prepared to give her positive strokes. The therapist tape-records all comments on her work, so that she can review them later. The supervisory group trades places with the therapy group after each piece of work.

WHAT ARE THE QUALITIES THAT ARE IMPORTANT IN A PSYCHOTHERAPY TRAINEE?

I don't find that degrees in the field are an indication of actual or potential skill. I wonder what goes on in graduate schools that people can finish a psychiatric residency, get a Ph.D. in clinical psychology, receive an M.S.W., and still know so little about curing people. I don't mean that they don't know our methods; I mean that they don't know anybody's methods for assisting people to change their lives! I feel sorry for these therapists when they arrive at our institute and watch some young trainee from the California Youth Authority, who has completed maybe two years of college, do a better job than they can do in spite of their beautiful degrees. I blame the schools.

At the same time, I remember that when I was getting my M.S.W., I read every book I could find on how to do therapy. I searched avidly for good therapists and

demanded to pick their brains. During my first year of field work, I found one probation officer who really knew what he was doing and one psychologist who liked to teach but worked at a different agency. I would phone him on the county hot line after each session and get his supervision. I spent my lunch hours and coffee breaks with the P.O. who was a natural at therapy. And when I got to the Alameda County psychiatric clinic, I didn't bother with the supervisors who were know-nothings. I found the people at the clinic who knew something. And I kept finding people and finding books. That's how I met Bob Goulding, who was the smartest therapist I'd ever run across! I still learn from books and from workshops and from participants at our workshops. Any therapist who wants to be a real artist can search for teachers and she'll often find the best teacher in an office right down the hall!

I think most fine therapists are also fine clients. They are willing to expose their own pathology, willing to label it pathology, and are willing and able to change within the therapy structure.

A good therapist doesn't have to be right and doesn't blame her client for any lack of success in their work together. For example, I am sure there are therapists who didn't get anything good out of the exercise presented earlier. There may even be some who found the exercise destructive. If so, I am sorry, and neither you nor I are to blame. What you and I did simply wasn't right for you today. I do what I can do, and so do clients. Sometimes we work miracles together, and sometimes we flop around and get nowhere.

I believe a good therapist loves the work—the mystery, the sameness and the uniqueness of each client, the sheer fun of being present at the moment of change. I love figuring out what to do and then waiting almost breathlessly for the client's next move. I love being a therapist! I have spelled this out in detail in "The Joy of Psychotherapy," in the book *Redecision*

Therapy: Expanded Perspectives (Kadis, 1985). The best trainees I know experience the joy of psychotherapy.

HOW HAS YOUR APPROACH EVOLVED AND WHERE DO YOU SEE IT EVOLVING? WHERE DO YOU SEE PSYCHOTHERAPY EVOLVING?

This year Bob and I celebrated our 20th year of working together. We began our partnership in 1966, using our own professional skills, plus what Bob had learned in his two years of individual training with Eric Berne and what he was learning from workshops and individual contact with Fritz Perls. We experimented with merging these two quite different forms of therapy, and we added imagery to make the clients' scenes more vivid. When we began doing weekend marathons, we were interested in people feeling intensely. Our clients, with our encouragement, had fantastic angers and sadnesses. Gradually, we have learned that catharsis is not necessary and that humor is, for us, a better treatment tool than suffering. Today we work more quickly and efficiently than we used to.

Pio Scilligo in Rome has an extraordinary collection of videotapes of the work of American therapists including, by the way, complete workshops that Jim Simkin did in Rome. In the spring of 1985, I asked him to compare my present workshop with my earlier workshops, which he and his students had been studying. He said my current work is much quieter, that I spend more time encouraging the client to think and less time encouraging the client to feel. He said I am wiser today and more willing to share my wisdom. He, too, of course, is older and wiser and continues to be a very gifted therapist.

I see psychotherapy evolving in many interesting directions. Therapists are combining Radix and bioenergetics and other body work with Gestalt and Transactional analysis. I love to watch them! Joen Fagan uses kinesiology with psychotherapy, and

Irma Lee Shepherd and many others are exploring spiritual parameters.

I applaud that therapists are recognizing the life-wrecking effects of trauma—in physical and sexual abuse of children, in rape and other violence against adults, and in war. I hope we will recognize the same life-wrecking effects that the trauma of incarceration has on criminals. Some day I hope we will offer special therapy for prisoners and ex-prisoners, spouses of ex-prisoners, and children and adult children of these prisoners. They are desperately in need of the best therapy we can give them.

I don't think we are doing enough when we learn how to treat the victims of trauma. I think we in the mental health fields must work to prevent trauma.

HOW DO I DEFINE MENTAL HEALTH?

In the 1960s, we had the flower children, the loving antiwar rebels, who did not take very good care of themselves but who cared desperately that war be abolished. We had therapists who worked all week with their clients and then spent their Saturdays marching for SNCC and CORE and marching against the war in Vietnam. Some of us met our clients on the picket lines, and we marched together. I think those Saturdays on the picket lines were at least as curative as anything we did in our offices.

During these same years, TA therapists brought "I'm OK, You're OK" balloons to conferences, dressed in wondrous robes, and frolicked in their newfound "Free Child" ego states. Overworked, desiccated therapists thought the Free Child was the answer to everything. This Child-we-never-quite-were, this wonderful Peter Pan in each of us, does have a place in our lives, but those of us on the picket lines knew this Free Child was not the ultimate in mental health.

I believe mental health is the desire and the commitment to love and to work not only for self and for family, but for all people. The goal of mental health is the development of a profound capacity for empathy and action in support of life, the ability to appreciate life, to appreciate self because I am, to appreciate others because they are. This is what is meant by the existential position "I'm OK, You're OK." This is what the Bible means by "Love thy neighbor as thyself." With this appreciation of self and others is also the appreciation of the world and the universe. With appreciation comes responsibility and action—action on behalf of self, others, and all of this universe.

I once had great hopes that we therapists could cure this world simply by making people personally healthy. I thought that when people learned to love themselves and care for themselves, they would almost automatically love and care for the planet Earth. I no longer believe this. I think we learn early to care for self and family and to barricade our minds against what goes on outside our homes. I don't think we therapists use therapy as we could to extend our caring and our client's caring beyond these barriers.

What are these barriers? When my grandson Brian was about three years old, I talked to him on the telephone almost every day. One day, he began the conversation with, "Grandma, did you know we eat pigs!" His voice was agonized. He had just found out that his good friend, the neighbor's pig, had been murdered and was going to be eaten. He was horrified to learn that the bacon he loved came from living animals.

I think we put up barriers in our brains when we are very young, when we find out that people eat pigs, for example. It is too horrible to know the worst of the world. We learn early not to look, not to see, not to hear, not to know. We redefine animals as meat rather than as living creatures. In exactly the same way, our slave-holding ancestors redefined blacks as non-human. Today we define human beings as communists and then set up "moral" rules that say it is commendable to kill them because they are subhuman or dangerous. We disregard tragedy that is not our own. I remember when my German-American grandparents listened to Hitler on the shortwave. My grandmother said he did not speak like an educated man and that was her only condemnation of Hitler. People in this country, as in Germany, guarded themselves against knowing about the genocide in Hitler's Germany while it was occurring. We pretended that there were not Jews who had escaped, had witnessed, and who did tell the world what was going on. Today we are guarding ourselves against knowing about the genocide of the Indian population in Central America, while we sell the arms and the expertise to carry out this genocide. We tolerate torture.

We are teaching our children that they do not have to submit to physical and sexual abuse; yet we allow them to be abused, neglected, and deprived. Welfare to families has been cut and cut again. Our children today are poorer, shabbier, hungrier than they have been in the past 50 years. Pay for foster homes is a disgrace; the traumas continue, while the children wait for homes. We are therapists and we know the lifelong effects of childhood trauma and neglect. How many of us are fighting for the right of our nation's children to be cared for adequately?

I have not noticed that "getting one's act together," "learning to love oneself," or any other happy result of psychotherapy has made people more active in fighting the horrors of this world. Eleanor Roosevelt and Norman Thomas, undoubtedly without the benefit of anyone's psychotherapy, are examples of passionate commitment to others, which is the part of mental health that I see underemphasized in the evolution of psychotherapy. I applaud the passionate commitment of many churches and congregations in the sanctuary movement. They are practicing mental health.

I believe any definition of health must include commitment beyond self and family. The therapy of the future must recognize that the exclusive emphasis on self and self-healing is a form of psychopathology, a modern-day narcissism. The world needs the virtue of unselfishness. Psychotherapy must include a commitment to world-change as well as self-change.

REFERENCES

Berne, E. (1966). *Principles of group treatment*. New York: Oxford University Press.
Goulding, M.M. *Who's been living in your head?* Watsonville, CA: WIGFT Press.

Goulding, M.M. & Goulding, R.L. (1978). *The power is in the patient*. San Francisco: TA Press.
Goulding, M.M. & Goulding, R.L. (1979). *Changing lives through redecision therapy*. New York: Brunner/Mazel.
McClendon, R. & Kadis, L.B. (1983). *Chocolate pudding and other approaches to multiple family therapy*. Palo Alto, CA: Science and Behavior Books.
Kadis, L.B. (Ed.) (1985). *Redecision therapy: Expanded perspectives*. Watsonville, CA: WIGFT Press.

Discussion by Jeffrey K. Zeig, Ph.D.

I first met Bob and Mary Goulding in 1973 when I sought them out for training in Transactional Analysis and group therapy. My friend, Ellyn Bader, who is currently President of the International Transactional Analysis Association, had suggested I get training from the Gouldings. At first I was a bit skeptical; TA sounded like too much of a fad. I had been trained in Rogerian methods and I knew that was the only "correct" way to do therapy. However, I spent an afternoon watching the Gouldings work. I found they were doing things that were creative, unique, and fun. I signed up for the program.

Bob and Mary have an excellent training model based on a combination of supervision, didactic training, and modeling. They treat therapists whom they train; part of the training is to participate in the group therapy sessions they lead.

My first afternoon in training was spent in a fishbowl supervision session. The student therapists formed a group, and one of the students was a group leader; the other members of the group were expected to get personal therapy on real problems. Bob and Mary each supervised a different small group.

I got to my first session just a bit late; they had already assembled but hadn't started. When I entered the room, Mary introduced herself and immediately asked if I would be the first therapist. I can say that I was more than a bit intimidated. But I was there for training, so I agreed.

After finishing 20 minutes of work with the group, I turned to Mary for feedback. She said, "Jeff, these are the things that you did right." And she listed them. Then she told me, "Here are some options for things that you could do differently." She listed those. Then, she said, "All right, now you go back into the group and somebody else will be the therapist."

I was shocked. Something was missing. I said, "Mary, what did I do wrong?" Mary looked at me quizzically and replied, "What do you want to know that for?" I said, "That's what my supervisors would normally have done. They tell me what I do wrong." Mary said, "It's not valuable information." When I reflected on her observation, I realized she was right!

I have recounted that anecdote in therapy sessions I have conducted, especially those involving parent/child problems. Also, I have come to subscribe to that philosophy as a supervision model. I tell my students what they're doing right, and then give them options for what they could have done differently.

Therefore, in making comments about Mary's paper, I would like to describe some of the things I think are right about Redecision therapy. (1) One of the important things I learned from Bob and Mary is that therapy can be fun. So many therapists (so many of the supervision voices in my head) make therapy a *serious* business. Bob and Mary were my first model of how humor could be used constructively in psychotherapy. It's not only good modeling for the patient, it's a great way of avoiding therapist burnout. (2) Another aspect I like about Redecision therapy is that, in general, the Gouldings follow Eric Berne's dictum of asking themselves, "What can I do to cure patients today?" Redecision therapy is a brief therapy. It follows Jay Haley's dictum that therapy is a problem, not a solution. The problem is that patients are in therapy. The solution is that you get them out of therapy, living their own lives independently of therapy as quickly as possible. (3) Redecision therapy considers psychotherapy to be an art. I do not think that therapy has a lot to do with science. Like the arts, therapy is a process of using a medium (in this case, communication) to help alter mood and perspectives. Because each person thinks, feels, and behaves differently, there is no way of quantifying psychotherapy. Neither is there any way to quantify other human influence situations of the same sort, for example, being a parent. (4) In Redecision therapy, Bob and Mary remind us about the importance of autonomy, especially in regard to feelings. Patients are not the victims of their feelings; rather, they are the authors of their feelings. The Gouldings regularly confront "make-feel" statements. They remind us that people don't "make me feel upset"; I make myself upset in response to something that happens in my environment. The idea of autonomy is one of the cornerstones of their work.

Next, I reiterate some of the important aspects of Bob and Mary's approach. Transactional Analysis and especially Redecision therapy are important developments that depart from Freud's basic concept of the unconscious as a seething cauldron of negative impulses. In Redecision therapy, the power of the conscious mind is emphasized. As a logical extension, the therapist uses contracts with his patients. Especially in the initial part of the therapy, the patient makes a contract or a clear agreement about change. Therapy no longer becomes archeology; rather, it is strategically directed toward a goal. Whether or not the goal is accomplished can be clearly determined. The Redecision approach deals with what the Gouldings call "stuck spots," or impasses. The patient is helped to get in touch with the impasses in his past and then cathartically resolve them in the present. To accomplish this, they conduct group therapy, using their own unique blend of Transactional Analysis and Gestalt.

The impasses have their origins in messages received in childhood (mostly from parents) and in the decisions made by the child about these messages. The job of the therapist is to help the patient get in touch with early decisions and to redecide in a way that fosters effective living.

In providing therapy, the Gouldings emphasize the idea that each person is responsible for deciding and redeciding. Most of the therapy is done at a conscious level. It is at this point that I tend to differ with them. Hence, I will offer some contrasts. Where Bob and Mary remind us that the "power is in the patient," which is true, they seem to be talking about the power of the conscious mind. My orientation is that the power is more in the patient's unconscious. All therapy involves redecision, but I believe that most redecisions (and most change) are decided on more of an unconscious level, in which case the use of multilevel techniques is necessitated.

When the Gouldings conduct therapy, ordinarily they use only direct transactions. Also, they ask their patients to keep their transactions direct. If one works on the direct conscious level, the use of confrontation is a logical option and Bob and Mary often use it in their work. Personally, I don't see that there is much possibility in keeping transactions direct because all communications contain multiple levels of meaning. As a logical extension, I use indirect techniques which are ways of establishing a context for patients to empower themselves. The use of indirect methods is a way of supporting patients. It is not that the therapist is doing something to the patient. It is like working with a broken clock. If you want to fix it, you can shake it or you can go around the back of the clock and do a little tinkering.

In Transactional Analysis terms, indirect technique would be considered "ulterior transactions." Unfortunately, that label has a pejorative connotation. However, Eric Berne pointed out that all communications have both a social level and a psychological level. Outcome is normally determined at the psychological level of the communication. If outcome is determined at that level, the therapy should be conducted at the level of experience at which the problem is generated. For example, early decisions are most often made at an unconscious level. Conscious children do not consciously say to themselves, "I am not going to exist." Consciously, redeciding is not necessarily conducive to change or is it a necessary precondition to change. Through the use of indirect technique, the therapist can guide the patient's thinking so that redecisions can be conscious and/or unconscious.

In the Ericksonian approach, we emphasize the benign unconscious. Conscious change is used. However, unconscious change is used to a greater extent. When one speaks about the unconscious (or in TA terms, one might say, "what goes on outside of Adult awareness"), one speaks to the issue of autonomy, one of the cornerstones of the Gouldings' work.

I differ with Bob and Mary a bit, in regard to their insistence on autonomy. It is true that no one can make another person feel something unless it's done through physical contact. Also, in general, individuals benefit by taking full responsibility for their feelings. However, it does not stand to reason that people take *total* responsibility for their feelings, nor is it necessarily beneficial that they do so.

Much of human behavior is autonomous and happens automatically. For example, we do not consciously think about walking, talking, laughing, thinking, digesting, and so forth. There are degrees of automaticity in human functioning. Feelings are somewhat autonomous by nature. They are not fully under conscious (volitional) control. It is both a charming and disarming aspect of feelings that they are not fully volitional.

It is a good idea to remind people that they have more control than they realize in regard to their feelings. However, to insist that they have total autonomy is neither reasonable nor helpful. The philosopher Santayana said, "Somebody comes up with a good idea, and somebody else is sure to overextend it."

The importance of autonomy and avoiding "make-feel" statements is central in Bob and Mary's work. They succeed beautifully. Others may not do it so easily. Personally, I haven't found it a helpful intervention to say to a patient, "You make yourself sad. So, instead of making yourself sad, make yourself happy." Nor have I found the power inside myself to immediately turn my anxiety into excitement.

Another area of contrast has to do with the process of therapy. In the Ericksonian approach, I emphasize what needs to be done before and after the main intervention, namely, seeding, moving in small steps, and following through. In the Gouldings' model, the main intervention is often redecision. In watching them work, one sees that it is how they set up the redecision and how they follow through after it that really adds power to their therapy. Similarly, when one reads about Milton Erickson, one perceives that the main interventions are clever and artful, but often the reader does not recognize that they draw their power from the setup and following through. As ingenious as Erickson was at devising creative interventions, he was even more ingenious about the process of therapy. It's like playing tennis. The approach and follow through are crucial. If you concentrate just on the period in which the racket hits the ball, you cannot be very effective.

In their future writings, I hope that Bob and Mary place more emphasis on the process of therapy before and after the redecision. Solely emphasizing redecision can lead to misinterpretation by the novice therapist who, for example, could take a nonchalant attitude, "If you don't redecide, it's your problem."

In summary, the Gouldings' therapy is based in helping people to get out of perceiving themselves as victims and take control of their lives. In Redecision therapy, change is rapid *and* enduring. The Gouldings remind us that we are paid not to make decisions for people, but to help people realize their own power to decide.

QUESTIONS AND ANSWERS

Question: Given Claude Steiner's work with scripts or Hedges Capers' work with the miniscripts, how do you see Redecision other than as a difference of just style of the therapist doing it?

M. Goulding: I see it primarily as a stylistic difference. I don't want to comment on that particular brand of work. I think their work is more Adult-Adult and I think we use more imagery and we use more being, more inducement to be little and to redecide within the context of being little. Certainly, we're working to have the person go very quickly into an early scene in an adaptive manner, feeling bad in the way they felt bad back then and feeling impotent in the way they felt impotent back then. And then the scene involves redeciding from a Child position, so it's not an Adult decision. I think that the

miniscript Hedges Capers did was lovely; he also believes in positive strokes. It's very, very similar. Claude did some nice work on looking at scripts and that kind of research is useful to all of us.

Question: You mentioned that every client wants in his own way to get well. What if his early decision had been, "I can only get help or attention when I am sick," or "No therapy is going to be more efficient if I am not efficient myself"?

M. Goulding: He still wants to get well. We all have a struggle in changing, of course, especially if the strokes are for being sick. Unfortunately, lots of strokes in therapy are for being sick. In your group, people may tell something pleasant they've done and everyone says, "That's fine. Now who suffers most? We can work with them." The therapist has to avoid falling into this trap and be creative in inventing ways of stroking health instead of stroking pathology. The client wants to be well just as you and I want to be thin and successful and loved.

Question: Can you say something about the difference in the transference in hypnotherapy and Redecision therapy? Would there be more dependence in Redecision than would be likely in hypnotherapy.

M. Goulding: I see dependence as something that the individual therapist either promotes or doesn't promote, whatever the type of therapy. If the therapist needs the client, the client will often need the therapist.

Zeig: I think it's the bane of analysts that life distorts the transference. I don't really know how to answer that question about the difference in transference. I think that it is such a vague term. If you talk about tranference in terms of the analyst being a shadowy figure who sits behind the patient and doesn't make much comment, then the patient can project an awful lot of things onto the analyst.

Question: The point was whether you think there is more of a tendency in hypnosis for the patient to see the therapist as an all-powerful figure and himself as a passive figure than there is in Redecision therapy where the patient is very overtly contracting with the therapist.

M. Goulding: No, I think those practicing Redecision therapy could set themselves up as very powerful figures and those doing hypnosis can do so as well. Patients in hypnotherapy can take different roles just as well as those in Redecision therapy. I think that what happens depends more on the particular therapist than on the model that therapist is using.

I would say that same thing about the automatic and the autonomous feelings. If the therapist is into being parental and putting a value judgment on the patient performing in the right way, then that becomes very destructive and after she snaps out of it, "That will be 5¢, please."

Question: I'm curious about the extent to which you see the differences between the Redecision method and the hypnosis or Ericksonian approach as substantive? Or do you think it is just a difference of semantics and how you define it? The extent to which it's substantive, when would you refer somebody to each other rather than take the patient on yourselves?

Zeig: I'll make a point on that. I don't solely do Ericksonian hynotherapy in my practice. I learned excellent skills in Gestalt and Transactional Analysis from Bob and Mary Goulding. I use them. For example, following Perls' dictum I learned from Bob and Mary that when people are in terror, play out the terrorizer. I will sometimes ask patients with phobias to do a Gestalt with two chairs. One part of them will be the terrorizer and I'll have them exaggerate terrorizing themselves with all of the horrors about the particular thing that they're afraid of—airplanes, dogs, or whatever it is they fear. I'll strategically use that technique of exagger-

ating to absurdity so that they themselves can start recognizing the absurdity of the way they are terrorizing themselves and be able to reclaim their own power and stop scaring themselves about something that has little likelihood of doing harm.

I will use that kind of therapy, but even though I learned a Redecision model from Bob and Mary, I don't often go back into stuck-spots and ask the patient to redecide from an early Child position. I haven't used that method much, although I did in the mid-1970s. Maybe it's not my style, just as it's not Mary's style to use paradoxical injunctions. I don't believe that you have to go back and resolve those impasses at that particular point. There are so many different roads to home—the process-oriented method of Virginia Satir, or going back into an impasse, bringing it into the present and resolving it, or a hypnotic-strategic technique, or others—that choice of method probably comes down more to a matter of style than substance. To my mind the issue is that therapy is no longer based on insight, but rather on helping people to empower themselves.

Question: You're creating the redecision, but with a different approach?

Zeig: Yes, it must be the patient's redecision. A decision has to come from the patient.

M. Goulding: I tend to refer to people whom I know to be good therapists. I think there are great differences between the way I work and the way I read that Milton Erickson worked. I see it as substance, I see it as process, I see what is very different. This does not mean that one is right and one is wrong, and I don't think it even means that one is better or worse for the particular client. I tend to refer to people I know *are* artists at their own way of working.

Question: So you wouldn't find a particular person with a particular type of issue more appropriate for a certain approach than another?

Zeig: Not ordinarily.

M. Goulding: Ordinarily I will say the best therapist I know in Phoenix is . . .

Zeig: But there are some things that I would use hypnosis more for, for example with somebody with a multiple personality. I have a hard time imagining how you could work with somebody who has a dissociative disorder without really understanding something about hypnosis. I'm sure lots of people do. I think that when you have a patient who goes into that kind of dissociative work, then I think that hypnotherapy is the treatment of choice. Most of the time, when I refer to somebody, I don't refer because he or she is an Ericksonian therapist or whatever. I refer because I know he or she is a good therapist and it doesn't matter what technique is used.

M. Goulding: I want to respond to that. As far as I know, successful cures of multiple personalities do involve the therapist being a good hypnotist who knows how to access within a light trance-state and then knows how to get the permission of the facilitator among the personalities and then knows when and how to merge the personalities. It's a specific skill. I've be-

come very interested in the subject, but I don't do it. Therapists do use Redecision therapy for this, group therapy, family therapy, everything there is. However, if you're not a good hypnotist, you can't treat for multiple personality; if you're not a good family therapist, you can't either. It's currently the most exciting new field because those who are successfully treating multiple personalities—and they do it within three to six months—know all of these skills. There are only a few of these people around the country and I would refer a multiple personality only to them.

Satir: I just wanted to say that the context for me often dictates some things. I was invited to one of the communist bloc countries to do two weeks of training and I knew I was in a situation which was very touchy. What I did was to use hypnosis in order to do the work that I needed to do so that there was nothing outward that could be utilized against the person I was treating. I also wanted to say that I think we're learning more and more about what and how change comes about in an individual. We haven't finished with that, and maybe we never will, but all the questions that you're asking say something about that. I feel very excited that we have so many different approaches serving as new eyes to look at the process of human beings becoming more fully human.

Group Therapy: Mainline or Sideline?

◆

Robert L. Goulding, M.D.

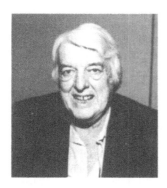

Robert L. Goulding, M.D.

Robert Goulding received his M.D. in 1944 from the University of Cincinnati and practiced general medicine until he switched to psychiatry in 1958. With his wife Mary, he founded the Western Institute for Group and Family Therapy in Watsonville, California, and authored two books. Dr. Goulding is a Distinguished Life Fellow and member of the Board of Directors of the American Group Psychotherapy Association. He served as president of the American Academy of Psychotherapists. An extraordinarily talented therapist, he has synthesized Transactional Analysis and Gestalt into his own model, Redecision therapy.

Goulding presents some of the history of group therapy and describes his own evolution as a practitioner of this method. The advantages of group therapy are developed, as are aspects of the Redecision model, especially as it can be used in working with phobics.

I want to divide my presentation into two parts: The first is my invited theme "Group Therapy: Mainline or Sideline?" and the second is my comments regarding Redecision therapy.

I have decided not to talk about the history of group therapy at length as there are many good books available, such as Powdermaker's and Sam Slavson's. The essential history of group therapy is going on right here—in this huge conference. In these huge halls, is one of the originators of group therapy in this country—Zerka Moreno, who with her husband Jacob were two of the early pioneers years ago. At the same time that Sam Slavson was forming the American Group Psychotherapy Association in New York, Dr. Moreno started the International Group Therapy Association, and the two went their own ways for all these years. Now, just recently, since both of these originators have died, there is beginning to be a joining of the two organizations, with many group therapists belonging to both of them, including those who are board members of both.

I think that in my own case I represent part of the history since the early days. I have been practicing group therapy in some way since my graduation from medical school in 1944. While I was in medical school and rotating internship in Cincinnati, I trained with John Romano and Milt Rosenbaum, as did Tom Szasz who was in my class in medical school; Tom and I had

300

not seen each other since, until this conference. We have gone different ways, even though we started in the same way, with a thorough understanding of some of the principles of psychoanalysis.

My history of group therapy began with working with alcoholics who had nowhere to go in the wild frozen northland of North Dakota. I started working with them because I had a good friend who was an alcoholic, and probably because I had some leanings towards alcoholism myself, as it turned out. I worked with alcoholics for ten years then, having them in a group and encouraging them to join and attend AA. I did not really know what I was doing, not having much trained experience except the analytic training that I got in Cincinnati, which didn't seem to help very much. I learned a lot about the psychodynamic process of groups by simply doing groups.

I also enjoyed obstetrics. I almost went into obstetrics when I quit general practice; it was the late hours that kept me out of it! I delivered over 2000 babies during my ten years in North Dakota. I used to have groups of pregnant ladies meeting once or twice a month. They talked about their fears of delivery, and I taught them the Reid method of relaxation and how to look forward to their delivery with excitement instead of anxiety, how to have their babies with joy rather than fear. So my experience in groups was one of experimentation for me, not knowing where to go to learn anymore.

Then I quit my practice and moved west again, back to my roots in California. After a few months of general practice there, I decided that I really did want to go back into psychiatry, which had been my original dream and intent. I took off to spend six months investigating residencies that fit where I was, at 40 years of age. I didn't want a residency that emphasized psychoanalysis; I already had studied that and wanted to go somewhere where I could learn about different kinds of therapy, including group therapy. I landed at the Perry Point VA Hospital, where I spent almost three and a half years and had a wonderful experience learning all kinds of different therapies, including group process.

One of my first groups was with veterans who were outpatients in the VA regional office in Baltimore. I still remember that group; one person was a multiphobic, an agoraphobic, who had been in the group since 1947, for 11 years. He was afraid to go out of the city of Baltimore and had not been out of Baltimore for all that time. There were several other patients who had also been in that group for 11 or 12 years. This was really an experience in learning how not to do group therapy, as these veterans had been there for a long time without changing anything. However, I learned a lot from these people about process group therapy and thought that a little experimentation was indicated.

It was obvious to me that I had to do something different with this group, so I arranged to meet them one night at a bar just inside the city limits. They agreed and we met there, and the next week we met at a bar across the street, outside the city. Then we met several blocks up the road. Finally, I told them that I had a lot of work to do the following week at the Hospital (about 40 miles from Baltimore) and asked them if they would be willing to meet me there. They agreed to do that for *me*—sometimes transference is wonderful, you know! Our phobic patient came along, although admitting he had some trouble crossing the city line. He cured himself of his phobia. So I did some Wolpe desensitization without having even read Wolpe!

I saw that, as an early experience in learning, it is OK to experiment in psychotherapy. We don't have to do exactly what the "experts" say to do. I thought that perhaps all of the belief systems of psychotherapy were not necessarily true and that it was OK for someone to look at them, to test them out. There was an adventure, an excitement, in doing things that people said we shouldn't do. I made friends with some of my patients, I worked with alcoholics again, I touched patients, and I studied what happened, what was good therapy and what got in the way.

When I finished my residency, I went to the Roseberg VA Hospital in Oregon for two years, which was only 600 miles from my family instead of 3000. I called to make an appointment with Eric Berne, with whom I had planned on finishing my psychoanalysis since my first two analysts in Baltimore had both died. During the intervening week between making the appointment and seeing Eric, I happened to read his first book on TA (*Transactional Analysis in Psychotherapy*, 1961) and reread it and reread it. I got so excited that someone was finally doing something different. I went to see Eric, at 11 o'clock on a Saturday morning. He asked, in his own inimitable drawl, "What can I do for you?" and I said, "Well, two things. I want to finish my analysis, and I want to learn TA." "That would be kinda sticky," he responded, again in his drawl. So I said, "Screw the analysis, I want to learn TA," and I spent two years with Eric, learning TA.

This was a very exciting time in California, during the 1960s. Don Shaskan, in San Francisco, the dean of group therapy in the West, led a one-week training session in group therapy every fall. I went to one of these sessions the first year I was at Roseberg. There I saw again my good friend Virginia Satir, whom I had first met in a family therapy training session at Temple University in Philadelphia. I learned from her a different kind of family therapy than I had learned from my first teacher in family therapy, Murray Bowen.

I learned TA from Eric for those two years (1962–1964). I learned about contracts—how to make firm, clear contracts that everyone understood. I learned how to treat people individually in the group. That, too, was a new experience; it was not what the process therapists did. During those two years and the year following, I experimented with the one-on-one approach in the group, primarily using

TA. Then Fritz Perls came to Esalen, and I was in one of his one-week workshops, along with Virginia, Irma Shepherd, Joen Fagen, Howie Fink, and others—a wonderful workshop. And I thought, "This is fascinating." One of the problems I had had with process therapy, and even with TA, was that it was too much head and not enough guts. The only "guts" in process therapy is anxiety—and they talk about anxiety for years! I began to learn from Fritz how to change anxiety to enthusiasm. For the next four or five years, I was around Fritz a great deal, as well as with Irma and Joen, Jim Simkin, and later the Polsters, and I began to assimilate Gestalt into my group practice.

Now, I'm still a group therapist. I believe that group therapy is the treatment of choice for everyone and that some also need individual therapy. But I started out moving from individual to group therapy because I had much more fun in group therapy and because I saw people changing much more rapidly. I also saw the patients having more fun in the therapy process—therapy didn't seem to be nearly as painful. Groups seemed to add a humanness to therapy that just didn't seem to be there in individual therapy. It was and is much easier to get patients to talk to an empty chair in the group, to do Gestalt experiments, where the patients have models, even if you have to bring in a shill to do the first experiments! That's a great way to get a group started, by the way—bring an old, experienced patient from another group, who is familiar with many of the techniques, such as talking to an empty chair.

Also, I started doing workshop therapy—marathon group therapy—at Esalen in 1962 or 1963. I did quite a few there, and then Virginia and I did a multiple family therapy one-week workshop there around Labor Day 1965. I began to see that marathon therapy was applicable for people in ongoing therapy as well as for new patients, and especially for couples and families. Frequently, a marathon experience got patients off to a new start without ongoing therapy. The intensity of the experience enables some patients to make lasting changes in a relatively short period of time—40 hours over a week often got more done than twice that many hours spread out over a year. Anyway, Virginia and I did that multiple family workshop, and I returned to Carmel excited, enthusiastic, turned on, about the possibility of doing training-treatment one-week workshops for the ever-increasing load of therapists I was training to do TA/Gestalt therapy.

It was after that famous week that I, high as a kite, first met Mary. We began to do more and more different things and to look at it all with a critical eye. What was happening in our groups that seemed to make people move much faster? We were using the groups for many different things. We were not using the process technique, except to know, from our psychodynamic training, what was going on. We were analyzing what was happening more in terms of TA. What were the transactions between patients? What kinds of Games were being played, and what could we learn about the origins of the psychopathology from the transactions and Games we saw going on in the here and now? What could we learn about where they were "stuck" in their lives? How could we learn about their scripts by observing the kinds of Games they played with each other, which was not as easy to see in individual therapy? Also, the workshop format gave us a chance to resolve critical impasses that we could never get to in the hour-and-a-half group. We began to realize that an hour and a half was really not enough. I never could figure out how the hour-and-a-half format got started, except that perhaps groups were first done by aged men whose bladders could not last any longer!

That, of course, brings me to the question raised for all of us to answer—what is psychotherapy? Mary has already answered that, and I would like to add just a little to her answer. Psychotherapy, to me, is more than an art; it is also a science, and I think the science can be taught to others. It is the science of personal change—change in thinking, feeling, behavior, and sometimes body. In our way of doing therapy, there is a certain consistent methodology in facilitating the process of change; the art is the delivery of that methodology—how the therapist facilitates the change from his or her own personality. Some of the constants in the science have to do with the patients changing their belief systems. For instance, most of us were taught that we were not responsible for our feelings, thinking, behavior. Our parents would say things like, "You make me feel angry," and of course we believed it. Our songs, our literature, are full of similar beliefs— "You made me love you, I didn't want to do it."

Thus, we convince ourselves that we are victims. Part of the science of change is the process of facilitating autonomy in the patients, so that people start to believe that they are in charge of self. The obsessive doesn't know that he is in charge of his thinking and talks about how thoughts "come to him." Nonsense! Thoughts are not shot into our heads from radar guns from the moon; we generate them.

Another of the processes of psychotherapy is the resolution of the impasse. All of us are struck somewhere in the past, or else we wouldn't be stuck in the present. Our books discuss the ways in which we get stuck; essentially, we think, feel, behave in response to parental messages. These responses seemed logical at that time and place; they seemed to be for psychological or physical or social survival. Now, these responses no longer serve us; rather we serve them from habit, from believing they are still appropriate. The science of psychotherapy here, then, is the refutation of those belief systems. Our group therapy methods are designed to help people make new decisions, redecisions, to anchor those redecisions in place, and to stroke positively for the changes. Behavior therapy works.

A great advantage to groups is the stroking that goes on, not just by the therapist but also by the other patients. I can't overstate the power of positive stroking in the group. Neither can I exaggerate the power that exists in seeing other patients change. I remember that when I was in my analysis I had no idea what other people in therapy with my analyst were doing because I never saw them—we walked in one door, walked out another, and never saw anyone else.

The group makes it much easier to talk about forbidden subjects; things that were hard to talk about in an individual hour become commonplace in a properly run group. It is far easier for a patient to tell about being seduced at age seven when the other group members do the same kind of talking, when the sympathy and the empathy of the other members are present, where relationships develop between the members that are trusting and warm and loving, and there is stroking, ever stroking, for change.

Another advantage to group therapy is the presence of others to facilitate action—to use the others in a psychodramatic way to represent family members from the past, people in the present, and so forth. Of course, the presence of others also adds immeasurably to the possibilities of people, especially withdrawn ones, learning how to relate. The increasing confrontation of denial is still another advantage, of great importance in treating addicts.

Yet another advantage is the economy of money and of time. I can teach eight people some of the facts of life, the autonomy, much faster together than I can teach each singly, and I can do it a lot cheaper. I just wouldn't do individual therapy anymore, except as adjunctive to group therapy. There are some people who need individual therapy—the schizophrenic, the borderline, the eating disorders, anorexia and bulimia; they all need individual time as well. But they do resolve the basic impasses much faster in the group experience and learn much better how to relate appropriately.

I am very tough about everyone being in the group, not just for all the reasons stated here but also because of the living experience they get in the group—an experience that they can take out to their family, their friends, their community. I am not particularly interested in their relating to me, but rather in how they relate to the other group members. I see myself primarily as a facilitator. I know that I am more than a facilitator. I know how Yalom, Lieberman and Miles (1972) saw me in the research reported in their book, *Encounter Groups—First Facts*. I was the leader of group #8; and if you read the italicized, opening paragraph in their description of group #8, it is obvious that I am more than a facilitator. I get involved in the therapeutic process. Now at our Institute we have people living with us for a month, swimming with us, playing with us, eating with us, as well as working with us in the group. They see us as models; they see us fight and resolve our fights and go on living with and loving each other. It's a real living experience and people make all kinds of moves in those four weeks—whether we do Redecision therapy or some other kind of good therapy—and they move faster. So I see group therapy as the mainline; and it doesn't have to be restricted to TA, or Gestalt, or psychodynamic, or psychodrama, or behavior, or any other kind of therapy, but it can be a combination of all therapies one knows how to do.

I *love* to cure phobias in a group. It's a joy you simply can't understand until you have seen it. Take water phobics, for example. We allow three or four days to let them develop trust, and then I take the four or five people who are water phobic into the pool. The rest of the crowd stands or sits around the pool to watch and cheer. I don't do fantasy work first with water phobias (we do use Wolpe desensitization with fantasy work with other phobias); I just take them into the pool water. Most of them are afraid of getting their faces in the water, or afraid to get water in their nose, or afraid to get water in their trachea—all infantile fears. So I take them into the water and have them gargle, and snuff water into their nostrils, and play spitting games with one another, spitting water at each other. They start to laugh, and a laughing Child Ego State has a hard time also being frightened.

Then I teach them how to float. Most people beyond the teenage years can float. I hold the phobics with my hands and teach them to put their hands over their heads *in* the water, to counterbalance their feet. Then I teach them to be aware of how they rise and fall off my hands with their deep breathing, and then I hold them with five fingers, four fingertips, three, two, one, and finally they rise off that one finger. As they experience that they really can float, their muscles relax, every cell seems to know that it can float, and they begin to drop their fear.

All this time the spectators are cheering madly with each step, and of course that stroking helps the phobics to start to enjoy the process, enjoy the feeling of floating in the water. Then I teach them a few simple strokes, backstroke first, then breaststroke, and I also teach them to float face down and then turn over and float on their backs. Once they have learned that and know that in any situation they can turn over and float, they drop the last remnants of their fear. It usually takes four or five minutes with each person. I have done this individually a few times, but the power of the group of phobics learning together facilitates each individual much more, as does the power of the applauding peers.

Height phobias we do first with fantasy. I take the people who are afraid of any kind of heights and ask them to sit on the floor looking out the sliding doors at the ladder leaning against the shed across the driveway. I teach them how to climb the ladder by taking them, in fantasy, one step at a time, in the classic Wolpe method, except that I use humor rather than relaxation. In the middle of climbing the fantasy ladder, I say, "And in comes your Mother, and what does she say?" Usually each one answers with, "Get down from there before you fall," or "Be careful,

you'll break you neck," or "What are you doing up there? Come down at once," or some other frightening statement. I then ask them to answer back with such statements as "I'm OK, I'm not going to fall or slip or slide or jump off this ladder." So, in addition to the desensitization I do some Redecision therapy when they are in their Child Ego State listening to the words of mother. Then I take them across the driveway to the ladder, and they climb in reality, get over to the roof, walk around the roof, climb to the peak, and look at the wonderful, marvelous view. The crowd below is cheering and taking pictures and holding the ladder for them, and the height phobics drop most of their fear. Then with the remaining specific fear of tall buildings or mountains, I do another piece of fantasy work, not unlike Wolpe's, except that instead of using a "safe place" I simply have them back up when they scare themselves, then do it slower, again and again. As the onlookers cheer, I ask them to do it somewhere nearby in reality that night or that weekend to anchor the new enjoyable experience.

OK. Enough about groups per se. Now I want to talk about Redecision therapy. Redecision therapy is not simply making a decision to be different. It is the process in which we facilitate the client getting into his or her Child Ego State. From that state he relives an old scene and changes his or her part in it. For instance, I am remembering a scene of my childhood when I was sent down to get a bottle of milk at the corner grocery. I am about five years old. I am walking home and I drop the damn bottle and it smashes. Milk is running all over the sidewalk. I can see it there and feel scared about coming home to catch hell. I can see the ice wagon dragging by with a horse pulling it and I can smell the hemp and spices and coffee from the docks only two blocks away. As I am remembering, I am there in the street. I can *smell* the damn coffee right here while I am talking to you and I am in my Child Ego State.

People ask me, "Isn't that just a trance

state?" I don't know whether it's a trance state or not—all I know is that when in that state, I and others remember and experience earlier scenes as if we were there at that time, while at the same time being aware of our present surroundings. I have learned over the years that we don't have to go into the past in order to facilitate a redecision—all we have to do is to get into the Child Ego State, with humor, with Gestalt experiences, with exaggeration, with repetition, or with countless other techniques.

The technique of getting into the Child in earlier scenes is similar to some of the hypnotherapy techniques. We facilitate the client getting into what Jeff Zeig calls *the unconscious.* I see the unconscious differently than Freud did; I see it as not *immediately* available, yet accessible with certain techniques other than free association. It is that which is suppressed enough to keep it from coming into immediate consciousness. There are many ways of accessing this unconscious; one of them is the use of clues. A client, for instance, made a contract to make friends with women; ordinarily he would find ways to get angry at them and distance himself. He started to become angry in the middle of a series of transactions between two other patients. So we asked, "What are you feeling?"

"Well, I'm feeling angry."

"What did you tell yourself in your head to make yourself angry?"

"He was talking about his mother's death and all of a sudden I thought of my mother."

"What did you tell yourself in your head about your mother?"

"I miss my mother."

"What else do you say about her?"

"She was such a wonderful woman and did so many things for me, and then she went away."

"Where did she go?"

"She had my brother."

"What is happening when your mother is gone and you miss your mother and you feel angry?"

"I feel like I'll never have her to myself again, that she doesn't love me anymore."

What we do is facilitate memory by giving enough clues to help the neurons close the synapses. We go around the resistance by going directly to the neuron pathways by giving the client back his own words. And he goes "click-click-click" and remembers. By the way, we never ask for the earliest scene, since most people don't ever remember immediately what the earliest scene was; we look for screen memories, which are just as valuable.

All along the way, we help people realize that they are responsible for themselves, for their thinking, their feeling, their behavior, their body. Unless we can get them to claim their own autonomy, there is no way for them to make a valid redecision. So we insist, and we teach, that each of us is autonomous, even though we might feel like a victim.

I do want to present briefly about some of the research that has been done. The first is the work done by Yalom et al. (1972) in *Encounter Groups—First Facts,* which is about my 30 hours of therapy. John McNeel did his Ph.D. dissertation on the outcome study of a weekend marathon, led by Mary and me. Ellyn Bader did her dissertation on the outcome study of Redecision therapy with a family in a workshop led by McClendon and Kadis.

REFERENCES

Berne, E., (1961). *Transactional analysis in psychotherapy.* New York: Grove Press.

Yalom, I., Lieberman, M. & Miles, M. (1982). *Encounter groups—first facts.* New York: Basic Books.

Discussion by Virginia M. Satir, M.A., A.C.S.W.

♦

As Bob Goulding was talking, I was having some strong feelings of gratitude, gratitude about how my life has been for me. I have had the privilege, and also the opportunity, to be with most of the people who started new things after 1900. I am going to be 70-years old on my next birthday. I started my career when I was 19-years old, when I got my first degree, and it was only in the last few years that I decided that I knew what I would do when I grew up. And what that means is that I think I discovered for myself living in a way I have never known before.

When Bob was talking, I was thinking back to extraordinary things that have come to human beings through the lips and through the energy and through the eyes of many people since 1900. I couldn't help but be also aware of some of my own evolvements. All I knew at one time was how to do one-to-one. I did good work one-to-one. As I did more of that, I began to be more aware of certain kinds of new possibilities that could happen. Then I learned how to do work with a pair. When I knew how to do work with a pair, some of those things I was missing but didn't know I was missing when I was only working with one came to my awareness. I can take no credit for knowing ahead of time what I should learn. I only know it in the process of things happening.

Well, when I knew about couples, I thought there are other things going on. Although I could have said to myself that I was doing good work, there was something in me that wanted to grow. Then I started working with families. All this is accidental, in one sense. When I started working with families, I understood some more things that were missing. And then I said, "Oh, I wonder what else there is?" I didn't know.

Then I said to somebody, I made a mistake and scheduled two people for the same time. You know, you can't do that with family. However, I thought, let's put them together. And so I did, and then I added more to that, and it was up to 20. And then I said to myself, "My goodness gracious, there is so much I can do here."

Now I did something which I'm pleased about for me. I am very slow to throw out the past until I'm really sure it no longer fits. What I was doing was building up in my mind a way of looking at people, and looking at more and more dimensions—not right or wrong, just more and more filled in. Then I began to see another piece, which was that therapists were either handling patients "in a parental position"—which was from the state of benign, malevolent domination—or being true facilitators. And then I realized that any transaction that was reminiscent of the old parental domination, whether it was I'm doing this for your own good or I'm doing this to get you in a decent place, didn't really matter because it could not work toward the empowerment of the person, which is what was necessary.

So as I look back at all the things I was doing, I realized that for me, however I did it, I was going toward the facilitation model. Then I realized that I had a viewpoint that I didn't see written about anywhere during those early days—that people have everything they need. It's a matter of accessing. And then I began to be aware that I didn't even know how to do this, but I decided to try and see what could happen. Then I became aware of the fact that in anybody's presence, whenever there were coping difficulties (I make a distinction between a difficulty and a difficulty of coping, because we all have difficulties), I found that what was basic to the coping difficulty were old messages that I had learned in the past and which were anchored in the security of my life at that time. They are the messages that you recall or talk about as the old messages that need to be redecided.

There is no way that I can come into this world, nor can you nor anybody else, other than helpless. Therefore, all the things we learn are like first learnings about anything and thus become a part of our warp and woof. Whenever I see a struggle or a coping, whether it's murder, attempted murder, rape, or just plain anxiety, I look for what that person has learned—what they're handling and keeping there, as Bob discussed—because it's what they learned that keeps them from utilizing other parts of themselves or other possibilities.

I developed something that's called family reconstruction, which enhances and deals with the same thing. And I think it deals with the same stuff that Jeff Zeig was talking about: How in your own head, do you begin to get a perspective on something that allows you to go beyond where you are? That's a hard thing to do because our reality is based upon whatever it is we've made it. So one of the things that's important, and I think both Bob and Mary Goulding accomplished it in a great way, is to be able to come up and do something like Edgar Mitchell the astronaut did when he was flying up from earth and could put the whole earth behind his thumb. It didn't invalidate anything on earth, because he could stand on the surface there and remember trees and all that. Yet the point when he could put the whole earth behind his thumb was the point at which he began to believe in new possibilities in reality.

Therapists also need other people from time to time. I do to help me see realities that I'm not aware of, not because I'm not smart, not because I'm not wonderful, but simply because we're all limited in terms of our own perspective. That's one of the very basic things.

By the way, I want to say that Bill Narron, who studied with me for a long time, has published a book called *Long Day's Journey Into Light* which has to do, basically, with the messages we learn as children, how they cripple us when they pop up in our present reality, and how we can change them. That is the reconstruction concept.

What I want to underscore is the importance for me of all the people like Fritz Perls, Eric Berne, Roberto Assigioli, Alexander Lowen, and others who put their noses into new places. I had the privilege of being there, of feeling them as people, and knowing that we were all forging something that was going to affect generations to come, because it was a new consciousness about people. To be able to relate to Bob Goulding, who has his lovely places about being crazy and not being ashamed of it, which I like, and is able to move forward, is a great joy. And this conference is a joy in that regard, because I feel that people are not saying, "You know, I got the word, kid." But I do think that central to all the things Mary and Bob Goulding were saying are two things: One is the respect and value we hold for the person we're dealing with, while having respect and value for ourselves; the other is recognizing the overwhelming potential of an old saying of mine which I love to repeat, "If my past is illuminating my present, hurray; if it is contaminating my present, let us look and let us release me."

QUESTIONS AND ANSWERS

Question: What I keep hearing over and over again is the importance of values. In what you said about mental health, you talked about values in a broader way than I've heard anywhere else. If everyone is in agreement that part of therapy is the relationship, then it seems that the values you bring to that relationship are paramount. I believe that one of the things totally lacking in the training of therapists is addressing those values and the way they drive us to be more creative or to hang in there with a client. Could you talk a bit about how you deal with these issues?

R. Goulding: Being here is one of our ways of dealing with those issues. Letting ourselves be out in front of the world and saying what we have to say, teaching the way we teach in our own place with our own treasures around us, with our banners and posters and freedom flyers and antiwar statements and Indian pots and all the things that have to do with us, these things are part of our own process of living. That's what we somehow pass along in our writing. You want to say something about that, Mary? On how we are for monogamy, that the screwing around that people do takes away from monogamy, takes away from the family, is an antimental health process. We've said that openly for many years and I think what we do, who we are, is not just what we do in the psychotherapy room but what we do in our living. That's how we pass along our model.

M. Goulding: I'm very active in the International Transactional Analysis Association, not because of the theory but largely because the majority of members do not reside in the U.S. At our next conference, about half the people will be from Europe, Central and South America, Japan, and Australia. A year from January our mid-winter conference will be in Singapore. Our summer conference last year was in Europe. To me it's tremendously exciting to know therapists from everywhere. Most of the Germans in ITAA are Green party members and many of them have been to jail to try to get our nuclear warheads out of Europe. It's exciting to me that the Israeli therapists and the German therapists are on the same side in terms of peace. So that's another answer.

Question: How do you know when it's not working, whether it's your impatience with yourself or with the patient, how do you decide when you've done what you can do and it's not working?

R. Goulding: "It's not working." I don't know what the "it" is. That's a good question and we'll answer it. One of the best things about what we do is the contract we start with. The contract is going to be specific on what people want to change about themselves, today, this week, this month, this year. If we don't fulfill the contract and work through the impasse, then it's pretty clear these people have not gotten what they asked to get. I think that making the contract the first portion of the work makes all the difference in the world in measuring whether we're moving to a desired goal or not. That's why we have contracts.

Now if I'm having trouble curing somebody—or rather, a better way of putting it is if I have trouble in facilitating their curing themselves—then I have to do what Eric Berne used to do and ask myself what can I do during this hour to change the process going on and facilitate this person making this change. If I don't know the answer to that question after a little bit of time, then I ask whether I know enough about my own skills and need to learn something else, or do I want to send the client to someone else because somehow there's some personal problem going on between us, transference, countertransference, whatever it may be. I keep learning from people; I started learning from Wolpe's desensitization when I wasn't curing phobias or redecision. That's what we do.

Satir: I'd like to say something else. Your basic contract is between yourself and someone you're working with. If your own value depends upon the client's response, then when something doesn't go on, you are unable to say openly, "You know what, I don't think this is working and I wonder if you see the same thing as I do," and then take it up as a transaction in a way that might be able to clarify some things. You might say, "Maybe we need to make some other kind of plans," and that can be done in a loving kind of open way because your value doesn't depend on what happened. I can't underscore that enough with the people I work with. If I undertake anything with somebody and there is the metamessage that what that person does reflects on me, I'm going to be in serious trouble. So I usually talk with people and say there's nothing wrong with failing. As a matter of fact, I often say to people that we have to get rid of both failure and success; that sounds a little bit contradictory, but it really isn't. If I can get rid of an endpoint and look at the *process* of what's going on, then I have a chance to take care of the things that are coming up and be alerted to them. When somebody talks about "curing" because they have a certain "I think," I have a different image. I always think of salt-cured pork because I was raised on a farm. That's probably not what you're talking about, but it could easily be that.

R. Goulding: I was thinking a little more about looking for other things. One of the things I was dissatisfied with early on was that we could do some great things at a workshop or marathon to facilitate people changing themselves, but we didn't know how to get that to stick, how to get them to hold on to those changes. That's a very important problem because people do make wonderful changes in marathons and intensive workshops, but they don't always last. One thing I did was to plan to come out to learn from Milton Erickson, whom Jeff Zeig called the only genius he ever met. Unfortunately, he died. Instead I came to the first Ericksonian conference here in Phoenix in 1980. One of the things I learned there after watching some of Erickson's tapes and listening to some of his disciples is that storytelling is wonderful. I put storytelling into my repertoire of things to do. I tell stories which help to anchor. Anchoring is a lovely word and I thank Grinder and Bandler for it because it's what we've done for a long time. Anchoring really puts it directly: How can

we anchor this person in this room today around this impasse so that the next time he gets into the same stress situation he can come back to this room rather than to his little child dropping the milk bottle? Storytelling is a great way of doing that. I thank Dr. Erickson for that.

Question: You spoke about the value of using individual therapy sometimes, adjunctively with the group, with people who have schizophrenic or certain characterological disorders. Do you see any value to using it adjunctively with people who have other kinds of disorders?

R. Goulding: Yes, there are a lot of things for which I would do individual therapy. For example, we have not been very successful with anorexics and bulimics in the way we have been treating them in the past in workshops. They need more follow-up than we've been able to give them. We get them off to a good start but we don't get them finished. I think they need a long time of good solid, supportive individual therapy as well as group therapy.

Question: You have mentioned the problem of maintaining positive changes. Could you comment on specific population groups? I do a great deal of work with sexually abused children and we have very limited time. Often the state will fund only six group sessions. Then the children are back into the system where the victim stance is again reinforced.

M. Goulding: I can't even imagine trying unless someone is doing something so that these children are not being victimized any longer in their home. I would see it as absolutely essential that parents belong to either an anonymous group, which seems to be effective in California, or a multifamily group meeting with therapists. I think it's criminal to treat children as if the treatment is going to do them any good when they go home to continue to be victimized. I just couldn't do it.

Question: That's not the type of victimization I'm talking about continuing. I'm talking about the attitude of friends at school, teachers, and others who continue to treat them like poor little abused children, and the whole facade.

Satir: Let me take a crack at that one because I've really worked with it a lot in the past and still do to some extent. First of all, I know of no way to guarantee anything. In our society today, teachers, preachers, priests, counselors of any sort are dispensing behavior messages by their communication. So one of the things that I try very hard to do is to equip people, even the kids themselves, to deal with it. I remember in certain schools where I worked with kids, there were some teachers I was not in a position to deal with, so I taught the kids how to respond. I used role-playing and taught them how to respond so that the whole burden was not on trying to do something outside but to help the victims themselves because this wouldn't be the only time they would have to deal with it. I remember working with kids as young as five, to help them understand what they could do.

It's really hard to meet all people however much I try to in the schools and other places. What we're going to take into our adulthood is our ability to do that kind of discrimination and learn that kind of judging. One sentence I use to give the kids to use was, "I hear you. Do you want to know how I feel about it?" The teachers would usually be taken so off guard that they would say, "yes." I taught the children how to say what they were feeling instead of what was wrong. That was just one piece that worked. It's not easy, for we live in a society that is not readily accessible to even being aware of what it does. So this is one piece that I deal with. Let's never underestimate the possibility of people being able to take care of themselves.

Question: I'm still curious about the issue of differentiating preferred modes of working. Could you speak to the question of when you would want to work in a family setting and when you might want somebody to work in a group, to take them away from their family and let them work in a new family to change some things?

R. Goulding: In two minutes, or less?! Trial and error is a great way of working. If something doesn't work, change it. I believe in not accepting contracts to fix broken marriages. I believe in taking contracts to fix the people who are in the broken marriage and so I'm going to do what I can so that everybody in the family group gets something out of it, out of life, together or separately. If it looks like they can get together, then it's important to work with them as a family unit. If it looks like they're not going to make it work together, then I would look at different options. How to say good-by constructively is something the lawyers haven't learned about yet.

Gestalt Therapy: Evolution and Application

◆

Miriam Polster, Ph.D.

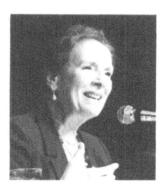

Miriam Polster, Ph.D.
Miriam Polster is Co-Director of the Gestalt Training Center in San Diego, and Assistant Clinical Professor at the Department of Psychiatry, School of Medicine, University of California, San Diego. Along with her husband, Erving Polster, she is co-author of a book on Gestalt therapy. She received her Ph.D. in Clinical Psychology from Case Western Reserve University in 1967.

Miriam Polster discusses the evolution of Gestalt psychotherapy from some of its theoretical and clinical antecedents. Principles that are the basis of present theory and practice are offered. Extending theory, she develops what she calls an "integration sequence"—the steps that one follows in integrating new behavior.

No theory springs full-blown from the head of its creator—and Gestalt therapy is no exception. Frederick Perls was as much a product of his times and experience as was Freud. And, as Freud was influenced by Charcot, for example, so Perls was influenced by others, including Freud.

I will begin with a short summary of some of the psychological and psychotherapeutic antecedents of Gestalt therapy, in order to illustrate both the impact of these theories and the brilliant ability of Perls and his wife, Laura, to synthesize, uniting disparate parts into a new formulation which reflected the contemporary needs and knowledge of a different generation. Following that, I shall discuss three concepts which are basic to the theory and practice of Gestalt therapy. I will

conclude by offering a perspective—consonant with Gestalt theory—which may illuminate certain essential sequences in the course of psychotherapy.

EARLY INFLUENCES AND PERLS' FORMULATIONS

First of all, anyone who does therapy today is hugely indebted to the insights provided by Sigmund Freud. The implications of his assertion that mankind was driven by impulses and motives which were not rational, or even conscious, shocked a generation that prided itself on its capacity to reason, and then to act in conformity with such rational decision. Into this smug society, Freud introduced the suggestion that much behavior which seemed self-crippling was the result of experience and impulse which were *not* under rational control; his therapeutic belief—and one to which Perls also subscribed—was that the cure resides in self-knowledge. Both Freud and Perls conducted "raids" on the unacknowledged and unrecognized determinants of neurotic behavior, trusting that this knowledge was essential to good function. Freud used the illuminating power of insight; the patient agreed to speak freely, to let his/her thoughts flow unhindered as much as possible, and the analyst facilitated self-discovery by the careful timing of interpretive statements.

The Gestalt equivalent to the analytic sequence of free association-interpretation-insight is the awareness continuum. The patient increasingly concentrates on the simple components of experience and it is this process of awareness, mediated by the patient him/herself, that culminates in self-knowledge.

Another important influence on Perls' formative experience was Carl Jung. Mystical, almost poetic in his conception of the struggle for individuation, Jung had confidence in the human impulse for expression. He differed from Freud, therefore, in his attitude toward patients' dreams. Freud saw in the dream an attempt of material from the unconscious to escape and dominate. In this struggle of the repressed against censorship, the dream was a battleground of disguise, evasion, and distortion. Jung, on the other hand, viewed the dream as a creative effort wherein the dreamer grappled with contradiction, complexity, and confusion, trying to express these dilemmas as fully as possible. The dream was not an attempt to disguise but rather to express. It was a creative urge, cunningly using symbolic representations of aspects of concern in the dreamer's life. Its aim was resolution and integration. Furthermore, Jung viewed each element in the dream as an aspect of the dreamer, and each person's individuation required a reincorporation of these projected qualities.

Perls advanced Jung's conception of the dream as projection by having a dreamer play out parts of the dream and, in doing so, reclaim what s/he previously disowned. In addition to reowning projected parts of the self, Gestalt therapy also conceives of the dream as a setting for making contact with others (Polster & Polster, 1973).

Another formulation of Jung's which is relevant to Gestalt therapy was his understanding of the polarities inherent in human nature. He cast these dualities in archetypal characters such as anima and animus, or in the concept of the shadow—the obscure but inevitable companion to the public persona. Otto Rank was influenced by Jung's concept of polarities and it was through his work that Perls became interested.

Perls' genius at extending what he learned from others led him to perceive the energy bound in the polar struggle and to devise a methodology—the use of dialogue and of the empty chair—to release this energy and put it at the practical service of the troubled individual. Perls' characterization of topdog/underdog can be seen as a more dynamic restatement of Jung's shadow versus the persona. The struggle between topdog/underdog also often appears similar to the clash between id and superego. Underdog speaks for the resentment, reluctance, and subversive impulse of the disrespected or disregarded aspects of the person. The enlivening addition of dialogue between these warring parts reveals the ways in which underdog subverts: through confusion, pseudostupidity, laziness, or just plain hostility. Through dialogue it is possible to reach a new level of respect and understanding which can resolve the debilitating conflict.

Two gifted and inventive divergences from classic Freudian thought also influenced Perls. Wilhelm Reich (1949) was actively curious about the *how* of human behavior. This resulted in his observations about the body as both the expressor and repository of the problems and experiences of the individual. The body incarnates habitual structures that reveal and record attempts to resolve these conflicts. Reich's view of the body was more real than Freud's, whose autoerotic zones are more concept than flesh and blood and deal primarily with only three bodily areas: the mouth, the anus, and the penis. Reich's theory depicts the sensate nature of the whole body and explores the relation of body armor to character armor. Perls' work advances this attention to the body, finding in gesture and posture relics of past experience, attending to them instead of ignoring them, permitting them to move past petrified habit into adaptive present activity.

Two more aspects of Rank's influence on Perls deserve mention. Rank respected creativity and perceived the creativity contained in the production of what other therapists labelled symptoms. He insisted that this effort deserved to be dealt with more respectfully—not as resistance to be exorcised—but as a creative function which represented an attempt to solve a dilemma. After all, the patient is not trying to create a symptom but an answer to a troublesome situation. This attitude finds its parallel in the Gestalt concept of creative adjustment (Perls, Hefferline, & Goodman, 1951), where the individual creatively balances personal needs and environmental opportunity.

Respect for the creativity of the patient also pervaded Rank's attitude about the nature of the therapeutic relationship. He was one of the early advocates emphasizing the importance of the relationship between therapist and patient. Instead of the distancing concept of transference and analytic neutrality, Rank held that therapeutic leverage depended, in large part, on the person-to-person interaction between therapist and patient. Gestalt therapy's emphasis on contact is a logical extension of this idea; it emphasizes the relationship of organism to environment and of patient to therapist.

Both Kurt Lewin and Kurt Goldstein were acutely aware of the importance of environmental and organismic influences on human behavior. Lewin masterfully explored the impact of the environment on the person. He did this in topographical representations of the individual in a life-space, in classic sociological experiments which investigated approach/avoidance conflicts and the influence of groups and group leadership on individual behavior (Marrow, 1969).

Goldstein (Hall & Lindzey, 1970) studied brain-damaged veterans of World War I and observed how the entire personality of the veteran reorganized itself to accommodate to his diminished capacities in dealing with his surroundings. He identified the *catastrophic reaction* and described some of its sequelae: increased psychological rigidity, greater emphasis on superficial orderliness, and a reduced capacity for abstract thought. All were attempts by the veteran to decrease the likelihood of surprise, of unpredictable or excessive environmental demand. Perls' concept of the *catastrophic expectation* of the neurotic can be seen as an extension of Goldstein's analysis. Here, psychological trauma replaces or accompanies physical trauma—and the incapacity may result from the *unwillingness* to confront troublesome issues, in addition to, or instead of, actual inability.

It was from the Gestalt psychologists that Perls learned of the powerful organizational skill underlying human perception. Their most basic principle was the organizing perception of figure and ground. A figure of interest invites the lively response of the viewer, and the background fades, supporting the current figure and offering a source for new figures yet to come. Perls extended this concept beyond purely perceptual behavior and expanded it into an analogy for units of human experience. From these, and other Gestalt principles of learning, Perls applied the activity of Gestalt formation as problem-solving efforts whose interruption springs from neurotic inhibition. A fixed Gestalt is a figure which is not surrendered by the perceiver. S/he insists on perceiving it as static, not risking the inevitable evolution into new figures because of a neurotic attachment to things-as-they-are. In this fashion, the individual's behavior remains archaic because it is not focused on actuality but is dominated by habitual coping with the painful past or the dreaded future.

Gestalt learning theorists also discovered the persistence in memory of experience which feels incomplete or interrupted. From this concept Perls developed his view of unfinished business and how its perseveration interferes with present experience. The person is so inhabited by past incompletions that s/he remains preoccupied with stale concerns. Until these persistent distractions can be resolved, for example, through dialogue reenactment or fantasy, they will continue to compete for attention and prevent full and satisfying engagement in the present.

BASIC PRINCIPLES IN GESTALT THERAPY

Gestalt therapy evolved from these traditions to an emphasis that insists on the relevance of the environment in any appraisal of individual behavior. In *Gestalt Therapy* (Perls, Hefferline & Goodman, 1951), the book which delineates his theory most completely, Perls et al. state:

There is no single function of any animal that completes itself without objects and environment, whether one thinks of vegetative functions like nourishment and sexuality, or perceptual functions, or motor functions, or feeling, or reasoning . . . every human function is an interacting in an organism/environment field, sociocultural, animal, and physical. (p. 228)

Gestalt therapy proposes that the relationship of the individual to his/her environment is growthful and exciting and that the basic element in this relationship is contact. Good function, therefore, can be assessed by the quality of contact, by the ability of the individual to respond flexibly and creatively, with persistence

and clarity within an environment that invites interest and is responsive to his/her needs. Perls et al. (1951) describe this process:

the materials and energy of growth are: the conservative attempt of the organism to remain as it has been, the novel environment, the destruction of previous partial equilibria, and the assimilation of something new. (p. 373)

This sequence is disrupted when there is an overpowering need for the person to perceive a situation as unchanging or as containing no novel elements. To foster this illusion, s/he then inhibits perception and remains stuck in past circumstances, viewing either him/herself as incapable of change or viewing the situation as equally intransigent. This situation is what Perls et al. (1951) called a *chronic low-grade emergency*.

In Gestalt therapy, there are three therapeutic instrumentalities to dislodge the psychological stand-off and to restore momentum and excitement to the stale situation. These are awareness, contact, and experiment.

AWARENESS

The fluidity of awareness is equivalent to the perceptual flow of figure/ground, where new figures succeed one another in effortless progression and the individual's experience is one of interested participation in a lively and engrossing environment. Ideally, awareness is determined by the individual's needs and moves sequentially between an internally mediated focus and responsive attention to the environment. It is in the nature of the individual to move energetically from experience to experience, reacting to what is novel—be it internal sensation or external event—and engaging with it as long as the interest or need lasts. This process is apparent as we watch any healthy infant. Neurotic interruption occurs when the individual has erroneously diminished faith either in him/herself or in his/her environment.

Recovery of the acceptability of awareness—no matter what it may reveal—is a crucial step along the road to the development of new behavior. For one thing, the willingness to be open to new experience, come what may, is already a new level of courage and a step out of stale habit. It is a return to the fluidity of experience, instead of the *fixed gestalt* that excessive or dysfunctional anxiety commands. This courage initially requires the assistance of the therapist in mobilizing the self-support system of the individual—a sequence which I will describe in greater detail later.

Awareness has three major characteristics. First, it is a continuous means for keeping up-to-date with oneself. It is an ongoing process, readily available when needed. The focus of one's awareness can range through the awareness of sensations, of feelings, of wants, of personal values, and of appraisals or expectations. The therapist can concentrate on these components of experience, staying with them and amplifying them until the patient moves organically into some form of expressive action.

The second characteristic of awareness follows from the first. It produces a build-up in arousal which demands expressive discharge, not merely on a cathartic level, although this is not to be dismissed lightly, but also in order to evoke a responsive echo from something or someone in the world outside. The person is impelled to a sense of mutual interaction in which s/he moves and is, in turn, moved by an event which includes, but is not limited to, the self.

Awareness has a third attribute. Not only does it lead to expressive and contactful engagement with what is outside the person, but it also caps or completes this sequence by sensing and registering that something did indeed happen. The confirming influence of awareness includes the recognition of success or pleasure, a sense of satisfaction. Completed, and rec-

ognized as complete, the individual is free to move into new experience, free to become interested in what comes next. The fixity which was required by the neurotic expectation of catastrophe and the excessive preoccupation with unfinished business is nudged back into movement. The self-imposed stalemate is eased out of familiar but unsatisfying territory, and the client begins to explore fresh experience— which might inspire fresh living. Awareness accompanies this movement; and one notes when the dreaded catastrophe did not materialize, or when it does, the person can note that s/he faced the catastrophe with ingenuity and courage. This cycle may have to be repeated many times in order to lay the unfinished situation to rest. Each time the process must be accompanied by awareness which will make it a vital experience, not just a stale rehash of previous events.

A young woman patient was all practical do's and don't's. There was hardly a statement in therapy that she didn't immediately make into an order or a recommendation for herself to carry out immediately. One session we spent most of the hour just attending to what she became aware of, reducing her experience to its simple essentials: what she was aware of sitting in her chair; what it was like for her to be in my office; what it was like for her to have her hand on her knee; what it was like to lean forward and move her head; and so on. She surprised herself by not moving immediately from awareness into giving herself orders to "do something" about it. Her delight in being able to notice what simple things were happening, without plaguing herself into making them productive in her accustomed fashion, was a joy to see. For her, it was an entirely new way to move about in her environment.

CONTACT

It is no news to anyone that life is full of paradox and that much of our energy goes into trying to resolve or, more realistically, to live with inconsistency and contradiction. In Gestalt therapy, paradox is apparent in the relationship between the organism and its environment. Perls et al. (1951) observed that every organism maintains itself in its environment by heightening and remaining acutely aware of its difference. Even so, the human organism is an open system, not at all totally self-sufficient, requiring for survival and growth that it receive sustenance—physical and psychological—from the world outside of itself. Air and food must be taken in, companionship must be provided, so that each human creature can flourish. Growth is therefore best understood as the interaction between the organism and its environment, whereby the organism assimilates the environment according to its needs and according to the generosity of environmental conditions.

Awareness is a mediating prerequisite in this sequence because it is through awareness that the environment is perceived as novel, as worthy of attention. This perception, while heightening the separateness of the perceiver, also draws him/her toward closer interaction, toward contact with this otherness, whatever it may be—an eclair, a sunset, an easy chair, or another person. This contactful interaction can take many forms: obstacles may be overcome or averted, nourishing objects are taken in and digested, useful information is heard and selectively adopted, dangers are rejected or shunned, appealing people are approached, while toxic or feared people are avoided, and so forth.

The concept of the contact-boundary is Gestalt therapy's formulation, recognizing the paradoxical nature of contact, where the organism maintains its separateness, while at the same time seeking assimilation and union. The contact-boundary is the *organ* (Perls et al., 1951, p. 229) of the meeting between the individual and his/her milieu, at which, in moments of good contact, there is both a clear sense of oneself and a clear sense of the other. The energy inspired and used in this meeting risks a momentary loss of self in order to make the meeting more poignant. This is not a decision deliberately made, but rather a merging into the surge of the moment when the union between self and other is irresistible. The clear sense of oneself can be risked precisely because, in the healthy individual, it is sensed as reliable and stable, and therefore recoverable. In contact, the energy of the individual is aimed at a satisfying completion of the interaction between self and other—completion, but *not* perpetuation (Perls, et al., 1951, p. 420).

Contact, then, is the continually renewed and renewing creative adjustment of the individual and his/her environment. It is through contact that novelty is responded to with interest and reworked into usefulness and relevance. Contact uses and produces excitement as the basic fuel which supports the individual during moments of strong concern. It is the lifeblood of growth, using all the responsive capacity of the individual. In good contact there is always "cooperation of sense and movement (and also feeling)" (Perls et al., 1951, p. 228).

When arousal is unwelcome there will be an attempt to subdue it, by constricted breathing, dulled vision, incomplete hearing, failure to understand, confusion, numbness, and so on. These inhibitions divert energy which could be available for rich contact and keep it bound up in maintaining the state of pseudo nonexcitement that neurotic self-regulation requires for reassurance. This is an artificial and uneasy calm, a stand-off, where the person deadens his/her responsiveness and devotes his/her energy to prolonging suppression and minimizing contact.

Every person decides what will be for him/her the limits of permissible contacts. This I-boundary (Polster & Polster, 1973) determines what psychological territory s/he is willing to venture into; where to go; whom to be with; what ideas to believe; what wishes to permit; what images to entertain—in short, how fully s/he will participate in those arenas where contact might contain threatening or unpredictable possibilities.

The I-boundary determines the selectivity about contact which governs a style of life—which actions are permissible and which are out of the question. For example, there was the young woman who was reluctant to appear as the stereotyped ninny-about-things-mechanical which she thought all men believed. As a result, she was uncomfortable about going into a service station and asking the attendant how to use the air hose to inflate the tires on her bike. Instead of viewing this as a chance to learn something she wanted to know, she saw it as an indictment of her character, and yet another chapter in her ongoing battle with know-it-all men. Her I-boundary required that she not appear stupid. The irony was that this requirement perpetuated her ignorance.

I-boundaries are the archeological record of the experiences of the person as s/he progresses to the present moment; the experiential background, if you will, for the figural present contact-possibilities. It is at the I-boundary where opportunities for growth are most probable. It is here also that improvisation and courage are often required because the circumstances are more likely to be unfamiliar and one's response is untried and risky. The spirit of improvisation which has been stifled by neurotic self-regulation needs to be activated to support more nourishing interaction between the individual and his/her world.

EXPERIMENT

Experiment is a Gestalt technique aimed at restoring momentum to the stuck points of a person's life. It is one way to recover the connection between deliberation and spontaneity by bringing the possibilities for action right into the therapy room. Through experiment, the patient is mobilized to confront the emergencies of his/her life by playing out troublesome situations or relationships in the comparative safety of the therapeutic setting. This is a safe emergency. Safety and emergency are actually components whose proportion can be calibrated to reflect the patient's needs at various points in the therapy, incorporating the advances made during the course of therapy and extending them into newer levels of experience. The therapist observes whether the experiment seems too safe or too risky and makes suggestions that change the ratio of safety to emergency. For example, to imagine doing or saying something to the therapist or to another group member is less of an emergency than actually doing it and may unearth some of the same information. Alternately, adding gestures and volume to something that was only muttered softly adds to the sense of daring and emergency.

There are several forms that a Gestalt experiment might take involving the enactment of an important aspect of a person's life: dramatizing the memory of a painful or profound experience; imagining a dreaded encounter; staging a dialogue between the patient and otherwise unavailable, but influential, characters in his/her life; playing one's father, mother, or some other person who is important to the patient; setting up a dialogue between isolated or disrespected parts of the patient; attending to an otherwise overlooked gesture, grimace, or posture and allowing it to evolve into broader expressive possibilities, and so on.

Dreamwork is another activity which Perls (1969, 1973) explored in his demonstrations and writings. The Gestalt view of dreams as projection, where the dreamer has cast him/herself into each of the constituents of the dream, is well known. These cast out parts of the dreamer must be reowned and assimilated as relevant information in the experience of the dreamer. There are other opportunities in dreamwork, however. The dream may contain representations of central people or concerns in the dreamer's life, so dreamwork may focus (through dialogue) on improving the contact between the dreamer and these figures (Polster & Polster, 1973).

The dream may be seen as a retroflective act where the dreamer, in a sense, communicates with him/herself rather than the therapist, and the process can be reversed by addressing the therapist directly (Isadore From, personal communication). The dream may be used as theater where the dreamer can, in a group, cast other members as parts of the dream, and its relevance may extend beyond the dreamer into the significance that the parts they have played may hold for the other participants. (Zinker, 1977).

THE INTEGRATION SEQUENCE

The process of growth is usually a fitful one, oscillating between rewarding experience—where advances in therapy are mirrored in successful consequences—and episodes of discouragement—where what has been accomplished in the therapy session appears to work badly or not at all when tried out in everyday circumstances.

It is important to pay attention to this uneven pattern of progress and identify some of the factors which may be at work during the gradual improvement that all therapists seek. I propose an orienting principle that I call *the integration sequence;* this is the sequence of stages that culminates in the integration of new behavior within the I-boundaries of the individual, where it becomes an indistinguishable "given" in the range of permissible experience; where the person feels whole or entire and the possibilities for fresh, unstereotyped interaction between the individual and his/her environment are increased.

DISCOVERY

The first part of this three-stage sequence is the phase of *discovery.* It is at this point that something novel occurs— a new realization about oneself, a novel view of a familiar situation or belief, or a new look at another person or event.

This realization often comes with a sense of surprise and a temporary absorption in the discovery, which momentarily blots out distracting perceptions and leaves the patient with a heightened sense of figural discovery but with a diminished awareness of context. The discovery is figural and the customary support system of the patient is caught by surprise, unprepared for the rush of excitement—either welcome or unwanted—that arises. This is what Perls et al. (1951) call an *aperiodic* process, occurring irregularly; as contrasted with periodic processes, such as hunger, which occur predictably and with regularity. In this condition the attention of the individual is withdrawn from the environment and focused instead on the body; the therapeutic focus is on the supportive functions that the patient can provide for him/herself and extends into the possibilities for environmental support of which he/she may not be aware at the moment.

The personal supports of the patient are threefold. First, the patient's breathing may be constricted or disrupted and therefore does not support the rise of arousal. Regular and rhythmic breathing must be established so that the patient's excitement is not only supported by the better supply of oxygen, but also because regular breathing can help to distribute the excitement throughout the body rather than limiting it to a narrowed and concentrated locus, for example, in the upper chest. This confinement contributes to a sense of strain and is experienced as anxiety. Breathing is also one of the most basic exchanges between the individual and the environment. It reflects a sense that the environment is safe to take in and to use for purposes of self-support. Finally, breathing is a subtly optimistic function. It implies that the person is going to exist a little while longer and it reestablishes momentum, if only for a moment. This is a nonverbal process—a metaphor. The resumption of regular breathing suggests a crisis has been met and is presently being traversed, the situation is in flux, it is not static. The customary stuckness is challenged.

Second, the patient needs to experience the support that his/her skeletal and muscular system can provide: to feel the support of his/her legs and pelvis, if standing; to feel his or her shoulders positioned so that the chest is not cramped; and to note that movement can be supported by muscular coordination and strength. This can involve the surprise of the return of sensation to a previously numbed or constricted part of the body or the extension of a gesture beyond the limited range it had been allowed. For example, a woman learns to feel the strength of her own legs as she plays out in fantasy a confrontation with her dictatorial husband. A young man discovers that he enjoys making broad sweeping gestures with his arms instead of trying to remain colorless and stiff— in contrast to his flamboyant but unreliable father.

Third of the personal supports is the cognitive ability of the patient. Perls (1969) noted that one of the main techniques of the underdog is to play dumb, to forget or deny some knowledge that might facilitate or support the patient in time of emergency. Therefore, a patient may feel overwhelmed by the realization that she wants to speak angrily to her mother and scared that she might come on too strong. The memory of what her mother has endured—being orphaned at an early age, coming to a strange and unfamiliar country as a nine-year-old immigrant, losing a baby, tending to a dying relative—can provide proportion that places an angry confrontation with a daughter a little lower on the scale. Perls et al. (1951) observed that "It is the accepted way of posing the problem, and not the problem, that is taken for reality" (p. 394). To get a fresh restatement of the problem, or a new way of looking at some of its features, to make new connections or deductions can prove supportive and encouraging in moments of discovery.

In addition, there are two sources of support from the environment in which

discovery is made. First, the therapeutic setting: the quiet and seclusion of the office or group meeting room, the confidentiality assured in the therapeutic contact, and the guarantee of time adequate to confront the arousal of discovery. These important elements can sustain the patient during a difficult time.

Second, there is the person of the therapist. In appearing to be a person of some scope and personal experience and in the sense of having seen other people through dramatic personal explorations, the therapist provides perspective and support, suggesting—not necessarily in words but often in spirit—that there will be a next moment, and then a next. . .

It is apparent that most of these elements have the power to restore momentum to the breathless instant of discovery, when it seems that time itself stands still. It may need to stand still, in order to experience and to plumb the significance that the moment of discovery holds. The restoration of momentum is a beginning of the movement to place that stand-out minute in time back into the ongoing chronicle of the patient's life.

ACCOMMODATION

The second stage of the integration sequence is the stage of *accommodation*. Therapists are unwilling to settle for exciting insights that occur only in therapy and have little to do with how the patient actually lives in the everyday world to which s/he returns after the session. The accommodation phase is that necessary step where the patient begins to behave in his/her actual world in accord with the discoveries made during therapy. This is the point at which the patient realizes some of the implications and consequences of the original discovery and makes further adjustments which could not have been predicted initially. The patient who discovers the depth of his/her own sexuality may begin to react differently to friends and acquaintances and evoke a different reaction from them. Their reaction—differing from the supportive or concerned response of the therapist—can call for the patient to improvise, faithful to the spirit of the earlier discovery, but moving beyond it into fuller discovery and exploration of its implications in his/her interactions outside therapy. People will respond uniquely and unpredictably, sensitive primarily to their own needs and not necessarily reacting as the patient may have predicted. In this stage the environment has expanded outside the therapist's office, it responds unexpectedly, and the patient is forced to improvise, for better or worse.

It is at this stage where behavior may be awkward and poorly coordinated, and the patient feels clumsy. There are distractions, as contrasted with the single-minded focus of the therapy session. The world is not as obliging as one might like: People have headaches or indigestion, or they have an appointment, or they may just be uninterested. The patient may manage this complication ineptly and become discouraged. The therapeutic task is to continue with the mobilization of the patient's self-support systems. Environmental supports at this juncture are often less reliable and the patient's ingenuity and adaptability are challenged. The physical supports mentioned earlier, breathing, posture, and movement, sustain the patient bodily, but now they serve an additional purpose. They help tolerate the excitement and, furthermore, they temper the disruptive effect of too much sensation. In doing this, the cognitive system of the patient, which is crucial to adaptability, is more able to cope with the present situation, improvising and varying behavior instead of being frozen into inaction or habit.

The support system must allow the patient to move past exclusive focus on him/herself—an indulgence granted in the therapy sessions—and to pay closer attention to the effect that his/her words and actions have on others. This sensitivity to circumstance makes for more effec-

tive and rewarding interaction, for better quality contact. Furthermore, it signals a move out of excessive preoccupation either with oneself or with one's stale concerns and greater accessibility for engagement with others.

The ability to identify and locate environmental supports may be part of the preparation in therapy for the accommodation phase of the work. For example, a young woman suffered from debilitating anxiety attacks whenever she went to eat in restaurants. In therapy we worked with her management of anxiety attacks: restoring her spasmodic breathing, identifying some of the background concerns underlying her anxiety, articulating how she scared herself and what she feared would happen in the restaurant. Then, we began to deal with her fantasies of going into a restaurant, identifying what she would need to feel more comfortable there. Her main fear was that her anxiety would be so severe that she would vomit and everyone would see her. The plan we arrived at was, first, that she would eat several times in a drive-in, where she could stay in her own car. The next step was for her to go to a regular sit-down restaurant and select a table near the women's room so that she could get there in a hurry if she had to.

ASSIMILATION

The third phase of the integration sequence is *assimilation* . What was at first a novel and innovative experience now seems more possible and representative; it is felt to be "like me" to do, think, or feel differently than before. At this stage, behavior is in the middle mode between spontaneity and deliberateness. The individual feels capable of dealing with the surprises that s/he might encounter—or even generate—and considers that the chances for a successful, or at least necessary, outcome are pretty good. The attitude combines an awareness of risk with a mixture of feelings ranging from optimism to determination. The patient's support system is sensed as dependable and his/her behavior has a range of inventiveness which will stand him/her in good stead.

Often the behavior at this stage is situation-bound; that is, it is in response to a certain individual—as when a 40-year-old man reacted differently to his mother's disapproval, or when a social worker recognized her own needs enough to tell her supervisor that she was getting inadequate supervision. Or it may be a reaction to specific circumstances—speaking up in class or at a staff conference or at a family dinner. Behavior at this stage may sometimes feel like "taking a stand."

INTEGRATION

Integration, or when the new behavior or attitude fits seamlessly within the person's I-boundaries, is the final result of a unit of therapeutic work. This is the stage when the individual is able to respond in effortless and unself-conscious involvement with the situation-at-hand. Behavior has the quality of undeliberate response, where situation and person seem mutually interactive and where the result is a reciprocal exchange of influence, with a minimum amount of preconceived conditions or restrictions. By effortless, I do not mean that there is no work or energy involved; but it will be the interaction that commands attention. Behavior is directed by the organismic ordering of the individual's needs, in concert with what the environment offers.

CONCLUSION

Many years ago I taught psychology at an art school. One of the questions raised by students who learned that psychology is a science was, "If it's so scientific, why are there so many theories of personality?" Obviously I could not avoid the issue

by merely pointing out that physicists have the same problem and they are workers in the hardest of the "hard" sciences. By way of introduction, then, one morning I asked my students to fantasize that there was a model for a life drawing class in the middle of our room and that in various parts of the room were Rembrandt, Modigliani, Gainsborough, Van Gogh, Picasso and Renoir, each painting from the model. Which one of the paintings would be the *true* one?

So it is with a theory of therapy. To claim that there is only one right way is presumptuous and, even more important, untrue. Each methodology evolves because its perspective illuminates some of the darker corners of contemporary existence and merges with the insights of theorists who have gone before. Gestalt therapy was born of the union between a fertile mind and a fertile milieu. What maintains the vitality of the theory is its growth in subtlety and application—through the enduring contributions of Perls and his colleagues, and through their students. It is a rich and elegant theory, providing orientation and range for therapeutic choice.

REFERENCES

Hall, C.S., & Lindzey, G. (1970). *Theories of personality* (2nd ed.). New York: John Wiley and Sons.

Marrow, A.J. (1969). *The practical theorist: The life and work of Kurt Lewin*. New York: Basic Books.

Perls, F.S. (1969). *Gestalt therapy verbatim*. Lafayette, CA: Real People Press.

Perls, F.S. (1973). *The Gestalt approach and eye witness to therapy*. Palo Alto, CA: Science and Behavior Books.

Perls, F.S., Hefferline, R.F., & Goodman, P. (1951). *Gestalt therapy*. New York: Julian Press.

Polster, E., & Polster, M. (1973). *Gestalt therapy integrated*. New York: Brunner/Mazel.

Rank, O. (1975). *Art and the artist* (reprinted). New York: Agathon Press.

Reich, W. (1949). *Character analysis*. New York: Orgone Institute Press.

Zinker, J. (1977). *Creative process in gestalt therapy*. New York: Brunner/Mazel.

Discussion by Robert L. Goulding, M.D.

◆

When the book of this conference comes out, take this chapter and read it again and again and again.

This is the very core not of Gestalt therapy but of therapy. The beautiful illustration of how we stick ourselves and of some of the ways in which we can get out of that stuck place could not be more elegant. This is a succinct paper. The thing I like about the Polsters' writing is that it is so literate. I don't know how many of you have read *Gestalt Therapy Integrated* (New York: Brunner/Mazel, 1973). As I read it, I thought I was reading Hemingway or someone who knows how to write. The Polsters know how to write.

I was delighted to hear something that Miriam said along the way. I worked with Fritz Perls quite a bit in the early days and I remember Fritz saying over and over, "Lose your head and come to your senses." And for years I had a picture, somewhat like Ichabod Crane, of my patients wandering around the world with their head underneath their armpit and I'm delighted that Miriam put the head back where it belongs.

One of the wonderful things about Gestalt therapy is keeping things in the here and now. I was delighted to see her put this meeting room back in the context in terms of the here and now of Gestalt therapy in dealing with the current problems as they arise.

I have some questions I'd like to raise. You mentioned how the Gestalt learnings theorist discovered the persistence in memory of experience which feels incomplete or interrupted. From this concept Perls developed his view of the unfinished business, how its separation interferes with present experience, and how the job of the theorist is to close the old openings of the unfinished gestalts. This is what I'd like to bring in our own framework. This is Redecision therapy—getting back to that stuck place, the impasse, and helping that patient to end, to close, to finish the unfinished business of that time. This is a beautiful help for me, this whole paper, helping to explain to people what we mean by Redecision therapy.

The question I have is about integration. One of the questions my own students raise is that Gestaltists say that everything should be integrated, but how do you deal with that when you talk about saying good-by to parts? For instance, a suicidal client is dealing with some of the early messages that he got from his parents where he experiences one of his parents as being angry with a scowling face. When he's sitting in the other chair, he's being that parent, saying, "I wish you were dead, I wish you'd never been born!" What is the response that succeeds in finishing that? I don't know how to integrate that part of the parent that is so scowling, murderous, disruptive. I teach my people to say good-by to that part. I would appreciate some kind of response from the Polsters on how they see that integration.

RESPONSE BY DR. M. POLSTER

The question is, "How do you integrate what you want to forget?" I suppose if I were paradoxically inclined I could say, "I want you to remember it and hold a memorial service for it once a week. Establish a nice ceremonial in which you do obeisance to the past, over and over again." That might make them sick enough of it to forget it. But I would also say, "Perhaps you don't need to forget it, perhaps you just need to assume that it is a piece of your life that has painful and prickly aspects. It's there but you don't have to go back to it over and over again. It may never be 'forgotten.' "

QUESTIONS AND ANSWERS

Question: I'd like to ask about a point you made almost in passing, but somehow to me it relates to what you were just discussing. You said that the relation between top dog and underdog was similar to the Jungian psychology of shadow and persona, which I think is more or less accurate. The other parallel that you made was between the Freudian superego and the id, which I believe is not as accurate. The way Perls formulated it was that if you have a superego you must have an infraego. This was the part that Freud overlooked, that the top dog and underdog are both together in authentic parts of the organism, rather than the id. If you want to use the Freudian formulation, the id is part of the original organism. What we have with top dog and underdog is an introject. An introject is not assimilable as opposed to an identification or something you can use and digest. I think that when you have something you're working on, some demand that the parents made upon you that is not assimilable, like "Don't be yourself," you have an introject that is not assimilable. With introjects, one does not get rid of one's parents but one gets rid of the demand not to be oneself. One spits it out.

M. Polster: As to the question whether the id is the underdog and the top dog is the superego, I was comparing it to polar struggles. There are certain classic polar struggles. In that sense, I was referring to one of the classic divisions that we find in individuals. There is also in *Gestalt Therapy* by Perls, Hefferline, and Goodman (New York: Dell, 1951) a strong description and a translation, if you will, of some of the original Freudian terms into the way Gestalt views them. The id in that definition was regarded as the back-

ground, the habitual, the state of the body on its own. The superego also can be construed as composed of the introject, the shoulds, the should nots. I would argue with you that the introjects have to be merely spit out. They have to be spit out, possibly reexamined and then redigested in a choiceful condition rather than the unchoiceful, force-feeding that accompanied their origin. What you might do with an introject is to spit it out, take a look at it, and swallow some of it back down again after reworking so it is appropriate to you rather than merely a rehash of the bromides you may have been given as a child.

Question: I wonder if you could comment or explain further the word need, as it is used in Gestalt, the fact that the organism moves toward fulfilling a particular need? It seems to me that is something that arises within the individual. I wonder, too, about behavior or interaction with something that is novel arising in the environment and how that is described? Isn't there something beyond need in the sense of lack?

M. Polster: Certainly we would start with some of the most basic survival needs, the need for air, the need for water, the need for food, the necessity to defecate, the desirability of companionship, some of the needs that we would feel make us healthy physically and psychologically.

As to the second part of your question, it is through this need for fascination, which is not necessarily a deficit need, that very exciting interaction with the environment is maintained. I'm reminded of the research by Harlow and Butler where monkeys would perform all sorts of complicated behaviors, the reward for which was the opportunity to look out of a window.

Question: You gave as an example a woman who had a problem with panic about vomiting and it seemed that you used a desensitization procedure. Is that really part of Gestalt?

M. Polster: Why not? I was paying attention to the quality of the contact as I did it.

Question: Could you say something more about the person of the therapist? How do you experience yourself and express that in the interaction with the client? As I look at Carl Rogers, I think about the congruent way of being, which has also been useful for me. How does the person as a therapist relate to restoring momentum and discoveries that you talked about earlier?

M. Polster: That's a very good question because we're getting here into a matter of taste, I think. Balance, proportion. What I sense about myself is that I am easier and easier with self-revelation, both verbalizing it and just presenting it, however I reveal myself, whether I'm talking or not. I am more and more at ease with that, but I am also more and more discriminating with it because there are times when it is distracting and intrusive and arrogant. So with that increasing willingness to be visible and present comes an increasing responsibility to temper it with a sense of where the person is and whether it's useful or not.

Question: One of the things I find difficult is to balance the support function as a therapist with the creative frustration. I'm aware that in myself I find it much easier and more natural and safer to offer my support. It is a little more scary to balance that with what Perls calls the creative frustration. I'd be interested in what you could say about that.

M. Polster: I do not, as a rule, try to frustrate somebody. The world is so accommodating in that way that I don't feel I have to add to it. I might pay very close attention to differentiating between support and problem solving. Thus, I may support a person in her own efforts at solving the dilemma without offering the solution to the problem. People confront us with so much frustration that, by and large, I'm unwilling to add to it. However, I will not give them the answers. For one thing, I don't have them. They know that situation better than I do, but I will accompany them as they search for the answer.

Question: So would that be the meaning of creative frustration, that you will resist the temptation to do that?

M. Polster: Yes.

Escape from the Present: Transition and Storyline

◆

Erving Polster, Ph.D

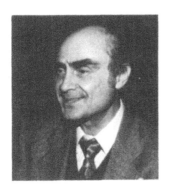

Erving Polster, Ph.D.

Erving Polster (Ph.D., Western Reserve University, 1950) is Director of the Gestalt Training Center, San Diego. He is also Associate Clinical Professor at the University of California, San Diego Medical School. Polster is co-author, with his wife Miriam, of an important text on Gestalt therapy, Gestalt Therapy Integrated.

Erving Polster discusses the place of the "here and now" in Gestalt therapy and practice. He also presents case reports that underline the importance of having patients flesh out their stories rather than merely providing the titles of their lives.

Theories of therapy require continual freshening up for at least two reasons. One is that their concepts spawn connotations which either corrupt or desert the original meanings. The other is that the concepts compete with each other for centrality and the winners in popular esteem may crowd out equally vital ones. With these sources of error in mind, I want to examine one aspect of Gestalt therapy, its here-and-now emphasis. This emphasis has been corrupted from its original intent and it has won out in centrality, crowding out other more important concepts. After

sketching the strengths and weaknesses of present orientation, I shall offer two correctives to this emphasis.

THE PRESENT AS A RALLYING POINT

For the psychotherapist, it seems only natural that the full dimensions of time and space be taken into account because things do obviously happen anytime or anyplace. It is therefore curious that the more narrow emphasis on here-and-now should have gained almost cult-like ascendancy over the past 35 years. Shortly after World War II, many people began to believe, with repercussions still going on,

---

This paper is composed of a mosaic of excerpts taken from a forthcoming book, entitled *Every Person's Life Is Worth a Novel.*

that the here-and-now was the center of psychological living. Although the reasons are not altogether evident, there are some obvious speculations. For one thing, the threat of a nuclear wipe-out offered a fearful justification for shunning the future. For another, new values concerning "relevance" were being adopted and high among them was the call for immediate gratification to replace the oppressively familiar delays for almost everything people did.

For psychotherapists, however, these common allures of the here-and-now were joined with some important technological advantages. What we found to be a therapeutic bonanza was the mind's extraordinary resiliency when it was freed to concentrate on only one thing. Focusing only on the present was a large step toward just such narrow attention. Kierkegaard (1948) long ago recommended that purity of heart was to will one thing and his credo—originally intended to invoke total attention to God—was then put to a more mundane practical application. It became clear that if you cut out all distractions, either internal or external, the resulting concentration would release new personal awareness and maximize function. Anybody studying for an exam or trying to pitch a strike in baseball knows this; yet, it is hard anyway to achieve such pointed attention.

The here-and-now emphasis served as a bridge to thorough absorption by underscoring simplicity in a world gone haywire in complexity. This narrowing of attention—dissociation, in a sense—helped to close off many debilitating habits of mind that normally fenced people in and made therapy slow going. It was an exciting turn of the psychological kaleidoscope. In this new mode, any single point of keen concentration might trip off a chain of internal events. As simple a sensation as an itch, for example, when receiving such concentration, might at first get stronger. Then it might move to another area of the body, then another, then back to the original place. In continued concentration each awareness might ignite the

next until the whole body would be warmed as though with a soft fire. The growth of sensation came like dominoes rising instead of falling, collecting waves of feeling which released pent-up energy, invigorating the person who originally only had an ignorable itch.

Such absorbing effects of simple sequences of sensation were comparably experienced in the more complex behaviors. Here-and-now dialogues with a visualized father were more dramatic than conversations *about* him, hitting pillows was more potent than telling *about* lost aggression opportunities, and expressing held back criticism right now to group members was better than discussing vague grievances. Uncounted exercises in immediacy were invented. These experiments led many people into previously unimagined highs in personal concentration. A new term, *peak experience,* became adopted as a nationally well known code word for total absorption and its scintillating consequences.

The impressive effects of concentration led to a widespread adherence to what was identified spuriously, I believe, as the power of the present. It was much easier to say *now* than *how;* and this emphasis on the present did indeed reduce the complexity of attention, fostering improved concentration. When the instruction to stay in the present caught on more readily than the more arduous mechanics of concentration, it was not long before there was a swelling of the numbers of people who endorsed the idea of living in the present. They had presumably come to realize how much they had lost by allowing their lives to be delayed and deflected. For them to put life on the back burner until some future time when they would graduate or get married or retire, understandably, was no longer acceptable. Nor was a brighter twenty-first century consoling to the underclass of the society. Many people came to believe that the present was all they had in life, the only reality.

Fritz Perls, among others, was unusually skilled in publicly demonstrating the power residing in simplified experience, and his followers were often amazed at the depths of the experiences he speedily induced. In his early theorizing, Perls (1947) emphasized the present as "an ever moving zero point of the opposites past and future" (p. 95), still recognizing the past and future as live reference points for the present. Though he never actually changed his mind, his penchant for communicating quickly and without qualification, especially when addressing mass professional audiences, led to oversimplification. Thus given over to sloganizing, Perls (1970) was moved later to write: "I have one aim only: to impart a fraction of the meaning of the word *now*. To me, nothing exists except now. Now = experience = awareness = reality. The past is no more and the future is not yet" (p. 14).

To make such distinct equations between now, on the one hand, and experience, awareness and reality, on the other, is excellent sloganizing but only loosely accurate. Since the present is simply a point on a time continuum, it is actually neither experience, nor awareness, nor reality. They are occurrences in time, not time itself, just as a jewel in a box is not the box. A person has the choice, on the one hand, to describe his sadness about his mother's death without caring about time; caring instead only about the sensations, thoughts, intentions, hopes that may enter his consciousness. On the other hand, he could also relate his sadness to time by saying that he is *still* sad about his mother's death two years ago or that he is sad because she is *soon* going to die. *All* details of experience exist within either time or space dimensions, and everybody is free to take account of these dimensions as he sees fit. Minds will not stay put and their freedom to roam over the years is self-evident.

Many of my fellow Gestalt therapists would cry foul at my sticking Perls with his own slogans. They would have a point. It is true that, in spite of its simplistic overtones, the here-and-now approach of Gestalt therapy was more comprehensive

from the beginning. A major provision giving equal billing to the there-and-then was the premise that remembering, imagining and planning are validly taken as present functions. This qualifier, though it supports illusory connotations about the present, does look beyond the present and it restores dimension. However, it suffered the fate qualifiers often do; it took a back seat. Unfortunately, the past and the future, though taken into account by most serious students of Gestalt therapy, were widely disregarded by those who were superficially knowledgeable—practitioners and lay people alike. The consequences of this misunderstanding are one element in the total cultural configuration that has popularized the notion that "the future is now."

Too tight a focus—with a highly concentrated emphasis only on the "here and now"—will foreclose on much that matters: continuity of commitment, implications of one's acts, preparation for those complexities that require preparation, dependability, responsiveness to the demands that people will assuredly be exposed to, and so on. When these inevitable requirements of living are chronically set aside for what should be only *temporary* technical purposes, alienation from large parts of the relevant society is one consequence; living life as a cliché is another.

PRESENT AS DISSOCIATION

One example of a person infected by the stereotypes about present experience will help show its *dissociative* effects. Abigail, a 25-year-old woman, was alienated from her parents who, for religious reasons, objected to her living with a man if they were not married. Though greatly distressed about her distance from them, Abigail stood firm on living with this man, whom she loved. She wanted urgently to reconcile with her parents, though not at the cost of her freedom of choice. In telling me her story, she spoke in the tone of a person younger than her 25 years, fighting her parents from a hopeless childlike position. She knew much more than they about contemporary living but she still spoke weakly. I asked her to talk out loud to her parents, imagining them sitting in my office. She said that they would ask her acidly whether she was going to get married. In response, she said she didn't want to talk about it. Normally, in actual contact with them, she would either melt while dripping tears or go into a catatonic-like paralysis. I encouraged her to be as generously verbal as she could, cashing in on her knowledge by saying what she knew to be true. Then, taking both sides, she played out the following dialogue between her and her parents:

Abigail: The reason we haven't gotten married is because we enjoy living together and I don't want to do something just because I'm supposed to . . . I have to feel like it's important inside.

Parents: (Caustically) Well, isn't the church a good enough reason for you?

Abigail: The church is very important to me. To me what is important is the spiritual part of it, to experience God. To me it's not just following the rules. According to our church, marriage is a sacrament. And I don't know why . . . I don't understand it at all. (Cries, looks confused again, resigned)

A crucial point was reached. For a moment, Abigail did well at stating her position clearly. Then, characteristically, she got confused. She couldn't make the shift from firmly knowing something in her current environment to knowing it also with her parents. Her own truths, though she believed in them, were dissociated, therefore inapplicable, when talking to her mother and father. They were from an alien world. She told me, as she visualized them, that they were looking at her critically, neither understanding her nor even attempting to. What she felt—common for her—was that she was doing something

wrong. In spite of her discomfort with her parents, she was still vaguely attached to her past, beleaguered like a punched-out fighter looking for his corner. She needed them not only for the relationship itself, but also because she felt isolated from her entire past. Her sense of disconnection was like an amputation, which cut her away from her supports, leaving her with a cosmic whine. To feel bereft about losing her parents was sad enough, but the malaise was multiplied when she invalidated her lifetime of experience, which, of course, was not owned by them.

At this point I told her she looked like she wanted to stop talking to them because she thought they wouldn't listen—but she may be stopping too soon. Whether they listen or not, she needed to get the clarity that words provide. When I asked whether she would be willing to go on with the conversation, she returned to it. Again, she played both parts, this time in a rather softer tone. Her parents told her how deeply hurt they were by her leaving the fold; they said they are worried about her wasting her life, that she has no future. In response Abigail replied,

I don't think that's the way it is. I have a darn good future. To me what's important is what I have right now, not 20, 30, 50 years from now. And it should be. I don't know what's going on that long. What I have right now has nothing to do with the future. This is the way I have chosen to live my life now—it may change, I don't know (starting to get a marked whine in her voice again and sounding contrived). What I know is that I am happy with today. (Unconvincing)

She seemed enmeshed in the liturgy about present experience. I explained to her that she started out saying she had a darn good future, then abandoned this belief by discounting the future entirely. I explained that she probably does have expectations about the future, some subtle and some quite evident. I suggested that her parents thought she was wrong when she told them the future doesn't count,

330 THE EVOLUTION OF PSYCHOTHERAPY

rather than, as she had started to say, that she merely had a different opinion about her future. She probably thought she was wrong, too, because the future does count. This was contradicted, however, by the people she associated with who were heavily present-oriented. Her confusion left her without a leg to stand on. At this point, I suggested she speak to her parents again, saying what was actually true for her.

Abigail: When you say I have no future, that has no merit, that if I'm not married it could end too easily and if I were married it couldn't and wouldn't. Nobody could just drop out of it . . . I don't think this is true . . . I believe we have a very strong commitment to each other . . . Whatever problems come up between us, we think in terms of long term, not in terms of it's good for now only and we'll not be married because it's easier to pick up and leave.

By this time, her voice had lost all trace of whining. She was clear in her gaze whereas, ordinarily, she had a questioning look on her face. She now seemed unconcerned with whether her parents accepted what she was saying. She obviously believed what she said and when I asked her how it felt to say it, she simply replied, "Clear." She now looked like she was well-grounded and later remarked about her lifetime of accumulated understandings, "It's a process of changing what I was taught and taking everything else I've learned and putting it all together."

What was apparent in Abigail's mindset was the ascendant place of the present. This focus permitted her to have a relationship that her background would not allow. Since she could not manage the contradiction, she had to cut out her parents' influence, unnecessarily also detaching from other large regions of her life. She had mistakenly equated her parents' influence with her past life. But her past—anybody's past—is much larger than her parents' attitudes and may remain as hos-

pitable background to her current life whether her parents accepted her or not. This whole interwoven mosaic of her past, present, and future became hopelessly confused, much as the state of the brainwashed person returning from Chinese internment to American culture. Putting it all together was not as hopeless a prospect as she assumed, once she recognized the truth in her own argument. Once she believed in her actual future instead of relying on dissociated jargon, her rights to her relationship to the man she loved were seen as a part of the simple continuity of her life.

To escape from the cramped scope of the here-and-now, I propose two remedies. One is to emphasize the transition point between now and next; the other is to accent the there-and-then by awakening the storytelling faculties inherent in all people.

TRANSITION AS THE CENTER OF FOCUS

First, the transitional experience: If we start by looking at the digital clock, we see an apt symbol of a fixed present. In the interests of simplicity, the digital expunges the context within which any specific time appears and it nullifies the visual experience of continuing transitional movement. For all but an infinite fraction of a whole minute, time stands still, and, always, whatever time the clock shows is the only time anybody can see. That this invention is more than a mundane convenience, representing larger social concerns, is illustrated by observations of a New Jersey educator (Jacabowitz, 1985), who noticed that children don't learn fractions as well as they once did. She wondered why and decided that, among other things, the digital clock deprives children of the direct representation of whole, part, half-past, and quarter-to, always previously visible in clocks. Nor do the digitals give any sense of before and after.

Standing against this illusory sense of

arrested time is our knowledge of the inevitability of time's passage. I propose that, built into this awareness of time's sequences, people have a surge to focus on the transition points between now and next. One simple representation of the excitement of this experience of transition is the thrill of traveling at high speeds, whether on a bicycle going downhill or in an auto going 90 miles an hour. Speed thrusts people into nextness, highly accenting the transition point, as it changes palpably in each instant.

For the reader to get a personal experience of comparably simple transitions, I suggest this experiment. As you continue to read, alter your focus slightly by attending not only to the present word but also by simultaneously anticipating the next one. Nextness is the key angle. You are always in between and always moving. Notice whether it makes a difference in your reading experience when you consciously lean into nextness. You will probably have tapped into a reservoir of your energy, creating alertness, excitement and fluidity. Leaning forward might also cost you a measure of comprehension, particularly if you move ahead more quickly than you can readily coordinate. If you have already been accustomed to focusing on the transitional, it is probably easier; many readers already do this spontaneously, actively anticipating nextness.

There may be some eyebrows raised by this perspective. Isn't this a frantic way to live, always alert to whatever is next, never settling into whatever is already going on, rushing headlong into the future? Though people may, of course, stumble over themselves trying to get ahead into nextness or trying to predict what is next, what is proposed here is nothing so clamorous as that. Rather it is a reminder of the naturalness of movement into the future—normally effortless and ingenuous. A telephone rings and we head toward it. A sentence emerges from a strung-out series of individual words. A question is followed by an answer. Events flow naturally, one after the other, just like the more primitive sequences of inhaling and exhaling or landing after leaping. Unless called to our attention, generally we don't even notice the relationship of one moment to the next.

This trip through continuity is, of course, not always so easy as these reflexive and peaceful sequences might intimate. Instead, the management of sequences often is filled with complexity or danger, which slows us down or even stops us. Every event, whether simple, like a single word or a flickering in facial color, or complex, like a policy announcement by the government, will point *arrows* into the future. As one illustration of the varieties of direction possible even in simple circumstances, note the headwaiter in a restaurant who says, "Your table is ready now." Almost always if you hear these words you will readily follow the waiter to your table. The choice of arrows is clearly made and you ride it happily forward. Even in this simple exchange, however, there may be elements which create greater complexity. You might have wanted a table outdoors and the waiter is leading you indoors; you might have waited an hour and feel either relieved or annoyed; or you might suddenly remember a phone call you must make. Nevertheless, in spite of unique personal possibilities, the direction of arrows most likely will move you toward the table.

Where there is a larger array of competing arrows, some luminous, some dim, a greater sensitivity will be required. Suppose, for example, that a friend says to me, "I want to call Henry." Simple words, leading to a simple act. If, however, I forsee unhappy implications of her calling Henry, I might warn against it. Or, I might remain silent, believing I shouldn't interfere and hoping it will not work out as badly as I suspect it might. Or, my friend's tone of voice may relieve me as I think she is at last going to call Henry and I may smile happily. Or, knowing my friend as I do, I may realize she doesn't really want to call Henry herself; that she would prefer that *I* do it. I then may offer to

332 THE EVOLUTION OF PSYCHOTHERAPY

make the call. Or, I may tell her to get on with it and do it. What I choose from among all the options is important because if I choose the wrong arrows from among diverse signs there will be interruptions in the grace of our movement. As my friend goes her way and I go mine, there may be a silent gnashing of gears. Sometimes this will provoke severe incompatibility. More commonly there will only be a vague sense of not getting anywhere. Unfortunately, just such missed connections will often decay relationships.

To further illustrate the surges imbedded in each expression, here is an example of a few short exchanges with a research biologist, who was a patient of mine. I was trying to influence him to talk more than he did about his activities—to the woman he lived with and to others. In response, he said, "It's a lot easier to talk about things I am excited about and that are going real well than if I was being really frustrated." From this sentence, there are a number of arrows which could give me an interesting ride into nextness. I wondered about his need for things to be *easy*. There was a whole story which could evolve about just that simple theme. I passed that one up. Then there was the word, *talk*. Did he prefer showing people things to telling them? Who listened when he talked and who pulled a veil over their faces? I didn't follow that arrow either. Then there was the word, *excited*. What excited him and what happened to him when he got excited? That didn't draw me either. Any of these might have been prime arrows for other people or for me at another time. This time, though, the arrow I rode was his difficulty telling about things which *frustrated* him. So I said to him, "Frustration is interesting too. Novels and movies are filled with frustrating events."

Then he told me about his work which was, according to him, "99 percent frustrating." I asked him what was so frustrating. After some generalizations, he went on to tell me about one of his experiments. In spite of knowing little about biology, I became engrossed in his descrip-

tion of working with two proteins which were similar but serve quite different metabolic roles. He gave details of his timebound struggle to crack the problem and how, after about a week of work, he "finally got very lucky and found a way to solve it." He told the story of his frustrating research well and, while telling it, presented any number of new arrows pointing toward new nextnesses. His allusion to luck was the one I rode.

Imbedded in this idea of luck are two contradictory possibilities. One was that he was blessed with nature's bountifulness, a lovely feeling to have, but not one which he ever exhibited. The other side was belittling himself, ignoring that his own strong hand created the solution. So, I said, "*Lucky* sounds like you had nothing to do with it. I'd like to know more about your luck." As he went on, he soon came to recognize that he had made a skillful guess in experimenting with proportions of the proteins and how they would affect each other. In further acceptance he also recognized that good research allows luck its best chance to work. That made him a partner of luck, rather than a passive recipient. In summary, during these simple sequences, he told a story with important elements of drama. The characters were chemicals not people, but he gave a lively account of how these characters related to each other and what happened to them in one or another set of circumstances. He allowed his frustration to be a part of his story, facing up to it and feeling the fun in it. He described the risk of making certain choices, and, as it happened, created a happy ending, though that would not be required. Furthermore, as a vehicle for personal message, the story gave him a good perspective on luck and a precedent for accepting his own good function.

STORYTELLING

The story which unfolded through riding the arrows from one in a series of units to another leads us to the second general remedy for the here-and-now emphasis, namely, storytelling, which is always composed of experiences of there-and-then. Each moment in a person's life is host to an infinite number of events, and as these events occur the raw material for stories is formed. However, the span of these events is wretchedly limited. Most are given no more notice than the effect of your car on the pavement. Some may be given unconscious notice, for example, continued resentment of forgotten insults. Even so, only a fraction remains in the mind's merciless exclusion of most of life's happenings. Those which live in memory and in story remain understandably dear; they are carriers of a personal sense of enduring reality, prime vehicles for linking together the selected survivors of personal experience. Without this linkage, only the most dim sense of reality would remain—isolated pulses, unmarked.

In Jean Paul Sartre's (1964, p. 39) novel, *Nausea*, through his character, Roquentin, a gloomy view is presented of the contradictions that may sabotage an enduring reality. His gloom is caused by the paradoxical clashes that are common to "living" and to "telling" about it. Though the dilemma is not as hopeless as he sees it, it is one which must be taken into account. Roquentin says, "Nothing happens while you live. The scenery changes, people come in and out, that's all . . . Days are tacked onto days without rhyme or reason, an interminable, monotonous addition." For him, the solution to this nihilistic state is to tell about these happenings and he even thinks "for the most banal event to become an adventure, you must (and this is enough) begin to recount it." He goes on, though, to add his seemingly hopeless contradiction, "But you have to choose: Live or tell." The implication is that if you only "live" there is nothing really there; the fleeting experience is nonsense, hardly worth the attention it commands. On the other hand, if you tell about it, it can, through the telling, be a vibrant, adventurous experience. But, once you start doing that, the living is over.

Paradox is no stranger to human existence, though, and this one is neither more nor less vexing or challenging than any other. Rather, it is illuminating because through Sartre's confrontation of the paradox between raw living—untold—and confirmed living—that which is told—he gives unaccustomed centrality to storytelling, normally accorded only a peripheral place in any person's life. Though it is, of course, difficult to live something out and tell about it at the same time, this seeming mutual exclusivity is served well by the remarkable integrative skills of the person. Integrative dexterity is evident everywhere, ranging from the crucial coordination of the disparate functions of the brain hemispheres to the frivolous trick of patting the head while rubbing the belly. This deftness is equally available for coordinating living and telling, a feat which, in spite of Sartre's Roquentin, we all accomplish everyday. It is, of course, evident that some people do it better than others. Some will be fooled into mistaking the tales for the events themselves, repeating them over and over as though that will restore the living referent itself.

All people vary in the proportions of attention they give to living and telling, as well as in how they time the telling or in the style of their interconnections between living and telling. For some people, telling a story enhances the living to which it refers; for others, it only distorts what actually happened. For some people, stories are marvelous elaborations on what is only a simple experience; for others, the most complex event will be worth only a grunt, the punctuation mark in a story to be fleshed out. Some people are wary about telling those things which they are afraid will make them look bad. On and on.

Much of what happens in life floats on the periphery of awareness. Jane may ask, for example, whether I thought Agnes was unfriendly to her; she had a hard time knowing. John seemed to talk more about his ex-wife than he recently had. Agatha vaguely sensed that there was more music in her life these days. These were all dim awarenesses, suggestive but undependable. In spelling them out by telling stories, details could be added giving broader perspective and greater clarity. Hints become realizations; bare facts, when recounted, expand like yeast; unvisioned feelings and their associations become revealed. When the poet is moved by seeing a tree, the tree is only the skeleton of what he wants to say. He fleshes out an outline with his personalized words. While telling about the tree he sees, he may say that it beckons him to climb it, or that he wants once again to pick its bark, or that its branches form an umbrella. He may become clear about fertility or gnarledness or grace. When people see trees casually, they are only trees. For those who tell about them, they may be much more, as they clarify what trees are like in their diverse characteristics and implications.

In psychotherapy, special attention is given to the elusiveness of experience. People want to change their lives but often can't put their fingers on just what it would take. One such person was Ingrid who, in her group, spoke about a general sense of shame, fear and self-criticism, untied to anything that would account for her feelings. She just thought she "should have it more together, more confident, more successful, more loving and more accepting." Her concepts didn't stand still long enough to hang a wish on them. When pressed further to spell out what she was ashamed of, it took her a while before she said that when she disagreed with people she got mad, gritting her teeth and becoming silently unyielding. That, she said, is what she was ashamed of—the dishonesty of her silence. Suddenly her shame seemed a little less elusive. She added that her mother always preached honesty at all costs, although when Ingrid practiced it her mother couldn't handle it. When lying was immoral and truth unpalatable, Ingrid, of course, found herself in a bind; she wound up silent over the years and forgot why.

In an attempt to flesh out the story, I suggested that, rather than stay stuck with the contradictions about truth, which only paralyzed her, she try an experiment in lying, assuring her it need be only for the moment. She got excited, transforming a worried look into one that was loose, even a little wild. Tongue in cheek, she told about the really tough week she had, working so hard around the house that her fingers split open and her nails crumbled. She "cleaned at the office, watered plants, did lots and lots of work and lots and lots of reports, lots of letters." At this point she was still caught in the phoniness of the lie. But she was getting warmer. There were giggles about all she had done for the people in her house, when suddenly she realized she was saying something true; truths she normally would not tell. Then she licked her chops and went further to tell a true story about how she recently entertained Norwegian relatives. Here is how it goes and clearly her experience by now is no longer elusive. She said proudly,

I cooked for these people, I entertained them, I listened to their problems, their frustrations, I poured them drinks, emptied their fucking ashtrays. I spoke Norwegian for them so they would like me and be entertained by me and I gave them all hugs and kisses and I cleaned the whole fucking house Norwegian style. I mean, I worked my fucking ass off. Then I set this beautiful table, with lace cloth and flowers and candles. I even asked my uncle to say a prayer before dinner, so they would feel at home and comfortable. Did this three nights in a row for three sets of people. I did an incredible job. . . . There is a lot of excitement to that.

She could go on forever, but she stopped herself at this point in her prideful account. As it happened, in her family, men were allowed to go on and on about their experiences, some tall stories included, but the women were supposed to serve and tone themselves down. This realization clarified her shame about not being *counted*. By now though, she *felt* counted and her shame simply evaporated.

To extract stories from people's lives, the therapist often has a mind-bending job, trying to lay bare the stories that actually count. On easy days these stories may be readily apparent and one may gather them like picking stones off the ground; at other times they are deeply imbedded in their host psyche. Only through sensitive, patient, and inventive efforts will the therapist recognize the signs of the story's existence and succeed in prying the right ones loose.

People often have difficulty telling these stories even when the outlines for them are already apparent. One woman spent her childhood getting beat up by her father but was reluctant to tell about it. For the listener the violence would have been absorbing but quite assimilable. For her, however, the extra stimulation of telling it might have drastic effects, like screaming or feeling as if her head might burst. She might also feel like a coward to have allowed the beatings or a wanton mischief-maker or a betrayer of her father, whom she also loved. Thus, the actual story may remain heavily veiled, but the story is always there, waiting for the right inspiration to bring it out into the open. As Loren Eisely (1975, p. 3), the noted scientist-writer, says:

Everything in the mind is in rat's country. It doesn't die. They are merely carried, these disparate memories, back and forth in the desert of a billion neurons, set down, picked up, and dropped again by mental pack rats. Nothing perishes, it is merely lost till a surgeon's electrode starts the music . . . Nothing is lost, but it can never be again as it was. You will only find the bits and cry out because they were yourself.

The difficulties in finding the story line are further exemplified in the writings of Proust (1924), as well as a number of other twentieth century writers, including Kafka, Joyce and Faulkner. Proust is especially well-known for obscurity in story line. He paradoxically tells about his own early enthrallment with the novel. He loved it because of the dramatic clarity with which it condensed a lifetime of gradualism. He saw the novel speeding up life's process, replacing life's gradualism with a "mental picture." Through ingenious acceleration of events, the novelist crams his pages with "more dramatic and sensational events than occur, often, in a lifetime."

In his actual writing, however, Proust frustrates this expectation that the novelist will rescue the reader from gradualness. Instead of providing an easy story line, he disseminates detail so luxuriantly that the elements of story line are veiled and only gradually revealed. The story is, of course, there but recognizing it may seem like finding faces hidden in a drawing. As a result, a legendary number of Proust's readers have been awed by his perceptual masterfulness while never finishing his novels. Though the ingredients Proust lays open are far more scintillating than the ordinary sensations which people regularly experience, his gradualness nevertheless requires the reader to be continually attentive with unusual perceptual acuity to ferret out the advances in plot.

The therapist must also attend carefully to the emergence of story lines by highlighting the patient's "mental pictures" which otherwise would remain either shadowy or concealed. What usually stands out for the patient, emerging from his almost undifferentiated gradualness, is a generalized theme that serves as a distant pointer to events long ago locked away yet still anxiously throbbing for a return to awareness. This thematic structure, often no more than a title, is a guiding factor in each person's orientation toward himself but making no greater mark in a person's life than the title of a novel will in the novel itself. Whereas a title without a novel would be absurd, people will often find it difficult to look beyond the titles that have been given up to the experiences in their lives.

One woman saw herself as having had a terrible sexual relationship with her ex-husband, but at first she could tell me nothing about it. All she knew was that she had a Terrible Sexual Relationship. She surely knew more than the title and it, alone, was too tight a summary. I pointed this out to her, saying she probably knew more than she thought she knew. Only when she talked more did it become clear to her that she actually knew much more but, oddly, hadn't realized it mattered. As she went on, she remembered that every night her husband would watch Playboy TV; he was no longer interested in her. That, by itself, added substance to her feeling degraded and dismissed. Getting warmed up to the details, she then found it worth telling me that he had herpes and was contagious two weeks out of four. Moreover, he wouldn't tell her when he was contagious, so she had to be personally on the lookout for it. Fortunately, she never caught it. In addition to these severe interruptions in accessibility, the pernicious effect on his self-esteem was great and he compensated by treating her with great disdain. Her Terrible Sexual Relationship, more than a title, evolved into a fleshed-out tale of misery.

Perhaps this may seem a special case of shame, preventing this woman from telling her story, but when she told it, she didn't seem prohibitively ashamed. Once started, she easily went into considerable detail, with little probing necessary. For her to limit herself to the titles of her stories was simply a familiar style; she merely was unaccustomed to spelling out the events which gave her life substance. This form of narrowing life was more than one woman's neurosis; abstractions are a common shorthand system through which people come to assume too much about themselves and know too little. Too often, the titles to the stories of life are given so prominent a position as symbols or guides that they come to be accepted as substitutes for the real thing. For someone to say he is country folk, for example, will not be as uniquely identifying as the details of the Baptist revivalist meetings he lived with, the games he and his friends played, the whippings he got, or getting lost in the woods.

Patients who come for therapy are commonly oriented to their own special abstractions, which title large sweeps of their lives—marital troubles, homosexuality, school failures or fear of elevators. These titles crowd their minds; only by unfolding the titles into the specific elaborations will the special qualities of each life be restored. Once actual happenings can be reexperienced for their own sake, the titles may change and their lives, too. Marital Discord may become Boiling in the Kitchen or The Homosexual Life may become Better Than to be a Boxer. Yet, no matter how intriguing the new titles may be, sometimes even helpful through the new perspective they give, they can never substitute for the story. Though many people hope they can change their lives by changing their titles, on such a wish hangs a multitude of fruitless searches.

It is also evident that Gestalt therapy, concerned with movement through time and with the entire range of a person's experiences, would be well-served to reexamine its title as a here-and-now therapy. With its revelatory technology having established the value of amplified existence, it seems timely now for a new phase of Gestalt therapy. Although a fundamentally broad-ranging approach from its beginnings, intending to widen the realms and fullness of human engagement, the emphasis on technique dramatically upstaged what was always methodologically crucial: the centrality of simple, high quality contact and the versatility of a person's awareness. These instruments of simple humanity can generate fascination. In concert with supporting technoloogy, they highlight the drama, therefore the reality, of each lived life. Such engagement includes much that is ordinary: support, curiosity, kindness, bold language, laughter, cynicism, assimilation of tragedy, rage, gentleness, and toughness. The principles of Gestalt therapy orient therapists to notice not only how people presently live, but also how they have lived, and will live, not only *here* but also *there*; not only *now* but also *then*.

REFERENCES

Eisely, L. (1975). *All the strange hours.* New York: Scribner's.

Jacabowitz, T. (1985, January 23). Letter to the editor. *New York Times Magazine.*

Kierkegaard, S. (1948). *Purity of heart is to will one thing* (rev. ed.). New York: Harper and Row.

Perls, F. S. (1947). *Ego, hunger and aggression.* London: George Allen & Unwin.

Perls, F. S. (1970). *Gestalt therapy now.* Palo Alto: Science and Behavior Books.

Proust, M. (1924). *Remembrance of things past.* New York: Random House.

Sartre, J.P. (1964). *Nausea.* New York: New Directions. (Original work published 1938)

Discussion by Carl R. Rogers, Ph.D.

I have a real double pleasure. I had the opportunity of reading Erv Polster's paper and then I've had the opportunity of hearing his presentation. There are a number of things I reverberated to. Let me stress particularly the natural corruption at the original intent. Have I experienced that! I feel that so much of what each of us does gets corrupted by people who seize upon some superficial aspect and turn it to their own purposes. So I reverberated to that.

I think what he's saying, what all of us try to do, is to bring together the living and the telling so that it isn't either/or. So that we can live and experience fully and yet be able to take account of it in our own experience.

And then I enjoyed all his case stories. There was a rich tapestry of interwoven ideas and then there would be colorful spots of the tapestry which were composed of the case stories and interviews. There were also flashes of humor that I just loved.

My comments are going to be brief because there is so much of what he said that I simply agree with. Like him, I deplore the present stress on the here and now. I don't know so much about it in Gestalt, but I think about it in our culture. It seems to me that many of us, and per-

haps young people especially, have become victims of the cult of the here and now. They want immediate gratification of all their desires. I think a lot of our middle- and upper-class youth are really spoiled children. They expect immediate gratification. The notion of working for something doesn't seem to fit the television ads. The process of trying to gain our ends by hard work and persistence and so on has lost a lot of the charm that it has in our experience.

I won't easily forget the metaphor of the digital clock. I've seen that in my great-grandchildren, the fact that they no longer can tell time by what I think of as a clock. They're accustomed to the digital clock and I do think that makes a difference, but it's a metaphor of our times. So that had meaning to me.

I was interested to learn recently that clients in therapy focus only on the here and now. That was news to me. I see it as deeply untrue, but it was interesting that we were classified in that category too.

I, too, dislike the lazy way in which oversimplification has become a part of our all too lazy culture. He stressed some of the slogans that have been a handicap to Gestalt therapy. I think oversimplification has become a mark of our culture.

It's evident at all levels and in a variety of ways. Our leader characterizes a whole complex culture as an evil empire and then has to back away from that when he finds there are human beings who live in that culture.

I think of the whole, impressive array of experiences under the heading of intensive group experiences. That can be scornfully tossed aside as a touchy-feely movement, along with the whole range of things from those that were ridiculous and absurd to those that were very meaningful and really changed lives. That's all categorized in one, easy sweep of the term, "touchy-feely movement."

I enjoyed the complexity of his listening. I particularly responded to that example of the research biologist where he could have focused on any one of a number of words. As I read the man's sentence, I believe that Erv was right because that frustration was the important element. Still it is true that in making our responses we do continually make very subtle discriminations. It's good to be aware of that and to be aware that someone else would respond in a different way and still be equally effective, but in a different fashion.

There was just once in reading the paper that I winced and I was so pleased that he didn't use this sentence when he gave the talk. What he said in the paper in talking about storytelling was "the therapist pries the right story loose." Pries the right story loose? I can't imagine Erv using a lever to pry the right story loose. I spoke earlier about the difficulty in sometimes getting people to tell their stories, but I'd be surprised to see any example of his prying the right story loose.

All in all, I was very pleased with the fact that he is broadening and deepening the concept of Gestalt therapy, getting it away from any narrowness that it might possess. As a result, I think, he is making the whole therapeutic approach more useful and deeper.

There's only one major point that I would like to make which I regard as a supplement to what he says, not a contradiction or an argument against it. I can

overstate it by saying that we do not know and cannot know the past. All that we can possibly know is the present perception of past experience. I think it's important to recognize that. Whether it's mine or yours or his or hers, we never know the past. All that we ever know is *my* perception of the past or *your* perception of the past or *his* perception or *hers*. We live in a perceptual reality. Perhaps we like to think that there is a real reality, but if there is we'll never know it. All that we know is our perception of the past. The same is true of the future. We perceive our future in different ways, but it is our perception of the future. I think Erv recognized that when he said, "Once actual happenings are reexperienced, the titles may change." That's when he was speaking about the titles of people's stories. In other words, perception of our past does change and we change the title of the story.

I am reminded of once hearing Alfred Adler talking about his own work and that of the people who worked with him. He told how one of their favorite procedures is to ask the person, "What is your earliest memory?" As therapy progressed, they would ask that again, and again when therapy was completed. The reason was that the earliest memory that seemed like a solid landmark when first told might change in different ways. It might be that the earliest memory became the memory of a different event or, very frequently, the same event now remembered with a very different flavor, a very different meaning, a very different emotional context and significance. Thus, we do change our perceptions of the past.

I want to give another example that tells of the infant boy with his mother in the park, feeding some pigeons. The small boy leaves his mother, goes towards the pigeons, and looks back. That could be interpreted as an anxious look. The child is feeling anxious and looks back for reassurance—is mother still there, is my life secure? Or he can be looking back for encouragement, for a sense of understanding. Does mother realize I'm being very bold? Is she with me in this new aspect of being a big boy? Either way can be true and the only way we could possibly know what that experience was would be to question the infant at the time. The trouble is that at that point in his life I doubt very much that he could inform us as to what his experience was. So we make our own interpretations.

Let us suppose that later in life, in therapy, he remembers that incident. I think it's quite possible that he may remember it as an anxious moment, a symptom of the insecurity that he feels now when he is concerned as to whether his mother would desert him if he left her, and so on. Or he can remember it as the first step toward being an independent individual, how proud he was, how proud his mother was of him. I think that the quality of the past changes very markedly, depending on the way that we receive it. I stress again that there may be a reality. All we can know is our perception of that reality.

To me it's very useful to realize that in all of our dealings in therapy and in life, we're dealing with perceptions of reality. To me, that gives the basis for a lot of living together, because if I think I know the reality, then I'll insist that you see it the same way. This is THE reality, why can't you see it? If I recognize this is my perception of reality, then perhaps I can be willing that you have your perception of reality and I can enrich my life by seeing the differences. What I think gives us the basis for reconciliation of differences, for mutual understanding between individuals, between cultures and races. If we can recognize that none of us knows the reality, but we can live with our differing perceptions of reality, we can come to accept those differing perceptions and to appreciate them and to appreciate the differences that reside in them.

QUESTIONS AND ANSWERS

Question: I work a lot right now with sexual abuse and incest, particularly with adolescent males who are sex offenders. I've found that to be a real difficult area; there's very little research, there's very little information. I feel that this issue has been ducked a lot at this conference. People have said, "Well, we don't work with those," or whatever. Have either of you two done any work in San Diego with Parents United or with incest families or any of this category? If so, could you give any feedback about strategies you've found effective working?

E. Polster: I have not worked with those organizations and I've not worked with adolescents for many years. I did at one time. The only experiences I have with working with incest problems are those relatively few times when the issue comes up in the lives of patients I work with. I would imagine that I would follow the general principles that I've been talking about in working with them, but I would not have the actual experience to relate to you. I could imagine problems of having freedom to be in a new nourishing and inspiring contact, flushing out the details of their lives, being able to tell something to me that they wouldn't otherwise be able to tell. The sense of vigor in the relationship and respect. But those are so general that they're hardly of any use. I don't have direct experience. I'm not sidestepping this issue, it's just that I don't have the direct experience.

Question: Dr. Polster, do you recommend the use of journals with your clients? I read something about journal writing and one technique is to outline chapters of your life. When you were talking about the titles that people put, do you use that technique with your clients?

E. Polster: Only occasionally. I don't have that as a common part of my repertoire. I think the idea is very good. I find that when I do suggest writing things that people may agree to do it but frequently don't do it. I think any avenue for expression that gets to the root of what one is experiencing and recognizes it and exercises it is useful. But I don't have that as one of my techniques.

Question: You talked about the title and the fact that we all have a title for events that have happened in the past, or a story. I believe we have stories about our dreams or stories about who we could be or our potentials. Do you do any work with telling stories about that?

E. Polster: Yes, I can remember one woman I worked with who wanted to be a great therapist; that was her dream. It was apparent in working with her that she had a greater need for privacy of her own experience than would be good in becoming a great therapist. So I worked with her in terms of her willingness to let certain areas of her life become known to others in the group she was in. She did this and it not only was important for her but also stimulated others to tell their stories. Thus, in a sense she felt her impact through that process of opening up her own life to others. That would be one example of a person with a dream telling a story connected with one of the characteristics necessary for her reaching the dream.

Psychodrama, Role Theory, and the Concept of the Social Atom

———————◆———————

Zerka T. Moreno

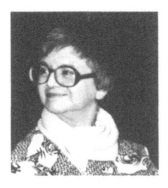

Zerka T. Moreno

The name Moreno is synonymous with psychodrama. Zerka T. Moreno is honorary president of the American Society of Psychodrama and Group Psychotherapy; president of the Moreno Workshops; and honorary member of the Board of Directors of the International Association of Group Psychotherapy.

Zerka Moreno is the author and co-editor of many books and articles in the field of group psychotherapy and internationally known as a teacher, therapist and lecturer. She is the widow and was for more than 30 years the collaborator of the late Jacob L. Moreno, M.D., who pioneered psychodrama.

Zerka Moreno presents the development of psychodrama, centering on the seminal contributions of J.L. Moreno. He is credited as one of the first action-oriented therapists, and as an originator of cotherapy and group and marital approaches. Moreover, he was one of the pioneers in treating psychosis. Not only is history presented, Zerka Moreno clarifies important psychodrama methods and concepts such as role and social atom. Cornerstones of this approach are the notions of spontaneity and creativity.

HISTORICAL BACKGROUND

J.L. Moreno first began his formal interest in psychology by observing and joining in children's play in the gardens of Vienna, Austria, in the first decade of this century. At the time he was a student of philosophy; he had not yet entered medical school. He was impressed by the great amount of spontaneity in children and became aware that human beings become less spontaneous as they age. He asked himself, why does this occur? What happens to us? The same process struck him when he started to direct the children in staged, rehearsed plays. At the first portrayal, whatever spontaneity was available to the children was mobilized. But the more the children repeated the performance, the less inventive, creative, and spontaneous they became. They began to conserve their energy, to repeat their best lines, movements, and facial expressions because these produced the greatest effect upon the audience. What resulted was a mechanical performance, lacking in reality. Clearly, this was the same phenomenon evident in aging and in certain types of emotional disturbances, where one finds repetition without relation to the current situation, a freezing of affect and of memory.

How could this process be reversed or slowed? Looking at the world at large—and it is notable that most of Moreno's theories and concepts were based on observations from life and were not limited to the clinical setting—Moreno conceptualized that what is of essence in human existence are the twin principles of spontaneity and creativity. The end products of these he called *cultural conserves*. They were attempts to freeze creativity and spontaneity of a past moment into a concrete product. He noted that conserved products are all around us, in music, in literature, art, religion, culture, technology, and even biology. The principle of energy conservation, the freezing of a past moment of creativity resulted in ubiquitous conserves.

Wanting to break these frozen patterns and try to redirect energy back to the source of creativity, Moreno asked himself, what is spontaneity? How does creativity emerge? He decided that spontaneity and creativity were inherent in the human organism, endogenous, but the conservation of energy can block them and turn them pathological under certain conditions. What are these conditions and how can lost spontaneity and creativity be revitalized? How does this loss affect our relations with one another? How does learning via play differ from learning via the intellect? This last question has since been elucidated by the studies of the left brain and the right brain, but this information was not yet at hand in Moreno's time.

In his magnum opus *Who Shall Survive?* (1934, 1953) he dealt with creativity and spontaneity as *the* problem of the universe.

The universe is infinite creativity. But what is spontaneity? Is it a kind of energy? If it is energy it is *unconservable*, if the meaning of spontaneity should be kept consistent. We must,

therefore, differentiate between two varieties of energy, conservable and unconservable energy. There is an energy which is conservable in the form of *cultural conserves*, which can be saved up, which can be spent at will in selected parts and used at different points in time; it is like a robot at the disposal of its owner. There is another form of energy which emerges and which is spent in a moment, which must emerge to be spent and which must be spent to make place for emergence, like the life of some animals which are born and die in the love-act.

It is a truism to say that the universe cannot exist without physical and mental energy which can be preserved. But it is more important to realize that without the other kind of energy, the unconservable one—or spontaneity—the creativity of the universe could not start and could not run; it would come to a standstill.

There is apparently little spontaneity in the universe, or at least, if there is any abundance of it only a small particle is available to man, hardly enough to keep him surviving. In the past he has done everything to discourage its development. He could not rely upon the instability and insecurity of the moment, with an organism which was not ready to deal with it adequately; he encouraged the development of devices as intelligence, memory, social and cultural conserves, which would give him the needed support with the result that he gradually became the slave of his own crutches. If there is a neurological localization of the spontaneity-creativity process it is the least developed function of man's nervous system. The difficulty is that one cannot store spontaneity, one either is spontaneous at a given moment or one is not. If spontaneity is such an important factor for man's world, why is it so little developed? The answer is: man *fears* spontaneity, just like his ancestor in the jungle feared fire; he feared fire until he learned how to make it. Man will fear spontaneity until he will learn how to train it. (p. 47)

Though approaching creativity from another aspect, Otto Rank had this to say in *Art and Artist* about its end products:

[the artist] desires to transform death into life,

as it were, though actually he transforms life into death. For not only does the created work not go on living; it is, in a sense, dead; both as regards the material, which renders it almost inorganic, and also spiritually and psychologically, in that it no longer has any significance for its creator, once he has produced it. He therefore again takes refuge in life, and again forms experiences, which for their part represent only mortality—and it is precisely because they are mortal that he wishes to immortalize them in his work. (1968, p. 39)

Clearly, one reason spontaneity is feared is because it is confused with irrationality and unpredictability. But anxiety and spontaneity are inverse functions of one another—the more anxious we are, the less spontaneous we become, and vice versa.

There seems to be a paradox in the notion of training spontaneity. If it is trained, can it still be called spontaneity? Perhaps a better designation would be the re-evocation and retraining of spontaneity.

Looking at some definitions of spontaneity and creativity, we note the following: Spontaneity derives from the Latin *sua sponte*, from within the self. The *Random House Dictionary* defines spontaneity as "coming or resulting from a natural impulse or tendency, without effort or premeditation, natural and unconstrained, unplanned, arising from internal forces or causes, self acting." The philosopher Charles Sanders Pierce (1931) spoke of spontaneity as having ". . . the character of not resulting by law from something antecedent. . . . I don't know what you can make of the meaning of spontaneity, but newness, freshness and diversity" (p. 232).

Creativity in the abovenamed dictionary is described as: "To cause to come into being, as something unique that would not naturally evolve or that is not made by ordinary process, to evolve from one's own thought or imagination, to make by investing with new functions, rank, character, etc."

For Moreno spontaneity was "a new response to an old situation or an adequate response to a new situation" (1953, p. 336), with creativity adding the element of inventiveness. Both Pierce and Moreno stress newness.

The question remains, by what route can we train spontaneity? When Moreno noted the children's repetition in a role, he instructed them to throw away the written script, to improvise within the rationale of the role and the interaction, to remember feelings, not the lines, and to practice newness. By cutting off the old route, he forced the actors to find within and between themselves new ways of sustaining their roles.

During the early 1920s Moreno began to apply his method to adult actors. Out of that experiment, the Theatre of Spontaneity as an art form was born. Moreno put his actors into a variety of situations, taking them by surprise and having them respond to one another. It was a freeing of their ability to act and interact on the spur of the moment—being accused of infidelity by a spouse, being fired from a job, being insulted or misjudged by a friend, and so forth.

He attempted to tap into the unconservable energy, spontaneity, from within the wellspring of the actor and to use it in the developing interaction, to see if some resolution could be found, either between the actors or within the actors themselves. The bonding which took place between them and which helped them to be more creative due to their co-creation he called *tele*. Tele goes beyond empathy and transference and may be thought of as two-way empathy. It is feeling into and appreciation of the reality of the other, mutually experienced and reciprocally involving. Tele is responsible for mutuality between persons, over and beyond their projections, and is responsible for interpersonal and group cohesion.

In a New York State training school for delinquent girls, a study was undertaken in which the residents were asked to indicate whom they wanted as dining room partners at tables seating four persons. The seating arrangement was carried out according to these choices. Mutual choices far outpaced what had been projected on the basis of chance. The factor responsible for these mutualities was revealed to be tele. Moreno decided that tele is the cement which binds people together in a reciprocally satisfying relationship.

Tele is found in several categories: mutual positive, mutual negative, positive versus negative, and neutral. The sense for tele develops with age. In general, it is weakly developed in children and grows with social awareness.

EMERGENCE OF THE THERAPEUTIC DRAMA, OR PSYCHODRAMA

While exploring the implications of his findings with his actors in the Theatre of Spontaneity, Moreno began to apply his ideas to interpersonal disturbances. He required his patients to show him, in action, how they had reached their current impasse, turning them into actors instead of reporters. He conceived of three intrapersonal phenomena: the director who tells the actor what to do, the actor who carries out the directions in action, and the observer who records, makes mental notes, and either encourages or discourages the action, interpreting what has occurred ex post facto. These could all be at odds with one another and thus disturb the smoothness of performance. In addition, each of these could be in discord with the others facing him, further diminishing spontaneity and increasing anxiety.

Moreno wanted to have the problem displayed in action for a number of reasons. There was often a discrepancy between the verbal representation and the actual action, and he wanted to reduce this. To a greater or lesser degree, patients display, as all humans do, incomplete perceptions of self and others, as well as perceptions which are lacking, weak, distorted, or pathological, and especially one-sided and subjective. Where perceptions

are clear and mutually confirmed, positive tele is at work. The enactment was for Moreno not merely a better diagnostic tool, but a more lifelike model, yet larger than life. Later he often called it "a laboratory for learning how to live." It incorporated not only action and interaction, therefore including the body which was left out of the verbal approach, but also speech, mime, music, dance, and the dimensions of past, present, future, and space.

He did not trust the verbal method to be the royal road to the psyche. There is no universal language; each is culture-bound. He observed that there are, in fact, language-resistant portions to the human psyche which can preclude or impede speech as when emotions are deep or in turmoil. And, he asked, if speech were the central and all-absorbing sponge of the psyche, why do we have the various forms of art? These communicate to us in ways which cannot be replicated in speech. Indeed, the verbal method requires a secondary process of interpretation, in itself a product of the therapist's own philosophical orientation. In the dramatic form, the patient was learning to interpret himself as well as the others with whom he was engaged.

Perhaps even more basic as a reason is that both ontogenetically and phylogenetically language is a fairly late development in man. However, we are in interaction from the moment of birth, and much learning goes on in the first few years in action without language. Moreno saw man as an improvising actor on the stage of life. He concluded that he needed to tap a more primary level than speech, that of action. Children and psychotics frequently devise their own language, incomprehensible to auditors, unless carefully studied, and even then it may elude interpretation.

Dramatic depiction allows for the uncovering of concurrent fantasies; and a number of techniques were devised to enable the actors to concretize them.

What other basis could there be for the need for psychodrama? It was noted that developmentally every human infant goes through a stage in the first few months after birth, in which it is not yet aware that there are other beings, outside of itself, around. It experiences itself as the totality of the universe, everyone and everything are extensions of its own being. Hangovers from this period may manifest themselves in children's play. It is called *normal megalomania;* the child uses it whenever it feels the need and this use may well be therapeutic in itself. This phenomenon is also related to Moreno's view of man as more than a biological being, reflecting his cosmic aspect. Here he approaches Rank who spoke of a lost union with the cosmos in which present, past and future are dissolved, and he hypothesized the trauma of birth as a final rupture of this union.

The child emerges gradually out of this state of all-identity into a state of differentiated identity, wherein other individuals and objects separate and become distinct from the self. This later stage leads to a complete breach, making the child aware that there are several kinds of experience, subjective and objective. This final breach, which is a universal phenomenon—the realization of the world within and the world without—is usually brought about by some traumatic experience, some deprivation. From this time onward every human being lives in these two spheres, subjective reality and objective reality, the world of fantasy and the so-called real world. If the essential nurture needs of the child are met, the child will learn about the two realms and, aided by spontaneity, will integrate and balance them. To the extent there is profound, continued deprivation or inadequate spontaneity, these two realms cannot mesh adequately. Then the child will withdraw into the subjective sphere which is once again the entire universe, all-powerful. The pathological seedlings planted there may eventually manifest themselves in various forms of intrapersonal, interpersonal, and socio-emotional disturbances. We all fall somewhere along this continuum; and as long as we are able to maintain our ho-

meostasis or sociostasis, we can remain functioning.

Moreno's attention was engaged particularly by the psychotic experience as one of the most advanced forms of this split and it challenged him to treat psychotics through psychodrama. He conceived this method to be the bridge between the two spheres. Treatment should result in greater flexibility and creative adaptability.

Rank had this to say about play, "In every case play, by diminishing fear, liberates an energy which can ultimately express itself creatively" (1968, p. 324). Through the dramatic format of a play we are able to enter into the subjective, albeit psychotic, reality of the patient-protagonist by using supportive actors known as auxiliary egos, who concretize with and for the patient all those personae, real and fantasized, who are needed to complete and enlarge the internal drama. The protagonist is seen as a creator whose self-creation has gone awry, his creativity has erred, and he is stuck in his creation. It may be pathological creativity, but it is creativity nevertheless. It is the therapist's task to turn it eventually into healthy creativity. To this end, helpers are needed, midwives, to bring the incomplete creation to birth. Then the patient can complete the work, develop distance from it and eventually release it. The midwives are the director, auxiliary egos and supportive staff. They are also the guides who bring the protagonist back into objective reality.

Rank also wrote, "A man with creative power who can give up artistic expression in favor of the formation of personality will remold the self-creative type and will be able to put his creative impulse *directly* in the service of his own personality. . . . The creative type becomes the creator of a self" (p. 430).

In the 1930s, psychotic patients were considered largely untreatable since they were unable to establish transference. In constructing a therapeutic approach, Moreno thought it more productive for the psychiatrist first to warm up to the patient, to establish the relationship by internally role reversing with the patient, and then with empathy and creativity to feel himself into the reality of the patient's subjective world and assess his needs. As there were multiple personae, real as well as hallucinatory or delusional, in the patient's world, the therapist needed helpers. Thus a team of co-workers emerged for the first time in psychotherapy. Up until that time it was deemed best for only one therapist to be actively involved in psychotherapy. It may be argued that active group psychotherapy was born here.

The auxiliary egos had to learn to put their own organisms at the service of the patient, his drama, and his world. For the patient this also represented the first step to resocialization. One remarkable aspect is the ease with which the patient is often able to accept the therapeutic helpers as representatives of the personae in his subjective system and is able to engage with them in interaction. The auxiliary egos had to develop spontaneity which helped them move fast along the axis leading from objectivity to subjectivity and back again.

The development of treatment teams was much like what had occurred in surgery. But is was a revolution in psychotherapy—previously only the therapist was supposed to have meaningful access to the mind of the patient. Moreno knew he could not influence a delusion or hallucination directly, but he hypothesized that such influence could be introduced through the relationship first established on the psychotic level. His auxiliary egos became the go-betweens; these he could direct. As the protagonist began to leave his subjective world, the auxiliary helpers were there to support and guide him into the larger world, on the basis of the trust established earlier. This pioneering effort took place in a small mental hospital in Beacon, New York, in the later half of the 1930s.

In addition to using psychodrama as a comprehensive tool for treating psychotic

and neurotic patients, before discharge their families were brought into therapy with them, to assist in achieving and maintaining more balanced interrelationships.

In 1937 Moreno started other innovations, using himself as a go-between in marital conflicts, as well as having both husband and wife in treatment together at the same time. Reports were published in 1937 in the journal *Sociometry* and later in the three volumes on psychodrama. In the September 1981 issue of *Family Process*, a Belgian psychiatrist, Theo Compernolle, published "J. L. Moreno: An Unrecognized Pioneer of Family Therapy," from which I quote:*

from his earliest writings in 1923 J. L. Moreno developed an interactional view of psychotherapy that in 1937 already resulted in formulations of a true systems orientation and very concrete ideas about marital therapy, family therapy and network therapy. He probably is the first therapist who actually involved a husband's lover in conjoint marital therapy. His general theoretical formulations about the pathology of interpersonal relations as well as his practical suggestions for their therapy seem to be insufficiently known to workers and researchers in the field of family therapy. (p. 331)

Compernolle's article contains the following (p. 331):

Then the momentary structure of the patient's life situation, the physical and mental makeup of his personality, and, most of all, how this operated and interacted with members of his family, and with various members of his network, was the information needed for diagnosis. . . . Considering the more complex forms of social neurosis, when two, three or more persons were to be treated simultaneously, the scenes enacted between them became a formidable pattern for treatment. Finally, all the scenes in their remote past, and all the remote networks, became important from the point of view of general catharsis of all the people involved. The solution was the resurrection of the whole psychological drama, re-enacted by the same persons in the re-creation of situations in which their association had begun. The new technique, if properly applied, aided the patient to actualize during the treatment that which he needed to let himself pass through in a procedure which was as close to his life as possible. He had to meet the situations in which he acted in life, to dramatize them, to meet situations which he had never faced, which he avoided and feared, but which he might have to meet squarely one day in the future. It was often necessary to magnify and elaborate certain situations which he was living through sketchily at the time or of which he had only a dim recollection. The chief point of the technique was to get the patient started, to get him warmed up so that he might throw his psyche into operation and unfold the psychodrama. A technique of spontaneous warming up of the mental states and the situations desired was developed. The spontaneous states attained through this technique were feeling complexes and, as such, useful guides toward the gradual embodiments of roles. The technique demanded usually more than one therapeutic aide for the patient, as aides in starting off the patient himself and as representatives of the principal roles the situation and the patient might require. Instead of one, numerous auxiliary egos were needed. Therefore it led to this: the original auxiliary ego, the psychiatrist, remained at a distance but surrounded himself with a staff of auxiliary egos whom he coordinated and directed and for whom he outlined the course and the aim of psychodramatic treatment.

The 1923 reference made by Compernolle was Moreno's first book dealing with problems of spontaneous production and improvisational drama, *Das Stegreiftheater*, translated into English and published in 1946 as *The Theatre of Spontaneity*, in which he dealt not only with the research aspect but also the therapeutic and philosophic areas. Again I quote,

But the true symbol of the therapeutic theatre is the private home. Here emerges the theatre in its deepest sense, because the most treasured secrets violently resist being touched and exposed. It is the completely private. The first house itself, the place where life begins and ends, the house of birth and the house of death, the house of the most intimate interpersonal relations becomes a stage and a backdrop. The proscenium is the front door, the window sill and the balcony. The auditorium is in the garden and the street.
Spontaneous role playing gives the "meta-practical proof" of a realm of freedom, illusion is strictly separated from reality. But there is a theatre in which reality or being is proven through illusion, one which restores the original unity between the two meta-zones— through a process of humorous self-reflection; in the therapeutic theatre reality and illusion are one.
Some of the most significant techniques refer to the domain of *forms*, of *interpersonal relationships*, of *presentation* and *the treatment of mental disorders*. (p. 89)

In psychodrama, repetition of a scene or interaction need not be deadly. Because it is impossible to reproduce life exactly, an element of newness is already introduced; it is living it again, but with a difference. The cultural conserve, on the other hand, such as the legitimate drama, does not allow for genuine deviation. But, states Moreno,

The cultural conserve is not an inescapable trap. Its stultifying effects can be corrected. Instead of making the machine an agent of the cultural conserve—which would be the way of least resistance and one of fatal regression into a general enslavement of man to a degree beyond that of the most primitive prototype—it is possible to make the machine an agent and a supporter of spontaneity. . . . Indeed, every type of machine can become a stimulus to spontaneity instead of a substitute for it. . . . The reproductive process of learning must move into second place; first emphasis should be given to productive, spontaneous-creative process of learning. The exercises and training in spontaneity are the chief subjects of the school of the future. (1946, p. 55)

Clearly Moreno's concern was not only with the treatment of mental disorders but also with a new model of education, from kindergarten on up.

In Goethe's play *Lila*, the heroine is treated for her insanity by having all the persons involved in her private life join her in her delusions, taking the roles as she envisions them. After having lived these out in life itself with her co-actors, she can now rejoin them; and thus she is cured and returns to reality. Goethe pointed out in a letter to the director of the royal theatre of Saxony on October 1, 1818, "The play *Lila* is actually a psychological cure in which one allows the madness to come to the fore in order to cure it. . . . The best way to attain a psychological cure is by allowing the madness to enter into the treatment in order to heal the condition" (1971, p. 14). Similarly, Moreno often spoke of psychodrama as a homeopathic remedy and as a "small injection of insanity under conditions of control." It is the control which is of importance, the madness being contained within it, with the learning taking place in a nonthreatening and protective setting. Family therapists similarly induce crises in order to treat the family in therapy.

THE METHOD

Psychodrama primarily uses five instruments: the patient or protagonist, the director or chief therapist, the cotherapists or auxiliary egos, and the group members, plus a space or theatre for the action.

Psychodrama sessions proceed in three stages: the warm-up and interview, the enactment and the closure. The warm-up is intended to prepare the group for the emergence of a protagonist or, if a protagonist has already been designated, to become more relaxed individually and more cohesive as a group. There are a great many warm-up techniques: some may be physical, such as doing exercises, some may be done with music or dancing, some with mingling, or with introductions by

name. Directors often devise new warm-up techniques on the spur of the moment. There are group-centered warm-ups and sessions as well as individual-centered ones. The warm-up is also to assist the protagonist in establishing some level of comfort within the group. Over the years, as patients become familiar with this type of treatment, they are often ready to start when they come into the session, having been warmed up by the psychodramas of other patients or by some recent happening in their own lives. As patients start trusting the method and the therapists, their warm-up time is reduced.

A further warm-up is the interview when the protagonist comes to the stage space. This interview is to elicit essential facts and to help the group become familiar with the patient's needs and mental set, as well as to prepare the protagonist for the forthcoming action. The interview is greatly reduced in the treatment of psychotics: as soon as the director, auxiliary egos, and group members become familiar with the patient's inner world, action starts almost at once. The interview should set the stage for the protagonist, the place, the time, and the persons involved as the action begins. It also enables the auxiliary egos to be ready to step into the action as needed. If the group is homogeneous in terms of diagnosis, for instance drug users or alcoholics, the group members may bring up a related or unrelated topic and the protagonists may be self-indicated or group-chosen. The enactment follows, incorporating self-presentation, role reversal, doubling, soliloquy; shifting to more relevant scenes—real or fantasized; returning to the past or projecting into the future, as seen essential by the director, all with the cooperation of the patient, or as indicated by the patient.

A special adaptation in psychodrama, called the mirror technique, is the enlistment of the patient as a colleague, an auxiliary ego in his own role, watching his behavior in relation to others, yet at the same time helping the director to guide the action. Another is role reversal with the director who becomes the patient, placing the protagonist in the role of the therapist. This technique has been taken over by individual therapists of various orientations. The patient can also be interviewed as a colleague and asked how this patient might be treated. One of the most useful role reversals is one in which the patient takes the role of the person with whom the conflict is to be explored and is then interviewed from that perspective. The amount of data and the sort of data which come out of this are frequently more valuable than the results of interviewing in the role of self.

One of the reasons why patients appreciate psychodrama is that their autonomy is mobilized, respected, and put to use in their own behalf, in a setting where mistakes, if any are made, are not punished but can be corrected on the spot, and where the possible consequences of their interactions can be tested out. Another reason is that it becomes obvious to patients that they know more about themselves than they realized and, especially in the beginning, more than the therapist. For example, their homes and the way they live with others are unknowns to anyone but themselves. This changes their status in relation to the therapist and makes them equal partners in an exciting process of exploration and learning. This experience is important for the patients to overcome their fears of acting, giving themselves away, and possibly losing control.

The function of director is complicated. It takes approximately two years to train a director, who must be a combination of scientist and artist. The more fully the director lives, the better he/she can fulfill this function. He/she has to be aware of cues of all sorts since action by itself may not be enough. Often a subtle cue must be followed up and the current scene dropped for a catharsis of integration to take place. My sense is that family therapists are so close to this role that they could easily incorporate psychodrama into their armamentarium.

The auxiliary egos have five major functions:

1. to embody the role required by the protagonist of either an absentee, a delusion or hallucination, an animal, an object, an idea or value, a voice, a body part, or as the double of the various aspects of the protagonist himself;
2. to approximate, in taking the role, the perception held by the protagonist, at least in the beginning;
3. to investigate the true nature of the interaction between the protagonist and the role being enacted by the auxiliary;
4. to interpret this interaction and relationship, and if possible, to bring that interpretation into the scene; and
5. to act as a therapeutic guide toward a more satisfactory relationship and interaction.

The first three functions are genuine additions to what the psychotherapist has been doing all along in points 4 and 5, but it is exactly the nature of the interactional process that refines the interpreting and guiding.

Because the auxiliary ego is closer to the protagonist in the action and because it serves as the agent of action on behalf of the director, the function of the auxiliary ego is the next important aspect. The auxiliary ego can assist the director in his own evaluation and guiding. The function of the auxiliary ego as a double to a psychotic patient cannot be overestimated; the more bizarre the patient is, the more a double can be effective in this process. Often a protagonist is unable to communicate what is going on inside and around him, but the double can, and does. Whenever possible, family members eventually are brought into the therapy. They, in turn, may become auxiliary egos for a while, or may be treated as co-protagonists, learning about what they may have contributed to the patient's difficulties. Auxiliary egos and directors are required to be protagonists in their own dramas during the course of their training, not only to develop as therapists and as people, but also to enlarge their role repertoire and to increase spontaneity. This becomes especially necessary when there is some aspect of the patient's psycho-drama that enmeshes the auxiliary ego in his personal psychodrama.

The first rule, therefore, for directors and auxiliary egos is: Be sure you are not doing your own psychodrama on your patients. There is always danger of this in any form of therapy; in psychodrama it becomes a little more evident since it takes place in a group. Such developments should bring the director and auxiliary egos to the stage as protagonists in psychodramas of their own. Whether to have patients present or not is a decision to be made. We have found it enormously useful for patients to attend such sessions because they learn that therapists, too, have their human problems. Prophylactic use of psychodrama sessions as a prevention of burnout is also to be recommended.

The final part of the session is sharing. This consists of bringing the protagonist back into the group circle and having group members identify with the protagonist or with another role represented in the psychodrama. Group members should speak about themselves, not the protagonist; here we share our common humanity. It is not merely that we are all more human than otherwise, as Harry Stack Sullivan declared, rather we are more alike than we are different. The differences do stick out, causing us often to forget our commonality. Dialogue, discussion or interpretation, and evaluation must come later, when the protagonist is not as vulnerable. At this stage he is, as in surgery, in recovery and must be handled gently, but firmly. The protagonist had denuded himself or herself before a group. This giving of self must be rewarded in kind, not by cold analysis, critique, or attack—no matter how shocking the revelations may have been—but by becoming once again a member of the group. Sharing has been found to be the most healing aftereffect; once sharing has taken place, analysis and interpretation can take place. However, these are best done by the protagonist. Many are eager to get this response so they can extract further learning, but it

is not the primary aspect of sharing, or rather, not the first step. Analysis leads to intellectualization. Healing comes from the revelation of others. Insight by itself rarely heals anyone. In any case, healing is more readily achieved after the emotions have been stirred and acceptance has been made manifest.

THE CONCEPT OF ROLE IN PSYCHODRAMA

In psychodramatic terms, the *role* is a final crystallization of all the situations in a special area of operations through which the individual passes in interaction with others who play complementary roles. A role does not take place in total isolation from the environment or from significant others. It is thought of as a functional or dysfunctional unit of interactional behavior. The role can be defined as the actual and tangible form which the self takes. Self, ego, personality, character, and so forth, are cluster effects, not roles in themselves. The role is a fusion of private and collective elements.

During the 1960's, an unfortunate connotation was attached to the term "role playing," wherein the enactment of roles was not seen as an inherent function of the human being, but as something dishonest, a mask over the real person. This is a complete misunderstanding of the role concept in therapy.

The dramatic format of the Theatre of Spontaneity led to the concept of the role and role formation. They are placed into three main categories: Psychosomatic Roles, relating body and psyche, Psychodramatic Roles or Fantasy Roles, and Socio-Cultural Roles. The role is not considered separate from a person's essence, like the clothes he puts on or takes off, but as an existential part of his being, the part that makes up his ego with other roles. The personality may emerge from the roles, since role enactment takes place before there is role perception. The psyche is an open system with the roles in various stages of development. It is not a container into which the roles fit, like pick-up sticks in a tube.

Every human being has a role repertoire far larger than normally used. There is great individual variation in the number of roles each one activates and in the value placed on them. Roles may be absent, latent, emerging or developing, incomplete, distorted, in full activation, descending, dying or burning out and replaced. They may be of central order or peripheral. Their condition and states are not fixed; they may move from one position to another. Inability to move, rigidity of roles, has to be attended to by therapy and/or retraining.

Rapid and extreme shifting of roles can create group upheaval. An example of this is Gauguin's life. In the midst of a successful career in the world of finance, he gave it all up for the role of the creative artist, thereby upsetting his family's lives—his wife moved back to Sweden with the children. The role of the artist has no counterrole except that of the art appreciator. It is probable that Gauguin was considered psychotic, since such a dramatic emergence of a hitherto latent role, along with the burning away of all the other roles, is frequently regarded as insanity by interactors in the person's previous role and by observers of the process because their own role responses and needs no longer fit. We see similar events today, though not always in such extreme forms, in the growing number of people who are giving up successful careers for a second or third one. If there is no support for these changes within the family or social setting, no effective counterroles, the protagonist must establish a completely new and different set of associates.

Our role repertoire is activated and enlarged as we develop, moving from the protection of the family into the larger world. Inadequate role development in a much-needed role can lead to unsatisfactory interaction.

Society rigidifies certain roles and we have to struggle to free ourselves of these preconceptions: male versus female roles, the older person in our society seen as a nonworker and a nonsexual partner, to mention but a few sources of societal disablement.

While certain roles develop and remain fairly stable throughout lifetime, changing only in frequency, duration, or intensity, such as the psychosomatic roles of the sleeper, the eater, and the walker, certain other roles cease to be as central. For example, the role of the protective parent changes gradually, as required by the growing child, into a relation of greater partnership. Failure for this to happen brings the growing child and the family into conflict. There are parents who so love small children and their own parenting that they cannot permit the small child to grow up. Infantilizing and overprotection result. If the child rebels, the parents feel threatened and react, often negatively. There are others who feel the burden of small children to be beyond their own role ability and they can become child abusers, or they push their children into early adulthood, sometimes requiring them to reverse roles with them, to become their ideal parent. Their own small needy child gets in the way because of its early deprivation. Such role distortions require attention. Role structure is a complex phenomenon.

An example of misperception of a sociocultural role was reported to me by a teacher. The first day of a first grade class one of the little girls did not sit down in her assigned seat but stood up, next to it, when the class began. Upon the teacher's request that she be seated she answered, "But I'm not tired." Evidently she had not perceived that in the classroom the teacher is the only one allowed free movement—students are required to sit and must ask for permission to move about. She stayed aloft all day. But the next day she had grasped the student role and sat down with the rest. This may be an example of spontaneous behavior; however, in the eyes of the teacher and the rest of the students, it was inadequate.

Changing roles in our society requires great strength of purpose and determination; and while such changes may be seen afterwards as worthwhile, the actors in the ongoing drama go through much turmoil in the process.

There are three levels in role playing: role enactment, role perception and role expectation. Discrepancies between any of these create interpersonal as well as intrapersonal disturbances. Certain roles, specifically psychosomatic ones, require specific changes in our society. For example, in the average middle-class household, eating is done in the kitchen or dining room, sleeping in the bedroom, the bathroom is for dealing with excreta and cleaning oneself, the den is for the family to gather in and watch TV. Deviations from this pattern can be greatly upsetting to the managers of the household. We even demand proper toilet training from our small children and our pets; if they fail, they are not housebroken. Wrong or rigid emphasis on the correct settings can lead to family turbulence.

The roles of the eater and the sleeper in children are often distorted because their interactional matrix is inequitable. A mother needs to have her child eat at a specified time and to eat the prescribed amount of food. This need may impose itself on the child's wants in ways that create a struggle between them. The same may be true for the need of sleep. Having the child asleep is often more the adult's need for rest and recuperation than the child's need. Problems at sleeping time may result. The stress lies in the varying enactments of the interlocking roles, needs, and perceptions, in terms of quantity, length, and time. Intensity, duration and timing all play a significant part in role interaction.

Sometimes a simple reorganization of the seating order around the table can resolve eating problems. The parents may not share each other's view of how the child's eating role should be handled. We have successfully managed such reorganization by having the siblings take over some of the supervisory functions and by increasing the physical distance between the parent and child. This indicates the importance of space in interpersonal role conflicts.

Instances of intrapersonal conflict between two or more psychosomatic roles are known to us all. The eater role, for instance, may thrust itself into that of the sleeper, awakening the sleeper and making it imperative that it be satisfied. The sleeper gets up, has a snack to satisfy the eater, and is once again able to return to the act of sleeping.

On the psychological or fantasy level, role conflicts are usually more difficult to resolve. There may be conflict between two or more roles in different categories. A familiar one to persons in the helping professions is the conflict between private and personal roles, that of the therapist versus that of the parent. A little boy of nine, the son of a psychiatrist, came to therapy and was a striking example of this. When confronted with a male auxiliary ego in the role of his father, he angrily stamped his foot and said, "I don't want to be your son. I want to be your patient. Then you'll pay attention to me." This was a self-fulfilling prophecy which could not, in the end, be fulfilled since the father was not able to treat his son. The entire family entered into treatment so that new interaction could create familial balance.

The auxiliary egos in such treatment are extremely valuable; they can double for each of the family members, assisting in the communication between them. Individual members can work with auxiliary egos to express safely their innermost conflict without fear of retaliation and with reduced guilt, since the offending family members are absent. If indicated, the partners in the conflict are treated first via auxiliary egos who become familiar with the conflict and represent the absentees realistically. Only when the various partners are able to enter into more open, honest contact with one another will they be brought together in treatment.

We note role deficiencies at times. One or another partner in a conflict may not have the particular role required by another in the repertoire, or may not give it the same centrality. This can be the cause of breakdowns in the relationship; the dissatisfied partner may search for substitution with another partner who has the required function and with whom interaction is more complete and satisfying. Role repair and substitution with another partner may lead to dissolution of the earlier relationship and they are often found in marital breakdowns. This does not refer only to sexual roles, although these may be involved; rather it is often a hitherto underdeveloped or ignored role that becomes dominant in one of the partners.

The designation of a person having a weak or strong ego beclouds the issue. No one has ever seen an ego. At best we can observe that a person has a weakly- or strongly-developed role. This allows the individual to realize what this structure does to the counterstructure in the partner or partners. Putting these structures in better balance may result in stronger partnership. There are few among us who are equally strong in a great many roles; they are the exception rather than the rule. The majority of us are deficient somewhere in one or another role relationship. Identification and training in these areas require spontaneity and creativity.

Anticipation of certain roles makes us anxious and insecure about entering situations where these roles will have to be embodied, such as the role of the lover, the spouse, the parent, the teacher, the employee, the traveler, etc. Desensitization is called for, along with some exploration of the earlier history that contributed to this anxiety, therefore requiring repair in the present.

Role structure and interaction can be plotted on diagrams for diagnostic and guidance purposes and are especially useful in the treatment of families and small groups. Such diagrams may be drawn by each partner and then compared with those of each of the other group members for discrepancies of perception and for further dramatic enactment and correction. Role reversal is the essential ingredient here. The more harmonious the interaction, the greater will be the areas of agreement as well as the number of roles perceived as mutually satisfying. These diagrams can vary from total disagreement to considerable overlap. If done longitudinally, they are good indicators of changes achieved and of those still needed.

THE CONCEPT OF THE SOCIAL ATOM

The position that emotional disturbance is largely a product of human interaction that is not restricted to intrapsychic phenomena led to the examination of the individual plus his relevant others, as well as of the relationships they shared. In the treatment of husband and wife, designated as the intimate social atom, the focus of treatment was upon three entities: the two individuals *and* their relationship. As with the psychotic patient, Moreno found it difficult to influence the psyche directly and thought it might be more effective to approach it through the relationship.

He applied this frame of reference to the study of a residential school for delinquent girls in upstate New York. His findings, published in 1934 in *Who Shall Survive?*, were the first sociometric investigation of an entire community. The sociometrist is not merely an observer-participant and interviewer; rather he elicits the active cooperation and collaboration of the group members. The group members become, in effect, co-researchers in the project. Out of this research came a large number of sociograms, or charts depicting the living, learning, and working space of the group members in interaction in these settings. From this study the concepts of the *social atom* and *social networks* emerged, among others. The structures around and between individuals, which tied them together, Moreno termed the social atom and their role relationships he termed the *cultural atom,* which complements the social atom on the role level. The social atom and the cultural atom are two formations within a more comprehensive one called the social network.

Definitions of the social atom are:

1) The nucleus of all individuals towards whom a person is related in a significant manner or who are related to him; the relationship may be emotional, social or cultural.

2) The sum of interpersonal structures resulting from choices and rejections centered about a given individual.

3) The smallest nucleus of individuals in the social universe who are emotionally interwoven, emotional because even the highest spiritual or intellectual relationships are meaningless without some feeling.

4) The center of attraction, rejection or indifference; the interweaving of emotional, social or cultural factors eventually takes the form of attraction, rejection or indifference on the surface of human contact.

5) The ultimate universal "common denominator" of all social forms, not normative like the family or an abstraction from the group like the individual.

6) An existential category, it consists of individuals. Once brought to cognizance it is in immediate evidence and cannot be further reduced. Contrary to it, the physical atom is not in immediate evidence and can be further reduced. It is not a reality but a construct. The term *atomos,* any very small thing, is a misnomer for the physical atom is not the smallest and simplest elementary particle of matter. Electrons, neutrons, protons, etc., are smaller and in the course of time still smaller particles may be found. But it cannot be imagined that at any time a smaller social structure than the social atom will be found, as it is nothing else but the most immediate social coexistence of individuals.

7) A pattern of attractions, repulsions and indifferences discerned on the threshold between individual and group. (Moreno, J. L., 1961, p. 36)

In terms of the cultural atom, according to Confucius there were five basic sets of human relations: Ruler versus Subject, Husband versus Wife, Father versus Mother, Older Brother versus Younger Brother, and Father versus Son. In our society there are additional ones which had no significance in the China of Confucius's time. Among these are: Employer versus Employee, Employee versus Employee, Stranger versus Native, Majority versus Minority group member, Government versus Citizen, Father versus Female Child, Father versus Middle Child, and so forth; and the same goes, of course, for the Mother-Child relationships and the Female versus Female and Female versus Male relationships.

Of particular concern to psychotherapists are six relationships uncovered in this microscopic overview. The dyad, or pair, is the smallest unit of social interaction. The family consists first of this pair. The dyad and its treatment, as pointed out earlier, encompasses three entities. These structures become far more complex in their interrelationships when entire families are involved (triangles, squares, pentagons, etc.), all considered with their substructures and bonds.

Within the dyadic organization the following are discernible:

1) Two healthy persons can have a productive relationship if it is mutually satisfying and growth-supporting; this is a reassuring finding even if somewhat rare.

2) Two otherwise healthy persons can have a disturbed relationship—with other partners they would be balanced, but together they contribute to one another's disequilibrium, disturbance, or destruction.

3) One healthy and one so-called sick person can have a healthy relationship— on this psychotherapy is based. This cannot last; it may eventually lead to an end, with release and independence of the dependent person. But it means a mutually beneficial and satisfying relationship.

4) A healthy person and an unhealthy one can have a pathological relationship, one which is mutually destructive.

5) Two so-called sick persons can have a healthy relationship when one of the partners is somewhat better integrated than the other, that is, well enough not to be disequilibrated by the weaker partner. Group psychotherapy and AA are based on this, as are all the mutual self-help groups, with each partner acting as therapeutic agent for another.

6) Two disturbed individuals can have a disturbed relationship in that they contribute further to the disturbance.

In psychodrama, after dealing with the dyadic organization, the social atom is studied not only from the perspective of the two central protagonists, for instance a couple, but also from the perspective of the children, in-laws from both sides, and siblings.

The effects of birth within the social atom are often profound. In addition to the exploration of these effects on the intimate, work, and socio-cultural atom, psychodramatists began to look at death within the social atom. In an aging population or in a network of dying, such as with AIDS, the deprivation by social and physical death becomes of major concern. Not only the aged are severely affected by death. Working with adolescents and young adults who have attempted or are depressed enough to contemplate suicide, treatment is directed at having the protagonist role reverse with a person whom they recently lost, either through the ending of a relationship or through death. In the latter case, we often find that the continued relationship with the deceased is more valued than one with anyone alive. Thus another subset of relationships was revealed, that of the Dead versus the Alive.

Here treatment consists in having the patient role reverse with the dead person and face himself portrayed by an auxiliary ego who firmly declares love for the deceased and the fervent wish to join the dead. In all cases treated in this way, the deceased did not wish the patient to join him in death. However, to complete the healing there must be a restoration of balance in the social atom of life, which must defuse the relationship to the dead person. Often patients are not aware that there is potential help around them. The way to reach for help is to ask the protagonist, who will be most hurt if you should happen to commit suicide? The person so selected by the patient becomes the next candidate for role reversal into that person learning of the patient's suicide. When one patient denied that anyone would care, the start of the psychodrama was with the person who would first discover her. This led to a chain of six persons, each of whose roles she embodied and each time the person was informed of her death. She did not have *psychodramatic shock* and full realization of the consequences her contemplated act would evoke until she became her own mother.

In another case, a teen-ager had made several such suicide attempts. In exploring what had happened to her in the last year, she set up seven empty chairs of persons whom she cared about, each of whom had died. Again, in the role of each one she did not give herself permission to die; instead, all encouraged and supported life, reminding her that she was a promising student and that she must live her life to the full. A lack of support was evident in her familial social atom. Although she and her father essentially had a caring relationship, it was her mother (who had been pyschotic before the daughter's birth) who was the center of her father's life. He was bound up in keeping his wife out of a mental hospital. Their relationship was so symbiotic that it excluded the children. The girl's only sibling, an older brother, had recently married and moved far away; they had been very close before this, being each other's mutual support. Here was, of course, another death in her life—the vital link to her brother. She felt he had to live his own life since he was newly wed; but when the protagonist was put into her brother's role, interviewed from that perspective, and asked if he would want to help his sister because the danger of completed suicide could be real, the role of the protective brother came to the fore. It was clear that the sister had never revealed her despair to him. In his role the protagonist felt dreadfully burdened, as if his new life cost the life of his sister. When asked if he was willing to pay that price, the protagonist was shocked and asked how he could help. It was suggested that perhaps his sister should inform him what she was going through and that she should ask if he would be willing to help her move close to him and continue her schooling there. The answer was distinct and positive. Ending the role reversal here, the ensuing interview dealt with the writing of a letter. After a few more sessions, the correspondence was revealed to go well and she eventually did join her brother. In that healthier setting she thrived and has gone on to higher education. In this case, the restructuring of the social atom (moving from a diseased family setting to a healthy one) was the necessary step, since the parents did not come for psychotherapy and were unwilling to do so. We think of such intervention as social atom repair.

If exploration of the social atom reveals pulls from the side of death, then pulls from the social atom of life have to be enhanced. The social atom is a rich source of diagnostic and therapeutic information; it can be used to help restore what is called *sociostasis*, homeostatic balance in the social atom. Homeostatic balance is primarily linked to stability of relationships and not to stability of the individuals involved, nor to their characteristics. In the study of the work and school social atom, it has been shown that proneness to illness, proneness to accidents and absenteeism in business and industry, as well as in school with children, are reflections of the lack of integration in the group, rather than characteristics which reside only in the individual personality.

In psychodrama, process is more important than content, even though the content is reconstructed—"How did this happen to you, show me" is the focus rather than "What happened to you, tell me." Patients frequently repress or forget what happened, both in and outside of therapy, but they rarely forget how they experienced it and how this experience affected them. Thus, we tap into the process and, remarkably, the contents begin to emerge again, within the flow of the process. Protagonists may fall temporarily out of a scene by stating, "Oh, I had forgotten, this and that occurred here," thereby amplifying and intensifying the re-enactment. Because it is a flowing, life-connected process, learning can be carried from therapy into life itself. It affects the protagonist on the level of action, fantasy, and reality. We start with the magic "as if," but after a while the "if" falls away leaving only "as."

Rank has this to say about play, "For play, after all, differs not only conceptually, but factually, from art. It has in common with art the combination of the real and the apparent; yet it is not merely fancy objectivized, but fancy translated into reality, acted and lived. It shares with art the double consciousness of appearance and reality, yet it has more of reality, while art is content with the appearance" (1968, p. 104).

In practical terms, psychodrama protagonists should speak in the present tense; verbs are action words. Placing protagonists into the present, no matter when the scenes actually happened, reduces the verbal reporting and turns them into actors. As Longinus in the first century A.D. wrote, "If you introduce things which are past as present and now taking place, you will make your story no longer a narration but an actuality" (1970, p. 71).

Psychodrama is a synthesizing process, putting together many elements, sometimes in disorderly manner; but, out of this disorder, some order eventually arises.

Returning to Rank, we find him saying, "The great artist and great work are only born from the reconciliation of . . . the victory of a philosophy of renunciation over an ideology of deprivation" (1968, p. 429). It strikes me that this applies to our patients who may have to reconcile themselves to a deprivation of their privacy to gain or regain themselves on another level and with larger dimensions. But to achieve this and not to feel deprived, they must find within themselves and their relationships, as artists find in their work, something of equal or greater value. Possibly some can even become artists at living. Our task is to guide them so that this can take place. Then they can achieve, as Eric Erikson put it in *Young Man Luther*, "This pure self is the self no longer sick with a conflict between right and wrong, not dependent on providers, and not dependent on guides to reason and reality" (1958, p. 265).

Moreno ventured a prediction in *Who Shall Survive?* He wrote:

When the nineteenth century came to an end and the final accounting was made, what emerged as its greatest contribution to the mental and social sciences was the idea of the unconscious and its cathexes. When the twentieth century will close its doors that which I believe will come out as the greatest achievement is the idea of spontaneity-creativity and the significant, indelible link between them. It may be said that the efforts of the two centuries complement one another. If the nineteenth century looked for the "lowest" common denominator of mankind, the unconscious, the twentieth century discovered, or rediscovered, its "highest" common denominator—spontaneity-creativity. (1953, p. 48)

REFERENCES

Blatner, A. (1985). The dynamics of catharsis. *Journal of Group Psychotherapy, Psychodrama and Sociometry, 37* (4), 157–166.

Buchanan, D.R., & Enneis, J.M. (1980). The central concern model: A framework for structuring psychodramatic production. *Journal of Group Psychotherapy, Psychodrama and Sociometry, 33*, 47–62.

Buchanan, D.R., & Enneis, J.M. (1984). Moreno's Social Atom: A diagnostic and treatment tool for exploring interpersonal relationships. *The Arts in Psychotherapy, 11*, 155–164.

Compernolle, T. (1981). J.L. Moreno, an unrecognized pioneer of family therapy. *Family Process, 20*, 331–335.

Diener, G. (1971). Relation of the delusionary process in Goethe's Lila to analytic psychology and to psychodrama. *Group Psychotherapy and Psychodrama, 28* (1–2), 5–13.

Erikson, E. (1958). *Young Man Luther*. New York: W.W. Norton.

Goldman, E.E. & Morrison, D.S. (1984). *Psychodrama: experience and process*. Dubuque: Kendall Hunt.

Hollander, C.E. & Hollander, S. (1978). *The warm up box*. Denver: Snow Lion Press.

Lieberman, E.J. (1985). *Acts of will, the life and work of Otto Rank*. New York: The Free Press.

Longinus. (1970). *Treatise on the Sublime*. In Walter Jackson Bate (Ed.), *Criticism: The major texts*. New York: Harcourt Brace Jovanovich.

Moreno, J.L. (1924). *Das Stegreiftheater*. Potsdam: Gustav Kiepenheuer Verlag.

Moreno, J.L. (1932). *Application of the group method to classification*. New York: National Committee on Prisons and Prison labor.

Moreno, J.L. (1937). Inter-personal therapy and the psychopathology of interpersonal relations. *Sociometry, A Journal of Inter-Personal Relations, 1* (1–2), 9–76.

Moreno, J.L. (1938). Psychodramatic shock therapy: A sociometric approach to the problem of mental disorder. *Sociometry, A Journal of Inter-Personal Relations, 2* (1), 1–30.

Moreno, J.L. (1939). Psychodramatic treatment of marriage problems. *Sociometry, A Journal of Inter-Personal Relations, 3* (1), 1–23.

Moreno, J.L. (1939). Psychodramatic treatment of psychoses. *Sociometry, A Journal of Inter-Personal Relations, 3* (2), 115–132.

Moreno, J.L. (1939). A frame of reference for testing the social investigator. *Sociometry, A Journal of Inter-Personal Relations, 3* (4), 317–327.

Moreno, J.L. (1940). Mental catharsis and the psychodrama. *Sociometry, A Journal of Inter-Personal Relations, 3* (3), 209–244.

Moreno, J.L. (Ed). (1945). *Group psychotherapy, A symposium*. Beacon: Beacon House.

Moreno, J.L. (1946). *Psychodrama, Vol. I*. Beacon, N.Y.: Beacon House.

Moreno, J.L. (1947, 1973). *The theatre of spontaneity*. Beacon, N.Y.: Beacon House.

Moreno, J.L. (1951). *Sociometry, experimental method and the science of society*. Beacon, N.Y.: Beacon House.

Moreno, J.L. (Ed.). (1956). *Sociometry and the science of man.* Beacon, N.Y.: Beacon House.

Moreno, J.L. (1957). *The first book on group psychotherapy.* Beacon, N.Y.: Beacon House.

Moreno, J.L. (1961). The role concept, a bridge between psychiatry and sociology. *American Journal of Psychiatry, 118,* 518–522.

Moreno, J.L. (Ed.). (1961). *The sociometry reader.* Glencoe, IL: The Free Press.

Moreno, J.L. (1971). Comments on Goethe and Psychodrama. *Group psychotherapy and psychodrama, Vol. XXIV.* Beacon, N.Y.: Beacon House.

Moreno, J.L., & Jennings, H.H. (1937). Statistics of social configurations. *Sociometry, A Journal of Inter-Personal Relations, 1* (1–2), 342–374.

Moreno, J.L., & Moreno, Z.T. (1959). *Psychodrama, Vol. II.* Beacon, N.Y.: Beacon House.

Moreno, J.L., Moreno, Z.T., & Moreno, J.D. (1964). *The first psychodramatic family.* Beacon, N.Y.: Beacon House.

Moreno, J.L., & Moreno, Z.T. (1969). *Psychodrama, Vol. III.* Beacon, N.Y.: Beacon House.

Moreno, Z.T. (1952). Psychodrama in a well-baby clinic. *Group Psychotherapy, A Journal of Sociopsychopathology and Sociatry, 4* (1–2), 100–106.

Moreno, Z.T. (1954). Psychodrama in the crib. *Group Psychotherapy, 7* (3–4), 291–302.

Moreno, Z.T. (1958). Note on spontaneous learning "in situ" versus learning the Academic Way. *Group Psychotherapy, 9* (1), 50–51.

Moreno, Z.T. (1958). The "reluctant therapist" and the "reluctant audience" technique in psychodrama. *Group Psychotherapy, 9* (4), 278–282.

Moreno, Z.T. (1959). A survey of psychodramatic techniques. *Group Psychotherapy, 12* (1), 5–14.

Moreno, Z.T. (1965). Psychodramatic rules, techniques and adjunctive methods. *Group Psychotherapy, 18* (1–2), 73–86.

Moreno, Z.T. (1967). The seminal mind of J.L. Moreno. *Group Psychotherapy, 20* (3–4), 218–229.

Moreno, Z.T. (1969). Moreneans, the heretics of yesterday are the orthodoxy of today. *Group Psychotherapy, 22* (1–2), 1–6.

Moreno, Z.T. (1969). Practical Aspects of Psychodrama. *Group Psychotherapy, 22* (3–4), 213–219.

Moreno, Z.T. (1971). Beyond Aristotle, Breuer and Freud: Moreno's contribution to the concept of catharsis. *Group Psychotherapy, 24* (1–2), 34–43.

Moreno, Z.T. (1972). Note on psychodrama, sociometry, individual psychotherapy and the quest for "unconditional love." *Group Psychotherapy, 25* (4), 155–157.

Moreno, Z.T. (1974). Psychodrama of young mothers. *Group Psychotherapy, 27,* 191–203.

Moreno, Z.T. (1978). The function of the auxiliary ego in psychodrama with special reference to psychotic patients. *Group Psychotherapy, Psychodrama and Sociometry, 31,* 163–166.

Moreno, Z.T. (1983). Psychodrama. In H. I. Kaplan & B. J. Sadock (Eds.), *Comprehensive group psychotherapy.* Baltimore: William and Wilkins.

Moreno, Z.T. (1985). Moreno's concept of ethical anger. *Group Psychotherapy, Psychodrama and Sociometry,* (In press). *38 (4).*

Moreno, Z.T., & Moreno, J.D. (1984). The psychodramatic model of madness. *Journal of The British Psychodrama Association, 1,* 24–35.

Moreno, Z.T., Moreno, J.L., & Moreno, J.D. (1955). The discovery of the spontaneous man. *Group Psychotherapy, 8* (2), 103–129.

Pierce, C.S. (1931) *Collected papers, Vol. I,* Cambridge: Harvard University Press

Rank, O. (1968). *Art and artist.* New York: A.A. Knopf. (Original work published 1932)

Starr, A. (1977). *Psychodrama, rehearsal for living.* Chicago: Nelson Hall.

Toeman, Z. (1944). Role analysis and audience structure. *Sociometry, A Journal of Inter-Personal Relations, 8* (2), 205–221.

Toeman, Z. (1945). Clinical psychodrama: Auxiliary ego double and mirror techniques. *Sociometry, A Journal of Inter-Personal Relations, 9* (2–3), 178–183.

Toeman, Z. (1947). The "double" situation in psychodrama. *Sociatry, Journal of Group and Intergroup Therapy, 1* (4), 436–446.

Weiner, H.B. & Sacks, J. (1969). Warm-up and sum-up. *Group Psychotherapy, 23* (1–2), 85–102.

Yablonsky, L. (1976). *Psychodrama, resolving emotional problems through role-playing.* New York: Basic Books.

Discussion by Carl A. Whitaker, M.D.

I've had a great time reading this paper and thinking about it, Zerka, thinking about the times when I visited Beacon, New York, and J.L. But I have a series of protests. One of them is that you're about the worst male chauvinist I've ever run into, and the thing that makes it impossible is that you love that old son of a bitch so much, that you won't let him die. And my craziness was that I would go and visit his grave with you and we would have a psychodrama and your arm would regrow. That's how crazy I can get. But, I thought, what would have happened if I had been in a stage in my life, that would have been about 1938 or 1940, to have stayed on at Beacon, rather than visiting and leaving.

Learning about psychotherapy is an impossible task; I've only been at it 45 years and it's like raising children. I keep thinking, next year, when my oldest gets 47, I will stop having problems being a parent. Anyway, here is a story about psychotherapy I got out of the newspaper. It's very simple and very humbling. It seems that there was this guy up on top of a high bridge who was about to jump off and commit suicide. The cop was trying to talk him down. He said something about your poor father, your poor mother, your wife, your kids, etc. and he had all the answers for that, fast and flat. Finally, the cop lost his temper, pulled his gun and said, "You son of a bitch, if you jump, I'll shoot ya." That was psychotherapy. The man came down.

As I was struggling this morning, my thought was that he lost his role, he suddenly became a whole person and it was the whole person's function. So I have some problem with the question of roles. And I don't know how to answer the questions because I keep feeling it's now 48 years and 3 months to the day since I

married and it feels as though the roles betwen Muriel and I keep getting weaker and weaker. Thank God the power gets greater and greater.

In reading Zerka (Moreno's) paper, I ran into a few dangers and a few glories and a few questions that may hopefully be some contribution to Zerka's complex and exciting way of understanding life and the effort to change.

One danger is that you will adopt the needy child who comes for help. I think we are characterologically defective, all of us. If we were disillusioned supermoms, we would have found a better way to earn a living. I think you need to be aware of this problem. I don't think you'll cure it. I've never been able to get over it, but I think it's a very important problem and one of the dangers of psychotherapy.

The second is role fixation, of becoming a dedicated missionary in the curing of human ills. I finally decided, I think on my 71st birthday, that there probably will be several families still sick after I die. Therefore, I should try to choose ones that are growthful for me, rather than buying the cultural illusion which they train us to augment. When someone comes into your office, you right off give him your right breast, and if they should happen to bite the nipple, you put it back in and give him the other one. I think I'm going to get over that insanity some day.

The third danger is that of all living becoming a drama, without an audience, even of yourself or even the invisible audience of those you wished or feared might be looking over your shoulder. The fourth danger is that you might try to be a J.L. Moreno or even, more powerfully, a Zerka Moreno. I suppose if I were a Zen master I'd say the first thing you ought to do if you want to be a Zerka is to cut off your right arm.

One of the nice things, I thought, was to try to utilize her thinking about the alter egos in my thinking about the co-therapist. My growing conviction is that so far there really is no such thing as a single parent. That single parent cultural monkey business is like other cultural conserves. You know, a cultural conserve is either in syrup or vinegar, otherwise it wouldn't be conserved.

The glory of the psychodrama movements, of the psychodrama process, I would say, is in the massive castration of words. We are haunted by the inadequacy of these feeble symbols we call words and our efforts to get past these symbols are very frightening. One way to get past it that was most helpful to me was my spending a solid year from 1941 to 1942 on a playroom floor with five or six little children, five days a week. If there is anything that will get you over making believe words say something, it's doing play therapy and nothing else.

One of the glories of the psychodrama patterning is the capacity for role reversal. This is one of the ways of breaking the illusion of grandeur that we live in, if you can move from what you and the patient are operating with into where it is in your life. (I sometimes call *meta-therapy*, when you talk about your suicidal impulses, your suicidal attempts, rather than making believe you had never had a suicidal thought, to say nothing about a murderous impulse. I wouldn't even tell you about the time I was 12 and stood behind my father, having gone to get the ax he needed, fantasizing sinking it down through his head and cutting him into two equal parts.)

Another attraction arises from the moments of wholeness in the psychodrama process. There's this situation in which you're out of your head, and if you don't get out of your head, I don't think you can become a real psychotherapist.

The third of the glories of her presentation and of the process of psychodrama is that psychotics do establish transference, except that the therapist wants to manipulate it. That's why psychotics know more about how to get out of it. They move into the transference and they get debunked by our inadequacy. The real problem with psychotics that I've had just such fun with is not that they're crazy but that we are all schizophrenics, in the middle of the night. When we're sound asleep, we're just as schizophrenic as hell and we wake up and make believe that we're just the person who dreamed he was a cockroach, not a cockroach who awoke and made believe he was a man.

The process of being schizophrenic is a process that we in the social, sociopathic lifestyle of living in groups with other people don't understand. We don't even know how to talk baby language with people who want to talk baby language. We make believe it's dumb of them. It isn't dumb of them, it's dumb of us. Anyway, the psychodramatist knows about psychotics being able to be human beings and the problem is that we are not able to be human beings. We're trying to be social robots.

The fourth is the concept of the social atom. Some philosopher, I think it was Hegel, said that there's no such thing as the dyad. That's merely the remnant of an extruded third. So the nice part about getting married, you know, is that you get rid of two mothers at once.

The fifth one is the creativity. It's the result of a union plus nourishing of the new weed, the investment of yourself in the process of joining with the other half of you, or with another, or with a whole organismic other we call a group or a family, or with 7,000 screwballs at this conference.

The final one is the funny kind of dialectic in my thinking about social status and role-less-ness. And I think the critical problem to me is that you can't win, either way: you can't be roleless, and you can't win by belonging only to the social group.

As for questions, I have only three, I'm sorry to say. Tillich's book, *Being is Becoming*, was for me a concept I've struggled with for years. It finally dawned on me that the other half is that *doing is to keep from being.* As long as you keep doing enough, you never have to be anybody. If that's true, then is all doing a role? And is role adequacy a way to avoid personhood? If you get good enough at roles, then maybe you never have to be anybody. I remember seeing a wonderful patient who said that she had such a marvelous network of people. She just met so many lovely people. She worked in a five-and-ten cents store, and she met beautiful people all day long. Some of them even stayed for three or four minutes.

The question is, "Is personhood only a role?" And a final question is, "Is there a difference between A and B, the man and the woman, the husband and the wife, the father and son, the employer and the employee, and the relationship between them?" In other words, there is a "we." And the reason this hit me is that it dawned on me one day, with a shudder, that if my wife, Muriel, dies, and she better not, it's not just losing her, I will have lost *us.* And I think *us* is probably more important than she is, although I wouldn't want to say that out loud.

QUESTIONS AND ANSWERS

Question: I have several questions for Dr. Beutler who read Dr. Lazarus' paper because he was detained en route to Phoenix. First of all, I think many of us probably know of therapists who use different forms of therapy in a very intuitive and subjective way and seem to get very good results. I wonder if Dr. Lazarus would agree that that happens and how he would explain it. Also, Dr. Lazarus seems to believe there's a great danger of running into hidden theoretical contradictions in using different schools of thought. Obviously, that can happen but it hasn't been my impression that it happens all the time or that it is an enormous problem. I wanted to question the example that he gave of the seeming contradiction between Dr. Adler's belief that the life plan is unconscious and

the concept of Lifescript of Eric Berne which was supposed to be conscious. I'm not an expert in Transactional analysis but it seems to me that Berne felt that it was primary unconscious. In the book *What Do You Say After You Say Hello?* (New York: Grove, 1972), he talks about the difference between script and nonscript as being a difference in awareness verses nonawareness. Is there in fact a contradiction here?

Beutler: Let me broaden my role a little bit and see if I can speak more comfortably for Systematic Eclectic therapists rather than specifically for Dr. Lazarus, although attempting to respond to the concern. I think that most of us who adopt a systematic eclectic point of view would confess that most of the benefits that we are currently able to document in psychotherapy come from the good sense of therapists and their intuitive ability to relate to their clients and patients. It is not a diminution of the importance of the art of psychotherapy. If there is a theme in the presentations here, I think it is about where we stand in this dimension of weighing the art against the science and the objectivity and the planfulness of psychotherapy. Many of us disagree as to just where that line is—not that both aren't important.

I think that the other aspect would be, however, that therapists are notoriously poor judges of their own effectiveness. In my own research over the past several years, I've had the opportunity of systematically studying over 300 therapists and I haven't found one who said that he or she was ineffective, although I can document that at least 10 percent have more failures than successes. The power of the intuitive process is fine for those who are good at it, but we are not always good judges of whether or not we are good at it. As for the question of discounting the intuitive ability of the therapist, I think Dr. Lazarus and I would say that what we attempt to do is to make therapists thinking therapists as well as just feeling therapists. We want people to learn when to apply what, to whom, under what conditions, in what circumstances, and what outcomes to look for. Once you know that, there's a certain advantage to forgetting it and thus entering into the therapy process spontaneously, with feeling and emotion and trust in your judgment, and knowing what kinds of outcomes to anticipate and when to apply what. As to the contradiction you raised about Adler and Berne, it has also been my understanding that Berne suggested that the scripts were largely unconscious.

Question: I thought Dr. Whitaker gave us a kind of teaser with his distinction between doing and personhood. I wonder if he would elaborate on the concept of personhood as distinguished from doing?

Whitaker: I think it's in direct line with the comment that anything that's worth knowing you can't teach. I've been preoccupied with another variant of that same process. If you follow someone who presumably knows—a supervisor or a mentor—you end up making believe you know what he knows so you never learn anything. I'm more and more convinced that you should give up trying to learn from somebody of a previous generation. Link up with a peer and start to learn by yourself. I dare not say that because all of us supervisors would be out of business.

The thing I was struggling with in this discussion was the process in which science and art go in opposite directions. I think it's the dialectic. Not only that, you can't win by just going toward science. Then you end up being made of stone. If you go the other way and are just an artist, you may end up as a blob of gluck. The problem is that the more you have of one, the more you can head for the other. The more scientific you are, the more artistic you can dare to be; the more artistic you are, the more you can struggle with science. The problem I have is that I can't stay interested in science. It's in the wrong side of my head.

Moreno: I think that in psychodrama we really do try to combine the two—science and art. But there is a story about a very clever student of mathematics who left the field. When asked why by his professor, he said, "Well, I wasn't poetic enough." He became an economist. I think we have to start thinking in terms of the new science, the new physics. I don't know how many people here have read Lawrence Leshan's *The Medium, the Mystic, and the Physicist* (New York: Ballantine, 1982). You can't tell by the way these people experienced the universe which of these models is speaking. They all come out with the same kind of experience. Only a physicist can tell that the physicist is speaking, or a mystic can tell a mystic is speaking, or a medium can tell a medium is speaking. Still, they experience the universe in very similar ways.

Now we are still dealing in social science with old material. We can't seem to get rid of that old junk that has nothing to do with social science and which isn't even scientific anymore. We must begin to think in terms of alternate realities. That's what we're dealing with. An example for this would be when the patient comes and says, "I'm having a terrible difficulty, I can't get my ex-husband to listen to me on the phone, I'm having some conflicts, I want some therapy for six months, I've been in therapy and I've broken off, and I have this little girl, and I'm not well enough." The whole story comes out about how she supported this man through medical school, an old story, and as soon as he got through medical school, he fell in love with someone else. Again this business of role expansion, role immersion, role death, and so on.

By the way, I don't always look at people as if they are roles or dying. I really do look at the totality of the personhood. I get a little disturbed by this separation of roles and personhood. Anyway, I asked "What do you want to do about this?" She said, "I want to telephone him and ask him if he and his new woman can take this child for six months so I can get my head together." "Well," I thought, "why don't we do that," you know, prescribe the symptom? "Let's go, what do you want to do?" "I want to phone him." "Right, why don't we do that?" We both get on the phone and in role reversal I take her role and she takes her husband's. It becomes quite clear that he's not going to impose this child of an earlier marriage upon his new relationship. "No, I can't do that." So we seem to have come to a terrible impasse. She's not going to get what she wants.

This is where we talk about intuition, the intuition that is related to what is happening in front of you. It seems to be coming out of thin air but something is not fitting here. Inside my head I'm thinking that the pieces aren't meshing. There is something wrong. What is it? Meanwhile, she's sitting on the stage, crying and weeping, "I did everything I could for him, right? I put him through school, right? I deprived myself, right? And finally we have a baby, right? I've been a wonderful wife." You can dispute all these things from the point of view of the husband but that's not the issue. I don't know where the intuition comes from, but suddenly I walk up to her, I pick up her face, and I say to her, "You want the child out of the way so that you can commit suicide." She said, "Ahhh, you heard me." I said, "What do you mean?" "I've told two psychotherapists that I was suicidal. The first one laughed at me and said, 'You can't be,' and the second one said, 'All you need is a new love affair. Why don't we start?' This happened to me within the last two weeks." I said, "Alright, let's deal with that. You want to commit suicide, that's your perfect right." I seem to be a specialist in suicide, by the way. All of us must be in some way. "Well, who is this going to affect?"

What I'm saying is that you can't eliminate intuition and you mustn't. Your intuition can mislead you and you always should check with your patient. She has the right to say "No, that's not where it's at."

Question to Cloé Madanes: When you spoke before in response to Dr. Lazarus' talk, you gave an example from Dr. Erickson where he was helping a young woman who was afraid to have children. And you were contrasting the psychoanalytic viewpoint with a systems viewpoint. For those of us who might not want to go the psychoanalytic route to help that patient but might not have the hypnosis skills to help that patient, what would you advise the therapist to do with that client?

Madanes: I think that you can accomplish the same that Milton Erickson described as accomplishing through hypnosis without hypnosis. I think that you can discuss the life of a patient and find good things in it and build on those memories and develop them so that the trance state and regression and the introduction of their totally new character in the life of the patient are really not necessary. You can build upon what's there because all of us, no matter how miserable a life we might have had, had some good things in it.

Question: I would like to ask Dr. Whitaker a question. Could Dr. Whitaker please expand on the notion of therapists learning for themselves rather than just doing therapy for the client?

Whitaker: You just have to be a little crazier than you're supposed to be judging by your training. Just mix in fragments of your own life which they are interested in. You can say things about your own life that they don't know what to do with. I'm an expert in suicide, too. I had the painful early experience of failing to do it and decided it was hopeless if I couldn't make it that time. But I have a whole list of wonderful ways to commit suicide and whenever somebody starts talking about it, I get going on my own suicidal impulses and they just are lucky if they can get back in. The best one I know is to jump out a 14th story window. It's a way of being certain. The problem with most suicide efforts is that it's always so half-hearted. You end up paralyzed from the neck down and you've ruined a good car.

But the process of getting out of this, all you have to do is violate the rules that are set up for you and be who you are for a moment. They'll take you back to get a family. They come in and you've taken this four-page history in the first interview and in the second interview they come and say, "Well, what should we talk about?" I say, "I don't care what you talk about." "Well, you asked all these questions. Don't you have any more questions?" "No, I've decided to quit!" "Well, what are we going to talk about?" "I don't know, whatever you want." "Well, what do you think is most important for us to talk about?" "I haven't the vaguest idea, I don't know how much guts you have or who you'd like to be mad at—be my guest." "Well, you're gonna have to tell us. We don't know how to do psychotherapy. You're the expert at it." I say, "Well, I'll tell you what, let's talk about me, 'I'm 73 and I was suppose to be retired and I don't know what the hell to do. I keep worrying whether I should move south or get a trailer and go visit my six kids who are all over the damn country, or turn my social security check back to the government because it doesn't help much." "Hey, look Doc, we're paying you good money, what the hell are you talking about yourself for?" "Well I was trying to help you learn how, you know." You're talking about the art of psychotherapy, obviously. I'm not sure that would work with everyone.

Question: Let me raise a question for all of the panelists. What is the relationship between how you think, your theoretical constructs, and what you really do?

Whitaker: I never have any theoretical constructs until I get here. When I see the family after the first interview, I'm pretty much free-floating. If something happens I enjoy it and if it doesn't happen, I'm New England enough to just sit there and wait.

Question (continuing): But you do that because of some reason. You have some theory—whether that's a formal theory or indigestion, I'm not sure.

Whitaker: I think I sit there because when I grew up on this farm up in northern New York, I would sit for an hour. Well, my father and a neighbor would sit there saying three words every five minutes. I was brought up to be like Calvin Coolidge, you know. He went to church when his wife couldn't go, came home, and she said, "Well what did the preacher say?" "Oh, I don't know." "What did he talk about?" "Sin." "Well, what did he say about it?" "He was against it." So I don't have to have any flow. My sociopathy developed later than my schizophrenia.

Moreno: May I say something about the loss of a person being not only the loss of a person but the loss of the relationship. I'm dealing recently with people in bereavement a lot, with people who have relatives dying of cancer, and I'm preparing them for this whole business of cleaning up the relationship and how they feel about it. I explain the loss, the sensation of bewilderment and confusion in loss, as a double loss. You're quite right. There is no such thing as a dyad in principle; there are always three there and it is the relationship loss that we focus on.

I explained it to them by giving them an image: It is like an emotional umbilicus which was linked to another person. That other person falls away, but you still have the umbilicus, you still have that bond, and it has no anchorages flailing. Have you ever had that experience when you've lost someone? It's flailing, it's wounded, it's throbbing, it's bleeding, your guts and your heart are in it, and it has no anchorage. Until that somehow shrivels up, or in some way dies out, is reintegrated into you, you can't get over that. When I had this terrible thing in my shoulder, no one knew what was wrong and I wrote a letter to a brother with whom I'm very close and said, "Sometimes I feel like giving up," because I was in terrible agony, was misdiagnosed by seven doctors, and walked around with a growing lump for 15 months. I got a letter back right away from this man who usually takes months to write me. "What do you mean you're giving up? I can't afford to lose you." He wasn't just saying he couldn't afford to lose me; he couldn't afford to lose our contact, our relationship. That's what we're dealing with.

Question: I think we're all experts in suicide or think we are. One of the things about this is that rather than kill ourselves, we get divorced because we don't have the guts to face our own suicidal impulses. I don't know why we don't, but something in our culture sanctions looking at it this way rather than taking the personal responsibility that we are talking about here.

Moreno: Yes, I think you're right. After my amputation, I was very heroic, but you know, this manic performance always brings you down into the depths. The following year I developed viral pneumonia strictly by neglecting myself. Any viral infection makes me suicidal. I want to jump into the first body of water and forget it. I was extremely depressed. I'm allergic to penicillin so I couldn't be treated with that. I had to stay in bed for 90 days and it was really like a living prison. I used to contemplate how I could do away with myself and not let anybody know I had done it. I thought of injecting an air bubble like they did when experimenting on people in concentration camps. It would have done away with all my survival guilt, of course. Well, I didn't know if I could get rid of the hypodermic fast enough and they would find it.

One day, my little boy walked into the room and the sun shone. This was in the wintry days around Christmas, dark and gloomy up north. My son walked in and with him walked in this ray of sun and I realized that for the moment he was standing in the room with me, I was not depressed—I was whole with him. When he left, I did my psychodrama. I sat myself down at the other end of the bed and said, "Now listen, sucker, this cannot go on. You cannot make that child, or for that matter any other person, responsible for your happiness. You've got to find a way to do that now." I think we all have these voices and I think that's what we're trying to use sometimes for ourselves, and sometimes successfully, too.

Whitaker: It's great to see a mother who gets over being mother. It's a disease, worse than being a psychotherapist. I think you're wonderful. The other thing that's weird about mothers is that they're beginning to give up mothering us men. If they do, this is going to be a horrible world. Men are nothing but tool experts. They don't know anything about human beings and I think they're hopeless unless some woman keeps babying them. I worry about the culture.

Moreno: But that's involved with a needy child. Isn't it within them?

Whitaker: Of course, but they never get over it. If I get to be God, you know if he retires and turns it over to me, I've got this plan that the man shall have the second baby. That's one of my theories.

Moreno: My husband said, "Why don't we have another child?" and I said, "If you will have it."

Question: I'm intrigued by the juxtaposition of the two papers—the Lazarus and the Moreno. What do you learn or experience from the juxtaposition of the two papers? This is for anyone on the panel.

Moreno: The issue of having a model, by the way, as a therapist or a director came up in Carl's discussion, too, and I appreciate him mentioning that. Of course, in any art we use a model first, we try to copy someone we respect and admire. I'm just learning to do oil painting and I'm looking at the Masters and copying some of their paintings. I'm learning enormously from it. I'm hoping that I'll evolve eventually. In fact, I'm doing portraits side by side so that I can try to evolve with my own master, or at least mature. That's the same thing. You use a model and then eventually you emerge beyond that model and become your own person. You can use a model, even several models, but the final product—who you are—has to emerge. It cannot be a copy of anyone else. It's impossible anyway—don't even try it.

Beutler: I want to comment again and I think we're in part addressing your question as to the significance of drawing together these two papers. I'm still struck by the fact that I primarily identify myself as a psychotherapy researcher/practitioner. Yet I'm very aware that in my hat as psychotherapy researcher I don't read the same literature or talk to the same people as I do when I wear my hat as practitioner. These are very different bodies of knowledge and it gives me some concern that they don't touch each other more than they do. We have something like 250 (Arnold Lazarus cited this in his paper) or now, I think, over 300, different psychotherapy theories. There is a very good array of many of these here at this conference. A few years ago, I did a systematic evaluation of psychotherapy studies, looking at different therapies. There were fewer than 50 and most of them fell into only two or three different types.

It gives me some cause for pause that there are such discrepancies between that left hemisphere and that right hemisphere. I think these two papers in one sense represents that difference. Lazarus has come at his model of multimodal therapy primarily through an empirical idea of what science is and the relationship with science to practice. Most of the representatives among the psychotherapies in this conference are those who have come at it through a clinician's wisdom and intuition. Cloé Madanes talked about spontaneity and the idea of happiness, for example, as an ingredient in psychotherapy effectiveness.

That isn't something we read about or talk about very much in the psychotherapy research literature. But I have no doubt that it's an important ingredient. There is a need here for some commonalities to be developed. I think it's nice to see these two sides of the hemisphere represented in juxtaposition.

Whitaker: I have a new research project for you. You compare the 300 theories of psychotherapy with the number of old fashioned religion sects and I think you'll be outnumbered.

Beutler: I think you're probably right—and which one's right, Carl?

Question: I'd like to add to that, to compare it with the theories of parenting in general. I'm struck by looking around the room here and thinking this is like a modern campfire scene—a bunch of tribal people sitting around and comparing their intuition and their introspections. Despite all the cognitions and the theories we're talking about today, what the audience seems to be reacting to is something they identify with—when the speaker digresses from the mental masturbation, for lack of a better term, and suddenly says, "This is what happens to me, and this is why I did what I did, and this is the suicidality that I experienced a few years ago, the pain and how I dealt with it." I guess what I'm asking is if we have 200 to 300 different kinds of psychotherapies because we're desperately trying to create the treatment before we understand the anatomy, physiology, pathology involved in what it is to be human. Maybe we should take a step backwards and say we're trying to understand people first and understand who we are. We sit around the room and talk about who we are, and then maybe, not in a theoretical way, but in more of a raw scientific, clinical observer way, just kind of put together what we know from introspection and as well as from observation.

SECTION VI

Ericksonian Approaches

Mind/Body Communication and the New Language of Human Facilitation

◆

Ernest L. Rossi, Ph.D.

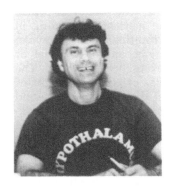

Ernest L. Rossi, Ph.D.

Ernest Rossi (Ph.D., 1962, Temple University) is in private practice in Los Angeles, California. He is the author of two books, one on dreams and one on the psychobiology of mind-body healing. Rossi has extensive experience in Jungian psychotherapy and has served on the certifying board of the C.G. Jung Institute of Los Angeles. He has written prolifically on the hypnotic approach of Milton H. Erickson and is the co-author, with Erickson, of three books. Additionally, Rossi edited four volumes of Erickson's collected papers and co-edited two volumes of Erickson's early lectures. He is editor of Psychological Perspectives: A Semi-annual Review of Jungian Thought.

Rossi presents the perspective that our 200-year history of psychotherapy can be understood as an effort to heal the artificial dichotomy between mind and body. His chapter consists of three parts. Part One outlines the history of rite, ritual, myth, religion, and philosophy as stages in the evolution of the concept of mind and psychotherapy. Part Two reviews the recent revolutionary research on mind/body communication that may become the basis for uniting all schools of psychotherapy into a single information-flow approach to human problems. Part Three presents an overview of how this new integration of mind and body as one information system is leading to the development of new languages for facilitating the evolution of consciousness identity, personality, and behavior in the growth-oriented psychotherapies.

PART I: THE MIND/BODY PROBLEM IN THE EVOLUTION OF CONSCIOUSNESS AND PSYCHOTHERAPY

The history of psychotherapy can be understood as a healing of the artificial dichotomy between mind and body that began sometime back in antiquity. This split between mind and body has been described as a necessary stage in the evolution of the concept of mind and psychology (Jung, 1963). Man came to know himself and to know that he knew himself. This self-reflexive understanding—to know that he knows himself—is the essence of psychology. It required some sort of division or split within the self to reflect the self, just as a mirror is needed to reflect our physical image.

Jung (1960), Neumann (1954), and Jaynes (1976) have described the entire history of man's rituals, arts, myths, philosophy, science, and psychology as stages in the evolution of the concepts of mind and psychology. According to their view, man's first glimpse of his mental or psychological nature may have come in the form of "gods" projected and reflected in the heavens, "spirits" that "animated" nature, and "forces" that "governed" the body from within. To grasp how the forces that governed behavior came from within was a crucial step in the evolution of our understanding of mind. However, still remaining was an artificial and troublesome division between mind and body.

This separation between mind and body reached its clearest expression in the acceptance of the philosophical views of Rene Descartes (1596–1650). The rise of science with its invention of physical experimentation led to a further reification of the *Cartesian dualism* of mind and body as separate entities or spheres of knowledge. I believe that our more recent 200-year history of psychotherapy, which began with the work of Anton Mesmer (1734-1815) and hypnosis, can be understood as an effort to heal this artificial split between mind and body.

The problem with the Cartesian dualism was that it led to an ever greater alienation and artificial dissociation between mind and body. This dissociation, when pushed to an extreme, resulted in the experience of various forms of psychopathology. In individuals, this psychopathology of dissociation became manifest as neurosis and "psychosomatic" problems. In society as a whole, the psychopathology of dissociation takes the form of all the political ideologies and systems that lead to the divisions and alienations between different groups of people. These ideological divisions into "them" and "us" eventually result in the striving for power and its natural consequent, the loss of human rights and, ultimately, war.

Since "dissociation" in one form or another is the psychological source of human problems, we can view the entire history of psychotherapy as a series of efforts to heal the artificial divisions in man's nature. Table 1 presents an outline of five stages in the evolution of psychotherapy, from the early spiritual/shamanistic approaches to modern depth psychotherapy of Freud and Jung, together with the more recent work of Milton H. Erickson on the psycho-neuro-physiological foundations of healing.

As can be seen in Table 1, the basic problem is always a dissociation or split that needs to be healed. In the earliest cultures, this split was described in one way or another as a division between the spiritual world and man's more physical nature. Man's spirit was portrayed in archetypal myths as being caught in the embrace of *physis*, the material world (Jung, 1959). The method of healing in the shamanistic traditions was to invoke spiritual power by means of a ritual or ceremony in order to heal the sick. The spiritual power was originally thought of as being outside the sick person; and therefore, the ritual was a means of constellating the spiritual forces so they could operate within the patient. The ritual or ceremony often took place in a magical circle that served as a *temnos* or vessel of transformation for the healing work. Sometimes the illness was conceptualized as a negative figure or force that was actually transferred from the sick person to the shaman or guru who would actually destroy it in his own body.

Anton Mesmer was the transitional figure between the ancient traditions of spiritual healing and the development of hypnotherapy and modern depth psychotherapy (Rossi, 1986; Rossi & Ryan, 1986). With the rituals that he and the early fathers of hypnosis developed, the frame of reference for healing shifted from the spirit/body dissociation to the mind/body dissociation. Rather than invoking spirits for healing, *direct suggestion* was used to facilitate *ideodynamic processes* whereby an *idea* communicated via words and verbal associations could stimulate the inner

Table 1: FIVE STAGES IN THE EVOLUTION OF PSYCHOTHERAPY

	Spiritual/Shaman	Early Hypnosis	Sigmund Freud	Carl Jung	Milton Erickson
Frame of Reference	Spiritual	Psychophysiology	Analysis	Synthesis	Utilization
Problem	Man/God *Dissociation*	Mind/Body *Dissociation*	Cs./Ucs. *Dissociation;* Repression	Ego/Self *Dissociation;* Complexes	Cs./Ucs. *Dissociation;* Learned Limits
Resource	Spirit	Ideodynamic Processes	Personal Unconscious	Collective Unconscious	Repertory of Experiential Learning
Method (Accessing)	Invoking Spirit	Direct Suggestion	Free Association	Active Imagination	Prescribing Symptom
Therapy (Reframing)	Ritual	Emotional Crisis	Catharsis; Transference	Amplification; Expanding Consciousness	Reassociation & Resynthesis of Learning

experience of sensations, movements, and psychophysiological responses that could resolve psychosomatic problems. The actual therapy often took the form of an emotional crisis that was safely contained within the *temnos* of the clinic or the doctor's consulting room.

With the evolution of depth psychology by Freud and Jung, there was a great increase in reliance upon words and verbal association to conceptualize and heal the divisions in man's nature. Freud used the terms *suppression* and *repression* to describe the dynamics of the dissociation between the conscious and unconscious minds. For his more sophisticated patients he found it more useful to create a new frame of reference for healing which he called *psychoanalysis.* He developed the technique of *analysis* to access the source of problems in the person's *unconscious.* In this psychoanalytic frame of reference, the patient now projected his early life conflicts and emotions onto the analyst—a process which Freud termed *transference.* A *transference neurosis* became the psychological *temnos* or vessel of transformation within which an emotional catharsis could safely take place in the medical consulting room.

Jung greatly expanded the conceptual world of depth psychology. He began by developing the word association test and found that there were patterns or covariations in a person's verbal associations. He called these patterns *complexes* and saw in them the basis of the autonomy of unconscious processes. It was this autonomous activity of the unconscious that led to dissociations and problems between people as well as within the individual.

Jung gradually developed the process of *active imagination* whereby he encouraged his patients to have an inner dialogue between these autonomous complexes. The inner dialogue was a therapeutic effort to unite the dissociated aspects of the mind. When Jung observed that patients were in danger of being overwhelmed by the emotions associated with their complexes, he had them channel these

emotions in the form of images in their imagination by doing actual drawings or

---

James Braid's Original Definition of Hypnosis

James Braid (1795–1860), a Scottish physician generally regarded as one of the founders of hyponotism, recommended that it be defined as follows:

Let the term *hypnotism* be restricted to those cases alone in which . . . the subject has no remembrance on awakening of what occurred during his sleep, but of which he shall have the most perfect recollection as passing into a similar stage of hypnotism thereafter. In this mode, *hypnotism* will comprise those cases only in which what has hitherto been called the double-conscious state occurs.

And, finally, as a generic term, comprising the whole of these phenomena which result from the reciprocal actions of mind and matter upon each other, I think no term could be more appropriate than *psychophysiology.* (Tinterow, 1970, pp. 370–372)

In the first part of the quotation, Braid defines hypnotism as a process that modern researchers would term *state-dependent memory and learning:* What is learned and remembered is dependent on one's psychophysiological state at the time of the experience. Memories acquired during the state of hypnosis are forgotten in the awake state but are available once more when hypnosis is reinduced.

In the second part of the quotation, Braid's use of the generic term *psychophysiological* to denote all the phenomena of "the reciprocal actions of the mind and matter upon each other" was another prescience of current thinking in the fields of medicine and psychology.

by modeling in clay or sand. We are all familiar with the more recent derivations of this aspect of Jung's pioneering work— today, they are called Gestalt Therapy, Transactional Analysis, Psychosynthesis, Art Therapy, Transpersonal Psychology, and others.

Jung called this inner work the *process of amplification* and believed it was based on our common psychobiological capacity for self-expression. He called this basic psychobiological resource the *collective unconscious;* it was essentially the same inner resource that spiritual healers called the *spiritual world.* Healing took place through an experience of the inner figures of the collective unconscious, cloaked as they were in the residues of our personal life experiences. A dialogue with these inner figures and complexes stimulated the evolution of the individual's conscious awareness of the "forces" that drove him. Once this awareness was achieved, the person had the ability to make the conscious choices to resolve the problems of life.

It could be argued that Milton H. Erickson's innovative approaches to psychotherapy are the most significant development in the field since the work of Freud and Jung. Like the works of both Freud and Jung, Erickson's work was entirely original and led to entirely new views and approaches to understanding human problems and facilitating their resolution (Erickson, 1980; Haley, 1985).

As is indicated in Table 1, we could summarize the unique contributions and differences of Freud, Jung, and Erickson as follows: Freud was a genius of *analysis;* Jung was a genius of *synthesis;* and Erickson was a genius of *utilization* (Erickson, 1985). When viewed from sufficient perspective, all the approaches in Table 1 supplement one another. Together, they present a well-rounded view of the entire field of psychotherapy in its current state of evolution. I would like to share with you something of what I understand about Erickson's utilization or *naturalistic approaches,* and how they may be of essence

in the creation of a new *language of human facilitation.* In order to accomplish this, however, first it is necessary to review recent research in the psychobiology of mind/body communication.

PART II: RECENT RESEARCH IN MIND/BODY COMMUNICATION

The clearest psychobiological evidence of the connection between mind and body is in recent research on the hypothalamus. The hypothalamus is an incredibly complex bundle of nerve centers located in the center of the brain. These nerve centers (or *nuclei*) integrate the higher cortical functions of "mind" with the memory and learning systems of the limbic system and the hypothalamic centers of virtually all the biological functions of the body. This central role of the hypothalamus in mediating mind/body connections is illustrated in Figure 1.* Figure 1 has truly revolutionary implications for the entire field of psychosomatic medicine and holistic healing. Until recently, it was thought that the major regulating systems of the body—the autonomic nervous sytem, the endocrine system, and the immune system—functioned independently of each other. It is now known that they are, in fact, all integrated into one single system of information communication, with the hypothalamus as a sort of "central control." Figure 2 illustrates some of the nuclei of the hypothalamus that regulate the autonomic, endocrine, and immune systems.

In the language of communication theory, the hypothalamus functions as a *transducer;* it converts the neural impulses of "mind" into the hormonal "messenger molecules" of the body. This is not speculation; this is fact that we can see under the microscope. Figures 3A and 3B illustrate how this process takes place

---

* All medical illustrations in this article are reprinted with permission from: Rossi, E. (1986). *The psychobiology of mind-body healing: New concepts of therapeutic hypnosis.* New York: W.W. Norton.

within single nerve cells of the hypothalamus; nerves from the higher centers of
mind connect with cells in the hypothalamus. Such cells convert the neural impulse of mind into "messenger molecules"
that stimulate the production of hormones
in the pituitary they are transmitted via
the bloodstream to all the other endocrine

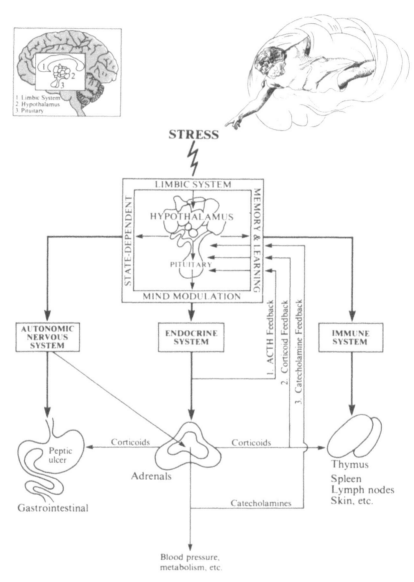

Figure 1
Selye's General Adaptation Syndrome updated to emphasize the mind
modulating role of the limbic-hypothalamic system on the Autonomic,
Endrocrine, and Immune systems. The state-dependent memory and
learning theory of therapeutic hypnosis is illustrated by the limbic
system "filter" (square box) surrounding the hypothalamus.

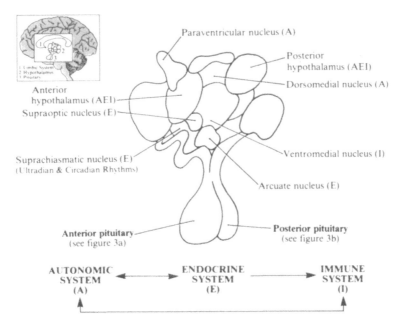

Figure 2
Some functions of the hypothalamus as the source of mind/body transduction to the Autonomic (A), Endocrine (E), and Immune (I) systems.

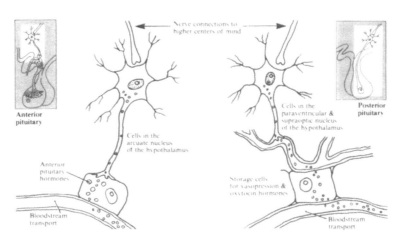

Figure 3A
Mind/body connections from higher centers of mind to hypothalamus, to anterior pituitary, and to remainder of body.

Figure 3B
Mind/body connections from higher centers of mind to hypothalamus, to posterior pituitary, and to remainder of body.

glands of the body that regulate metabolism, growth, sexuality, and so forth.

In my recent volumes on mind/body communication in hypnosis (Rossi, 1986; Rossi & Ryan, 1986), I present a detailed discussion and illustration of this entire process of information flow between mind and body, down to the level of molecular processes within the cells. I am reproducing one of these illustrations here as Figure 4, showing the process of information transduction from mind to the genome. Stress and emotions experienced on the level of mind are transduced into body processes by the hypothalamus-pituitary-endocrine system route. Steroid hormones of the endocrine system, the thyroid, the adrenals and the sexual glands, for example, enter individual cells of the body and direct the genes to produce messenger RNA that in turn directs the ribosomes in the cytoplasm to produce the proteins and "messenger molecules" described above. Figure 4 thus illustrates a process of information flow between mind and gene that functions automatically on an unconscious level. The goal of mind/body healing work is to make these processes available to conscious modulation.

There are two basic pathways for information transduction in mind/body healing. One involves the production of neurotransmitters that mediate information flow between the synapses of neurons; information is typically transmitted through the central nervous system (including the autonomic nervous system) by this route. The other more recently discovered process involves accessing genes to produce "neuropeptides." Neuropeptides are the hormones or "messenger molecules" that mediate the flow of information through the bloodstream to virtually all the cells of the body; information is typically transmitted via the endocrine and immune systems through this route.

It is important to understand the distinction between information transmitted by neurotransmitters and neuropeptides. Neurotransmitters usually transmit information between nerves and are therefore limited to the classical pathways of the central and peripheral nervous system. This process is "hard wired" or fixed and does not change as a function of life experience. There are some exceptions, but this is still the general rule. Neuropeptides, on the other hand, are transmitted through the bloodstream so that they can reach virtually any cell of the body. This system turns out to be highly flexible; it can change easily as a function of life experience and of the images, thoughts, and moods of mind. The most well-known of these neuropeptides is endorphin; its pervasive role in mind/body communication is illustrated in Figure 5.

One of the basic mysteries of mind/body healing is that it does not always follow the classical pathways of the nervous system. A person with a hysterical anesthesia or paralysis of some part of the body (such as an arm or a leg) is having an experience that frequently contradicts the actual pattern of nerve pathways. The nerve pathways illustrated in medical textbooks (as dermatomes or maps of nerve distribution) are irregular and never confined to only an arm or leg. Our picture of an "arm" or "leg" is a "mental map" that does not correspond to the actual distribution of the body's physical nerves. I have recently presented the lines of evidence (Rossi, 1986) that support the view that the mind's "mental image" is transmitted through the limbic-hypothalamic system to the body via the messenger molecules of the neuropeptide system. This is illustrated in Figure 1 as the "state-dependent memory and learning system" that serves as a "filter" for the mind modulation of virtually all the biological processes of the body.

THE STATE-DEPENDENT MEMORY AND LEARNING THEORY OF MIND/ BODY HEALING

In order to fully appreciate the scope of this state-dependent theory of mind/body healing, it will be necessary to re-

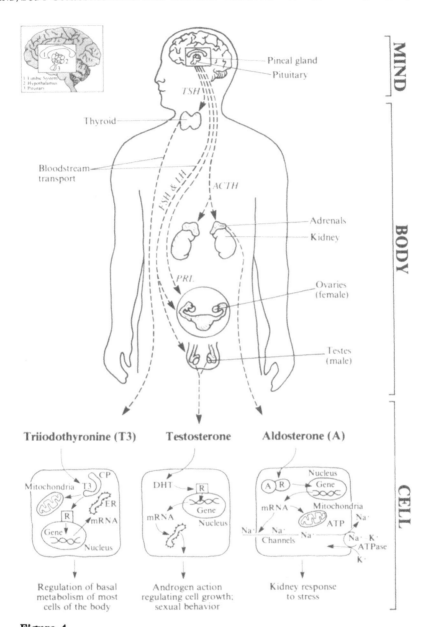

Figure 4
Mind modulation of the Endocrine System, with three examples at the
cellular level of the still theoretical "Mind/Gene Connection."

view its evolution as outlined in Table 2. The basic idea gradually developed in my mind over the past fifteen years as I studied with Erickson and attempted to integrate his hyponotherapeutic work with basic theory and research in psychology and psychosomatic medicine. The first breakthrough came in 1980 (Rossi, 1981, 1982) when I personally experienced and recognized the similarities between the

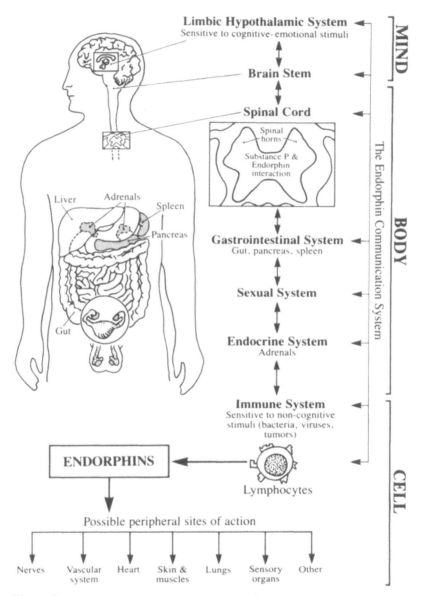

Figure 5
The nodal or focal areas of the neuropeptide communication system.
The central role of the endorphin neuropeptides in mind/body regu-
lation is emphasized.

psychobiological characteristics of ultradian rhythms (psychophysiological
rhythms involving many parasympathetic
and right-hemispheric functions with a 90-
minute periodicity throughout the 24-hour
day [dreaming, hunger, activity levels,

etc.]) and the *common everyday trance*
that Erickson utilized for hypnotherapeutic healing. Extensive reviews of the research literature (Kripke, 1982) indicated
that the suprachiasmatic nucleus of the
hypothalamus was probably a major reg-

ulator of these rhythms that were sensitive to learning and conditioning by both psychological and physiological factors. An independent verification of these findings came when I accidentally stumbled upon the remarkable work of Werntz (1981; Werntz et al, 1981) who found experimental evidence for the role of the hypothalamus as the source and mediator of ultradian rhythms in cerebral dominance, breathing, and autonomic system integration.

The second breakthrough came about two years later when I read McGaugh's (1983) review of recent research on the neurobiology of memory and learning which found that hormones released during stress modulated memory and learning

Table 2: EVOLUTION OF THE STATE-DEPENDENT MEMORY AND LEARNING THEORY OF MIND/BODY HEALING

1. Braid (1843, 1889) . . . . Dissociation manifest as *reversible amnesia* is the "psychophysiological" basis of hypnosis.

2. Janet (1889, 1907) . . . . Dissociation manifest as the block (or reversible amnesia) between the conscious and unconscious is the source of psychopathology that can be accessed and healed by hypnosis.

3. Selye (1936, 1982) . . . . Original research on the "stress hormones" of the *hypothalamic*-pituitary-adrenal axis that are essential mechanisms of psychosomatic illness.

4. Erickson (1943a,b,c,d) . . . . Demonstrated how traumatic amnesias and psychosomatic symptoms are psycho-neurophysiological dissociations that can be resolved with utilization hypnotherapy.

5. Overton (1968, 1972, 1973) . . . . Reviews 40-year literature which establishes state-dependent memory and learning as a valid experimental basis of dissociation in many paradigms of drug and psychophysiological research.

6. Fischer (1971a,b,c) . . . . Statebound information and behavior are conceptualized as the psychophysiological basis of "altered states," dissociations, mood, multiple personality, dreams, trance, religious, psychotic, creative, artistic, and narcoanalytic phenomena.

7. Hilgard (1977) . . . . Formulates the neodissociation theory of hypnosis which implies that state-dependent memory and learning are the same class of psychophysiological phenomena as hypnotic dissociation.

8. Rossi (1981, 1982) . . . . Formulates ultradian theory of hypnotherapeutic healing: (1) The source of psychosomatic problems is the stress-induced distortions of normal periodicity of ultradian psychobiological rhythms source in the suprachiasmatic nucleus of the *hypothalamus*; (2) Erickson's "utilization" hypnotherapy normalizes these ultradian rhythms with autonomic system balance.

9. Werntz (1981; Werntz et al., 1981) . . . . Correlation of ultradian rhythms in nasal cerebral hemispheric dominance is centrally controlled by *hypothalamus* mediating autonomic system balance.   *(continued)*

10. Benson (1983a,b) . . . . The "relaxation response" in yoga, meditation has its psychosomatic healing source in "an integrated *hypothalamic* response resulting in generalized decreased sympathetic nervous system activity."

11. McGaugh (1983) . . . . McGaugh's neurobiological research validates the role of "peripheral hormones" of the adrenals in modulating memory and learning in the limbic-*hypothalamic* system. Rossi recognizes the state-dependent memory and learning nature of these effects.

12. Rossi (1986, Rossi & Ryan, 1986) . . . . Integrates all the above into a general theory of healing by accessing and reframing the state-dependent memory and learning "filter" of the limbic-*hypothalamic* system that encodes symptoms and problems.

in the limbic system (specifically, the amygdala and hippocampus). I immediately realized (1) that these were the same hormones of the hypothalamic-pituitary-endocrine system that Selye found to be the source of stress-related psychosomatic problems and (2) that the new neurobiological research on memory and learning and Selye's classical psychosomatic research were both essentially state-dependent memory and learning phenomena.

A careful comparison of the details of the work of Selye and Erickson (Rossi, 1986; Rossi & Ryan, 1986) indicated that they were both dealing with the same basic phenomenon of "state-dependent memory and learning" in the genesis and resolution of psychosomatic problems—Selye from the perspective of physiological research and Erickson from the psychological perspective. Neither, however, was apparently aware of the concept of state-dependent memory and learning and how it could serve as the common denominator of their work.

A further search of the literature for possible antecedents of the *state-dependent memory and learning theory of therapeutic hypnosis* turned up Hilgard's remarks made about ten years earlier that implied an identity between the phenomena of hypnotic dissociation and state-dependent memory and learning. The work of Overton (1968, 1973), Fischer (1971a,

b, c), Orr, Hoffman, & Hegge (1974), and Benson (1983a, b) was then integrated as supporting evidence (Rossi, 1986). All together, these diverse lines of theory and research lead to one overall hypothesis: *The key to mind/body healing is to access and reframe the state-dependent memory and learning systems that encode symptoms and problems.*

If we take these views of recent psychobiological research to their logical conclusion, we have a pragmatic solution to the centuries' old mind/body problem—a resolution of the Cartesian dualism of mind and body. Mind and body are not separate, one being spirit and the other material. They are both aspects of one information system. Life is an information system. Biology is a process of information transduction. Mind and body are two facets or two ways of conceptualizing this single information system.

Mind and *body* are both rather old-fashioned and misleading terms. They were useful in the past; but with our current level of development, they unfortunately lead to dilemmas, problems, and paradoxes. They now exacerbate the formation of artificially separate frames of reference, domains of knowledge and language that inhibit the free flow of information between mind and body.

As indicated earlier, these blocks in the free flow of information have been conceptualized as *dissociations* in the history of psychotherapy. Dissociation is the basic

---

Hypnosis and Statebound Information and Behavior

After a long period of abeyance, Pierre Janet's (1859–1947) concept of mental dissociation as the source of psychopathology (a view adopted by Freud as the basis of psychoanalyisis) has found new life in Ernest Hilgard's *neodissociation* theory of hypnosis (1977):

Another approach to dissociated experiences is the peculiar action of certain drugs upon the retention and reinstatement of learned experiences, leading to what is called state-dependent learning. If learning takes place under the influence of an appropriate drug, the memory for that learning may be unavailable in the nondrugged state, but may return when the person is again under the influence of the drug. This occasionally happens with alcohol: the drinker forgets what he said or did while intoxicated, only to remember it again when intoxicated. Because memory is stored, but unavailable except under special circumstances, this phenomenon has some characteristics of hypnotic amnesia. Presumably, when the site and nature of these effects become known, they may have some bearing on the physiological substratum for hypnosis . . . *The concept of dissociation employed by Overton (1973) is consonant with neodissociation theory. That is, two types of behavior may be isolated from each other because of differently available information.* [Italics added] (pp. 244–245)

The theoretical integration of the concepts of therapeutic hypnosis and state-dependent memory and learning that is proposed in this paper is an extension of these intimations by Hilgard.

"mental mechanism" that was said to account for virtually all the problems of psychopathology. Dissociation is the basic mechanism that the early Mesmerists, spiritual healers, and fathers of hypnosis used to explain everything from "demonic possession" to psychosomatic illness. Freud and Jung used the phenomenology of dissociation to conceptualize the *functionally autonomous unconscious* as the foundation of psychoanalysis and psychotherapy. In the next part of this paper, I will outline how the language of dissociation, psychopathology, and psychoanalysis can be reframed into a more adequate *language of human facilitation* by utilizing our new understanding of the mind/body information system.

PART III: THE NEW LANGUAGES OF HUMAN FACILITATION

In the first part of this paper, I outlined how the entire range of mind/body healing, from the ancient spiritual/shamanistic traditions of ritual and ceremony to modern depth psychology, can be understood as different frames of reference that support essentially the same process of therapy. Mind/body healing, whatever its "method," always involves *accessing* the dissociated source of a problem and then *reframing* it in a therapeutic manner (Table 1). I believe all schools of psychotherapy are different languages for accessing and reframing the many different aspects of life that are called behavioral, psychological, and emotional problems. Each school of psychotherapy developed a different language of human facilitation to deal with what have been perceived as the different problem areas of mind and body. Although these different languages of human facilitation were needed in the early stages of the evolution of psychotherapy, I believe that our newly emerging conception of mind and body as being one information system will soon lead us to a single, more comprehensive language of human facilitation that will enable all therapists to communicate more easily with each other.

A beginning has already been made by a number of workers who are exploring the implications of state-dependent memory and learning in hypnosis (Erickson, Rossi & Rossi, 1976; Erickson & Rossi, 1979), in psychotherapy (Reus, Weingartner, & Post 1979; Peake, Van Noord, & Albott, 1979), and in counseling (Gunnison, 1985; Gunnison & Renick, in press; Rogers, 1985). The work of these clinicians is focusing on the insight that the psychotherapeutic process is itself naturally generative of an altered state of awareness because of the special context of the relationship with the therapist, the approach to the subject-matter discussed, and the special setting of the therapeutic situation. These workers are exploring the areas of equivalence between the concepts of state-dependent learning, Tart's state-specific knowledge (Tart, 1983), Fischer's statebound learning (1971a, b, c), and the general approaches of counseling, meditation, biofeedback, and drug-oriented psychiatric therapies.

The limited scope of this paper does not allow us to go beyond suggesting how many of the fundamental concepts of psychoanalysis and psychotherapy can be more adequately conceptualized in terms of state-dependent memory and learning and its natural consequent, statebound information and behavior (Rossi & Ryan, 1986, in press):

Terms such as *ego, id, superego, complex, archetype, attitude, role, state of development, personality trait, habits, sets, imprinting, fantasy, obsessions, compulsion* and *transference* can all be understood as statebound forms of information, behavior, and phenomenological experience that have heuristic value from a psychotherapeutic point of view. The classical psychoanalytical mechanisms of defense such as "regression, repression, reaction-formation, isolation, undoing, projection, introjection, turning against the self, sublimation, and reversal" (Freud, 1946, p. 47) are all cognitive strategies for coping with the basic processes

of statebound information in their relationships to the associative structures competing for conscious awareness. From this point of view, we could hypothesize that so-called "psychological conflict" is a metaphor for competing patterns of state-dependent memory and learning. Reframing therapeutic concepts in terms of statebound patterns of information and behavior renders them immediately (1) more amenable to operational definition for experimental study in the laboratory, and (2) more available for active, therapeutic utilization. The traditional process of "analysis" and "understanding" unfortunately does not always lead to the desired goals of problem-solving and behavior change (Erickson & Rossi, 1979; Rossi & Ryan, 1985).

From the point of view developed in this paper, the "creative unconscious" could be conceptualized as *the repertory of state-dependent patterns of memory and learning that can be made available for problem-solving.* Erickson termed this inner repertory, "experiential learnings." His "suggestions" were usually designed to access the memories of past experience and utilize them for current therapeutic needs (Erickson, 1985). For example, in one case in which he was attempting to relieve a woman of a terminal cancer pain no longer responsive to morphine, Erickson proceeded as follows (Erickson & Rossi, 1979, pp. 133–134):

I didn't want to try to struggle with her and tell her she should go into a trance, because that would be a rather futile thing. Therefore I asked her to do something that she could understand in her own reality orientation. I asked her to stay wide awake from the neck up. That was something she could understand. I told her to let her body go to sleep. In her past understanding as a child, as a youth, as a young woman, she had had the experience of a leg going to sleep, of an arm going to sleep. She had had the feeling of her body being asleep in that hypnogogic state of arousing in the morning when you are half awake, half asleep. I was very, very certain the woman had some understanding of her body being asleep. Thus the woman could use her own past learnings. Just what that meant to her, I don't know. *All I wanted to do was to start a train of thinking and understanding that would allow the woman to call upon the past experiential learnings of her body.*

In this case, Erickson used the state-dependent nature of comfort associated with the body being asleep to relieve the woman of her pain. Researchers (Hilgard, 1984) have wondered just exactly what Erickson meant by the term, "creative unconscious." I believe that *state-dependent memory and learning* is an adequate experimental analogue for his use of "experiential learnings" of the creative unconscious for hypnotherapeutic problem-solving.

Erickson's approach to many problems that ranged from pain control to psychosis was the utilization of what is now being called *symptom prescription* (Erickson & Zeig, 1980). A patient who had a pain or any form of behavioral or psychosomatic symptom first was asked to "make it worse" (Rossi, 1986). This has been described as a form of "paradoxical suggestion." From the mind/body approach being developed here, however, we can understand how *"making it worse" is actually a very direct means of accessing the state-dependent memory and learning systems that encode the problem.** As is the case with biofeedback, the patient's conscious mind often does not know how it is accessing the psychophysiological source of the problem to make it worse. Once the person has made it worse (on a subjective scale of one to ten [Tart, 1972]), however, the therapist can then introduce many strategies that can help the patient attenuate, transform, and *reframe* the symptom or problem (Erickson & Rossi, 1979; Rossi, 1986) to make it better.

---

* It would be an interesting study to determine the degree to which all of the so-called paradoxical approaches are actually paradoxical only from a rational, logical point of view. From the psychological point of view, they all may be the most direct means of accessing and activating the state-dependent memory and learning systems that encode a "problem" so that it can be engaged and resolved.

In my training with Erickson, he continually emphasized the principle that in order to resolve an intrapsychic problem, we always needed to access or activate it as a current experiential reality. Only then could we explore with patients just how their inner resources could engage and resolve the problem. Erickson never used "suggestion" to program the person with his view of the solution. I now believe that all effective "suggestion" is this process of accessing and activating the mind/body state-dependent memory and learning systems that encode a problem so that the patient's inner resources can be mobilized to reframe and resolve it.

In contrast to the symptom-based approach, I would now like to illustrate how the mind/body communication approach discussed in this paper can be useful in the growth-oriented psychotherapies in which the goal is to facilitate the evolution and expansion of personality, individuality, and consciousness. Figure 6 is reproduced from my book, *Dreams and the Growth of Personality: Expanding Awareness in Psychotherapy* (Rossi, 1985b). I now conceptualize all the dimensions shown in Figure 6 as more-or-less autonomous, state-dependent memory and learning systems that are all interacting with one another in the creative processes of daily living, as well as in dreams. The basic work of the growth-oriented psychotherapist is to help the client access, engage, and utilize these intrapsychic processes to reframe "problems" in ways that maximize their psychological development.

I can illustrate how this approach proceeds with an example from the dreams of an unusually gifted, 23-year-old woman whom I called "Davina" (Rossi, 1985b). In the following quotation, she describes an emotional problem of "frustration" which she is able to resolve by allowing herself to "take-a-break" and utilize the ultradian rest rhythms (see Table 2) (Rossi, 1982, 1985a). Her description is of a dream-fantasy taking place during a spontaneous altered state in which she was

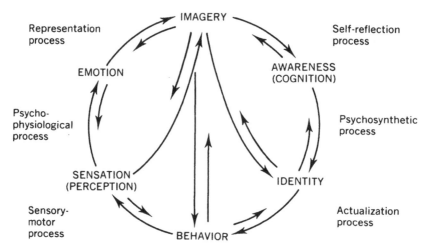

Figure 6
Some basic processes of psychological change evident in dreams, self-development, and creativity.*

* From: *Dreams & The Growth of Personality: Expanding Awareness in Psychotherapy* 2nd ed., by Ernest Lawrence Rossi, Ph.D., New York: Brunner/Mazel, 1985.

able to access and transform her frustrating *emotions* into *images* that then provided her with the basis for *self-reflection* and *new awareness* (Rossi, 1985b, pp. 90–94):

Circumstances: Lost, lost I felt, frustrated and alone. My husband, enmeshed in his graduate studies, with final exams coming up, felt tied up in knots, and so nervous that I, too, became depressed . . . Overall, my feeling is to bash my brains in!

At work, I can't seem to do a thing. Luckily I'm pretty free of pressure on my job of arranging manuscripts so I just sit and pull at my fingernails now! I force myself to work, but tears well up all on their own. Inwardly I can't stand it anymore. But I don't feel like running away anymore—I feel heartbroken, paralyzed, sad deep into my bones.

Finally, crying silently, I close my eyes to contain the tears. There in the depths of my imagination a fantasy takes shape.

Fantasy: In the "City of 23 Years" I find myself again; sad, droop-shouldered, tear-stained.

There in the center of a forest of rain clouds and deep green pine trees, a huge towering monster appears!

This creature is a mass of tangled, alive and hissing snakes, of branches, twigs, green leaves, crushed flowers, and in the center of it all is a huge eye, imprisoned. The whole thing writhes in agony, crying, screaming!!!

The *imprisoned eye* sees me, and speaks out—"*Oh, help me!* I am *Frustration*, ever doomed and fated to writhe in agony and pain, unless you help. I can't control this tangled mass alone! I am the Frustration of ages of tension, caught, helpless. Please help me!"

I am terrified at meeting the monster Frustration like this. I tell her I am weak myself, sad and afraid. "*What can I do to help you, I need help myself!*"

"Please don't fail me," she cries out. "You will be rewarded if you set me free. It will take you a long time, but you are the only one to help!"

Sadly I promise I'll try and then I, myself, cry out in agony for help!

Then my *old woman Sophia appears*. She sees me crying, downfallen, and scolds me for such weakness. When she sees how sad and pitiful I am, she then speaks softly, patting my hair with her old wise hands!

I point to the monster Frustration and tell Sophia of my promise to help.

At that Sophia smiles and says, "Good, you are to accept this challenge. Not many would. Most would give in to their fear of Frustration and run away!! But you will untangle it. What a task, though!"
"Tell me how I can do it!" I plead.
Sophia speaks—*"First you must find the Queen of the City, Patience!* She doesn't look regal of dress, but her eyes are emeralds, carved with tears, and her dress is rags and ashes. When you find her, hold her hand, and beg her to come with you to help untangle Frustration. She must travel with you, but she is very shy and brooding and will slip away from you, for Patience usually lives alone, hidden deep in the bowels of the earth. But she has the only power to untangle the snakes of Frustration, and set the Great Eye free. *You must call out for Patience* at every place in this city, *you must sing songs so beautiful* that they will lure her out to come and live with you, to travel with you—for *Patience loves beauty* and they go hand-in-hand together.
"Good luck my child." Sophia then stood up. Then Sophia kissed my forehead and vanished. I sat there, tearfully, singing. Then I got up, and began my journey to find the Queen of Patience.
In this fantasy-dream where her emotional state of frustration is personified in the form of an imprisoned eye we observe a striking phenomenological shift from emotion to imagery and awareness. In her current fantasy her emotional state of frustration is itself represented as an image (imprisoned eye) which Davina can then engage in dialogue. Thus [see below]:

. . . .The psychological value of experiencing emotion as imagery and new patterns of awareness is obvious: The images and new patterns of awareness function as containers or labels that enable her to structure and transform the intense but diffuse emotions that threaten to overwhelm her. The personification of the psychological states of Frustration . . . and Patience and her relation to them is another instructive aspect of this fantasy-dream. Her active participation is needed to free the eye, the organ of light and consciousness, from the toils of Frustration. She is learning to take a more active stance in controlling the emotional storms that tend to take over her mind. She could easily have given into frustration and hopelessness at this point. Many people do and end up "mentally ill," sick with psychosomatic problems, or unable to carry on their life effectively as they project the source of their frustration to the outside world. The key to mental health and psychological development lies in the individual finding an active way of cultivating the emotions, images and thoughts that develop within rather than allowing their behavior to become a captive of whatever [state-dependent learning and memory systems that] arise.

The *phenomenological equations* outlined above are typical of the way I now view the processes of psychological growth and the evolution of consciousness in dreams, fantasies, and hypnosis. The equations conceptualize a process of psycho*synthesis* that can supplement the tra-

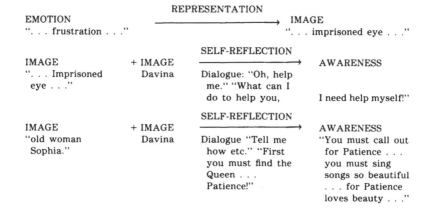

		REPRESENTATION	
EMOTION		⎯⎯⎯⎯⎯⎯⎯⎯⎯⎯→	IMAGE
". . . frustration . . ."			". . . imprisoned eye . . ."
		SELF-REFLECTION	
IMAGE	+ IMAGE	⎯⎯⎯⎯⎯⎯⎯⎯⎯⎯→	AWARENESS
". . . Imprisoned eye . . ."	Davina	Dialogue: "Oh, help me." "What can I do to help you,	I need help myself!"
		SELF-REFLECTION	
IMAGE	+ IMAGE	⎯⎯⎯⎯⎯⎯⎯⎯⎯⎯→	AWARENESS
"old woman Sophia."	Davina	Dialogue "Tell me how etc." "First you must find the Queen . . . Patience!"	"You must call out for Patience . . . you must sing songs so beautiful . . . for Patience loves beauty . . ."

ditional approaches of psycho*analysis*. They represent a new language of human facilitation that ultimately may be broad enough to integrate the entire range of our understanding from molecule to mind—and perhaps beyond.

REFERENCES

Benson, H. (1983a). The relaxation response and norepinephrine: A new study illuminates mechanisms. *Integrative Psychiatry, 1,* 15–18.

Benson, H. (1983b, July). The relaxation response: Its subjective and objective historical precedents and physiology. *Trends in Neuroscience,* pp. 281–284.

Braid, J. (1843). *Neuryphology.* Revised as *Braid on hypnotism,* 1889. Reprinted in 1960 by Julian Press (New York).

Erickson, M. (1980). *The collected papers of Milton H. Erickson on hypnosis.* (Vols. 1–4). Edited by Ernest Rossi. New York: Irvington.

Erickson, M. (1985). Memory and hallucination, Part I: The utilization approach to hypnotic suggestion. Edited with commentaries by Ernest Rossi. *Ericksonian Monographs, 1,* 1–210.

Erickson, M., & Rossi, E. (1979). *Hypnotherapy: An exploratory casebook.* New York: Irvington.

Erickson, M., Rossi, E., & Rossi, S. (1976). *Hypnotic realities.* New York: Irvington.

Erickson, M., & Zeig, J. (1980). Symptom prescription for expanding the psychotic's world view. In E. Rossi (Ed.), *The collected papers of Milton H. Erickson on hypnosis: Vol. IV. Innovative hypnotherapy* (pp. 335–337). New York: Irvington.

Fischer, R. (1971a). Arousal-statebound recall of experience. *Diseases of the Nervous System, 32,* 373–382.

Fischer, R. (1971b). The "flashback": Arousal-statebound recall of experience. *Journal of Psychedelic Drugs, 3,* 31–39.

Fischer, R. (1971c). A cartography of ecstatic and meditative states. *Science, 174,* 897–904.

Freud, A. (1946). *The ego and the mechanisms of defense.* New York: International Universities Press.

Gunnison, H. (1985). The uniqueness of similarities: Parallels of Milton H. Erickson and Carl Rogers. *Journal of Counseling & Development, 63,* 561–564.

Gunnison, H., & Renick, T. (in press). Hidden hypnotic patterns in counseling and su-

pervision. *Counselor Education & Supervision.*

Haley, J. (1985). *Conversations with Milton H. Erickson.* (Vols. 1–3.) New York: Triangle Press.

Hilgard, E. (1975). *Hypnosis in the relief of pain.* Los Altos, Calif.: Kaufman.

Hilgard, E. (1977). *Divided consciousness: Multiple controls in human thought and action.* New York: Wiley.

Hilgard, E. (1984). Book review of *The collected papers of Milton H. Erickson on hypnosis. The International Journal of Clinical & Experimental Hypnosis, 32*(2), 257–265.

Janet, P. (1889). *L'automatisme psychologique.* Paris: Alcan.

Jaynes, J. (1976). *The origin of consciousness in the breakdown of the bicameral mind.* New York: Houghton Miflin.

Jung, C. (1959). *The archetypes and the collective unconscious, Parts I and II. Vol. IX. The collected works of Carl G. Jung.* (R.F.C. Hull, Trans.) Bollingen Series XXX. Princeton, N.J.: Princeton University Press.

Jung, C. (1960). *The structure and dynamics of the psyche. Vol. VIII. The collected works of Carl G. Jung.* (R.F.C. Hull, Trans.) Bollingen Series XXX. Princeton, N.J.: Princeton University Press.

Jung, C. (1963). *Mysterium coniunctionis.* (R.F.C. Hull, Trans.) Bollingen Series XX. New York: Pantheon Books.

Kripke, D. (1982). Ultradian rhythms in behavior and psysiology. In F. Brown & R. Graeber (Eds.), *Rhythmic aspects of behavior.* Hillsdale, N.J.: Erlbaum & Associates.

McGaugh, J. (1983). Preserving the presence of the past: Hormonal influences on memory storage. *American Psychologist, 38*(2), 161–173.

Neumann, E. (1954). *The origins and history of consciousness.* (Vols. 1–2.) New York: Harper & Row.

Orr, W., Hoffman, H., & Hegge, F. (1974). Ultradian rhythms in extended performance. *Aerospace Medicine, 45,* 995–1000.

Overton, D. (1968). Dissociated learning in drug states (state-dependent learning). In D. Effron, J. Cole, J. Levine, & R. Wittenborn (Eds.), *Psychopharmocology: A review of progress, 1957–1967.* Public Health Service Publications, 1836. U.S. Government Printing Office, Washington, D.C., pp. 918–930.

Overton, D. (1972). State-dependent learning produced by alcohol and its relevance to alcoholism. In B. Kissen & H. Begleiter (Eds.), *The biology of alcoholism. Vol. II. Physiology and behavior* (pp. 193–217). New York: Plenum.

Overton, D. (1973). State-dependent learning produced by addicting drugs. In S. Fisher & A. Freedman (Eds.), *Opiate addiction: Origins and treatment.* (pp. 61–75). Washington, D.C.: Winston.

Overton, D. (1978). Major theories of state-dependent learning. In B. Ho, D. Richards, & D. Chute (Eds.), *Drug discrimination and state-dependent learning.* (pp. 283–318). New York: Academic Press.

Peake, T., Van Noord, W., & Albott, W. (1979). Psychotherapy as an altered state of awareness: A common element. *Journal of Contemporary Psychotherapy, 10*(2), 98–104.

Reus, V., Weingartner, H., & Post, R. (1979). Clinical implications of state-dependent learning. *American Journal of Psychiatry, 136*(7), 927–931.

Rogers, C. (1985). Reaction to Gunnison's article on the similarities between Erickson and Rogers. *Journal of Counseling & Development, 63,* 565–566.

Rossi, E. (1981, March). Hypnotist describes natural rhythms of trance readiness. *Brain/Mind Bulletin,* p. 1.

Rossi, E. (1982). Hypnosis and ultradian cycles: A new state(s) theory of hypnosis? *The American Journal of Clinical Hypnosis, 25,* 21–32.

Rossi, E. (1985a). Altered states of consciousness in everyday life: The ultradian rhythms. In B. Wolman (Ed.), *Handbook of altered states of consciousness.* New York: Van Nostrand.

Rossi, E. (1985b). *Dreams and the growth of personality: Expanding awareness in psychotherapy.* (2nd ed.). New York: Brunner/Mazel.

Rossi, E. (1986). *The psychobiology of mind-body healing. New concepts of therapeutic hypnosis.* New York: W.W. Norton.

Rossi, E., & Ryan, M. (Eds.) (1985). *Life reframing in hypnosis. Vol II. The seminars, workshops, and lectures of Milton H. Erickson.* New York: Irvington.

Rossi, E., & Ryan, M. (Eds.) (1986). *Mind/body communication in hypnosis. Vol. III. The seminars, workshops, and lectures of Milton H. Erickson.* New York: Irvington.

Rossi, E., Ryan, M., & Sharp, F. (Eds.) (1983). *Healing in hypnosis. Vol. I. The seminars, workshops, and lectures of Milton H. Erickson.* New York: Irvington.

Selye, H. (1936). A syndrome produced by diverse noxious agents. Cited in *The stress of life.* (1976). New York: McGraw-Hill.

Selye, H. (1974). *Stress without distress.* New York: Signet.

Selye, H. (1982). History and present status of the stress concept. In L. Goldberger, & S. Breznitz (Eds.), *Handbook of stress.* New York: Macmillan.

Tart, C. (1972). Measuring the depth of an altered state of consciousness with particular reference to self-report scales of hypnotic depth. In E. Fromm & R. Shor (Eds.), *Hypnosis: Research developments and perspectives* (pp. 445–477). Chicago: Aldine-Atherton.

Tart, C. (1983). *States of consciousness.* El Cerrito, Calif.: Psychological Processes.

Tinterow, M. (1970). *Foundations of hypnosis.* Springfield, Ill: C.C. Thomas.

Werntz, E. (1981). Cerebral hemispheric activity and autonomic nervous function. Doctoral dissertation, University of California, San Diego.

Werntz, D., Bickford, R., Bloom, F., & Singh-Khulsa, S. (1981, February). *Selective cortical activation by alternating autonomic function.* Paper presented at the Western EEG society Meeting, February 12, Reno, Nevada.

Discussion by Lewis R. Wolberg, M.D.

◆

Dr. Rossi's paper brings to mind an experience that the former dean of the Postgraduate Center for Mental Health in New York City told me about. His friend, the Bishop of Utrecht, told him, "Since the dawn of time, man has always tried to place the mind or soul in one or another principality. Abraham put it up in disguise in God, who ruled all of mankind. Moses put it in the Ten Commandments that had been handed to him on Mount Sinai by the Creator. Descartes put it in the pineal body within the brain. Karl Marx put it in the stomach, the seat of his economic concerns. And," continued the Bishop with a twinkle in his eyes, "you know where Freud put it."

Now, listening to Dr. Rossi, one might asume that he's taken it from where Freud put it and put it in the hypothalamus, which is really almost as close to the main station as we can project today. Certainly, it's closer than anything speculated before. Dr. Rossi has spoken about the relationship of the mind to the body and one can get a better picture from a historical perspective of the concern that scientists have had with this problem.

A great deal of controversy has taken place about this point. On the one side, there were those, usually philosophers who call themselves dualists, who contended that the physical stuff of the brain was completely separate from the thinking stuff of the mind. On the other side, the Monists, firmly contended that they were part of the same process. The most ancient of the dualists was the Greek philosopher, Anaxagoras, in 500 B.C., who thought that the mind was the core substance that brought order to the universe, and that it was completely separate from the physical self. His dualistic idea was popularized by Plato and later endorsed by many religious authorities since it confirmed the traditional belief in the immortality of the soul or the spirit which could live on forever after the physical body had perished. The church, therefore, had an investment in keeping the spirit or the soul a separate entity from the perishable container, the body.

In the centuries that followed, factual knowledge about biology intensified the mind/body paradox and conflict developed in the attempt to reconcile scientific and religious ideas. Controversy reached a climax around the seventeenth century with the dualism of René Descartes who conceptualized the physical self as a closed system, solely governed by physical laws.

The mind, or psyche, on the other hand, was not explicable in physical terms. Even though Descartes claimed the soul was located in the pineal body, a small conical substance in the brain, he avowed that it would work independently of the brain, without the aid of any other part of the body or of the senses. "Man's will" Descartes wrote, "is so entirely free, that it can never be constrained."

The dualistic philosophy of Descartes was supported by a large body of followers who inevitably got tangled up in the contradictions of the system. Disagreements broke out regarding such things as whether animals have souls or could reason. Most Cartesians contended that animals were like machines and could function without souls or reason. They called this "animal automatism."

Another point of dispute was whether mental processes control the body or the body controls mental processes. Those who insisted that the soul existed as an immortal entity, apart from a mortal body, tried to explain the destiny of the soul when it left the body after death. A great deal of philosophical speculation resulted, with a number of movements emerging such as epiphenomenalism and occasionalism. It was contended that while God was the only true cause of things, man could make mistakes apart from the mischief caused by the devil. If mind and body were so dissimilar, how could they possibly influence each other, except through the direct participation of God's will? How did such entities as finality and purpose enter into the mind/body interaction. Was the soul naturally incorruptible, since it was of divine origin?

The rationalism of Descartes could not explain all these points, but attempts were made to tie the loose ends together by revealed Christian dogma. However, religious conclusions about how the mind and body interacted were vigorously disputed by a factious group of dissidents who claimed that the nexus between body and mind needed more material explanation. A rich resource in counteracting the claims of the dualists was an old monistic theory of substance, originally promoted by several ancient Greek philosophers and later refined by Spinoza and Hegel, which insisted that nothing in the world was independent of anything else. This included the body and mind. The one could not be divorced from the other.

There were many who followed the empirical ideas of Francis Bacon, Locke, Berkeley, and Hume, opposing rationalism and arguing that the theoretical dualism of Descartes could not be substantiated by experience. Mental operations were closely tied to bodily reactions, and vice versa. The manifestations of mind were escalations of physiological processes. This point of view was reinforced by Darwin's evolutionary doctrines related to the descent of man and by later developments in neurophysiology, psychosomatic medicine, and psychodynamics.

Dr. Rossi joined the ranks of the monists, as do most scientists, who see a unity between the mind and the body. Dr. Rossi holds that by utilizing models from information theory, the stress hypothesis of Selye, and modern neurophysiological concepts, we can get a much more complete idea of how the mind and body operate. He tries to explain how attitudes, ideas, and other operations of the mind influence body reactions.

Problems, he believes, developed when the flow of information is blocked. He calls this "difficulties in transduction." He states, "All human problems can be conceptualized as blocks in the free flow of information between and within the mind, body and society. Information becomes statebound." Stress activates physiological patterns of the general adaptation syndrome, with psychosomatic symptoms resulting. In therapy, he claims, we must access and liberate and utilize and reframe the statebound information because learning of neurotic patterns during certain states, such as alcoholic and drug intoxification or exposure to traumatic situations, consolidates and encapsulates the patterns. Thus, statebound learning results frequently cannot be recalled except by recreating the original state in which they were acquired, or by accessing them vicariously through such tactics as imagery and hypnosis.

Now, the description of blocked memories and their consequence that Rossi gives us, you will recognize has been excavated before, utilizing somewhat different language. The traditional analytic model, for example, is that certain experiences and memories are shunted from awareness because their revival creates anxiety. In other words, they are repressed. This stops the flow of information, which, if we use Rossi's terms, becomes statebound. The blocked-off information is stress-activating and produces physiological patterns and psychological defenses in the form of symptoms. Analysts attempt to access this blocked-off or statebound information and bring it to awareness with various techniques that Freud gave us.

The original technique was hypnosis, which Freud utilized and then abandoned in favor of free association, dream interpretation, and imagery. Later, he recognized that he could, through transference, actually create a state similar to the state that existed when traumatic happenings originally existed with caretaking agencies, thus restoring the early memories. This is exactly what Dr. Rossi has told us from another frame of reference. Rossi believes that the concepts he describes "more adequately conceptualizes the experimentally reverified data of state-dependent memory and learning" and he has done a considerable job of integrating a tremendous amount of material, particularly in describing the neurophysiological correlates of learning, memory, and hypnosis.

Researchers do find that the metapsychological language of classical analysis is difficult to work with and learning theorists certainly are justified in trying to translate this language into terms that can more easily be utilized for experimental studies. These studies are difficult enough, heaven knows, without being complicated with labyrinthian linguistics. However, in substituting one language form for another, we should be very wary of complicating matters even more. Some of the concepts of the intrapsychic structure are simply not convertible into the syntax of learning theory or neurophysiology or biochemistry. Can research help resolve some of the dilemmas of the mind/body problem? At the present time, research is definitely impeded by the fact that thinking, reasoning, remembering, and other mental operations contain many hypothetical assumptions that cannot be completely validated experimentally. It is difficult to apply to the events of mentation the precise principles on which scientific measurement is based, namely, the unprejudiced compilation of facts and information, the formulation of reasonable hypotheses, the subjection of these hypotheses to objective testing utilizing controls and the continuing of experiments with the idea of replicating the results. Eventually, we may hope that our methodology will be sufficiently refined that we can better understand the true relationship between body and mind. In the meantime, work such as Dr. Rossi is doing will bring us closer to this objective.

QUESTIONS AND ANSWERS

Question: How would you apply this knowledge to preparing for childbirth?

Rossi: That's really, really wonderful. In the first place, the whole general conception of the reality of the mind/body connections can help you with childbirth. Historians of medicine used the concept of iatrogenic illness. This concept goes way back to the time of the Greeks. Before we had the germ theory of disease, a doctor would, unfortunately, unknowingly transmit physical diseases from one patient to another. This was called iatrogenically induced disease. Iatrogenic means the doctor caused it. In modern medicine we don't

have too many iatrogenic physical diseases anymore because we understand, with the germ theory, how to prevent that—sterilization and so forth. However, the problem in the modern world is that we have a plague of iatrogenic psychological diseases. We have so many concepts that give us mental troubles, that divide us, that divide the spiritual, psychological, physical facets of our nature. A simple understanding of the reality of these mind/body connections, I believe, is a step for iatrogenic health.

To appply this to childbirth, simply knowing that your emotional state will affect the development of your baby can be a profound help to the whole process of childbirth, the whole process of the development of the fetus. We know that the mother's emotions do affect the development of the fetus. The mother can be calm, loving, generative, supportive of the new life that is developing within her. This is going to generate the neurohormones and neurotransmitters that are going to make the internal environment more conducive for optimal development. On the spur of the moment, therefore, my first answer to that question is that moving toward iatrogenic health by just understanding the reality of what you do with your mind is going to affect the overall development of your body.

Question: Dr. Rossi, would you care to comment at this point on the impact that your philosophy may have on the traditional symptom-based medical practice?

Rossi: Yes. You may have recognized that in the first slide I presented what was characteristic of Erickson's approach and many others is what we call *Symptom Prescription*. I remember when I was first in practice, I was following the model of being a psychoanalyst and I loved the ideas of psychological growth, transpersonal psychology, and so forth, but I was in mortal terror anytime someone came to me with a physical symptom that was suppose to have a psychosomatic source.

The traditional psychoanalytic model said that you had to analyze and that took years to uncover the sources of a physical symptom. When I began working with Erickson, the reverse was the case. The symptom became the starting point, the way of accessing what I now called the state-dependent memory and learning systems of the body. Using that simple idea of prescribing the symptom in many, many ways, no matter what the symptom, Erickson would try to get the person to exaggerate the symptom. That can be called paradoxical therapy only from a logical point of view. Actually, by accessing, by making the symptom worse, the person was accessing, making alive, making present, refloating the psychophysiological processes of the symptom. These can then be attenuated or reframed with other, what he would call indirect suggestions and that I now call the "language of human facilitation." So the symptom, which we can turn on or off, is a way of accessing the psychophysiological processes involved.

As far as traditional medicine goes, there's a marvelous new book that's just come out, *Placebo: Theory Research and Mechanisms* by Leonard White (New York: Guilford, 1985), where one paper describes how no matter what the medication is, no matter what the procedure is, surgery or whatever, 55 percent of the therapeutic effect is a placebo effect. Of course, formerly they thought the placebo was a nuisance variable. They tried to eliminate it from their experiments. A new definition of placebo that I would formulate as a function of this new theory is that a placebo is any procedure that evokes the natural healing mechanisms of the mind/body.

What this all means is that 55 percent of healing has a mind/body connection, that is 55 percent of the results of any analgesic, of practically any medication are actually due to the person's belief system—the interactions that take place between the person and the doctor. Actually, one of the interesting things about this research is that the more potent the medicine is on a physical level, the more potent is the placebo effect. This is not to say that placebos or the mind/body connections or psychotherapy will ever replace physical medicine; rather it will always potentiate, maximize, facilitate all drugs and medical procedures and aid our efforts to help nature heal herself.

With the state-dependent memory and learning theory, we're seeing the actual mind/body connections where we can help nature through either the psychological variables or physiological variables. The symptom is the key to accessing the state-dependent, memory-learning-healing systems.

Therapeutic Patterns of Ericksonian Influence Communication

◆

Jeffrey K. Zeig, Ph.D.

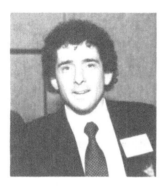

Jeffrey K. Zeig, Ph.D.
Jeffrey K. Zeig (Ph.D., 1977, Georgia State University) is the Director of The Milton H. Erickson Foundation in Phoenix, Arizona. He organized the International Congresses on Ericksonian Approaches to Hypnosis and Psychotherapy held in 1980, 1983, and 1986. Zeig serves as adjunct Assistant Professor of Clinical Psychology at Arizona State University. He received the Milton H. Erickson Award from The Netherlands Society of Clinical Hypnosis for outstanding contributions to the field of clinical hypnosis and the Milton H. Erickson Award of Scientific Excellence in Writing in Hypnosis from the American Society of Clinical Hypnosis. Zeig has authored one book and edited four volumes, all on the hypnotic psychotherapy of Milton H. Erickson, M.D.

Building responsiveness (especially the responsiveness to minimal cues) and accessing resources are two important aspects of effective hypnotherapy. Ten principles of Ericksonian influence communication are presented and described.

INTRODUCTION

The thesis of my chapter is that change does not necessarily happen because therapists communicate things that are meaningful. Often it happens because therapists communicate meaningfully.

A ruler, a scholar in a remote desert land, brought together international scholars from many disciplines and asked them to summarize the acquired wisdom of the field of psychotherapy. After some time of diligent study, they came back with more than a score of volumes they had written on the subject. The regent said, "No. Work further to distill the essence of the field." Eventually they returned with one volume but found it was considered unwieldy. Additional labor led to one chapter that was judged lengthy. Even one paragraph and one sentence were rejected as being too long.

Finally, the potentate was presented with one phrase. He looked at it and said, "This truly must be the essence of psy-

Note: The author is appreciative of the efforts of Deborah Laake, Stephen Lankton and Bill O'Hanlon who read drafts and provided comments which were incorporated into the manuscript.

chotherapy." The phrase read, "Accessing resources for change."

But then the monarch had an important question. He asked the assembled scholars, "If the task of psychotherapy is to access resources for change, how does one accomplish that?"

In answer, a hypnotic voice resounded from the panel of experts. It said, "Social influence."

THE ERICKSONIAN APPROACH

The characteristic that most distinguishes Ericksonian psychotherapy from other approaches is an emphasis on social influence—using communication for specific therapeutic effect.

This goal-directed methodology is atheoretical and based on ascertaining and modifying existent maladaptive patterns. Promoting change takes precedence over clarifying the past or gaining insight into the existence, meaning, or function of symptoms. It is a radical departure from traditional methods of psychotherapy.

Not only does Ericksonian therapy depart from traditional psychotherapy; but it also departs from classical hypnotic methods that use techniques to "program" a passive patient in an attempt to remove specific symptoms. In the Ericksonian model of hypnotherapy, clinicians do *not* program; they structure communication to have maximum effect so the patient can change many aspects of life, not merely the presenting symptom.

To enhance therapeutic influence, clinicians center on two processes: *building responsiveness* and *accessing resources*. The therapist promotes patient-based change by meeting and engaging the client at his frame of reference, and by using individualized multilevel therapeutic communication to build constructive interpersonal responsiveness and especially to identify, elicit, develop, recombine, and utilize existent patient resources.

When one considers the evolution of psychotherapy, be it traditional or Erick-

sonian, individual, group, couple, or family, there are two apparent stages: namely, diagnosis and utilization (intervention). In Ericksonian approaches, diagnosis is as brief as possible and merely serves the forces of constructive utilization. Therapy is mostly a process of accessing and utilizing resources.

In traditional therapy, however, diagnosis often appears to be an end in itself. The therapist provides treatment by making a diagnosis and then uses it supportively to clarify, interpret, and confront. The goal is to uncover and understand previously unrecognized aspects of life— to promote the patient's awareness of the influence of the past or the structure of the present. Patients are encouraged to learn diagnostic insight into their patterns and/or relationships and are expected to gain from insight the ability to alter their conduct and/or experience. Insight-oriented psychotherapy has essentially been stuck in a phase of "diagnosis."

The fact is that insight is neither necessarily a precursor of change nor is it necessarily a by-product. Change can be independent of understanding. One of Erickson's enduring contributions is that he liberated change from the shackles of insight. That is not to say that at times Erickson did not use insight. Insight is one of a number of methods that can be used to promote change. Erickson used insight only when it was likely to lead to change; however, many other techniques can promote therapeutic change more effectively.

The shift in Ericksonian therapy towards utilization is neither subtle nor philosophical. It is quite profound. It is the difference between a "companion traveler," with whom one can discuss aspects of present, past, or future trips, and a tour guide. A perceptive companion can point out some things that are interesting, but a tour guide knows the territory and can help get you there. The shift is from scrutinizing the psyche of the patient or family to the task of the therapist in relation to the patients.

When a therapist wants to learn therapeutic utilization, he will profit from studying hypnosis because hypnosis is based in thinking strategically toward a goal.

HYPNOSIS

Ernest Rossi has characterized hypnosis as the mother of psychotherapies (personal communication, March 1985). Starting with Freud, many theorists initiated their psychological inquiries by studying hypnosis. Subsequently, they departed from hypnosis to develop their theories of personality or their techniques of psychotherapy. Now psychotherapists from all disciplines are learning about hypnosis. As Watzlawick (1985) put it, "[hypnosis is no longer] the court jester in the solemn halls of orthodoxy."

To Erickson, hypnosis was not merely a trance state within a person; it was a special context for communication and an individualized interpersonal process. Erickson's hypnosis varied from patient to patient. Unfortunately, much traditional work in hypnosis has emphasized the subject's intrapersonal processes and/or the operator's technique.

The literature on traditional hypnosis abounds with reports of technique: techniques of induction, techniques of utilization with particular patient groups, methods of terminating hypnosis, techniques for dealing with resistance, and so forth. The emphasis on technique is stultifying and is part of the reason that hypnosis has been ostracized from mainstream psychotherapy. Also, more often than not, techniques are used across patient/groups without much attention to individual differences. Ericksonian hypnosis departs from classical methods in two ways—by emphasizing flexible individualized treatment and by addressing the interpersonal aspects of hypnosis.

Unlike traditional approaches, Ericksonian hynotherapy is used diagnostically to help the practitioner ascertain aspects of the patient's interpersonal responsive-

ness. *A central aspect of hypnosis is to elicit and develop inherent interpersonal responsiveness.* Through hypnosis a therapist can learn the limits of the patient's responsiveness and the patient's style of responsiveness; he can then help the patient develop responsiveness. The success of the therapy can be proportional to the degree of developed responsiveness, since if there is no responsiveness, there is no psychotherapy.

In building interpersonal responsiveness, it is not enough merely to elicit responsive behavior. *With hypnotherapy, one induces responsiveness to the therapist's minimal cues.* The use of indirect (multiple-level) technique is integral to achieving this goal. Let us understand this idea of responsiveness to minimal cues. If within the frame of hypnosis the patient is told to lift his right arm and he merely lifts it, that response is not necessarily hypnosis. However, if the therapist says to the patient, "I would like you to truly realize in a way that is *uplifting* that hypnosis is really an experience that is *right* for you in a way that you can find *handy*," and *then* the patient lifts his right arm, that is considered a hypnotic response.

Alternately, if the therapist says, "In hypnosis I would like you to really understand that you can find yourself *headed down* into a comfortable state," and the patient moves his head down in disassociative (automatic) response to the implied injunction, that is judged as hypnosis.

Before proceeding with complex therapeutic suggestions, Erickson usually worked with the person to establish to the best of their mutual ability—to the best of the patient's intrinsic limits—a responsiveness to minimal cues. Responsiveness to minimal cues is not only integral to hypnosis; it is the key that unlocks the door to the constructive unconscious. In Erickson's psychotherapy, responsiveness to minimal cues was the ground in which future suggestions were planted. They were placed in a fertilized bed of responsive behavior. Unfortunately, many psychotherapists are unaware of the existent potentials for interpersonal responsiveness. Studying hypnosis helps one to learn about responsiveness—especially responsiveness to minimal cues.

The degree of responsiveness to minimal cues varies among individuals. Thus, it makes sense that with Ericksonian hypnosis individual differences are stressed and the rote application of technique to different individuals is antithetical. Individual differences also exist in regard to inherent resources and how resources can be accessed. Once a patient's responsiveness has been established, the therapist's efforts are directed toward eliciting resources. This is basically a matter of looking into the reality situation for aspects that can be used in the process of achieving therapeutic goals. As will be seen, often trance phenomena are resources that are ascertained hypnotically. Also, resources can be found in the external environment and even in the presenting problem.

Another aspect of hypnosis is that it is used to frame the therapy, to create an "aura of influence." The frame in which therapy is presented is crucial. The hypnotic frame tells the recipient of the communication that more is being offered than just the words; gestures and verbal and nonverbal implications are being used as directives. In fact, one way to define "trance" is to call it that period in which the recipient of the communication perceives that there is more to the communication than just the detonation of words. Erickson understood this to the point that he could be considered the poet laureate of psychotherapy. Like fine poetry, each image, each element of the communication was chosen with care for multilevel effect.

What Erickson accomplished with his precision should focus all therapists on the importance of their communication. In fact, sometimes I think hypnosis is more helpful to the therapist than it is to the patient, because it makes the therapist really look at *perceiving* the effect of his or her communication. At this point of awareness the therapist is only a journeyman. A journeyman psychotherapist can recognize the effect of his communication; a master begins to anticipate some of the responses of the patient.

Here is a case that illustrates the ideas of developing responsiveness to minimal cues and using patient resources.

THE CASE OF FRANK: INCREASING SIGNAL, DECREASING NOISE

The case of Frank illustrates the way an Ericksonian therapist might think and practice. Frank was a blue-collar worker in his mid-50s who was plagued with anxiety and obsessed with his own well-being. Recently discharged from a psychiatric hospital, he reported for therapy in 1982 complaining of multiple fears and a sleep disturbance. The basis of the therapy was to abreact hypnotically. This was framed as a way of "releasing tension." Frank responded well and therapy was terminated after 15 sessions. Subsequently, he returned to treatment at infrequent intervals to surmount circumscribed problems.

Approximately two years after he initiated treatment, Frank requested hypnosis because he was bothered by noise in the factory-like environment in which he worked. At times his tension seemed unbearable to him.

Now, how might a therapist aproach this kind of a problem? Analyzing possible causes or speculating about underlying issues might not lead to change. Moreover, this was a man who wanted results. He was a person who was not interested in analyzing.

In approaching this problem, I looked for parallel life examples of problems and solutions and for usable resources in the reality situation. The patient was overly focused on one particular aspect of his environment and this focused attention induced discomfort. But we all have that kind of experience in our own lives. For example, when one enters the dentist's office the environment creates a subtle pressure for a person to focus attention on his mouth and the possibility of ensuing pain. There are many other things on which to focus both in the external and internal environment of the patient. Yet, dental patients often become fixated on pain or the possibility thereof.

However, focused attention can be a resource as well as a detriment in that focused attention can lead to comfort as well as discomfort. We have an ability for selective awareness and also for altering sensory experience. For example, when reading a book, one might not pay attention to the pressure of sitting in a chair. Concomitantly, the perception of time can be distorted. However, oftentimes in a situation such as the dentist's office, people become myopic and fail to recognize they can make themselves feel better through the same mechanisms they use to make themselves feel miserable.*

My therapy with Frank was to remind him of his latent capabilities, his unrecognized resources—his ability to be plastic in his perception, to block out and alter sensory experience. However, it would not have been adequate therapy to approach Frank directly about his resources. It would not have made much impact if I had said, "Frank, recognize that you have in your own personal history demonstrated an ability for constructive selective awareness and distorting sensory input." Rather, I indirectly led him to these understandings, bypassing conscious insight in the process, because conscious insight might have focused his attention in the wrong direction and precluded productive change. The first step, however, was to develop responsiveness to minimal cues.

As I elicited a hypnotic trance in Frank (I prefer the word "elicit" to "induce"; it is more accurate. The hypnosis comes from

the patient, not the therapist.), I indirectly suggested arm levitation. I did not talk directly about the idea of levitation, but Frank responded automatically to my minimal cues. Once he responded, I began weaving the utilization which consisted of stories about mundane aspects of life—common everyday examples.

I told him a series of six vignettes. One had to do with the experience of watching television and not seeing anything in the room except the screen. Another contained the theme of wearing clothes and yet not noticing the sensations of the clothing on one's body. A third had to do with driving in a car and not paying attention to the sound of the engine.

In between each story, Frank was presented with the task of creating and focusing on a symbolic hypnotic sensation. These elicited sensations were basically trance phenomena—simple sensory hallucinations that most hypnotic subjects can create. For example, he was asked to experience coolness around his temples, a layer of insulating dullness around his body, numb sensations at the tips of his fingers, light sensations around his shoulders, and so forth. Each of the symbols had ambiguous meaning that could be relevant to the solution of the problem.

In other words, counterbalanced were two strategic goals: (1) I subtly reminded him of his capacity to ignore steady-state information, and (2) I reminded him of his ability to distort sensory input in a positive fashion and then focus on it. These concepts were presented contiguously. Moreover, they were presented within a frame of responsiveness to minimal cues and under the aura of hypnotic influence. The hypnosis added power to the therapy. I would have been hard-pressed to conduct the same therapy in the waking state.

Treatment was successful, and Frank continues to work in an environment that previously was considered uncomfortable. He cannot say why the therapy worked. I did not tell him I was helping him construct a reservoir of positive associations. I did not tell him that I was associating

---

* It could be considered an axiom of Ericksonian therapy that the mechanism used to create or maintain the problem is the mechanism to be used for solution. Most strategies are intrinsically benign and can be used destructively or constructively. Actually the patient's problem is another resource in disguise.

him to previously unrecognized resources. I did not tell him that focused attention was not only a problem, it was also a solution. He knew why he was there, and he could take the resources that were elicited and developed and apply them himself (albeit unconsciously) to the problem state.

With Frank, formal hypnosis was used. However, this is not always the case. Ericksonian practitioners often take techniques of hypnosis and use them naturalistically, that is, without a formal induction ritual. In fact, Erickson only used formal hyposis 20 percent (Beahrs, 1971) of the time. Some of the cases in the next section on "aspects of influence" illustrate this modern use of Ericksonian hypnotherapy.

ASPECTS OF INFLUENCE

When one decides to communicate for effect, there are certain necessary preconditions on the part of the therapist. These are empathy, genuineness, and positive regard. The patient needs to bring to the consulting room, motivation, trust, and belief in a positive outcome. Because these aspects are well developed in other sources, I merely mention them here. They are not to be underemphasized; neither are they the be-all and end-all of psychotherapy.

When one is out to therapeutically influence, a different and more comprehensive type of thinking about psychotherapy ensues. I would like to share some of the things I have learned about hypnotic influence. Rather than presenting specific techniques, I will discuss attitudes—directions that one takes if he is interested in therapeutic influence. Although these ideas come out of my study of hypnosis, it is unnecessary to limit oneself to using these ideas under formal hypnosis; they can be used naturalistically.

Influencing is difficult business. I am in agreement with Carl Whitaker (personal communication) who mentioned that one

of the difficulties of psychotherapy is getting enough power. At the same time, I am amazed at people's malleability in response to social influence.

I will present ten aspects of influence here, all of them are important techniques for utilizing and dispelling resistance.

I) MEET THE PATIENT WITHIN HIS FRAME OF REFERENCE

This is one of the cardinal principles of psychotherapy. People are influenced best from within their own value system. A therapist must recognize and be ready to develop the individuality of the patient.

I know two particularly good examples that elucidate the principle of meeting the patient within his frame of reference. The first is from Erickson (1964a).

The Case of Ma K.: The Admonitions of the Past

Ma K. married at the age of 15 and came from a farm family that did not believe in education for women. However, Ma K. was ambitious; she wanted to learn to read and write.

Ma K. came upon the idea of trading room and board to country school teachers in return for personal tutoring. However, she never learned to read and write because she still lived under her early family prohibition that women do not learn reading and writing. And we all know that the admonitions of the past become the limitations of the present and the programs of the future.

Erickson saw Ma K. when she was 70; he was a medical student. He told the teachers that he would help Ma K. to read and write and that she would be reading the *Reader's Digest* within three weeks. It was quite presumptuous on his part.

Erickson said to Ma K., "Let's sit down on the floor, Ma K. Any ignorant little baby that can't read or write can sit on the floor." Then he gave her a pencil and said, "Now any ignorant baby can hold the pencil this way or this way. Hold it any old way." Ma K. took the pencil.

Erickson told Ma K. that a child could wriggle a pencil in any way and Ma K. agreed. Erickson then told her to do as much as any little child could do, make crooked marks on a piece of paper. Then Erickson said, "That's fine Ma K. Now you can write." Ma K. looked at him as if he should see a psychiatrist. She knew she couldn't write.

Then Erickson reminded Ma K., "You grew up on a farm and lived on a farm all your life until you retired and came to town. You know what a fence post is. Take the pencil and make a fence post. Now you can also draw a short board and a long board. The west side of the barn roof goes this way. The east side goes this way. Now make a long thin board lying flat on the ground. Draw a doughnut."

Having established the preliminaries, Erickson started to direct things therapeutically. He told her, "Let's take the fence post and stand it on end, and let's nail a short board across the top of it. You know some people call that a "T," but we will call it a fence post with a short board on top. Now if you take the east side of a barn roof and the west side of a barn roof and nail a short board across the middle, some people would call that the letter "A," but let's you and I call it a barn roof with a short board nailed across it."

Through this method, Erickson interested Ma K. in *building* letters and *building* words. He never told her that she was writing. He told her that she was *building* names. Erickson then showed her a dictionary indicating that is was a book of names. She could look into the book to learn various names. Three weeks later, Ma K. was reading the *Reader's Digest*.

Erickson presented ideas that she couldn't dispute, that she couldn't argue with, that she couldn't fear, even from some archaic part of herself. Ma K. suffered 50 years of frustration trying to learn to read and write, going against the teachings of her family. She couldn't vi-

olate those teachings. However, Erickson didn't ask her to violate any of her personal understandings. She could understand a fence post and a short board, and she could understand a barn roof with two slanted sides. Erickson used Ma K.'s own frame of reference, to influence her and to break through a limiting habitual frame of reference.

The Case of John: Crazy Talk

Here is another example, one from my own practice:

In working with John, a paranoid schizophrenic patient, I had a co-therapist, one of my residents, also named John. We worked for a number of weeks and got the patient to the point where he was communicating directly much of the time. One day, he came in speaking in garbled, unintelligible schizophrenese. It was as if he had regressed to his chronic state and our previous therapy was for naught.

I tried a number of ways to influence him to speak directly but none of these were effective. Then, I hit upon an idea. I turned to John-The-Patient, and said, "Let's have a crazy talking contest. I will talk crazy with you for five minutes and John-The-Resident will be the judge as to who does a better job."

John-The-Patient and I talked crazy for five minutes and then we both turned to John-The-Resident who looked up at me and said, "Sorry Jeff, John won." I indicated I was a little off that day but I could accept it graciously.

Next I turned to John-The-Patient and said, "Let's try it again. I will be the judge and let's have the two Johns talk crazy for five minutes."

I signaled when the time was up. They both turned to me. I expressed my regrets to the patient, saying, "Sorry John, John won." In fact, John-The-Resident did a better job of talking crazy.

Then I said, "Fair is fair." I took off my watch and gave it to John-The-Patient and said, "Now John-The-Resident and I will talk crazy and you be the judge as to who does the better job."

The patient looked carefully at his watch and parodied being a timekeeper. After the time was up, he looked at me and said his first coherent sentence of the day, "Sorry Jeff, John won." Subsequently, the patient spoke at a more coherent level and we were able to make better contact.

So if your patient speaks schizophrenic, then why not influence him from within his model by speaking schizophrenese—playfully? One doesn't need to push at the patient with admonitions to "talk straight." Rather, one utilizes what patients bring and one influences them from within their values. The best psychotherapists have the flexibility to influence patients from within their own frame of reference. Also, note how the patient's problem contained and was used as a resource.

2) EMPHASIZE THE POSITIVE

When attempting to influence therapeutically, it quickly becomes clear that people are best influenced by emphasizing and starting from their strengths. Influence does not have much to do with analyzing deficits. One starts with what is being done right. Consider the following vignette from Erickson (1964a).

The Case of Robert: The Right Spell

As a grade school boy, Erickson's son Robert explained that two of his friends were having difficulties with spelling. He asked his father to teach them how to spell. Erickson pointed out that Robert's friends' parents did not request assistance, and if he took time to work with the boys to teach them how to spell, their parents might see it as interfering. Also, the teacher might see it as interfering.

With that in mind, Erickson told Robert that he would come to the school. Robert was to see to it that his friends were there

waiting, and that they all had their spelling papers with them. Erickson arrived at the school and inquired about the boys' classes. Then he asked for Robert's spelling paper. Robert had 100. Erickson told Robert he did "a pretty good job." Then he turned to Robert's friends and asked for their spelling papers. Quite embarrassed, they handed them to Erickson. He looked at one and said, "Good heavens, do you realize what you've done here? Here's the word "chicken" and you've got the c and the k right together and they are the two hardest letters! You have got them side by side! Let's see how you did on some of the other words."

Erickson and the boy searched and found other words where the two hardest letters were together. He used a similar procedure with the second boy. Erickson indicated that he "sent the boys home with a different attitude toward their spelling because they could do the two hardest letters in any word that came along."

A few weeks later, the boys showed Erickson their spelling papers and they had good grades. There were no further difficulties. Erickson's comment on the case: "All I did was use a good hypnotic technique of centering their attention on one particular part of a word to emphasize that in a positive fashion. I gave them a sense of pride and enjoyment and satisfaction."

Erickson did not use hypnosis in terms of "look-at-the-pendulum-and-go-deeper-and-deeper-asleep." It was a naturalistic method based on focusing attention and emphasizing positive aspects of the reality situation.

3) USE INDIRECTION TO GUIDE ASSOCIATION

Indirection was one of the hallmarks of Erickson's technique. That is not to say that he could not be direct; he used direct technique when the situation called for it. Indirection is not therapy in and of itself;

it is only of value in the relationship to the patient. I have described what I believe to be one of the principles that Erickson used: "The amount of indirection is directly proportional to the perceived resistance" (Zeig, 1980a). In other words, it doesn't pay to be indirect if direct techniques will accomplish the goal. In general, I begin therapy by being direct and then I become indirect in proportion to the resistance I encounter.

Let us consider this principle in relationship to therapy. If the patient presents a phobia, the best possible common sense advice is to tell him, "Relax. Do not think about your fear. Change your reaction to or change your perception of some aspect of the situation." However, for the most part, patients do not respond well to that sort of direct intervention. Therefore, under the aura of hypnotic therapy, we present back to the patient, relevant common sense ideas, and we empower them to realize that they can be in a situation without incapacitating fear. In that spirit a therapist can begin to be indirect.

The literature on indirect technique in hypnosis is considerable. For example, Erickson, Rossi & Rossi (1976) and Lankton & Lankton (1983) described and categorized formal techniques of indirect suggestion. The Lanktons have done some excellent work with the particular indirect technique of multi-embedded metaphor (1983). Much of this early work is directed to classifying, clarifying, and developing indirect forms of suggestion. However, as those authors warn, it can be limiting for practitioners to think in terms of technique. The response of the subject is more important than the cleverness of the technique.

Erickson did not often talk about how to construct therapeutic implications. Rather he seemed to think, "Where is the patient in relation to therapeutic goals? How can I create a context that can help the patient achieve the goals?" Usually the prepared ground was comprised of fertile indirect suggestions.

I think that it is more important for a practitioner to get into the spirit and attitude of being constructively indirect than it is to know specific techniques. Techniques follow from the therapist's attitude. The best attitude is one in which the therapist has a goal in mind, such as relaxation, distraction, or distortion. Then the therapist creates communication (which will usually be indirect or "one-step removed") which helps the patient to associate to his or her power to achieve the goal.

Here is an example of a case in which indirection was used to guide associations and drive behavior. It uses an indirect metaphoric technique I learned from one of my early teachers, Eric Greenleaf, a talented psychologist in Berkeley, California.

The Case of Jack: Exploring the Dresser

Jack was a patient who returned to therapy because of low sexual desire. He recently had a urinary tract infection and subsequently had difficulty becoming interested in sex. To help with this problem, I used metaphoric therapy within hypnosis.

After eliciting responsive behavior, I told him a story about a walk in the desert and explained that after a while he would come to a cottage. Then I created comparisons between the cottage and his wife. For example, I talked about the dark-colored roof on top of the cottage in a way that was analogous to his wife's hair. I told him he *could go* into a special room inside the cottage. At first he might encounter difficulty, but pretty soon he could enter the room in a bold and forthright way. Inside the room there was a special piece of furniture, a dresser, that he could explore. He could touch the sides and feel the sleekness of the lines because it was attractive, and he would put his hand inside the drawers and find surprises to delight him inside the drawers. He could also play with the knobs.

The metaphor continued along these lines. It emphasized symbolic ideas that had ambiguous references. Jack was straight-faced and deeply absorbed in the trance. One of the advantages of using hypnosis in this case was that I was able to remain straight-faced.

In this type of technique metaphor is used to instruct the patient how to do things differently. Common sense ideas are presented indirectly to make them come alive. Associations are elicited and the patient can build up a wealth of positive associations that will generate new, more effective behavior.

4) CHUNK AND SEED

Another method is characterized by seeding future suggestions and building responses in small steps. First let us take the idea of chunking. As Erickson put it, when you divide, you conquer. If a patient presents the problem of losing 40 pounds, Erickson would quickly reorient the patient to losing one pound. The case of Ma K. was an excellent example of building responses in small, directed steps. Let us consider a case reported by a student of Ericksonian therapy in San Diego, Michael Yapko (personal communication):

John was frustrated at an early age from pursuing a career in art; instead he was encouraged to study math and science. Perhaps this was a factor in the development of his aloof, intellectual, and perfectionistic style. Not surprisingly, one of his problems was that he suppressed his artistic interests.

As part of the therapy, John was directed to paint every morning but to complete only three-quarters of the picture. He reported feeling good about painting but was frustrated with stopping prior to completion. In a subsequent session he was directed to complete the pictures but not to sign them. Next he was to surreptitiously give the paintings to neighbors. He reported an enjoyable sense of mischief. Finally, he was to complete the pictures and sign them if he wished. As a by-product of this procedure, the patient developed an awareness of his neighbors and even initiated friendly contact with them. He entered art competitions and won prizes.

This sequential step-wise approach is characteristic of good therapeutic influence. It is a matter of building change in minimal strategic steps.

Seeding is another important aspect of therapy. If a therapist can predict subsequent steps, he can seed these steps prior to presenting them. This is essentially a matter of priming responsive behavior. Erickson must have found seeding to be quite important. He regularly seeded concepts prior to presenting them. This technique is akin to the literary technique of foreshadowing.

For example, when using a fantasy rehearsal technique under hypnosis with a phobic patient, Erickson involved her in the fantasy of taking an airplane ride; he also conspicuously asked her to look at the mountain scenery. Subsequently he had her imagine the feared situation of being on a suspension bridge. The reference to mountains was purposeful. It was meant to orient her to the idea of heights. It foreshadowed that idea.

Seeding also can be used to build responsiveness. For example, if a goal is to elicit arm levitation, early in the process of eliciting a trance I might make tangential reference to the idea of movement and getting feelings of movement that just seem to happen. I might touch the arm lightly to orient the patient to those feelings.

The possibilities for seeding are numerous and Erickson was ingenious in using this method. Developing and clarifying therapeutic uses of seeding is a fruitful area for future investigation.

5) USE ILLOGIC AND CONFUSION

Upon initial observation, it would seem that illogic and confusion are antithetical to therapy. A primary "rule" for therapists has been to communicate clearly and directly.

It is unnecessary for therapists always to be clear. Illogic and confusion can be powerful therapeutic methods. Erickson often used illogic and confusion, mainly to disrupt maladaptive habitual sets. (For additional information about the use of the confusion technique, see Erickson, 1964b.) Patients bring irrational problems to the consulting room. Prior to seeking out the assistance of a professional, they battled their problems with rational logic. Since the use of logic was unsuccessful, the application of additional logic is illogical; more of the same seldom leads to success. If therapists limit themselves to logical approaches, they limit their effectiveness in providing treatment. Besides, why waste good logic on an illogical problem?

An excellent example of an irrational solution is contained in *A Teaching Seminar with Milton Erickson* (Zeig, 1980). The patient presented a phobia. (This is the same patient with whom Erickson used the previously mentioned seeding technique.) Actually, when one thinks about it, phobias are irrational. It makes no intellectual, logical sense to be paralyzed with fear by something that has little likelihood of causing harm. But this is the type of mechanism that can be utilized. If a patient uses illogic ineffectively, a therapist can use it therapeutically.

Erickson's solution in this case was to get the patient to move her phobia from her body into the chair beside her. This was accomplished through hypnosis. Erickson neither desensitized the phobia, nor did he modify it. He merely moved the phobia a few inches.

At first blush, this seems quite extraordinary. However, prior to moving the phobia, Erickson masterfully used hypnosis and techniques of seeding and building responses. Even so, it seems illogical that a patient would respond to a suggestion to "move" a phobia. But, as it turned out, the patient responded to the illogical solution and moved her phobia out of the way. Obviously, she was not concerned with the degree of rationality of the ther-apy; she was concerned with the degree of relief.

6) ACTIVATE CONSTRUCTIVE EMOTIONS TO MAKE THINGS MEMORABLE

Erickson often used drama, humor, and the unexpected to activate constructive emotions to focus the patient's attention and make things memorable. (For additional information on using drama, see Lankton & Lankton, 1983 and Yapko, 1985.) Erickson frequently accessed emotions and associations through dramatic anecdotes, riddles, and puzzles meant to effect change on multiple levels. An example provides clarification:

I had a patient who was making things unnecessarily complex. My goal was to get the patient to be parsimonious. I could have confronted the patient and told him that he was creating difficulties for himself. Instead, I added drama by using an analogy I learned from Erickson (personal communication). I did this without hypnosis; rather I just directed his attention and used common everyday trance. I provided the following riddle: "What do you call a cat that has five toes on its front left paw, six toes on its front right paw, four toes on its back left paw and six toes on its back right paw?" He considered the question and offered, "You call it an unbalanced cat."

I said, "No."

He tried again. "You call it a 21-toed cat with an asymmetric distribution of toes."

"No."

"Well, I wonder if there are historical examples that would give an indication of a proper name for this phenomenon."

"Yes. You call it 'a cat.'"

The goal was to remind the patient not to get lost in obscure details. However, confrontation or interpretation might not have led to change. Therefore, in a more dramatic fashion I presented an analogy that could make the understanding memorable and get the patient to enliven experientially his own understandings.

7) USE AMNESIA AND RELATED ASPECTS OF MEMORY

In influencing people, emphasis should be placed on what is stored in memory, how it is retrieved, how it influences behavior, how memory can be therapeutically modified, and how information can be presented so it is not consciously memorable but still influences behavior.

Traditionally, therapists have not placed much emphasis on human memory. However, patients can be empowered by things that they recall, by things that they do not recall, and by things recalled at a later time that were not remembered consciously at the time they were experienced.

Erickson was a master at amnesia. He used it often, both in social settings and with hypnosis (Haley, 1982). One of the more spectacular techniques that he developed to effect memory was named *structured amnesia*. This entailed abruptly ending an activity, presenting therapeutic suggestions, and then resuming and completing the activity as if the intervening suggestions had never been offered. One way of accomplishing structured amnesia is to disrupt a habitual task. For example, Erickson invented the handshake hypnotic induction. In one case, he worked with a woman using a hypnotic technique of deepening called *fractionation*, which involved evoking trance, partially waking the patient and then reestablishing trance. The process can be conducted repeatedly to intensify the hypnotic experience.

Each of the three inductions with this woman was tied to levitation of her right arm. After Erickson felt that the hypnosis had been completed, he asked the woman if he could shake her hand. He took her hand; but instead of shaking it completely, he used minimal cues, mostly nonverbal, to reestablish arm levitation and thereby

revivified trance. Subsequently, he gave the woman some therapeutic suggestions. Then Erickson again took her hand, as if the recently presented therapeutic suggestions had not been offered, and shook it and ended the trance, continuing his handshake where he had previously left off.* The purpose of this technique was to induce amnesia for the interspersed therapeutic suggestions. Actually, he also used a process of seeding and setting up responses.

Therapeutic amnesia is not an isolated technique or phenomenon; it is an integral part of the response to indirect suggestions. When responding to indirect suggestions (minimal cues), patients do so without full consciousness of the suggestion and/or the response (for further information on amnesia see Zeig, 1985 and Erickson & Rossi, 1976).

I predict that the therapeutic use of amnesia and related human memory processes will be an important area for therapists to explore in the future.

8) GET PATIENTS TO DO THINGS: PROVIDE THERAPEUTIC TASKS

Patients often learn more from what they do than from what they hear. Erickson knew this, and he was one of the first therapists to take therapy out of the consulting room and put it back into the patient's life situation. A number of therapists have emphasized Erickson's use of therapeutic tasks (see C.H. Lankton, 1985). Often Erickson's tasks were symbolic.

In one of his famous cases (Zeig, 1980a), he instructed a couple that requested marital therapy to separately climb Squaw Peak, a small mountain in Phoenix, and to go to the city's Botanical Gardens. (This case is discussed as an example of symbolical symptom prescription in Zeig, 1980b.) The husband reported that Squaw Peak was wonderful. The wife complained of being bored at the Botanical Gardens.

---

* The videotape of this session is available from The Milton H. Erickson Foundation.

Subsequently, the husband was instructed to visit the Botanical Gardens and the wife was told to climb Squaw Peak. Their reactions to the second task were similar: the husband was positive, the wife, derogatory.

The third task was for each one to pick his or her own task and do it separately. The wife embarrassedly reported that she climbed Squaw Peak again. The husband again enjoyed the Botanical Gardens. At this point, Erickson terminated the therapy and sent the patients back home. Even though they divorced, in the long run, both agreed that their experiences with Erickson had been positive. They both referred patients to him.

In discussing his technique, Erickson explained that the wife was climbing "the barren mountain of marital distress, day after day, feeling a brief sense that, 'Alas, that day is over'" (Zeig, 1980a, p. 147). Therefore, he gave her the symbolic task of climbing a barren mountain. Also, he symbolically suggested that they take separate paths. Erickson never discussed divorce with them, but through his tasks he gave them an opportunity to highlight and recognize their differences.

I often use symbolic tasks in my own practice. I remember one middle-aged woman who had a weight problem. During therapy, she unexpectedly got in touch with some feelings of grief about her mother, who had died years earlier.

Because the patient was an artist, I gave her the task of getting a rock and painting it in some way to represent her mother. After carrying the rock in her purse for one week, she was to find a place to put it to rest. She had difficulty with the task; she needed to find the "right place" to put the rock, a place that was peaceful and uncluttered.

Finally she found a location for her rock. It was the front yard of a stranger's home. Late one evening she "snuck out" and placed the rock.

This symbolic task was successful in absorbing her feelings of grief. It gave her a feeling of power over her circumstances.

She was actively involved in resolving the grieving. It gave her something concrete to do. No longer was she passive and "helpless" in the face of her feelings.

9) USE SOCIAL SYSTEMS

Erickson was a premier social psychologist, perhaps the best social psychologist to practice individual therapy. Also, he was keenly aware of the systemic reverberation of individual change. Erickson did not regularly see families as a whole. However, he was aware that a change in an individual could lead to change in the individual's social system.

Recently therapists have been incorporating hypnosis into family therapy (Aaroz, 1985; Ritterman, 1983; and Lankton & Lankton, 1983). In fact, the use of Ericksonian techniques in family therapy currently seems to be the growing edge of both fields.

Patients are influenced positively and negatively by their social environment. Change can happen not only by altering (manipulating) aspects of a patient's psyche; change can also happen by manipulating context.

Take, for example, a case in which Erickson worked with a couple that was involved in a long-standing power struggle (Haley, 1973, p. 225). The wife complained bitterly about the necessity of being involved in the family business because she also had to work hard at home. However, she thought that her husband was incompetent; the family business could not survive without her.

Erickson met her within her frame of reference. He explained that she must be tired from working so hard and that she deserved a rest. When she agreed, he told her that she should come to work 15 minutes late. Her husband would open the store, and he couldn't possibly do much damage in 15 minutes.

The woman went to work 15 minutes late and found, to her surprise, that her husband had done a competent job. After a while, she came half an hour late, then an hour late. Subsequently the marriage improved.

Simple alterations in social systems can be influential in promoting change. Especially in situations were there are symmetrical power struggles, discussion does not seem to have much effect. Psychotherapy should be conducted at the level of experience at which the problem is generated. If the problem is generated at the level of social interaction, discussion might not help. Rather, this is the time for therapy that influences the social system. Often it is also the time for tasks.

10) TAKE A TELEOLOGICAL ORIENTATION

Erickson admonished his students and patients that life was lived in the present and directed toward the future, and that therapy is lived in the present and directed toward the future. Ericksonian therapy is geared to the future. Goals are established and treatment is directed toward accomplishing strategic goals.

I remember an example of Erickson's future orientation. During a mutual discussion of one of his inductions (which is reported as an appendix in the Teaching Seminar, Zeig, 1980), Erickson reminded me that shortly before the discussion began, I took a picture of him holding his 26th grandchild, Laurel. Erickson would not take the picture until he also held the ironwood owl that he gave to Laurel as a present on the day she was born. It should be noted that the ironwood owl was a symbolic gift. Roxanna, Laurel's mother, nicknamed Laurel "Screech" because she had a powerful cry.

During the discussion with me, Erickson brought up the picture. He said that in 16 years, when he was long dead, Laurel would look at the photograph. She would see the baby and the smaller ironwood owl. This would mix together with her feelings of being grown up and in high school. He advised me to notice how memories were put together. Erickson noted that the ironwood owl added "a tremendous amount of humanness to that picture."

There was Erickson planning an intervention that would not take effect until 16 years later. That certainly is an orientation into the future.

Planted seeds do not immediately bear fruit, rather they need to mature over time. Being a "farm boy," Erickson understood the maturation process of seeds.

SUMMARY

This chapter presented some fundamental aspects of Ericksonian therapy. It is suggested that therapists assume a posture of influence toward their patients. This will entail using hypnosis and hypnotic technique. Two important issues are building responsiveness and accessing latent resources both in the patients and in the reality situation. Ten aspects of influence have been presented, many of which are based on indirect techniques that utilize patient values to accomplish strategic therapeutic goals.

REFERENCES

Araoz, D. (1985). *The new hypnosis*. New York: Brunner/Mazel.

Beahrs, J. O. (1971). The hypnotic psychotherapy of Milton H. Erickson. *American Journal of Clinical Hypnosis*, 14, 73–90.

Erickson, M. H. (Speaker). (1964a). *Hypnosis in education* (Cassette Recording). Phoenix, AZ: Archives of Milton H. Erickson Foundation.

Erickson, M. H. (1964b). The confusion technique in hypnosis. *American Journal of Clinical Hypnosis*, 6, 183–207.

Erickson, M. H., Rossi, E. L. & Rossi, S. I. (1976). *Hypnotic realities*. New York: Irvington.

Haley, J. (1973). *Uncommon therapy, the psychiatric techniques of Milton H. Erickson, M.D.* New York: W. W. Norton.

Haley, J. (1982). The contribution to therapy of Milton H. Erickson, M.D. In J. K. Zeig (Ed.), *Ericksonian approaches to hypnosis and psychotherapy* (pp. 5–25). New York: Brunner/Mazel.

Lankton, C. H. (1985). Generative change: Beyond symptomatic relief. In J. K. Zeig (Ed.), *Ericksonian psychotherapy, volume I: Structures* (pp. 137–170). New York: Brunner/Mazel.

Lankton, S. & Lankton, C. (1983). *The answer within: A clinical framework of Ericksonian hypnotherapy.* New York: Brunner/Mazel.

Ritterman, M. (1983). *Using Hypnosis in family therapy.* San Francisco, CA: Jossey-Bass Inc.

Watzlawick, P. (1985). Hypnotherapy Without Trance. In J. K. Zeig (Ed.), *Ericksonian psychotherapy, volume I: Structures.* New York: Brunner/Mazel.

Yapko, M. (1985). The Erickson Hook: Values in Ericksonian Approaches, In J. K. Zeig, (Ed.), *Ericksonian psychotherapy, volume II: Clinical applications.* New York: Brunner/Mazel.

Zeig, J. (1980a). *A teaching seminar with Milton H. Erickson.* New York: Brunner/Mazel.

Zeig, J. (1980b). Symptom Prescription and Ericksonian Principles of Hypnosis and Psychotherapy. *The American Journal of Clinical Hypnosis,* Volume 23, 16–33.

Zeig, J. (1985). The clinical use of amnesia: Ericksonian methods. In J.K. Zeig (Ed.), *Ericksonian psychotherapy. Volume I: Structures.* New York: Brunner/Mazel.

Discussion by Murray Bowen, M.D.

◆

I was completely intrigued by Dr. Zeig's paper. He's defined it and put it into words and put it into simple language. But as I listened, I was having a hard time distinguishing between the patient and the therapist. I was wondering who's who around here.

This notion of communicating on multiple levels is as old as mankind. I think one of the things that Dr. Zeig does, and Ericksonian approaches add to it, is systematizing this old, old thing of communicating on different levels. And I don't think he can say he can communicate on two levels. I think it's simplistic to say that. I know Gregory Bateson made a big deal out of the double bind, which is always there. But I used to say about the double bind, "You should never use a double bind when you can use a triple bind." That is a way to keep things in equilibrium, not letting anybody mess you up. That's what the world is about.

The Ericksonian technique of communicating in multiple levels is a part of the human experience. That is a way of responding, of picking up what was said or done. It doesn't have to be just said; you can do it. One of the beautiful things about Zeig is that he doesn't say it, he does it. But picking up the communication is not an unconscious act; a lot of this is automatic and just happens. Thus, somebody comes at you on a conscious level and you just relate back on another level. This has some pretty good things about it. It keeps the other at bay. It makes the other listen to you and, most important of all, causes the other person to think. They either say you're pretty good or call you crazy. People do call you crazy for these things, but that is a way to make the other think. There are an awful lot of things in what psychotherapists do that accomplish that. We do it all the time in our relationships with people. They come in at one level and you go back on another. You're protecting you, and you're also helping them.

One of the important things Dr. Zeig mentioned, more by implication than by stating it directly, is that anything that has to do with this kind of psychotherapy has to do with the relationship between the therapist and the patient. The patient relates with his time-honored way of relating which he developed from the far distant past.

Another element I think is important in this is the fact that some people are more capable of doing it than others. This has to do with the basic level of orientation of people. Dr. Zeig would warn against putting in another level until the patient's defense system can handle it, which is a very important factor and has to do with relationships with all the people the patient knows. You don't put in the crazy stuff, you just put it in a little bit at a time. You want to be heard, you don't want to be called crazy. And if you put in enough of it and they call you crazy, you have missed it. But if you put in just enough of it to make them think, now you're doing OK with it.

Another good aspect Zeig referred to is the concept that this kind of psychotherapy is helpful not only to the patient but also to the therapist because if the therapist is going to stay on top of it, he's got to be doing a lot of thinking about himself. Any thinking he does about himself is good for the therapist, for the patients, and for the therapist's family as well. So that is the big dividend which goes far beyond what the therapist does for the patient per se.

Another point to consider is the fact that the more anxious the patient gets, the more immature he is, the more he is going to look at things close to him, lacking the ability to back up and take a long look. One of the things about Ericksonian therapy is that it helps people to take a long look. We all get caught in situations when it's difficult to take a long look. One of the most beautiful examples is the one about people who get carsick. They need the ability to take a long look and Erickson would tell them to look at the mountains. Naturally, if they look at the mountains, they are in equilbrium with the universe

and are better able to handle themselves. If they look at the plain, they are shaken up and down in all kinds of ways.

This reaction is more common in seasickness. The individual who gets seasick is in the position of being jostled around and looking at the dashboard. If the person at sea looks at something fixed, like the horizon, or the stars, or the sun, she is more fixed in her environment. And if she looks at herself, and that self is going up and down and in all kinds of directions, she gets sick. Anther factor that gets into this is medication that counters seasickness. Somebody who is seasick, and is looking at the dashboard, turns to a drug to get out of it. But it takes more and more drugs and she gets sicker and sicker. If you could help her see the horizon or see something fixed, she would get better.

Another important point that Zeig mentions is taking therapy out of the office and returning it to life. I think it desirable if the situation that is occurring in the office can be transferred by the patient to daily life. If the therapist gets too important in this operation, then the patient has a problem with the therapist. He gets addicted to the therapist, which is highly undesirable. Therefore, if the therapist can help the patient remove the problem from the original fixation, whether it started in the family or anywhere else, and if the patient can help the therapist move it back to life, then the result will be a successful one.

QUESTIONS AND ANSWERS

Question: Dr. Zeig, suppose I wanted to begin incorporating some of the principles you describe into a non-Ericksonian therapy that I have been doing. I think that my clients would balk if I begin telling stories with these vague "uplifting," "right hand," and other indirect references. Do I need to do some kind of preparation with them such as implying to them that there is more going on than is just in the words I am saying. Do I need to create some kind of an aura like Erickson had or that a hypnotherapist has even though I don't call myself a hypnotherapist and don't know how to do hypnotherapy?

Zeig: That is an excellent question and a complex one to answer. Some people would say that ethically it is the responsibility of the therapist to inform the patient, "Right now I am going to be influencing you on multiple levels, so you should be aware of the fact that my communication is going to be more than the words." But when you think about it, what is part of the charm of doing psychotherapy? It is that your patient comes to you and tells you stories. Most of us like to listen to stories and it is not illogical or different for us to respond to the patient in kind. When the patient tells you a story, you can tell the patient a story. When the patient tells you a dream, you can tell the patient a dream. It seems unnatural only because we are programmed to the idea that psychotherapists only make clear and concrete statements or that psychotherapy consists of doing certain specific procedures. But what you are really doing is responding in kind. Jay Haley has talked about Ericksonian therapy as being a therapy of politeness in that you respond to the patient in a manner similar to the way that the patient responds to you. Therefore, I don't think it is necessary to inform patients that you are going to be telling them stories. Patients are glad to listen to stories.

As for the concept of responsiveness to minimal cues, that is something that is integral to studying formal hypnosis. However, you don't have to do that with formal hypnosis. It is an attentiveness that you learn as a therapist. For example, you sit down across from your patient, adjust yourself and say," "Let's become comfortable." Then you put your hands on your lap and watch the patient. Is he very vigilant, watching you? Is he immediately responsive and mimicking your behavior? Does he do something opposite to what you did? As Dr. Bowen aptly pointed out,

you are always communicating on multiple levels. Hypnosis may help us focus on the effect of our multilevel communication, but this is not something we ignore in any event. This is a tiring process because you have to stay alert. In fact, one of my students said after watching one of the videotapes of Erickson, "That is the most awake human being I have ever seen." That seems an odd thing to say about somebody who spent 50 years of his life saying, "deeper and deeper asleep." But Erickson was very alert and alive to his communication and the effect it had. Thus, in that sense it is not necessary to do formal hypnosis in order to elicit responsiveness to minimal cues, since you are always giving out minimal cues. Be aware of the effect. When I do psychotherapy, I especially try to be as aware as possible of the effect.

Question: Let us say I tell a story and the client tells a story. What happens if my concern is she asks, "Why are you telling me that?" or says, "This isn't helping me"?

Zeig: I have had that happen, but very infrequently, and usually it happens because of using the wrong technique. Recently I was working with a man who was an engineer and very concrete in nature. Early in therapy I told a metaphor under hypnosis to help him with his problem, but it didn't affect him even though he could understand some of the references. He said, "I understand that you are saying things to me that are relevant to my life, but it really doesn't connect to me." I understood then that I was seasoning my communication with too much indirection, so I stopped and became more direct. I explained that in such and such a situation, you do this. He responded to this and continues to respond to more concreteness. I had miscalculated the therapy.

I was thinking about whose comments, direct or indirect, I remember most vividly. I have a deep affection for Carl Whitaker. I recall that I would say something and Carl would respond with a little bit of a metaphor, a little bit of a something with an ambiguous reference, or a little bit of a symbol that he had free associated to in his right hemisphere way. This is what stuck with me. I can remember very vividly many of the interactions I had with Carl. They weren't so logical and if you looked at them you would say that it was a little absurd to respond in that free association way. However, you then start to catch on to the relevance and work to find that relevance in your life.

This also has to do with the comfort level of the therapist. If the therapist is uncomfortable using the technique, he shouldn't be doing it. If you are uncomfortable telling your patients stories, don't. But when you are comfortable telling stories to your patients, when you are comfortable doing hypnosis with your patients, enjoy it and they can respond and energize the situation and empower themselves thereby.

Question: Where in this system is there a place to build self-determination in the patient? We may tend, as therapists, to think of sheep and shepherd and we are the shepherd to the sheep. My concern always is to build self-confidence for our clients to become shepherds.

Zeig: Great point. That is a Bowenesque triple bind, I think. Bob and Mary Goulding wrote a book entitled, *The Power Is in The Patient* (San Francisco: TA Press, 1978), I could not agree more. The power *is* in the patient. It is the patient's individuality that needs to be affected. Therefore, you want the patient to realize more of who they are and it has got to be done in a self-determining way. Paradoxically, in this Ericksonian attitude, you become a sort of benevolent, authoritarian persona who is giving directives.

Now, I don't really believe in forming a fully I-Thou relationship and just having an existential encounter with the patient. I don't consider that to be psychotherapy. In psychotherapy, the psychotherapist operates on the experience of the patient. Just having an experience might be charming and build self-esteem. However, the patient can have experiences without paying someone lots of money and should have experiences like that. But I am very conscious of wanting to empower my patients. It is the patient who will do the work. Self-esteem comes from the patient taking on the challenges of life and learning that it is just as easy to cope and be happy as it is to cope and be miserable. Patients have to find that within themselves. I do take the role of being the shepherd, but at the same time it is directed to empower people to be their own shepherd.

SECTION VII

Counterpoint

Justifying Coercion Through Theology and Therapy

◆

Thomas S. Szasz, M.D.

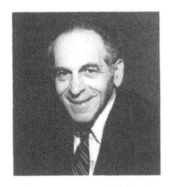

Thomas S. Szasz, M.D.
Thomas Szasz (M.D., University of Cincinnati, 1944) is Professor of Psychiatry at the State University of New York, Upstate Medical Center in Syracuse. He is recipient of numerous awards, including the Humanist of the Year Award from the American Humanist Association and the Distinguished Service Award from the American Institute for Public Service. He has received a number of honorary doctorates and lectureships, and serves on the editorial board or as consulting editor for ten journals.
Szasz has authored approximately 400 articles, book chapters, reviews, letters to the editor and columns. He has written 19 books.

Presenting historical examples, Szasz draws parallels between religion and psychiatry warning about the abuses of social control in the name of dogma perceived as truth—be it revealed or discovered ("in the name of God" or "in the name of science"). He argues against concepts such as "mental illness" because they can be used to justify coercion. Szasz argues for the primacy of individual rights and for individuals freely contracting with others for services.

I

Because human life is basically social, every group possesses certain methods for ensuring the role-conformity of its members. Because human behavior is basically goal-directed, there are two fundamental methods for encouraging or enforcing role-conformity: the carrot and the stick, reward and punishment, blandishment and coercion. Although coercion is, accord-

ingly, one of the most important facts of life, modern psychiatrists prefer to avert their eyes from it.*

The concept of coercion implies two closely related notions, namely, power and freedom. One person, A, cannot coerce another, B, unless A has power over B; the

---

This chapter has also been accepted for publication in the *Journal of Humanistic Psychology*.

---

* For the sake of economy and clarity, I shall, throughout this essay, use the masculine pronoun to refer to both men and women, and the terms "psychiatrist" and "patient" to refer to all mental health professionals and their clients. I believe there are more effective ways of advancing the dignity and liberty of women and non-physicians than by the now-fashionable flaunting of linguistic deformations.

weak, in other words, cannot (literally) coerce the strong. Conversely, one person, B, cannot be coerced by another, A, unless B has certain aspirations and desires, typically to go on living, to be free, to possess property, and to "pursue happiness." The person devoid of all wants—indifferent to whether or not he lives or suffers—cannot be coerced. This is why, in the West, people have sought to protect themselves from coercion by political means—principally by restraining the powers of the state (limited government)—and why, in the East, people have sought to protect themselves from coercion by spiritual means—principally by limiting their own desires (nirvana).

II

Since Western ideas about freedom and power derive in large part from Jewish and Christian religious traditions, I shall begin with some brief remarks about these creeds. Viewed as a literary and political document, one of the striking features of the Old Testament is its preoccupation with power and powerlessness, that is, with God's power to create, to destroy, to control and with man's powerlessness as person vis-à-vis God and as slave vis-à-vis his master. It is here, at its very roots in the Judeo-Christian heritage, that an important ambivalence—or double message—about domination and submission enters the picture. One message is that God's total power and man's complete submission to Him is a good thing; the other is that man's power over his fellow man—in particular, the power of the Egyptian Pharaohs over their Jewish slaves—is a bad thing. The story of Exodus may thus be viewed as, among other things, an expression of the fundamental aversion human beings experience when other human beings deprive them of their power of self-determination.

Yet, it would be wrong to say that the Old Testament story condemns slavery as such, that is, as a social arrangement or institution. Exodus implies only that slavery was wrong for the Jews at that particular time in their history. Not only is there no principled condemnation of this institution in the Bible, but, on the contrary, it is tacitly approved as a divinely ordained arrangement (an idea greatly emphasized later by Christian slave-traders and slaveholders). Lending support to this view is the fact that the ancient Israelites could not free themselves from slavery by their own efforts and needed divine assistance to do so.

Although Judaism was—and in some ways still is—a proselytizing religion, its record on rejecting the use of force to convert the nonbeliever is remarkable indeed. According to *The Encyclopedia of the Jewish Religion,* "The forced conversion of the Idumeans (Edomites) to Judaism by John Hyrcanus (135–105 B.C.E.) is the only such recorded case in history" (Werblowsky & Wigoder, 1965, p. 97). No other Western monotheistic religion can make such a claim. In view of the long history of Judaism, this is an especially remarkable record of nonviolence in the name of God. Perhaps it helps if God has no name.

It helps, too, that Judaism is a nonuniversalistic religion; the doctrines of Judaism do not imply, much less proclaim, that it is the right religion for everyone. In contrast, a universalistic faith—let us keep in mind here that the root meaning of Catholic is "universal"—implies that it is good for everyone. (A universalistic science similarly implies that it is true for everyone.) Why is this distinction—between the unlimited scope of what is Catholic and the limited scope of what is Jewish—so important? Because, given the human propensity for domination and coercion, it is but a small step from asserting that "X is true or good for everyone" to insisting, by force if necessary, that everyone accept X as true or good. This formula has justified forcible religious conversions in the past, and it now justifies a broad spectrum of psychiatric interventions.

Although a monotheistic God's power is necessarily total and unlimited, an earthly ruler's is not—a distinction that was apparently never lost on the Jews. Hence, perhaps, their simultaneous worship of both a fearsome, all-powerful God and of a Law that keeps Him in His place. Indeed, it would be no exaggeration to sum up the difference between Christians and Jews by saying that the former worship the icons of divinity whereas the latter worship the divine law. The holiest object in a Catholic church is the figure of the crucified Christ; in a Jewish synagogue, it is the Scroll. It is no accident that the Christian embraces the use of force in the name of God, whereas the Jew eschews not only the use of such force but the very use of God's name.

Contrast this particularistic—exclusivist, elitist—posture of the Jew and the psychoanalyst* with the universalistic—catholic, scientific—posture of the Christian and the psychiatrist. Christians believe that their ideas about religion are true not only for themselves but for everyone. Psychiatrists believe that their ideas about psychopathology and psychotherapy are true not only for themselves but for everyone. The former attitude—as we know all too well—led to the forcible spread of the Christian faith and to the glorification of this practice. The latter attitude—though it is generally denied, especially by psychiatrists—led to the psychiatric campaigns of forcibly imposing "mental healing" on unwilling subjects. Because the "goods" represented by Christian salvation and psychiatric cure have been considered superior to all others, their adherents have felt justified in suspending whatever value they reposed in the principle of limited power or the rule of law. To spread the benefits of Christianity and of psychiatry, no laws or limits need be observed—the end is so

lofty that it justifies any means. How else can we account for Christians killing heretics with the love of Jesus on their lips? How else can we account for psychiatrists imprisoning "mental patients" with the love of Mental Health on their lips?

III

How did it come to be that—over long stretches of history and in some parts of the world even today—religious ideas have justified the most absolute, unlimited uses of power? Although the details of the theological justification of repression are numerous and complicated, they all come down to a single, rather simple, image, namely, to a monotheistic, male God who rules from Heaven over all mankind, just as a father on earth rules over his children.

A classic exposition of this religious perspective on power is Sir Robert Filmer's treatise tellingly entitled *Patriarcha* (Filmer, 1640). This work, with its arresting subtitle, *A Defence of the Natural Power of Kings Against the Unnatural Liberty of the People*, was made famous by John Locke's satirical attack on it. Locke (quoted in Schochet, 1975) ridiculed the author for trying to "provide Chains for all Mankind," which Filmer in fact did quite well. But what should interest us, and perhaps also should have interested Locke a bit more, is how Filmer justified the benefits—one might now say "cures"—which redounded to those enlightened enough to fasten the chains on themselves or others.

What Filmer provided in his book was nothing novel but was nevertheless important, namely, a patriarchal—and specifically Judeo-Christian—justification of political authority. Filmer maintained that kings were entitled to absolute power over their subjects who, in turn, owed their rulers absolute obedience. Why? Because both the king's wielding of power and the subjects' yielding to it were decreed by God, the divine lawgiver. How did Filmer

---

* The would-be Jew, says Finkelstein, "must demonstrate that his desire is based on no mundane motive" (Finkelstein, 1960, p. 1741). *Mutatis mutandis*, the would-be psychoanalytic patient must demonstrate that he is "analyzable."

know this? The Bible told him so. Until God created Adam, God Himself ruled. With Adam, God created a paternal authority to rule in his place. This argument, writes Gordon Schochet, "implied that government—and monarchy in particular—was a natural institution and that the burden of proof was on anyone who claimed that there were justifiable, enforceable limits to political authority" (Schochet, 1975, p. 45).

A number of concepts and images come together here, such as patriarchalism, paternalism, the divine rule of kings (or other sovereigns), absolutism, slavery, and, last but not least, revealed religion (in particular Judaism and Christianity). What characterizes all of these ideas and images is that each sees the political order as "naturally" hierarchical, familial: On the one side is the father, or Father, or Lord, or God, or his vicar on earth, king or pope; on the other side are the people seen as children, or slaves, or sinners, or a flock tended by a shepherd. In such an image, Schochet reminds us, "Childhood was not something that was eventually outgrown; rather it was enlarged to include the whole of one's life" (Schochet, 1975, p. 15).

It might be unseemly, and unnecessary, to belabor that this basic image of what life is and ought to be, of how power ought to be distributed among human beings, is what informs the Jewish and Christian worldviews. God is our Father in heaven, the priest is called "Father," we are "His" children. Just a metaphor you might say. But a master metaphor that continues to pack a powerful wallop of real, literal power. The fact is that for millennia there were no individuals. As Sir Henry Maine observed, ancient law "knows next to nothing of Individuals. It is concerned not with Individuals, but with Families, not with single human beings, but groups (Maine, 1861, p. 250).

IV

Clearly, our rhetoric justifying the use of power not only reinforces our image of it but also ultimately determines how, or whether, we try to limit it. Thus, if God is seen as all-powerful, demanding total submission to His will, and if power is wielded in the name of such a God, then not only will the wielders of power demand total submission, but those subject to such authority and sharing its claim to legitimacy also will be eager to totally submit to it. To be sure, they may chafe under the yoke, but their complaints, couched in terms of misrule, will not challenge the principles legitimizing their own submission. Similar considerations apply to psychiatry and mental health as legitimizing images and principles.

It is important to emphasize, in this connection, that the great historical struggles for religious liberty, in Europe and especially in America, antedate the modern struggles for national independence. Sadly but not surprisingly, liberation from oppression by the priest led, in most cases, to oppression by the politician—the interests of the State replacing the interests of God as the leading symbol for sanctioning power. I shall not be concerned here with this tragic but perhaps often inevitable metamorphosis in the grand human drama of domination and submission. Instead, I want to comment briefly on the specifically American historical experience vis-à-vis the problem of religious oppression and religious liberty.

Leaning heavily on the great thinkers of the European Enlightenment, the men of the American Enlightenment saw their task clearly. Simply put, it was this: For centuries, the soil of Europe was bathed in bloodshed in the name of God. Catholics persecuted Protestants, Protestants persecuted Catholics, and both persecuted the Jews. For men who worshipped liberty as well as a loving God, it was not a pretty sight to behold. Because in these persecutions the use of force was justified by appeals to gods and churches, and because the actual use of force making the persecutions possible rested on an alliance between priest and king, the mechanism for controlling this sort of violence seemed obvious enough—separate church and state, (spiritual) authority and (secular) power. The great writings of Thomas Jefferson and James Madison are sharply focused on this one theme—taming the abuse of power justified by faith. Their words are as true and timely today as ever.

It is error alone [wrote Jefferson] which needs the support of government. Truth can stand by itself . . . The way to silence religious disputes, is to take no notice of them . . . It does me no injury for my neighbor to say there are twenty gods, or no God. It neither picks my pocket nor breaks my leg . . . Constraint . . . may fix him obstinately in his errors, but will not cure them. (Jefferson, 1781, pp. 276–77)

Madison was equally firm in repudiating clerical coercion. In 1785—when he was only 24 years old—he wrote:

. . . we hold it for a fundamental and undeniable truth that . . . the Religion then of every man must be left to the conviction and conscience of every man . . . Who does not see that the same authority which can establish Christianity, in exclusion of all other religions, may establish with the same ease any particular sect of Christians, in exclusion of all other sects? (Madison, 1785, p. 10)

For Jefferson and Madison, and their spiritual friends and allies, religious freedom—that is, freedom from constraint or coercion of any kind enforced in the name of God—was the crux of the struggle for personal and political freedom in general. This fact is familiar enough to historians and educated persons generally. What I think is less familiar is that Jefferson and Madison also clearly recognized that so long as a people want to submit themselves to a higher authority, whether it be Pope or King, Church or Crown, their struggle for freedom is doomed to failure by their own refusal to accept the indivisibility of rights and responsibilities across as many areas of human concern as possible.

So inspired, the founders of American freedom did two historically monumental things. First, they undermined and destroyed the idea of God as a morally legitimate sanction for the use of force, enshrining this bold proposition in the First Amendment to the Constitution of the United States. Second, they foresaw the danger to liberty that lurks in the nation-state itself and sought to fashion protections against it, enshrining this bold vision in a constitution explicitly delegitimizing total power. In short, the Founding Fathers rejected the religious, theological sanctioning of unlimited power by appeals to an approving deity, embracing instead the rational, prudential principle that since, unlike God, government cannot be perfect, its power must be limited.

V

We are ready now to draw some further parallels between religion and psychiatry, by focusing on the ideas and acts most abhorred by each of these systems of belief and social control. The core act of deviance in religion is blasphemy or heresy; in psychiatry, it is delusion or psychosis.

To appreciate the similarities between blasphemy and psychosis, we must first consider the idea of freedom of speech. Commentators on First Amendment freedoms often cite one of Justice Oliver Wendell Holmes' striking phrases to illustrate what this principle ought to mean. "The principle of the Constitution that most imperatively calls for our attachment," said Holmes "is 'not free thought for those who agree with us but freedom for the thought that we hate' " (quoted in Levy, 1981, p. x).

Here, then, is a short list of some of the typical utterances that people hated and still hate. In the past, those who uttered them were denounced as blasphemers; now they are diagnosed as psychotics.

"Jesus is the son of man, not of God."
"I should kill myself; my life is worthless."
"The government is violating my human rights."

The person who uttered the first statement was considered to be a blasphemer in medieval Catholic countries because he was said to deny the divinity of Jesus. The person who utters the second and third statements is considered to be a psychotic in the U.S. and U.S.S.R. because he is said to deny reality—namely, that life is good and that the state is good. Two more examples should be enough.

"The consecrated bread and wine of the Eucharist are the body and blood of Jesus."
"My wife is putting poison in my food and making me impotent."

The person who uttered the first statement was considered to be a heretic by certain Prostestants. The person who utters the second statement is considered to be a psychotic by psychiatrists.

It is false and foolish to try to dismiss such cases as instances of religious or psychiatric "abuse." On the contrary, they are typical examples of religious and psychiatric persecution—justified by "blasphemy" against the sacred beliefs of religious and psychiatric authorities and made possible by the blind adherence of the masses to the belief that such deviance amply justifies controlling the deviants. This persecutory position may be best appreciated in contrast with the position explicitly rejecting the use of force for the expression of opinion, as exemplified in one of Thomas Jefferson's letters to his grandson, written in 1808:

When I hear another express an opinion which is not mine, I say to myself, he has a right to his opinion, as I to mine, why should I question it? His error does me no injury, and shall I become a Don Quixote, to bring all men by force of argument to one opinion? If a fact be misstated, it is probable he is gratified by a belief of it, and I have no right to deprive him of the gratification. If he wants information, he will ask it, and then I will give it in measured terms; but if he still believes his own story, and shows a desire to dispute the facts with me, I hear him and say nothing. It is his affair, not mine, if he prefers error. (Jefferson, 1808, p. 249)

Consider that but one century before Jefferson —only a little more than 300 years ago (in 1648, to be exact)—the Parliament of England enacted "An Ordinance for the punishing of Blasphemies and Heresies," the punishment, in each instance, being death (Levy, 1981, p. 208). What were the acts so punished? They were such things as asserting:

that there is no God . . . that the Son is not God, or that the Holy Ghost is not God . . . or that Christ is not God equal with the Father . . . or that the Holy Scripture is not the word of God . . . or that the Bodies of men shall not rise again after they are dead. . . . (Levy, 1981, p. 208)

Some of these utterances are, of course, still offensive to many people. Suffice it to add here that the long history of persecution for blasphemy was based on the biblical injunction that "You shall not revile God" (Exodus 22:28). Since the writers of Exodus did not say which God, this phrase was equally useful for Catholics and Protestants. Jefferson, who did not mince words when it came to denouncing religious bigotry, spoke contemptuously of "the incomprehensible jargon of the Trinitarian arithmetic, that three are one, and one is three" (quoted in Levy, 1981, p. xii).

Enough, then, of religious blasphemies, that is, of the thoughts that the devoutly religious hate. What about psychiatric blasphemies, the thoughts that the devoutly "rational" hate? Psychiatrists have long had their *Index of Prohibited Behaviors*, called psychiatric diagnoses. In 1982, the American Psychiatric Association published its current catalog of blasphemies, punishable with involuntarily imposed or otherwise unwanted psychiatric interventions and a broad range of other social sanctions, especially when associated with the additional "crime" of "dangerousness to self or others" (American Psychiatric Association, 1980). A few examples of these "offenses" must suffice here:

Elective mutism: [a blasphemy usually committed by children, manifested by] continuous refusal to speak in almost all situations, including at school . . . School refusal . . . and other oppositional behavior . . . (p. 62)
Anorexia nervosa: [manifested by an] intense fear of becoming obese . . . [and] refusal to maintain minimal body weight (p. 67)
Tobacco dependence: [a blasphemy, we are warned, that is] obviously widespread (p. 176)
Pathological gambling: [Uneducated persons tend to confuse this with bad luck, or may overlook it as "losing," just as they tend to confuse the disease of "kleptomania" with the crime of "theft"] (p. 291)
Transsexualism: [manifested by] a persistent wish to be rid of one's genitals and to live as a member of the other sex . . . Atypical gender identity disorders or paraphilias [manifested by the subject's reports of] unusual or bizarre imagery or acts necessary for sexual excitement. (p. 261)

What makes many of these psychiatric blasphemies especially odious is that "frequently these individuals assert that the behavior causes them no distress and that their only problem is the reaction of others to their behavior" (pp. 266–267).

Why do we need this master list of contemporary blasphemies and heresies? What are these categories for? The compilers are eager to tell us. The purpose of the list is to help the sinners repent. "Making a DSM-III diagnosis represents an initial step in a comprehensive evaluation leading to the formulation of a treatment plan" (p. 11). There are three important ideas implicit in this smug claim: First, every "disorder" assembled by the compilers is a *bona fide* illness; second, every such illness is remediable by means of a *bona fide* treatment; and third, the treatment to be applied to the blasphemer ought to be chosen by the psychiatrist, not the patient. But surely, if a man has a right

to declare that there are three gods, or thirteen, or that there is no god, then he must also have the right to declare that he has three personalities, or thirteen, or that he belongs in the body of a person of the opposite sex, or that he is god, or any other idea that we may deem to be true or false, religion or heresy, reality or delusion, depending on whether we agree or disagree with him.

But we cannot simply leave it at that. We know that human beings are incapable of forming even a small group—much less a large, complex society—without resorting to some use of force. The practical question before us comes down to choosing between those uses of force of which we approve, and those of which we disapprove. Since the use of coerced psychiatric interventions and their justification on the grounds of therapy bear an alarming resemblance to coerced religious observances and their justification on the grounds of theology, I reject the psychiatric use of force. On the other hand, to those who believe that health is more important than freedom, coerced psychiatric practices will be justified by their therapeutic rationale, just as to those who believe that faith is more important than freedom, coerced religious practices are justified by their theological rationale.

VI

Before concluding, let us return once more to the similarities between religious and psychiatric coercion. What lessons can the history of absolute power justified by the absolute authority of God teach us about the problems of absolute power justified by the absolute authority of Science or pseudoscience? (It really does not matter which.)

The Reformation was fueled in large part by the dissatisfactions of Catholics, some of them priests, with the "abuses" of then prevailing religious practices. Protestantism is thus intimately connected with the development of fresh ideas about both limited government and religious freedom. The battle over blasphemy then entered a new phase. Some of Martin Luther's views are especially pertinent in this connection.

Early in his career as a critic of clerical "abuses," Luther advocated complete religious liberty—in effect, a separation of church and state. "Every man," he wrote in 1523, "should be allowed to believe as he will and can, and no one should be constrained [for religion]" (quoted in Levy, 1981, p. 127). He was fierce in his opposition to the Inquisition, declaring that "one could not be a Catholic without being a murderer," adding proudly that "We do not kill, banish, or persecute anybody who teaches other than we do. We fight with the Word of God alone" (p. 127). However, as Luther's power grew, he changed his tune, ending his life urging that Jewish synagogues and prayerbooks be burned, that rabbis be forbidden to teach, and that the Jews be forcibly converted to Christianity. He also insisted that the Catholic Mass was blasphemous and urged its suppression by the government (p. 129).

Interestingly, a number of elements in the Protestant-Catholic relationship, and especially in Luther's criticisms of the Roman Church, have re-emerged, in different terms, in the relationship between contemporary critics of psychiatry and conventional psychiatrists. To begin with, there were two distinct aspects to the Reformation protest against Catholicism. One had to do with the nature of God: Was He a single God or a Trinity? The other had to do with the power of the Church: Should religious deviance be punished by means of secular power or should religious differences be tolerated? The original Protestant position on the first question was to reaffirm the monotheistic definition of God given in the Old Testament. This is how, in the sixteenth century, the term *antitrinitarians* came to be applied to some Protestants. Protestants might have responded by asserting that they were not antitrinitarians but only *unitarians*—that is, monotheists.

Because I don't accept the expanded *(multitarian)* definition of disease, I have been accused of "denying the reality of mental illness' and called an antipsychiatrist. Actually, like the Protestants who reembraced the strict, unitarian-monotheistic definition of God, I have simply reemphasized the strict, unitarian-materialistic definition of disease (Szasz, 1961). It is important to note in this connection that people did not find it very interesting that the Jews had always rejected the doctrine of the Trinity. But people began to find it very interesting, indeed, when Christians—indeed Catholic priests—began to reject this idea and reembraced an earlier and stricter definition of a non-trinitarian deity.

It is no secret that most physicians—that is, real doctors, not psychiatrists—have always maintained, and still maintain, that mental patients are not really ill, that mental illnesses are not real illnesses, and that psychiatrists are not real doctors. To be sure, "real doctors" say such things only derisively, in jest; yet, much of what I have written about mental illness and psychiatry is similar to what internists and surgeons have long maintained. But when I, a professor of psychiatry in a medical school, rejected the idea that there existed illnesses of the mind or psyche—not to mention the terrible "mental" illnesses that affect whole nations, societies, cultures, or mankind itself—and reemphasized the definition of disease as a bodily, material phenomenon, people began to find this very interesting indeed. In short, my claim that mental illness is an oxymoronic fiction is similar to the claim that a monotheistic trinitarian God is an oxymoronic fiction.

The second parallel between the antitrinitarians and my criticism of psychiatry is equally striking. What animated the critics and criticisms of the early Protestants? It was the fraud and force, the deceptions and coercions, that had come to pervade the practices of the Catholic clergy and the Roman Church. In other words, the Protestants—the name is important—protested against two things: indulgences and the Inquisition. The former symbolized fraud, the latter symbolized persecution, both practiced, of course, in the name of God. The Reformers insisted that buying indulgences did not ensure salvation and that the Word of God could not and should not be spread by force.

What has animated me and my criticisms of psychiatry? Again, it is the fraud and force, the deceptions and coercions, that pervade psychiatric practices. I insist that a decent and honorable ("mentally healthy") life cannot be achieved by buying (or otherwise receiving) psychiatric "treatments"—because problems in living are not diseases that can be "cured," whether by drugs, electricity, or psychotherapy (Szasz, 1978). And I maintain that involuntary psychiatric interventions are not cures but coercions, and I urge that psychiatrists reject such methods (Szasz, 1963, 1977). However, although I condemn the "therapeutic" rape of the patient by the psychiatrist, I defend the legitimacy of psychiatric practices between consenting adults—not because "psychiatric help" is necessarily beneficial for its recipient (though it may be)—because infringing on people's freedom to give or receive such help, like infringing on the freedom to give or receive religious help, constitutes a crass violation of inalienable human rights.

These parallels between religion and psychiatry, between the use of fraud and force in the name of God and in the name of Mental Health, bring us full circle to the problem of unlimited power and the mechanisms for limiting it. The unlimited power of the Church rested on two pillars: God, the grand legitimizer, justifying the use of any means in His name, and the State, the ultimate repository of power, possessing the means for controlling deviants. When these two forces were allied, the result was total power wielded irresistibly by a totalitarian system. Similar considerations obtain for Mental Health, the grand legitimizer of our present age, and its alliance with the State. Thanks to this historical parallel, we need not invent a new mechanism for limiting the power of this new alliance between Psychiatry and the State.

Today, the psychiatrist is empowered not only to provide services to those who want them but also to persecute, in the name of mental health, those who do not want them. Faced with this situation, we have three basic options: We can take away the psychiatrist's power (to incarcerate the innocent or exculpate the guilty), we can take away his tools (lobotomy, electroshock, or neuroleptic drugs), or we can leave things as they are. Taking away the psychiatrist's power would be like the Founding Fathers' abolishing priestly power: Psychiatric help, like religious help, could be given to anyone who wants it; but it would no longer justify the use of force. Taking away the psychiatrist's tools would be like the communists' abolishing various religious practices: People would be "protected" from psychiatric "abuses," albeit paternalistically, since they would be treated like children who need the state's protection from their wicked "exploiters" and their weak selves. Leaving things as they are would be like continuing to support a status quo of forcing "help" on people in the name of God: We would continue to prattle about the "rights of mental patients," as if heretics could have rights in a theocratic society; and we would congratulate ourselves on our humanitarian laws guaranteeing the "mental patient's right to treatment," as if inquisitors had ever wanted to deprive heretics of their right to worship the God of their persecutor.

By separating church and state, religion was deprived of its power to abuse the individual and the state was deprived of one of its major justifications for the use of force. The upshot was a quantum jump toward greater individual liberty, such as the world had never seen. By separating Psychiatry and the State, we would do the same for our age: At one fell swoop psychiatry would be deprived of its power to abuse the individual and the State would be deprived of one of its major justifications for the use of force. The result would be another major advance for individual liberty—or, perhaps, the advent of another system of justificatory rhetoric and persecutory practice, replacing both the religious and psychiatric systems.

VII

I have presented certain facts and reflections about freedom and power and the role of psychiatry in the grand human drama of regulating behavior. I have argued that our basic psychiatric problems are not scientific, medical, or technical, albeit that is how they are now usually made to appear. Instead, these problems confront us, in ever-changing new cultural forms, with age-old problems of political philosophy—in particular, the justifications for maintaining and supporting a particular social institution and, more specifically, for its use of force. The basic formula is this: Acting as the agents of a dominant social institution, men always claim to be using force "to do good." The justificatory image and idiom for "doing good" thus typically covers both consensual and coerced actions. Therein lies a gigantic logical error and ethical mischief that we must expose and reject.

In a free society, acts between consenting adults are permissible (in a sense, "good") because they betoken the freedom of the actors, not because the consequences of the acts are necessarily beneficial to them. We can sell cars, vacations, and stocks regardless of whether buying them benefits the purchaser. Nor do benefits justify coercion: We could not force a person to buy stocks or bonds, even if we could prove that it was good for him because he would make a profit on the purchase.

The logic and ethics of paternalism—especially psychiatric paternalism—entail altogether different rules and standards. Thus, in their dealings with voluntary patients, psychiatrists typically deemphasize the issue of whether their clients *want*

their services and instead they dwell on the beneficial effects of their "therapy." Similarly, in their dealings with involuntary patients, psychiatrists justify their coercions, especially nowadays, by insisting on the therapeutic—indeed, lifesaving—powers of their practices. This perspective is sometimes referred to as the "thank-you theory," because it refers to the idea that the recovered "psychotic's" gratitude for getting involuntary electroshock or neuroleptics is an adequate justification for these coerced psychiatric practices.

What I am suggesting is that all of our traditional efforts to bring about "psychiatric reforms" have been misconceived and misdirected, as have our present preoccupations with "psychiatric abuses." We stubbornly conflate and confuse two different problems and questions. One question is, what are the proper or improper uses of psychiatry? The other question is, should psychiatric practice be based on the principle of paternalism (legitimizing virtually unlimited psychiatric power) or on the principle of contract (rendering such power illegitimate)?

Psychiatrists who like to debate the problem of "psychiatric abuses"—especially American psychiatrists who glory in righteously condemning psychiatry in the Soviet Union—are, without exception, psychiatric paternalists and totalitarians. The premise behind their posture is that if only psychiatry were practiced "properly" and not politically "abused," then psychiatric paternalism would be a valid principle for the practice of the profession and there would be no need to limit the powers of psychiatrists. But this is a tragically false and futile position. To begin with, it is impossible to know, or establish in a morally and politically unbiased way, what is or is not "psychiatric abuse." As all history teaches us, oppressors tend to view their use of power as good, whereas the oppressed tend to view their coerced conditions as bad. Thus, American psychiatrists calling Russian psychiatric practices "abuses" is but a feeble and ironic echo of American mental patients calling psychiatric practices in the United States "abuses."

In addition, we know, as Lord Acton emphasized, that power corrupts and that absolute power corrupts even more. We also know, as Thomas Jefferson never tired of telling us, that if men were angels there would be no need for limited government, or for any kind of government. My point is that the currently fashionable effort to combat psychiatric "abuses" is either a stupid and misdirected enterprise, or a ploy to preserve unlimited psychiatric power, or both. The only way to limit psychiatric abuses is by limiting psychiatric power, that is, by curtailing the power of psychiatrists. And that puts the problem of psychiatric power back where it squarely belongs, in the realm of religion, morals, and law—in a word, in the realm of politics.

Although my reflections might seem far-ranging, they come down to reenforcing an old adage, namely, that the pen is mightier than the sword. For our present purposes, I would rearticulate this observation as follows: Power is force that people wield over other people. Since those who wield power are always fewer in number than those over whom power is wielded, no person could rule, much less govern, without his power being credibly legitimized by certain ideas. It is these ideas that sanction some to use power and require others to submit to it. In the end, the whole structure of power—religion, politics, psychiatry, call it what you will—rests on certain ideas packaged in the master metaphors of our language. As psychiatrists, psychologists, and professionals in allied disciplines, it behooves us to scrutinize our own ideas—particularly the ideas of mental health and mental illness—which we must judge, of course, by their uses and consequences. I, for one, find these ideas wanting not only as conceptual aids but, more importantly, as sanctioners of violence against those who act or think differently than we do.

I have said it before and will say it again: Actions speak louder than words. Violence is violence, regardless of how we explain it or explain it away. We in the West have long repudiated the legitimacy of violence in the name of God. So long as we do not similarly repudiate the legitimacy of violence in the name of Mental Health, the very term "psychiatric help" will carry an impossible load of ambivalence, rendering it useless, if not obscene.

REFERENCES

American Psychiatric Association. (1980). *Diagnostic and statistical manual of mental disorders* (3rd ed.). Washington, D.C.: APA.

Filmer, R. (1640). *Patriarcha*. Quoted in Schochet; all references to *Patriarcha* and Filmer's work are based on this study.

Finkelstein, L. (1960). *The Jews: Their history, culture, and religion* (3rd ed.). New York: Harper & Row.

Jefferson, T. (1781). Notes on the state of Virginia. In A. Koch & W. Peden (Eds.) (1944), *The life and selected writings of Thomas Jefferson* (pp. 185–288). New York: Modern Library.

Jefferson, T. (1808). "Letter to Thomas Jefferson Randolph," November 24, 1808. In W. Whitman (Ed.), *Jefferson's letters* (p. 249). Eau Claire, Wisc.: E.M. Hale & Co.

Levy, L.W. (1981). *Treason against God: A history of the offense of blasphemy*. New York: Schocken Books.

Madison, J. (1785). Memorial and remonstrance against religious assessments. In M. Meyers (Ed.), (1973). *The mind of the founder: Sources of the political thought of James Madison* (pp. 8–16). Indianapolis: Bobbs-Merrill.

Maine, H. (1861). *Ancient law*. London: J.M. Dent & Sons.

Schochet, G.J. (1975). *Patriarchalism in political thought*. New York: Basic Books.

Szasz, T.S. (1961). *The myth of mental illness*. New York: Hoeber, Harper; rev. ed., (1974), New York: Harper & Row.

Szasz, T.S. (1963). *Law, liberty, and psychiatry*. New York: Macmillan.

Szasz, T.S. (1977). *Psychiatric slavery*. New York: Free Press.

Szasz, T.S. (1978). *The myth of psychotherapy*. Garden City, N.Y.: Doubleday.

Werblowsky, R.J. & Wigoder, G. (Eds.). (1965). *The encyclopedia of the Jewish religion*. New York: Holt, Rinehart & Winston.

Discussion by James F.T. Bugental, Ph.D.

◆

It is a pleasure and a challenge to comment on Dr. Szasz's stimulating, exciting paper. I have the feeling that he calls our attention, as well it needs calling, to an issue confronting not just the mental health discipline, but the human condition at this time in history. And that is the issue, fundamentally, of the individual as individual versus the individual as a part of a corporate body. We don't know how to do that. We don't do very well at it. And throughout human history we have not done well at it. It is not unique to our particular time, it is not unique to psychiatry or mental health. It is not a cop out to say that we can easily dismiss the issue; rather it puts it in the broader context of what is the human condition and what is the human problem. How can we live together in relative harmony with some degree of rationality, with some degree of humanity, toward ourselves and each other?

I want to now move to a different angle, to frame it by speaking of the individual and what we do as individuals in order to make life sustainable. That is, we need to create a world, a personal identity. We arrive in a world that is constantly evolving, and we arrive at a particular time. Rollo May speaks of our destiny, the destiny of the individual being the time, the epoch, the culture, and the subculture into which that person is born. The person that I am as I experience at this moment is very different than if I had been born in southeast Asia, Uganda, or someplace like that. Destiny affects our being, but we still, wherever we are born, whatever our

Note: Rollo May missed his flight and James F.T. Bugental, Ph.D., substituted.

destiny, have to create a world and a definition of who or what we are. As we do that, we make life sustainable.

The spiritual tradition talks about the importance of transcending the ego, but as Krishamurdi reminds us, you have to have an ego to get to the bus. We have got to have some way of getting around in the world as given. And nation-states are the same way. We need some structure. We arrive at some degree of consensus about what the world is, how we will live in it, what we will do in order to be effective in it, and how we will govern ourselves and each other. Those self and world construct systems that nation-states create become laws, become religious traditions, become the general mythology of the culture, and so on. These, too, are necessary to hold the corporate body together. Yet, again and again history demonstrates that over time they become crystallized and rigidified and what once was a method of freeing or preserving liberties can easily become a way of constricting or denying liberties.

There are many points at which we then find ourselves coming up against the borders of our self-definition, of our corporate definition of what the world is and how it should operate. I will cite just a few examples that fit in with what Dr. Szasz has been telling us. One is the issue of the church and the state: Must they be separate or can they be incorporated, can they be together? In the United States we have the tradition of separating them. Dr. Szasz quoted Jefferson and others who pointed out the necessity of that. We will return to the significance of that in just a minute. But in other countries it is not so. I was astonished the first time I taught a workshop in a Canadian university to find that on the state campuses there are religious schools teaching the various denominational viewpoints. That somehow seemed wrong to me. That is not my worldview. The church-state division and the church as the spokesman for what is right—that division becomes very important.

Another place we find this issue occurring is in the realm of advertising, propaganda, and public relations where the question is how legitimate is it to bend truth, however defined, in order to accomplish the purpose, whether it be the purpose of selling underarm deodorant or a presidential candidate. Here, again, is the problem of trying to decide what is the structure that we will accept as our corporate way of doing business, so to speak.

Let me speak for myself. A place I find myself much caught on this issue is in the realm of child pornography, which to me is one of the most unacceptable forms of abuse of the liberties granted by our Constitution. I find it very hard to accept this as something that has any defense whatsoever. However, the cry is that if we begin to control there, put on limits, then who knows who will be making limits, who will say this is too much, and so on? So we fear to restrict any form of expression under the notion that the freedom is more important than the restraint.

For 40 years or more I have been a member of the American Civil Liberties Union. Although once I dropped out and wanted to write a letter because I found at times the absolutism of their stand on some of these issues almost as repugnant as that which they opposed.

The corporate versus the individual. What can I accept as opposed to you or what can most accept, what can our agencies accept? We have to recognize that we are not going to come to a resolution of these issues. We are going to live with them throughout our time. These are the human issues. To try to say that this or that law or constitutional amendment, divine edict or ecclesiastical edict is going to solve this issue of the relation of the individual and the corporate is to be quite naive. Rather, we must find out how we as individuals and how we, in our relationships, can come to terms with those issues. And that is where Dr. Szasz is particularly directing our attention to what happens with psychiatric coercion. What is the role of the mental health professions in grappling with this larger, but very important issue?

He points out that coercion is one of two ways of influencing people. The other is blandishments, the carrot or the stick. If I have one point of difference with Dr. Szasz, it is his notion of power as punitive and attacking, as something that always subjugates another. As a psychotherapist, I have power with my patients. They grant that in realistic ways and in transferential ways, but I regard that gift or endowment of power as an opportunity to evoke from the client that which will empower the client, that which is already the client's, to help the client find his/her power so as to reduce that differential between us. That is, I exercise my power well, it is not forced on anyone or coercing in that sense, but is evoking the client's own power so that we can become true companions rather than dominator and submissive one. Perhaps there is a model there that can be of some use to us in thinking about this whole issue I am trying to point to— the relation of the individual and the corporate. If we can be wise enough to develop more ways of eliciting the power resident in each of us, drawing it forth, giving it form, giving it vehicles, then we may in some degree lessen this point of conflict between the group and the individual.

Therapy can provide, then, a kind of model of a use of power which is not coercive. But what do we do about those who are blasphemers, in Dr. Szasz's view? Those who say the things that are forbidden by DSM-III? That is a tricky problem and I think it is a good example of where the use of the corporate power becomes more crystallized. It tries to deal with more and more issues and oversteps its bounds. Let me see if I can make that a little clearer.

When we try to deal with some issue by legislation, whether it be the legislation in Congress or the legislation of a committee writing DSM-III, we try to reduce things to objective terms. We try to state them as if we had discovered universal laws, natural laws. If thus and so occurs, therefore thus and so should follow. However, when we do it, we begin to crystallize and rigidify. We may control the things we are trying to control, but in the process we control too much more. We overstep. There is no way to avoid it as long as we try to objectify, particularly if we are dealing with subjective phenomena. We make laws and each new law creates the need for three more new laws. It is a snowballing effect. Rather than a simple nomenclature that might give us a dozen, at the most, examples of conditions which constitute clear and evident danger to the person and to those about him, we end up with 227 pages more or less, listing in paragraph after paragraph all types of blasphemy.

Maybe we need to turn back on ourselves, turn back on our own efforts to control everything by legislative efforts, and begin to try to find ways of evoking power rather than restricting power. I wish I had the wisdom to tell you how to do that. I don't. But I think that may be a direction in which we need to go.

Barbara Tuchman, in a book I recommend to you, *The March of Folly* (New York: Knopf, 1984), traces the sad history of efforts of human beings to govern themselves and the corporate experience. She contrasts two things that sort of go with some of what Dr. Szasz said: Wisdom and Woodenheadedness. Wisdom, she says, is the exercise of judgment, acting on experience, common sense, and available information. Wisdom cannot be put in a DSM-III or a body of laws of any kind. Wisdom is a subjective thing and we have

to regain our trust of the subjective. Woodenheadedness, she said, is assessing a situation in terms of preconceived notions while ignoring or rejecting contrary signs. Too often, woodenheadedness would characterize our efforts to deal with the corporate.

QUESTIONS AND ANSWERS

Question: You very clearly showed the connection between the coercion of religion and how psychiatry has absorbed that. It is beautiful to understand that. However, would you comment on the victimization when the victim is the therapist? A former patient comes into my office with a gun and puts two bullets into me and says this is going to hurt you. Do you view it as victimization only when the victim is the patient or can the patient's coercion make a religious victim of the therapist?

Szasz: I appreciate that question very much because it gives me a chance to restate something which is obvious, but is also quite different from the prevailing view. I don't believe in mental illness. I don't believe in mental health. I don't believe in patients. I don't believe in therapists. I believe in human beings with equal rights and responsibilities. Obviously, if somebody shoots somebody, it doesn't matter if it is the psychiatrist shooting the patient or the patient shooting the psychiatrist. So your question is in some ways self-liquidating. Of course, it is not a nice thing when one human being injures another and I think people who injure other people should be dealt with by whatever mechanism society evolves. Your question really highlights the fact that therapists also feel endangered now, especially by patients. As you know, the danger of physical injury in the mental health profession is much greater than it is for gynecologists or dermatologists. Why is this? This is what I have been talking about for 40 years. It is because the relationship is certainly a combination of cooperation and antagonism, and nobody quite knows which is which and when.

Question: Do you believe that the mental health professional has the duty to protect the psychotic individual by coercion against harm either to himself or to another person—to protect him by confinement in a hospital; if he clearly says he is going to kill himself or his wife or someone else?

Szasz: I had a conversation with a friend this morning who kept telling me how I have been answering this kind of question in a bad way, by antagonizing the questioner. But you see, you have built into your question several problems I have been trying to clarify, namely that this person who is talking to you is psychotic. Can you give me an example? Who is this person and how come he is talking to you? Maybe I should get it that way.

Question: Okay, suppose you are talking to me and I am psychotic and I am saying I have been your patient for some time and I have been severely depressed and, finally, I am going to go out of this office, go home, and hang myself. Do you have a duty to do anything in a protective way?

Szasz: Oh, yes. That is easy. If you have been my patient and you come in and tell me this, obviously you are telling me this because you want to talk about it. Also, if you have been my patient, you will know what sort of things I do and don't do. Therefore, you will know that I am giving you a promise: never under any circumstances to betray your confidences or to do anything to you that you don't want done. Therefore, I would say, "Well, obviously you still haven't hung yourself. Therefore, you must be somewhat ambivalent about it. Why don't you go and check into a hospital? Why don't you do something so that maybe this will pass and you will preserve your life?" In other words, I will explore this question with you. What is it you want to do? If you said that you would really like somebody to protect you, then I would say, "By all means, here is the phone. Call up Dr. Jones and go down the hall. He will be very happy to hospitalize you in the proper psychiatric wing and take care of you." Psychiatrists do this. I do not do this type of thing.

Question: But you would not intervene if the person left the office and went home?

Szasz: Here English is important. Dr. Bugental alluded to some difference between us. Actually, I distinguish very sharply between coercion and the power that comes out of having some kind of authority or trust. A patient wouldn't be talking to me if I didn't have some power over him, so obviously he wants something from me. I would have a moral obligation to use that power in his interest and in the sense that I think is right, but I would have a moral obligation, also, not to use coercion. By coercion I mean the legal power given to me by virtue of the fact that I am a licensed M.D. and can do certain things that you can't do. I have abjured. Again an analogy would be the best one. I am like a former English nobleman in Virginia who has given up slavery and the Virginia gentleman's life and become a businessman in Boston. You come to me as a black and you say, "Wouldn't you make a slave out of me under some circumstances?" I would say, "No. I would do anything for you, but I wouldn't make a slave out of you."

Question: Dr. Szasz, I felt compelled to make a comment about some of the contrasts you made between the United States and Russia. There is a tribe of Indians in northern Arizona who are served by the Indian Health Service but have for several years been trying to contract their own mental health program. They feel that the care they receive may not be inadequate, but at times is inappropriate. They would like to play a greater part in directing it but the implied message is that you don't understand your own mental health needs although you have lived here for a thousand years. It seems that the attitude of mental health professionals is that the Hopi Indians can sit on their mesas and herd sheep or they can come down and have color tvs, but they can't manage both. It is attitudes like this that need to be squelched within our own country, not just in other nations of the world.

Szasz: You have raised a point about which I don't feel particularly despite my interest in religions. I think in some ways a mental health ideology (I am using words carefully now, as a mental health ideology is actually probably the greatest threat to the First Amendment, to freedom of religion, and so for American institutions) is one of the ways in which this encroachment occurs. What is interesting is that the established religions have completely coopted psychiatry, particularly the Christian and Jewish churches. They are completely in bed with the mental health establishment, agreeing as to what is moral and mentally healthy. I can only agree with your point. I assume that you know more about this than I do.

One thing I feel very strongly about is the fact that ideas have consequences. And the idea of mental health and mental illness as analogous to physical health and physical illness is an idea as powerful as the idea of Christianity in the sixth or seventh centuries. There are very few people, even in this room, who would say that some illiterate Indian or non-Indian or anybody else would know better than the professor of medicine what his child should take for a strep throat. That is a matter of science and you couldn't argue, even though some herbal medicine may be better for strep throat than something else. But when it comes to mental health services, it is an entirely different sack of potatoes.

What are we talking about here? We are talking, as Dr. Bugental said, about how we should live. But this becomes confused with physical health and this even becomes confused with certain ceremonial things, like should you use peyote, or should you use some other drug as a ceremonial thing which then becomes illegal because somebody else says this can't be used. Then you see that there is a collision course here because the Founding Fathers were quite paranoid about state power, as psychiatrists would now put it, and rightly so. They anticipated every possible problem, in particular problems from religious sources and from various political corruptions. That is why their assumption was that one corrupt politician should balance another one. They did not and could not anticipate what did not exist then—the rise of a mental health establishment. This, I think, is now the number 1 threat of the American system of government. Thank you very much, your question is enormously important.

Question: Dr. Szasz, I would respectfully admonish you on one thing. Ideas are important and do have impact. You, through your rhetoric and rational thought, have a lot of power. What I would point out is something I heard today about anorexia. I think your characterization of it is a dangerous use of your power, in that I think it was inaccurate. One of the reasons for anorexia is the social pressure placed on the young girl. It is easy for you to focus the power on the psychiatric and mental health community, but this is inaccurate and detracts from the actual issue of why that woman or girl was anorexic. Just because one social pressure forced someone into a life-threatening position, do you truly scoff at the concern of another social body to maintain a minimal body weight for that person to live in order to undo the previous social pressure?

Szasz: You are not being fair to me. You are implying that I am opposed to someone showing concern. I am distinguishing between concern, care and compassion and coercion. I think there is no need to coerce people if you show enough compassion and spend enough time. If you would only spend enough time, if parents would spend enough time with the children, then they could talk them into eating. There is a reason why some young woman does what she does and not even the most hard-boiled psychiatrist claims that the young person who is anorexic is irrational. Actually, it has been well described and I have had many such "patients." These are particularly intelligent young people. So if it is a question of the problem, then why not use the Jeffersonian model and tell them, "Now look, Miss Jones, you are now down to 80 pounds. If you lose any more weight, it is not going to be good for you." Now what else do you want? What other power do you want to give? This is opening the door, and not just for nervosa. Why not for something else, too?

Question: I am just addressing the comment you made with the example you made.

Szasz: Well, that was not directed toward not being compassionate and noncaring. You said I implied that somebody shouldn't care. It is coercion. Now are you in favor of coercion for these women, yes or no? If you are, that is a respectable position, mind you. I respect it.

Question: If rational concern would not work in the few days that I have for someone who has gone to 50 pounds, I would probably resort, unfortunately, to coercion. Then, when she is able to live, I would give her the choice of doing what she would like. If she would like to die, I would not get in her way.

Szasz: Well, I wish you would let me take another two minutes because this is very important. This gentleman is beginning to talk the rhetoric of psychiatric emergency, but there are no emergencies in human life unless you let them develop. Before you are 50 pounds, or 80 pounds or 90 pounds, there is a young woman and a mother and a father and friends, and so forth. That is when you should do something. There is an old joke about a stockbroker in the depression years. The stockbroker jumps out of a 100-story skyscraper. As he goes past the 50th floor, he has changed his mind and he shouts into an open window, "Stop me." Well, it is too late when you are falling. A psychiatric emergency is justification for psychiatric coercion and no one can deny it. But there is an old saying in English and American law, "Desperate situations make for desperate measures." So the thing to do is to avoid desperate situations.

Question: Dostoevski in *The Grand Inquisitors* suggested that people are sheep that like to be led. That that might be one aspect of human nature and I respect you very much for pointing out and exposing the cynical exploitation of that aspect of human nature. Ironically enough, I also see you as very idealistic because I am wondering what kind of society you envision that would address itself to that aspect. If Dostoevski is right at all, then it is not the powerful who are coercing the powerless; it is the powerless who are inviting this action by the powerful. Your vision of human nature is uplifting, a vision of all of us equally participating in a democratic society. I am not sure if that can ever work. I am not cynical myself, but I do want to be realistic.

Szasz: Well, what can I say? That is a nice point.

Name Index

Abrahms, E., 113, 118, 120
Ackerman, N., 8, 9, 10, 14
Adler, A., xviii, 98, 108,
   111, 115, 129, 132, 144,
   165, 166, 338, 361, 362
Adler, C., 137
Adler, M., xviii
Aichhorn, A., 224
Ainslie, G., 117
Albott, W., 382
Alexander, F.G., xxvii, 93,
   94, 251, 252, 267, 269,
   274, 275
Allen, F., 6, 8
Ames, A., 102, 103
Anderson, J., 183
Andrews, G., 134, 137, 146
Araoz, D., 404
Ascher, L.M., 137
Assiogli, R., 308
Auerswald, D., 8, 9
Austin, J.L., 97, 98, 100
Azrin, N., 137

Bader, E., 294, 306
Balint, M., 94
Bard, J.A., 112
Bateson, G., xxiv, 8, 9, 10,
   11, 13, 17, 18, 29, 30,
   47, 92, 99, 103, 229, 406
Baumann, D., xviii
Bavelas, A., 20, 21, 22, 30
Beahrs, J.O., 397
Beatty, J., 137
Beck, A.T., xxviii, 112, 113,
   131, 132, 135, 149, 274,
   275, 281, 282
Becker, A., 109, 118, 120
Bell, J.E., 5
Bender, L., 7
Benson, H., 380
Bergin, A.E., 134
Berman, J.S., 118
Bernard, M.E., 109, 118,
   120, 131
Berne, E., 108, 117, 129,
   130, 166, 285, 286, 292,
   295, 296, 302, 308, 309,
   361, 362
Bernfeld, S., 224

Bettelheim B., xv, xviii,
   xxii, xxiii, xxviii, 7, 215,
   219, 223, 229, 231, 232,
   233, 234, 235
Beutler, L., 361, 366
Bickford, R., 379
Bieber, I., 122
Bingham, T.R., 118, 127,
   131
Bion, W., 253
Bloom, F., 379
Blos, P., 239
Borkovec, T., 137
Bowen, M., xxiii, 7, 10, 11,
   12, 32, 34, 41, 42, 43,
   44, 45, 247, 248, 302,
   406, 408
Bowlby, J., 45
Bowman, K., 251
Bown, O.H., 194, 195
Brady, J.P., 134, 137, 139,
   140
Brody, M.W., 138
Brody, N., 29
Brougham, L., 137
Brown, G.S., 96
Bruch, H., 13
Budzynski, T., 137
Bugental, J.F.T., 424, 427,
   428
Burnstein, E., 138
Burns, D., 112

Canter, A., 127, 137, 248
Capers, H., 297
Castaneda, C., 205
Clarkin, J.F., 256
Colapinto, J., xxv
Compernolle, T., 346, 347
Coyle, L., 138

Davenloo, H., 148
Demost, V., 45
Dewey, J., 112, 113
DiGiuseppe, R.A., 113, 118,
   120
Dittman, A.T., 143, 147
Dryden, W., 108, 113, 120,
   122
Dubois, P., 115

Dymond, R.F., 184

Eggeraat, J.B., 115
Eisely, L., 335
Ellis, A., xviii, xxiv, xxvii,
   xxviii, 84, 88, 89, 90,
   107, 108, 109, 110, 111,
   113, 115, 116, 117, 118,
   119, 120, 121, 122, 125,
   126, 127, 128, 129, 130,
   131, 132, 135, 155, 165,
   276, 279
Elster, J., 95
Emmelkamp, P.M.G., 115,
   137
Erickson, E.M., vii, x, xvii
Erickson, K.K., vii, x, xvii
Erickson, M.H., vii, viii,
   xvii, xix, xx, xxii, 11,
   13, 17, 18, 27, 29, 31,
   56, 97, 101, 103, 174,
   175, 179, 180, 181, 182,
   183, 184, 185, 186, 188,
   205, 296, 297, 298, 310,
   363, 369, 370, 373, 377,
   378, 380, 382, 383, 390,
   391, 392, 393, 394, 395,
   397, 398, 399, 400, 401,
   402, 403, 404, 405, 407,
   408
Erikson, E., 229, 357
Eysenck, H., 30, 134

Fagen, J., 292, 302
Fairbairn, W.R.D., 253
Fay, A., 164, 169
Feifel, H., 218
Ferenczi, S., 93, 165, 252
Filmer, R., 415
Fink, H., 302
Finkelstein, L., 415
Fischer, R., 380, 382
Foa, E.B., 137, 167
Folkman, S., 112
Ford, F., 81
Ford, J., 11
Foster, T., 165
Foucault, M., 203
Frances, A., 256
Frank, J., 30, 134, 278, 282

431

142, 146, 147, 266, 274, 275, 276, 277, 278, 280, 281, 282
Marrow, A.J., 314
Maslow, A., 60, 117, 174, 218
Masters, W., 144
Masterson, J., 41, 45, 125, 126, 236, 237, 240, 242, 243, 244, 246, 247, 279
Mathews, A., 137
Maturana, H., 30
Maultsby, M., 113, 120, 121
May, R., xvi, xxii, 60, 212, 217, 219, 220, 424
McClendon, R., 290, 306
McGaugh, J., 379
McGovern, T.E., 118
McLaren, L., 137
McNally, R.J., 135
McNeel, J., 306
McPherson, F.M., 137
Meichenbaum, D., 113, 118, 131, 172
Menninger, K., 212
Meredith, R., 137
Mesmer, A., 370
Meyer, A., 256
Milby, J., 137
Miles, M., 304, 306
Miller, A., 195, 196
Miller, N.J., 118, 120
Miller, R.C., 118
Miller, T.I., 29
Minuchin, S., xxiii, 5, 14, 15, 16, 28, 90
Mitchell, D., 137
Mitchell, K., 137
Montalvo, B., xxiii, 8, 11
Moreno, J.L., 14, 15, 300, 341, 342, 343, 344, 345, 346, 347, 348, 353, 354, 357, 359
Moreno, Z.T., 14, 300, 341, 359, 362, 364, 365
Murdock, M., 29
Murray, G., 213

Narron, B., 308
Neumann, E., 370
Norcross, J.C., 166, 265
Nunn, R., 137

Orr, W., 380
Overton, D., 380
O'Hanlon, W., vii, 392

Papp, P., 13
Parloff, M.B., 143, 147
Paterson, C.H., 134, 184
Paul, G.L., 134, 135, 137, 146, 170

Peake, T., 382
Penn, P., 13
Perls, F., 165, 292, 298, 302, 308, 312, 313, 314, 315, 317, 318, 319, 320, 322, 323, 324, 325, 327, 328
Perry, S., 256
Peters, S., vii, x, xvii
Philips, C., 137
Piaget, J., 94, 95, 101, 127, 131
Pierce, C.S., 343
Pitkin, W.B., 117
Polster, E., 69, 90, 302, 312, 313, 317, 318, 323, 326, 337, 338, 339, 340
Polster, M., xvii, 198, 202, 302, 312, 313, 317, 318, 323, 324, 325, 326
Popper, K., 92, 99, 109
Post, R., 382
Powell, J., 118, 130
Prigogine, I., 98
Prioleau, L., 29
Proust, M., 335

Rabinowitz, C., 8
Rachleff, O., 117
Rachman, S., 137
Rado, S., 266
Raimy, V., 276
Rank, O., 93, 165, 215, 313, 314, 342, 343, 345, 356, 357
Rappaport, A., 102
Reason, R., 197
Redl, F., 199, 226, 227
Reich, W., 165, 253, 313, 314
Renick, T., 382
Reus, V., 382
Riesman, F., 16
Rinsley, D., 240
Ritterman, M., 404
Rogers, C., xv, xviii, xix, xxiii, xxv, xxvii, 60, 84, 102, 110, 117, 129, 165, 179, 180, 181, 182, 183, 184, 185, 186, 188, 190, 191, 192, 193, 194, 195, 196, 197, 198, 199, 200, 201, 202, 325, 337, 382
Romano, J., 300
Rosen, J., 18
Rosenbaum, M., 300
Rosenhan, D., 56
Rossi, E.L., 100, 184, 369, 370, 376, 377, 380, 382, 383, 384, 387, 388, 389, 390, 394, 400, 403

Rossi, S.I., 184, 376, 380, 382, 400
Rotter, J.B., 131, 134
Rowan, J., 197
Russell, B., 109
Ryan, M., 370, 376, 380, 382

Sagan, C., 33
Salter, A., 165
Salzman, L., 92
Sanford, R.C., 186, 188, 195, 197, 198, 199, 200, 202
Sartre, J.P., 220, 333
Satir, V.M., xviii, xxii, xxiii, 9, 58, 69, 70, 71, 72, 73, 89, 174, 298, 299, 302, 303, 307, 309, 311
Schimmel, A., 100
Schlien, J.M., 201, 202
Schmideberg, M., 138
Schochet, G.J., 415, 416
Schotte, D., 135
Schwinger, J., 57
Scilligo, P., 292
Selesnick, S.T., xxvii
Selvini-Palazzoli, M., 13
Selye, H., 60, 380, 389
Shasken, D., 302
Shepherd, I.L., 292, 302
Sichel, J., 121
Sifneos, P., 148, 279
Silverman, M.S., 118
Silverstein, O., 13
Simkin, J., 292, 302
Singer, B., 137, 146
Singh-Khulsa, S., 379
Skinner, B.F., xix
Slavson, S., 226, 300
Sloan, B., 144, 146
Smith, D., 165
Smith, M.L., 29, 137, 144, 146
Sonnemann, U., 217
Spurzheim, 164, 165
Standal, S., 195
Stark, C., 121
Steiner, C., 297
Steinmark, S., 137
Stekel, W., 165
Steketee, G., 137, 167
Stern, D., 45
Stolorow, R.D., 179
Stotland, 229
Stovya, J., 137
Strupp, H., 134, 144
Stuart, R.B., 137
Suinn, R.M., 137
Sullivan, A., 223, 224, 225

Subject Index

Abreaction, 159, 161, 272, 278
Accessing resources, 392, 393, 405
Accommodation, 320, 321
Activating Events, 111, 112, 114, 116
Activity scheduling, 156
Actualizing tendency, 180, 181
Affect, 168, 279
Agoraphobia, 137, 138, 157, 301
Agraphia, 207
Alexia, 207
Alienists, 35
Altered consciousness, 200
Amnesia, 26, 175, 403
Anorexia, 207, 304, 428, 429
Anorexia nervosa, 43, 158, 419
Anorexics, xxiii, 13, 30, 310
Anxiety, 23, 36, 43, 49, 56, 81, 107, 113, 116, 126, 131, 135, 136, 137, 138, 139, 144, 149, 150, 151, 153, 154, 155, 157, 160, 162, 167, 171, 206, 213, 214, 218, 238, 254, 257, 261, 262, 273, 278, 279, 282, 302, 316, 321, 343, 395
Anxiety disorder, 154, 155, 158, 160, 161
Aperiodic process, 319
Archetypal characters, 313
Archetype, 382
Art therapy, 272, 373
Assimilation, 95, 315, 318, 321, 336
Automatic thoughts, 136, 155, 157, 159
Auxiliary ego, 345, 346, 347, 348, 349, 350, 352
Awareness, 27, 313, 315, 316, 317, 321, 327, 333, 334, 335, 336

BASIC I.D., 164, 168, 169, 170, 171, 174
Behavior therapy, xix, 22, 28, 92, 104, 115, 133, 134, 135, 136, 137, 138, 139, 140, 142, 143, 144, 145, 146, 147, 148, 159, 161, 162, 255, 258, 260, 265, 268, 269, 270, 271, 272, 273, 278, 279, 303, 304
Behavioral rehearsal, 156, 270
Bibliotherapies, 122, 272
Bioenergetics, 61, 292
Biofeedback, 137, 171, 382, 383
Bio-psycho-social family, 76, 78, 85
Borderline, xxiii, 42, 125, 169, 170, 238, 239, 240, 241, 242, 243, 245, 247, 248, 253, 287, 304
Brief therapy, 25, 37, 44, 117, 282, 295
Building responsiveness, 392, 393, 394, 395, 401, 402, 405, 408
Bulimia, 257, 304
Bulimics, 310

Cartesian Dualism, 370, 380, 388, 389
Catastrophic expectation, 314, 316
Catastrophic reaction, 314
Child Ego State, 305, 306
Chunking, 401
Client-centered therapy, xix, 118, 157, 165, 179, 184, 188, 189, 190, 191, 192, 194, 196, 202, 271
Coercion, 413, 414, 417, 419, 420, 421, 422, 423, 425, 426, 427, 429
Cognition, 116, 149, 150, 153, 155, 161, 162, 168, 171, 262
Cognitive behavior therapy (CBT), 112, 113, 114,

115, 118, 119, 121, 131, 158
Cognitive errors, 155
Cognitive insight, 270, 271
Cognitive model, 150, 151, 153, 274, 281
Cognitive schemas, 132, 152, 153
Cognitive therapy, xix, xxiv, 112, 115, 120, 131, 135, 149, 150, 154, 155, 156, 157, 158, 159, 160, 161, 162, 163, 257, 258, 265, 272, 273, 274, 279, 280
Cognitive triad, 151, 152
Collaborative empiricism, 156
Collective unconscious, 200, 201, 373
Complexes, 372, 373, 382
Compulsions, 89, 127, 262, 382
Congruence, 183
Conjoint therapy, 161, 272, 273
Contact, 314, 315, 316, 317, 318, 321, 325, 336, 339
Contact-boundary, 317
Contract, 286, 287, 291, 295, 298, 302, 309, 311
Contractual therapy, 285, 286
Corrective emotional experience, xxi, 269, 270, 271, 272, 274, 275, 277
Countertransference, 35, 36, 37, 42, 201, 242, 268, 309
Creative unconscious, 382, 383
Creativity, 341, 342, 343, 345, 346, 347, 353, 357, 360
Crisis intervention, 37, 118, 251
Critical parent, 290
Cultural atom, 354
Cultural conserves, 342, 347, 360